ADVANCES IN THE DIAGNOSIS OF CORONARY ATHEROSCLEROSIS

Edited by **Suna F. Kiraç**

Advances in the Diagnosis of Coronary Atherosclerosis
Edited by Suna F. Kiraç

Published by InTech

Janeza Trdine 9, 51000 Rijeka, Croatia

Publishing Process Manager Sandra Bakic

Technical Editor Teodora Smiljanic

Cover Designer InTech Design Team

Additional hard copies can be obtained from orders@intechopen.com

Advances in the Diagnosis of Coronary Atherosclerosis, Edited by Suna F. Kiraç
p. cm.
ISBN 978-953-307-286-9

For EU product safety concerns:
IN TECH d.o.o., Prolaz Marije Krucifikse Kozulić 3, 51000 Rijeka, Croatia,
info@intechopen.com or visit our website at intechopen.com.

Meet the editor

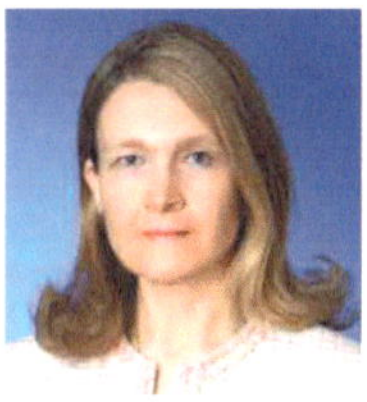

Suna F. Kıraç, MD, Prof, FASNC, completed her post graduation in three steps. First, she got a title of internal medicine specialist and then she educated in nuclear medicine. Later, she studied in nuclear Cardiology Lab in Yale University Medical School, USA and got nuclear cardiology certificate. Prof. Kiraç is a fellow of ASNC. She is generally interested in nuclear cardiology and cardiac imaging. Currently she is the editor in chief consultant of Anatolian J Cardiology and is responsible for ethical issues, in addition to being a part of the editorial boards of medical journals. Prof. Kiraç contributed as an attendant, presenter and speaker to national and international congress, symposium and courses on nuclear medicine, cardiology, nuclear cardiology and other related subjects.

Her publications in the national and international journals are on general nuclear medicine and cardiac imaging subjects. She has five printed books and book chapters one of which got mansion award from The Turkish Academy of Sciences in 2011.

Contents

Preface

Coronary artery disease (CAD) and its consequences are the most important morbidity and mortality reasons in the developed and developing countries. Advanced imaging techniques (intravascular ultrasound, MR and CT angiography, SPECT/CT, PET/CT, PET/MRI) and novel serologic biomarkers (C-reactive protein, interleukin 6, matrix metalloproteinase, P-selectin, intracellular adhesion molecule 1 and tumor necrosis factor α) provide early diagnosis of CAD and protect patients from hard cardiac events. Non-invasive techniques are being widely used in the diagnosis and management while conventional CAG is still the most commonly performed test in the cases at high risk. Following the first cardiac catheterization performed, first selective CAG has been reported at the end of 1950's. Patient specific and procedure-related complications range widely from minor ones with short term sequelae to life threatening events that may cause irreversible end-point if urgent treatment is not adequately provided. The important risk factors for complications are older age, renal insufficiency, uncontrolled diabetes mellitus, morbid obesity, and iodine allergy. However, operator skills and the type of invasive procedure being performed remain as the most important predictors to undesired outcomes. The risk-to-benefit ratio of the CAG should be considered carefully on an individual basis.

Coronary CTA and CMRA among advanced imaging systems offer anatomical informations not only for coronary vessels but also for peripheral vascular structures, and assessment of the left and right ventricular functions is possible in same image series. Quantified coronary artery calcification and many post-processing images (2-D images and the different 3-D rendering images such as volume rendering, multiplanar reformation, partial maximum intensity projection, curved multiplanar reformation) should be evaluated to increase diagnostic accuracy. High calcification level signs atherosclerotic changes in the coronary arteries, but is not specific for luminal obstruction. Because the absence of detectable calcium deposition has a high negative predictive value for CAD, CAC value is a significant predictive determinant for prognosis in asymptomatic patients. As with coronary angiography, myocardial perfusion abnormality may not be detected even there is coronary lesion causing a luminal narrowing of greater than 50 % defined by CTA and MRA. In asymptomatic and intermediate likelihood patients, assessment of myocardial perfusion by single photon emission computed tomography (SPECT) or positron emission tomography (PET) appears to be valuable even when coronary arteries are normal in angiography.

If gated study is added, left ventricular systolic and diastolic functions can be investigated simultaneously with myocardial perfusion. This field includes a overview of molecular targeted imaging, permeability of the coronary vessel wall, and interventional coronary MR. Recent developments in the field of ultrasonography have allowed us to objectively quantify global and regional ventricular function, and also, to get real-time evaluation of coronary walls and calcium load of atherosclerotic plaques. While we achieve more knowledge about atherosclerotic lesions by IVUS, tissue Doppler imaging has attempted us to assess myocardial function.

On the other hand, radiation exposure is the most limited factor for CTA and MPS gated SPECT procedures and needs particular attention. Ionizing radiation doses, hazardous effects and general radiation protection principles should be known for optimal protection of the patients. Mainly radiation safety rules, various techniques and equipments that may be used to reduce patient and staff radiation exposure during diagnostic and therapeutic procedures especially cardiac interventional fluoroscopic procedures have been detailed discussed in this book. In this field cardiac MR, which is a powerful non-invasive technique for the simultaneously assessment of coronary artery anatomy and function, has a great promise as a radiation-free method. But, it currently lays behind CTA for noninvasive coronary angiography because of some limitation factors such as metallic implants and equipment design.

Selection of the most appropriate diagnostic test in special situations such as chronic kidney disease (CKD) and diabetes mellitus is an other important issue. Although coronary angiography is a valuable tool, the major challenges with coronary angiography relate to when it is appropriate to perform and what the risks are associated with the procedure. Because renal function may be more and more impair with contrast agents used during CAG, and sometimes dialysis may be needed. Therefore, stress echocardiography, MRA and nuclear cardiac tests are often recommended to rule out the presence of CAD in those patients and the presence of any risk factor must be assessed on an individual basis in order to prevent for a soft or hard local or systemic complications. Contrast induced nephropathy (CIN) remains an important clinical issue in these patients, pre-treatment with theophylline combined with volume expansion using sodium bicarbonate; acetylcysteine; use of the lowest possible dose of contrast material (CM), and ISO-osmolar CM or low osmolar CM are advised to prevent CIN. Contrast induced nephropathy is diagnosed if a rapid renal dysfunction is occurred after CM administration without obviously any other cause of acute kidney insufficiency. Serum creatinine (sCr) is the standard marker for detecting CIN; however little changes in sCr after CM exposure may be seen but it is not considered clinically relevant. Therefore, glomerular filtration rate which usually measured by creatinine clearance is usually accepted as the most accurate method for the assessment of kidney function. But, even in patients with stable sCr the GFR may significantly be declined. Recently more sensitive markers (Cystatin-C and Neutrophilic gelatinase associated lipocaline) than sCr for GFR have been developed and validated. Cystatin-C is presented as more accurate marker than sCr for predicting renal function. Readers will get detailed discussions about advantages, disadvantages and possible complications of invasive and non-invasive cardiac procedures, and test selection criteria based on patient's characterizations, mechanism and definition of contrast induced nephropathy (CIN) and preventive therapy models in one more chapters of this task.

Consequently, this book summarized the clinics of atherosclerotic heart diseases, pathogenesis covering possible genetic factors and risk factors, a current view on new biomarkers as a diagnostic, prognostic parameters and future complications, novel diagnostic imaging modalities for CAD, and their advantages and disadvantages. Insight to molecular basis of CAD in a special chapter focusing on the role of on TRAIL (Tumor necrosis factor (TNF)-related apoptosis-inducing ligand) in the cardiovascular disease is really interesting and useful to understand how atherosclerotic plaques occur and what the importance of administration of recombinant TRAIL in protective therapy as a powerful approach.

Suna F. Kıraç
Pamukkale University, Faculty of Medicine, Denizli
Turkey

1

Mechanisms of Disease: Novel Polymorphisms in Coronary Artery Disease

Asghar Ghasemi[1], Morteza Seifi[2] and Mahmood Khosravi[3]
[1]*Tabriz Health Center*
[2]*Department of Iranian Legal Medicine Organization*
[3]*Hematology Department of Medicine Faculty, Ahvaz University of Medical Sciences*
Iran

1. Introduction

Coronary artery disease (CAD) is one of the most common cardiovascular diseases and has a high incidence of morbidity and mortality. CAD is a major public health problem in developing and developed countries and its increasing prevalence is a cause of considerable concern in the medical community worldwide (He et al., 2005). CAD involves genetic and environmental factors and their interaction with each other. Traditional risk factors account for at most one-half of the prevalence of CAD (Zdravkovic et al., 2002). Despite attempts to establish the molecular and genetic determinants that could account for variations in CAD (Zdravkovic et al., 2002), the etiology and complex multigenic basis of atherosclerosis is still not completely understood.

Completion of the sequencing of the human genome was a monumental achievement (Venter et al., 2001). Molecular researchers now take for granted the information provided by the sequence, however the clinical applications are not immediately obvious. A limitation of the Human Genome Project was that it produced only a single "reference" sequence. But in order to identify new disease causing mechanisms and cures for disease, we need to go beyond the "reference" and characterize the differences between our genomes, and in turn the effect that these differences have. The Human HapMap consortium (Frazer et al., 2007) and recent genome-wide association studies (GWAS) have set out to capture the interindividual differences that are associated with disease processes, including coronary artery disease.

The association between genetic variations and CAD have been reviewed in several previous manuscripts (Lanktree et al., 2008), but in our knowledge so far there has been no study in the field of association between novel gene variations and CAD; therefore we focused on introducing some novel polymorphisms and their relationships with CAD.

2. Genetics of coronary artery disease

2.1 Genetic architecture of CAD

The success of CAD gene mapping is dependent on its genetic architecture which refers to the number of disease genes that exist, their allele frequencies, the risks that they confer, and the interactions between multiple genetic and environmental factors (Wright & Hastie, 2001; Reich & Lander, 2001). Although the total genetic contribution to CAD risk can be quantified, the determination of the size and number of contributing effects is impossible without identifying all CAD susceptibility genes. The multiple risk factors for CAD themselves have their own genetic architecture. The heritabilities of some of the risk factors for CAD are considerable - total cholesterol (40 to 60%), HDL-cholesterol (45 to 75%), total triglycerides (40 to 80%), body mass index (25 to 60%), systolic blood pressure (50 to 70%), Lp(a) levels (90%), homocysteine levels (45%), type 2 diabetes (40 to 80%), fibrinogen (20 to 50%) (Lusis et al., 2004). Also, as CAD is rare before the age of 50 yr, it is unlikely to have an effect on reproductive success and hence less likely to have been subject to direct evolutionary selection pressure. Variants that confer susceptibility or protection for CAD might therefore have evolved neutrally in the past, and so could present at a wide range of frequencies.

This is the basis of the Common Disease/Common Variant (CDCV) hypothesis which holds that the genetic variants underlying complex traits occur with a relatively high frequency (>1%), have undergone little or no selection in earlier populations and are likely to date back to >100,000 years ago (Lander et al., 1996).The other competing model is the Common Disease Rare Variant hypothesis, with an inverse relationship between the magnitude of genetic effect and allele frequency (Pritchard et al., 2001). This model argues that diseases are common because of highly prevalent environmental influences, not because of common disease alleles in the population (Wright & Hastie, 2001). A review of candidate gene associations and recent genome wide association study results support the importance of common alleles in CAD. At odds with this, rare allelic variants of three candidate genes (ABCA1, APOA1, LCAT) that influence HDL levels, were jointly found to make a substantial contribution to the population distribution of HDL levels (Cohen et al., 2004; Frikke-Schmidt et al., 2004). The most likely scenario would be that the allelic spectrum of the disease variants is the same as the general spectrum of all disease variants. Under this neutral model, although most susceptibility variants are rare with minor allele frequencies (MAF) <1 per cent, variants with MAF>1 per cent would account for more than 90 per cent of the genetic differences between individuals. It is plausible that these common variants might contribute significantly to those common diseases in which susceptibility alleles might not be under intense negative selection.

2.2 Linkage and association studies

The 2 general types of studies that evaluate the relation between gene polymorphisms and disease are linkage analysis and association studies. Linkage analysis investigates the cosegregation of polymorphic DNA markers with inheritance of disease in families and has been highly successful in the detection of monogenic disorders. However, it is a tedious and complicated undertaking in the investigation of polygenic diseases such as CHD. Association studies provide an alternative method for dissecting genetically complex diseases and typically use the candidate gene approach for their investigation. Based on the known pathophysiologic characteristics of a disease, assumptions are made about the genes involved in its processes and the hypothesis of the association of these genes with the disease is then tested. For a disease such as CHD it makes sense to analyze genes that contribute to lipoprotein metabolism, blood pressure, and to diseases such as diabetes mellitus, among others.

This approach is more directed than is the genome-scan linkage approach, but it is limited by our incomplete knowledge of disease mechanisms and thus may miss important causative genes. It is worth noting that whereas in linkage analyses "disease" alleles are tracked in families, genetic association is a phenomenon of populations and association studies compare populations of subjects with and without the disease of interest (Bernhard et al., 2000).

2.3 Linkage studies

Previous methods for determining genetic linkage of a complex disease relied chiefly upon the technique of genome wide scanning of microsatellites (short tandem repeat sequences). This required the laborious selection of hundreds of families, particularly sib pairs with MI or CAD. Using around 400 microsatellite markers distributed evenly across the genome, the goal was to identify a significant linkage peak defined by a logarithm of odds ratio (LOD) greater than 3.5 corresponding to a p<10-6 indicating a gene that is in linkage disequilibrium (LD) near or even within the microsatellite region. However, identifying disease causing genes interspersed within microsatellites has proved to be quite difficult and studies from different centers reported varying results - Finland (2q21.2-22 and Xq23-26) (Pajukanta et al. 2000), Germany (14q32.2) (Broeckel et al., 2002), Iceland (13q12-13) (Helgadottir et al., 2004), US (1p34-36 ,3q13 and 5q31)(Hauser et al., 2004) and UK (2p11, 17p11-17q21) (Farrall et al., 2006; Samani et al. 2005). Genomic regions identified in the published linkage studies as being correlated with CHF are largely non-overlapping, suggesting genetic and/or phenotypic heterogeneity. Two genes, *ALOX5AP* and *MEF2A*, have been identified by fine mapping studies following the original linkage analysis. The Icelandic locus was replicated in population-based studies from Iceland and England, with different haplotypes of the *ALOX5AP* gene (encoding 5-lipoxygenase activating protein) associated with CAD in the two countries, and the Icelandic haplotype was also associated with stroke in Iceland and in Scotland (Helgadottir et al., 2004; Helgadottir et al., 2005). MEF2A (myocyte enhancer factor 2A) a transcription factor expressed in coronary artery endothelium was identified by linkage analysis in a pedigree in which 13 members had CAD, nine of whom had MI (Wang et al., 2003).

2.4 Genome-wide association studies

Genome-wide association studies (GWAS) became possible after the publication of the International Haplotype Map Project (HapMap) (International HapMap consortium, 2005; International HapMap consortium, 2007) and the development of array-based platforms that enable the investigation of up to one million variants in cases and controls of a certain disease (or other phenotypic traits). The HapMap was a large collaborative project that described the frequencies of genetic variants with a minor allele frequency above 5% in four distinct populations: Han Chinese, Japanese, Black African from Nigeria, and Caucasian of European ancestryfrom the USA (International HapMap consortium, 2005; International HapMap consortium, 2007).

The first GWAS to be conducted under these modalities was a large case-control study by the Wellcome Trust Case-Control Consortium (WTCCC), in which 14,000 cases affected by 7 among the most common complex diseases (CAD, arterial hypertension, rheumatoid arthritis, Crohn's disease, bipolar disorder, and diabetes mellitus types I and II) were compared with a set of 3,000 healthy controls. (Wellcome trust case control consortium,

2007) The WTCCC study identified 24 genetic variants associated with at least one of these complex diseases and helped to clarify key methodological issues, setting the stage for the more than 400 GWAS that were to follow. These GWAS have so far identified more than 250 loci at which common variants influence the predisposition to diseases that are common (i.e., diabetes, autoimmune diseases, and several types of cancer), an achievement that by far outweighed that of the previous decade of genetic studies. Results are available in the catalogue of published GWAS prepared by the National Cancer Institute (NCI)-National Human Genome Research Institute (NHGRI). (Hindorff et al., 2010) The genetic variants that can be identified by GWAS are common variants (with at least 5% frequency in the population) and have a low effect size; the conferred relative risks, as expressed by odds ratio, usually range between 1.1 and 1.5. These results confirm the views that the genetic predisposition to common diseases consists of the combined effect of numerous common genetic variants, each of a small effect size. However, it should be noted that GWAS identify regions of the genome (loci) rather than variants of specific genes. Indeed, the specific variant(s) identified by GWAS may simply represent the signal of one or more hidden variant(s) (not typed in the arrays used in GWAS). Limitations of GWAS need to be mentioned. First, these studies need very large samples of cases and controls. Second, DNA and data quality control procedures and statistical analysis need to be carried out by expert centers. Third, the overall cost of GWAS, ranging from hundreds of thousands to millions of US dollars, is prohibitive for most research groups worldwide. And finally, even after and in spite of all quality control procedures, there is still the chance that the results of GWAS include false-positive results, so that an independent replication of these results is still important even after testing thousands of individuals (Pier et al., 2010)

3. Candidate genetic factors

CAD is a complex, multifactorial disorder in which interactions among various genetic and environmental influences play an important role. Many genes are likely to be involved in some way in the process for CAD (Table 1). Some genetic studies have suggested that several gene polymorphisms, including those in the genes for angiotensin-converting enzyme (Samadi et al., 2009) and paraoxonase (Fallah et al., 2010) increase the risk for CAD. Polymorphisms in the genes for insulin-like growth factor-I and lipoprotein lipase have been shown to increase the risk of both CAD and type 2 diabetes (Wang et al., 1996; Vaessen et al., 2001).

There are certain genetic defects that affect activities of some enzymes (cystathionin β-synthase, methyltransferase and 5, 10-methylenetetrahydrofolate reductase) which may lead to homocystinuria. Heterozygosity for deficiency of cystathionin β-synthase is known to be linked with arthrosclerosis and thrombotic disease including CAD (Bakir et al., 2001).

Adiponectin gene locus, chromosome 3q27, is the candidate site for CAD. Adiponectin I164T mutation is associated with the metabolic syndrome and coronary artery disease. The I164T mutation in the adiponectin gene is reported to be a common genetic background associated with the metabolic syndrome and CAD in the Japanese population (Ohashi et al., 2004)

The Von Willebrand factor (VWF) may be causally associated with coronary heart disease or merely be a marker of endothelial damage. The G allele of the -1793 C/G promoter polymorphism in the VWF gene has been associated with higher plasma levels of VWF. Van der Meer et al., (Van der Meer et al., 2004) found a clear association of G allele of the -1793 C/G polymorphism in the VWF gene with an increased risk of Coronary heart disease.

Location	Gene name/Polymorphisms
17q23	Angiotensin-Converting Enzyme insertion/deletion (intron 16)
1q42-q43	Angiotensinogen Met235Thr, −6G/A
3q21-q25	Angiotensin II type1 Receptor 1166A/C
8q21-q22	Aldosterone Synthase (CYP11B2) −344T/C, Lys173Ar
14q32.1-q32.2	Bradykinin B2 receptor gene −58T/C
6p24.1	Endothelin-1 Lys198Asn
7q36	eNOS Glu298Asp, −786T/C
17q21.32	Glycoprotein IIIa P1A1/A2
5q23-31	Glycoprotein Ia 807T/C
17pter-p12	Glycoprotein Ib*α* Thr145Met
4q28	βfibrinogen −455G/A
11p11-q12	Prothrombin 20210G/A
7q21.3-q22	PAI-1 4G/5G (promoter region)
7q21.3	Paraoxonase1 Arg192Gln, Leu54Met
8p12-p11.2	Werner Helicase Gene Cys1367Arg
1p36.3	Methylenetetrahydrofolate reductase 677C/T
16q24	NADH/NADPH oxidase p22phox242C/T, 640A/G
5q31.1 CD14	Monocyte Receptor −260C/T
11q22.3	Stromelysin (MMP3) 5A/6A (promoter region)
20q11.2-q13.1	Gelatinase B (MMP9) −1562C/T
19q13.2	ApolipoproteinE E2/E3/E4
16q21	Cholesteryl Ester Transfer Protein (CETP) Ile405Val
9q31.1	ABCA1 gene Ile823Met
3p25	PPAR-gamma Pro12Ala, Pro115Gln
20q13.11-q13.13	Prostacyclin synthase gene

Table 1. The common genetic polymorphisms which are thought to be associated with myocardial infarction or coronary artery disease.

4. Novel genetic risk factors

4.1 MLXIPL

Triglycerides are produced from either fatty acids obtained directly from the diet or synthesized *de novo* when excess carbohydrates are consumed. Genes that respond to glucose contain a specific regulatory site, the carbohydrate response element (ChoRE), in their promoter regions. To date, ChoREs have been mapped within the promoter regions of the liver-type pyruvate kinase (PK), S14, fatty acid synthase (FAS), acetyl-CoA carboxylase 1 (ACC), and thioredoxin-interacting protein genes (Towle et al., 2005; Minn et al., 2005).
ChREBP is a basic helix-loop helix/leucine zipper transcription factor involved in mediating glucose-responsive gene activation (Yamashita et al., 2001). Mice with a disruption of the

ChREBP gene or hepatocytes treated with siRNA to reduce ChREBP expression cannot induce lipogenic gene expression in response to carbohydrate (Iizuka et al., 2004; Dentin et al., 2004). In hepatocytes prepared from ChREBP null mice, the induction can be restored by the addition of a ChREBP expression vector (Ishii et al., 2004). Thus, ChREBP is essential for regulating lipogenic gene expression. However, it has previously reported that ChREBP requires an interaction partner, Mlx, to efficiently bind to ChoRE sequences and exert its functional activity (Stoeckman et al., 2004). Mlx is a basic helix-loop helix/leucine zipper protein that heterodimerizes with several partners, including ChREBP; MondoA, a paralog of ChREBP expressed predominantly in skeletal muscle; and the repressors Mad1, Mad4, and Mnt (Billin et al., 2000; Billin et al., 1999; Meroni et al., 2000). Expressing a dominant negative form of Mlx in hepatocytes completely inhibits the glucose response of a number of lipogenic enzyme genes, including PK, S14, ACC, and FAS (Ma et al., 2005). This inhibition is rescued by overexpressing ChREBP but not MondoA. Therefore, Mlx is an obligatory partner of ChREBP in regulating glucose-responsive lipogenic enzyme genes.

Recently, SNPs localized within the MLXIPL (MLX intracting protein like; ChREBP, carbohydrate response element binding protein) loci have been associated with plasma triglycerides (Kooner et al., 2008; Kathiresan et al., 2008). The most significant association was described for the rs3812316 SNP (C771G, His241Gln); the CC genotype was associated with elevated TGs. The identified SNP is located at evolutionary conserved domain responsible for glucose dependent activation of MLXIPL. After activation and binding to the MLX, the complex increases the transcription of genes involved, among others, in lipogenesis and triglyceride synthesis. Since, elevated plasma triglycerides (TG) are an independent risk factor for cardiovascular disease development (Sarwar et al., 2007) and MLXIPL loci have been associated with plasma triglycerides, this gene might be a novel genetic risk factor for coronary artery disease (Pan et al., 2009)

4.2 Resistin

Resistin is a 10 kDa protein composed of 94 amino acids. It was cloned in 2001 and was shown to be a thiazolidinedione (TZD)-regulated cytokine expressed in adipose tissue (Wolf et al., 2004). The effect of resistin on insulin action has been extensively investigated in laboratory models. It was shown to be involved in hepatic glucose and lipid metabolism and appears to play a pivotal role in hepatic insulin resistance (IR) induced by high-fat diet (Rajala et al., 2003). Resistin was suggested to affect endothelial function and the migration of vascular smooth muscle cells (Cohen & Horel., 2009), which are regarded as key pathophysiological mechanisms of atherosclerosis. Further, resistin has been noted to play a vital role in increasing the level of very low density lipoprotein (VLDL) and low density lipoprotein (LDL) in an obese person (Rizkalla et al., 2009) which is directly atherogenic. Resistin induces increases in MCP-1 and sVCAM-1 expression in vascular endothelial cells which suggest a possible mechanism that contribute to atherogenesis (Cohen & Horel., 2009). Recent reports indicate that resistin promotes proliferation of VSMC that occurs through both ERK 1/2 and Akt signalling pathways (Calabro et al., 2004). Thus resistin is noted to enhance VSMC migration, which is a known component of athermanous plaque synthesis (Verma et al., 2003). Resistin promotes foam cell formation via dysregulation of scavenger receptors (SR-A) and ATP-binding cassette transporter-A1 (ABCA1) (Lee et al., 2009) through PPAR gamma. In atherosclerosis, increased level of resistin causes elevation of soluble TNF-_ receptor 2, IL-6 and lipoprotein-associated phospholipase A2 (Lp- PLA2) (Reilly et al., 2005).

With respect to the reported resistin variants, the mostly extensively studied has been the promoter variant SNP-420C>G. Functional binding studies have been done with stimulatory proteins (Sp)-1 and 3, which bind to the promoter. Their binding has been described to be influenced by SNP-420C>G. Sp-1 and 3 were discovered to bind efficiently only to the G-allele sequence and after binding to increase the activity of the promoter. (Chung et al., 2005). It seems likely that the more active promoter with the SNP-420C>G G allele is the reason for several observations of higher plasma resistin concentration in the G allele carriers (Yamauchi et al., 2008). However, in contrast to these studies, it has also been reported that the genotypes of SNP-420C>G do not influence the plasma resistin concentration in Italian subjects (Norata et al., 2007). Furthermore in a small study of polycystic ovary syndrome patients noassociation was detected between SNP-420C>G genotype and the serum level of resistin (Escobar-Morreale et al., 2006).
Recent studies have shown that the resistin levels are significantly correlated with coronary artery calcification and are predictive of coronary atherosclerosis in humans (Mohty et al., 2009). Previous studies described the association among this -420 (C>G) polymorphism, the resistin levels and cardiovascular risk factors (Ukkola et al., 2006; Norata et al., 2007) However, the association between the serum resistin levels and CHD seemed to be negative, and might be controversial for this polymorphism and CAD. (Norata et al., 2007; *Kunnari et al.* 2005) Differences in the cohorts might explain the different results, depending on which ethnic group was tested (Menzaghi et al., 2006; Hivert et al., 2009). Indeed, methodological limitations in the commercially available ELISA assays might also result in variations among serum levels, which might cause difficulties when comparing results from different publications.

4.3 Renalase

The kidney, in addition to maintaining fluid and electrolyte homeostasis, performs essential endocrine functions (Peart et al., 1977). Patients with end-stage renal disease are at high risk for cardiovascular events, even when provided optimal renal replacement therapy (Go et al., 2004; Anavekar et al., 2004). It has been suggested that failure to replicate the endocrine functions of the kidney may contribute to this risk, in association with heightened sympathetic tone (Joles & Koomans 2004; Neumann et al., 2004; Wolfe et al., 1999). Renalase, a flavin adenine dinucleotide-dependent amine oxidase that is secreted into the blood by the kidney, metabolizes circulating catecholamines, and is deficient in chronic kidney disease (Xu et al., 2005). Excess catecholamines promote the activity, secretion, and synthesis of renalase, providing a novel pathway of negative feedback homeostatic control (Li et al., 2008). In rodents, parenteral administration of renalase lowers blood pressure, heart rate, and cardiac contractility (Xu J, Desir GV 2007). During cardiac ischemia in rats, infusion of recombinant renalase reduces myocardial infarct size whereas neonatal nephrectomy leads to elevated sympathetic nervous system activity, renalase deficiency, and cardiac hypertrophy (Desir 2008; Ghosh et al., 2008). Human renalase is encoded by a 311Kbp gene with 10 exons located on chromosome 10q23.33. The major isoform of renalase contains 342 amino acids comprising a signal peptide (amino acids 1–17), a flavin-adenine dinucleotide (FAD) binding domain (amino acids 4–45), and a monoamine oxidase domain (amino acids 75–342). Evidence exists for at least four alternatively- spliced isoforms of renalase (Desir, 2009). The most common isoform (renalase1) is encoded by exons 1–4, 6–7, and 9. It is the predominant human renalase protein detectable in plasma, kidney, heart, skeletal muscle, and liver. The functional significance of the spliced isoforms is not known. It has weak AA similarities to MAO-A and MAO-B and distinct substrate specificity and inhibitor profile, which indicates that it represents a new class of FAD-containing monoamine oxidases. MAO-A and MAO-B are FAD containing, mitochondrial enzymes that metabolize intracellular catecholamines. MAO-A and MAO-B have overlapping substrate specificity; catabolize neurotransmitters such as epinephrine, norepinephrine, serotonin, and dopamine; and are specifically inhibited by clorgyline and deprenyl, respectively. Polyamine oxidase, the other known FAD-containing oxidase, is an intracellular oxidase that metabolizes spermine and spermidine and regulates cell growth (Jalkanen & Salmi, 2001). Unlike MAO-A and MAO-B, which are anchored through the carboxyl terminus to the outer mitochondrial membrane (Binda et al., 2002) and confined to intracellular compartments, renalase is secreted into the blood, where it is detectable by Western blotting. Amine oxidase activity has been measured in human plasma and is believed to be mediated by vascular adhesion protein 1 (VAP-1), a copper-containing semicarbazide-sensitive amine oxidase that is secreted by smooth muscle cells, adipocytes, and endothelial cells (Salmi & Jalkanen, 2001). VAP-1's substrate specificity and inhibitor profile are very different from that of renalase. It metabolizes benzylamine and methylamine and is inhibited by semicarbazide and hydroxylamine. Therefore, renalase is the only known amine oxidase that is secreted into blood and that metabolizes circulating catecholamines. While the hypotensive effect of renalase can be fully accounted for by the observed decrease in contractility and heart rate, we cannot categorically exclude the possibility that renalase's effect may be partly receptor mediated.

A common missense polymorphism in the flavin-adenine dinucleotide-binding domain of human renalase (Glu37Asp) has recently been described. This is the only reported common coding single-nucleotide polymorphism in the renalase gene, and was recently found to be associated with essential hypertension (Zhao et al., 2007). Whether common genetic variation at this locus affects cardiac structure, function, and ischemia in humans is not known.

4.4 P-selectin

P-selectin (GMP-140; granule membrane protein-140) is an adhesion molecule which mediates the interaction of activated endothelial cells or platelets with leukocytes. The selectin family of adhesion molecules also comprises E- and L-selectin. The genes coding for the three selectins are clustered on chromosome 1q21–q24 (Watson et al., 1990). The P-selectin gene spans >50 kb and contains 17 exons, most of which encode structurally distinct domains. P-selectin is stored in a-granules of platelets and the Weibel–Palade bodies of vascular endothelial cells (McEver et al., 1989) it rapidly shifts from the membranes of secretory granules to the surface of platelets and endothelial cells upon stimulation by oxidized low density lipoprotein (LDL) (Vora et al., 1997), oxygen radicals (Patel et al., 1991), thrombin (Lorant et al., 1991), cytokines and various other stimuli (Zimmermann, et al., 1990). P-selectin is required for efficient recruitment of neutrophils in acute and chronic inflammation (Johnson, R.C., et al. 1995) and recently has been shown to bind T cells on vascular endothelial cells. These properties suggest that P-selectin could contribute to atherogenesis (Hansson, G.K. , 1989, Libby, P. and Hansson, G.K.,1991). Actually, P-selectin expression has been demonstrated to be significantly increased in endothelium overlying atherosclerotic plaques, and it is focally expressed in the aorta of hypercholesterolemic

rabbits. It has been reported that P-selectin-deficient mice on an atherogenic diet develop significantly smaller fatty streaks than non-deficient mice (Johnson, R.C., et al. 1997). In humans, plasma P selectin levels have been shown to be increased in diabetic patients, in patients with unstable angina, post-angioplasty restenosis and after coronary artery spasm (Kaikita, K. , 1995).
Recent study that genotyped 5 single nucleotide polymorphisms (SNPs) in P-selectin (*SELP*) (V168M, S290N, N592D, V599L, T715P), 2 SNPs (M62I, S273F) in P-selectin glycoprotein ligand-1 (*SELPLG*), 5 SNPs in *CD40LG* (−3459A>G, −122A>C, −123A>C, 148T>C, intr4-13T>C), the H558R SNP in *SCN5A*, and rs2106261 in *ZFHX3*. In addition, length polymorphisms in *SELPLG* (36bp-tandem repeat) and *CD40LG* (CA-repeat) were genotyped by PCR methods. None of the gene polymorphisms showed significant differences between AMI patients and healthy controls. Among patients with a history of VF (Ventricular fibrillation), however, the SELP 168M variant showed a significantly higher prevalence as compared with patients without VF. This was the first description of an association of the SELP gene variant 168M with primary VF during acute MI. This variant may be a novel polymorphism for evaluating the susceptibility for VF in the setting of acute MI. (Elmas, 2010)

4.5 KDR

Kinase insert domain-containing receptor/fetal liver kinase-1, also called VEGFR2 (KDR), is expressed in a wide variety of cells such as endothelial progenitor cells (EPCs), endothelial cells, and primitive and more mature hematopoietic cells. Kinase insert domain-containing receptor/ fetal liver kinase-1 is required for the differentiation of EPCs and for the movement of EPCs from the posterior primitive streak to the yolk sac, a precondition for the subsequent formation of blood vessels (Shalaby et al., 1997). Studies with *KDR* knockout mice have found that KDR plays critical roles in the development and formation of blood vessel networks (Fong et al., 1995). Vascular endothelial growth factor binds to 2 tyrosine kinase receptors, VEGF receptor-1 (VEGFR1, Flt-1) and KDR, in endothelial cells. The mitogenic and chemotactic effects of VEGF are mediated mainly through KDR in endothelial cells VEGF receptor signal transduction which is activated through autophosphorylation of tyrosine residues in the cytoplasmic kinase domain of KDR. This event is followed by activation of downstream signaling pathways such as mitogen-activated protein kinases, Akt and eNOS, which are essential for migration and proliferation of endothelial cells, thereby stimulating angiogenesis (Matsumoto & Claesson-Welsh, 2001). After vascular endothelial growth factor (VEGF) binding to KDR, multiple early signaling cascades are activated in EPCs and in endothelial cells. An array of biological activities are subsequently elicited in vivo and in vitro, including angiogenesis, endothelial survival, proliferation, migration, and increased production of nitric oxide and prostaglandin I2 (Gerber et al., 1994). Dysregulated vessel growth is implicated in the pathogenesis of a wide variety of diseases, including proliferative retinopathies, tumors, rheumatoid arthritis, atherosclerosis, as well as CHD. (Dimmeler et al., 2001; Rehman et al., 2004; Werner et al., 2002). The variation of *KDR* gene may change the biological function of KDR. Bioinformatic analysis showed that the single nucleotide polymorphism (SNP) -604T/C (rs2071559) leads to structural alteration of the binding site for transcriptional factor E2F (involving in cell cycle regulation, interacting with Rb p107 protein) in *KDR* gene promoter region, which may alter KDR expression. Exonic polymorphisms SNP1192G/A (rs2305948, in exon 7) and SNP1719A/T (rs1870377, in exon 11) are located in the third and fifth NH2-terminal IG-like domains within the extracellular region, which are important for ligand binding, and result in nonsynonymous amino acid changes at residue 297V/I and 472H/Q, respectively. It is showed that patients carrying the KDR mutations are more susceptible to CHD. The higher CHD risk could be due to downregulation of the VEGF/KDR signaling pathway. However, the angiogenesis preceded by VEGF/KDR signaling pathway could be decreased due to low KDR activity. The SNP-604T/C decreases mRNA levels of KDR and both SNP1192G/A and SNP1719T/A resulted in slight but significant decrease in the VEGF binding efficiency to KDR. One can speculate that the decrease in KDR function is correlated with vascular dysfunction, including endothelial cell damage, impaired endothelial cell survival, decreased antiapoptotic effects of VEGF, and abnormal vascular repair. All of these can promote the progression of atherosclerotic disease. A previous study has suggested that -907T/C, -11903G/A, and -18487A/T (now called SNP-604, SNP1192, and SNP1719, respectively) have no significant association with the development of coronary artery lesion in Japanese subjects with Kawasaki disease (Kariyazono et al., 2004). The differences between the studies could be due to the different pathologic mechanism between the coronary artery lesion with Kawasaki disease and CHD, different genetic background of the populations as well as the sample size in different studies. (Schmidt-Lucke et al., 2005). The genotype frequencies of the 3 SNPs from the HapMap data were similar to others. The rs2071559 can capture rs7667298 (exon_1, untranslated). No linkage disequilibrium was found in rs2305948 with other SNPs in HapMap CHB data. The rs1870377 (exon_11) can capture rs10016064 (intron_13), rs17085265 (intron_21), rs3816584 (intron_16), rs6838752 (intron_17), rs1870379 (intron_15), rs2219471 (intron_20), rs1870378 (intron_15), rs13136007 (intron_13), and rs17085262 (intron_21). The results showed that 2 blocks were captured by SNP-604 (rs2071559) and SNP1719 (rs1870377), respectively, and SNP1192 (rs2305948) were associated with CHD.

5. Other novel polymorphisms

Asymmetrical dimethylarginine (ADMA), an endogenous arginine analogue, inhibits nitric oxide synthases and plays an important role in endothelial dysfunction. The results suggest that the DDAH1 (dimethylarginine dimethylaminohydrolase 1) loss-of-function polymorphism is associated with both increased risk of thrombosis stroke and CAD (Ding et al., 2010). Growing evidence has shown that inflammation plays crucial roles in the development of coronary artery disease. Interleukin-16 (IL-16), a multifunctional cytokine, is involved in a series of inflammatory disorders. One finding indicates that *IL-16* may be used as a genetic marker for CAD susceptibility (Wu et al., 2010). Two single-nucleotide polymorphisms (SNPs), rs1746048 and rs501120, from genome wide association studies of coronary artery disease map to chromosome 10q11 ~80 kb downstream of chemokine *CXCL12*. Coronary artery disease risk alleles downstream of *CXCL12* are associated with plasma protein levels of CXCL12 and appear to be related to *CXCL12* transcript levels in two human cell lines. This implicates *CXCL12* as potentially causal and supports CXCL12 as a potential therapeutic target for CAD (Nehal et al., 2011).

6. Conclusion

Studying only one SNP may be an overly simplistic method in investigating a complex disease such as CAD. Complex traits such as CAD, more large databases of high-quality genetic and clinical data need to be established and since genes and environmental factors are both involved in this disease; environmental causes and gene-environment interactions must be carefully assessed. These results will provide clues to the involvement and investigation of novel candidate genes in association studies. Large replication studies with different ethic samples are needed to investigate whether there are ethnic differences in the influence of novel polymorphisms on coronary artery disease. This issue should be investigated with different ethnic samples in the future. Therefore studies with large sample size of coronary artery disease and different ethnicity will be welcome to help elucidate the interconnection between novel genetics and pathogenesis of coronary artery disease.

7. Abbreviations

ABCA1: ATP-binding cassette transporter 1
ACC: acetyl-CoA carboxylase
ALOX5AP: Arachidonate 5-lipoxygenase-activating protein.
APOA1: Apolipoprotein A1
CAD: Coronary artery disease
LCAT: Lecithin-cholesterol acyltransferase
CHD: Coronary heart disease
ChoRE: Carbohydrate response element
ChREBP: Carbohydrate response element binding protein
ELISA: Enzyme-linked immunosorbent assay
EPCs: Endothelial progenitor cells
ERK 1/2 : Extracellular signal-regulated kinases1/2
FAD: Flavin-adenine dinucleotide
FAS: Fatty acid synthase
GWAS: Genome-wide association Studies
HDL: High-density lipoprotein
KDR: Kinase insert domain-containing receptor
Lp- PLA2: Lipoprotein-associated phospholipase A2
Mad1: Mitotic arrest deficient-like 1
Mad4: Mitotic arrest deficient-like 4
MAO-A: L-Monoamine oxidases A
MAO-B : L-Monoamine oxidases B
MEF2A: Myocyte enhancer factor 2A
MlX: Max-like x protein
PPAR: Peroxisome proliferator-activated receptors
PK : Pyruvate kinase
siRNA: Small interfering RNA
SNPs: Single nucleotide polymorphisms
Sp1: stimulatory proteins 1
SR-A: Scavenger receptors A
TNF: Tumor necrosis factors
VAP-1: vascular adhesion protein 1
VCAM-1: Vascular cell adhesion protein 1
VF: Ventricular fibrillation
VLDL: Very low density lipoprotein
VWF: Von Willebrand factor

8. References

Anavekar, N.S. (2004). Relation between renal dysfunction and cardiovascular outcomes after myocardial infarction, *N. Engl. J. Med.* 351:1285–1295.

Bakir, I., Zarzou W and Herrmann, W. (2001). Genetic Polymorphism of 5,10-Methylene-tetrahydrofolate Reductase (MTHFR) as Risk Factor for Coronary Artery Disease, *Arab Journal of Pharmaceutical Sciences* 1: 41-50.

Berliner J.C. (1997). Induction of P-selectin by oxidized lipoproteins. Separate effects on synthesis and surface expression, *Circ. Res.* 80: 810–818

Bernhard, R., Winkelmann, Joerg Hager, William, E. Kraus, Piera Merlini, Bernard Keavney, Peter, J., Grant, Joseph B. Muhlestein, and Christopher B. Granger. (2000). Genetics of coronary heart disease: Current knowledge and research principles, *Am heart J* 140: 511-526

Billin, A. N., Eilers, A. L., Queva, C., and Ayer, D. E. (1999). Mlx, a novel Max-like BHLHZip protein that interacts with the Max network of transcription factors, J. Biol. Chem. 274: 36344–36350

Billin, A. N., Eilers, A. L., Coulter, K. L., Logan, J. S., and Ayer, D. E. (2000). Mondo A, a Novel Basic Helix-Loop-Helix-Leucine Zipper Transcriptional Activator That Constitutes a positive Branch of a Ma-Like Network, *Mol. Cell. Biol.* 20: 8845–8854

Binda, C., Mattevi, A., and Edmondson, D.E. (2002). Structure-function relationships in flavoenzyme dependent amine oxidations: a comparison of polyamine oxidase and monoamine oxidase, *J. Biol. Chem.* 277:23973–23976.

Broeckel, U., Hengstenberg, C., Mayer, B., Holmer, S., Martin, LJ., Comuzzie, AG., et al. (2002). A comprehensive linkage analysis for myocardial infarction and its related risk factors, Nat Genet 30: 210-4.

Calabro, P., Samudio, I., Willerson ,JT., Yeh, ET. (2004). Resistin promotes smooth muscle cell proliferation through activation of extracellular signal regulated kinase 1/2 and phosphatidylinositol 3-kinase pathways, *Circulation* 110: 3335–3340.

Chung, SS., Choi, HH., Kim, KW., Cho, YM., Lee, HK & Park KS .(2005). Regulation of human resistin gene expression in cell systems: an important role of stimulatory protein 1 interaction with a common promoter polymorphic site, *Diabetologia* 48: 1150–1158.

Cohen, JC., Kiss, RS., Pertsemlidis, A., Marcel, YL., McPherson, R., Hobbs, HH. (2004). Multiple rare alleles contribute to low plasma levels of HDL cholesterol, *Science* 305 : 869-72.

Cohen, G., Hörl, WH. (2009). Resistin as a cardiovascular and atherosclerotic risk factor and uremic toxin, *Semin. Dial.*, 22: 373-377.

Dentin, R., Pegorier, J. P., Benhamed, F., Foufelle, F., Ferre, P., Fauveau, V., Magnuson, M. A., Girard, J., and Postic, C. (2004). Hepatic glucokinase is required for the synergistic action of ChREBP and SREBP-1c on glycolytic and lipogenic gene expression, *J. Biol. Chem.* 279: 20314–20326

Desir, GV. (2008). Renalase deficiency in chronic kidney disease, and its contribution to hypertension and cardiovascular disease, *Curr Opin Nephrol Hypertens* 17: 181–185.

Desir, GV. (2009). Regulation of blood pressure and cardiovascular function by renalase, *Kidney Int* 76: 366–370.

Ding, H., Wu, B., Wang, H., Lu, Z., Yan, J., Wang, X., Shaffer, JR., Hui, R., Wang DWA. (2010). Novel loss-of-function DDAH1 promoter polymorphism is associated with increased susceptibility to thrombosis stroke and coronary heart disease, *Circ Res.* 106(6): 1019-21.

Escobar-Morreale, HF., Villuendas, G., Botella-Carretero, JI., Alvarez-Blasco, F., Sanchón , R., Luque-

Norata, GD., Ongari, M., Garlaschelli, K., *et al.* (2007). Effect of the -420C/G variant of the resistin gene promoter on metabolic syndrome, obesity, myocardial infarction and kidney dysfunction, *J Intern Med* 262: 104–112.

Fallah, S., Seifi, M., Ghasemi, A., Firoozrai, M., Samadikuchaksaraei, A. (2010). Matrix Metalloproteinase-9 and Paraoxonase 1 Q/R192 Gene Polymorphisms and the Risk of Coronary Artery Stenosis in Iranian Subjects, *J. Clin. Lab. Anal.* 24: 305–310,

Farrall, M., Green, FR., Peden, JF., Olsson, PG., Clarke, R., Hellenius ML., et al. (2006). Genome-wide mapping of susceptibility to coronary artery disease identifies a novel replicated locus on chromosome 17, *PLoS Genet* 2: e72.

Fong, GH., Rossant, J., Gertsenstein, M., Breitman, ML,. (1995). Role of the Flt-1 receptor tyrosine kinase in regulating the assembly of vascular endothelium, *Nature* 376: 66 – 70.

Frazer KA, Ballinger DG, Cox DR et al. (2007). A second generation human haplotype map of over 3.1 million SNPs, *Nature* 449: 851-861.

Frikke-Schmidt, R., Nordestgaard, BG., Jensen, GB., Tybjaerg-Hansen, A. (2004). Genetic variation in ABC transporter A1 contributes to HDL cholesterol in the general population, *J Clin Invest* 114 : 1343-53.

Gerber, HP., McMurtrey, A., Kowalski, J., et al. (1998). Vascular endothelial growth factor regulates endothelial cell survival through the phosphatidylinositol 3=-kinase/Akt signal transduction pathway: requirement for Flk-1/KDR activation, *J Biol Chem* 273: 30336–43.

Ghosh, SS., Krieg, RJ., Sica, DA., Wang, R., Fakhry, I., et al. (2009). Cardiac hypertrophy in neonatal nephrectomized rats: the role of the sympathetic nervous system. *Pediatr Nephrol.* 24: 367–377.

Go, A.S., Chertow, G.M., Fan, D., McCulloch, C.E., and Hsu, C.Y. (2004). Chronic kidney disease and the risks of death, cardiovascular events, and hospitalization, *N. Engl. J. Med.* 351: 1296–1305.

Hansson, G.K., Jonasson, L., Seifert, P.S. and Stemme, S. (1989) Immune mechanisms in atherosclerosis. *Arteriosclerosis* 9: 567–578.

Hauser, ER., Crossman, DC., Granger, CB., Haines, JL., Jones, C.J, Mooser, V., et al. (2004). A genomewide scan for early-onset coronary artery disease in 438 families: the GENECARD Study, *Am J Hum Genet* 75: 436-47.

He, J., Gu D, Wu X, Reynolds K, Duan X, Yao C, Wang J, Chen CS, Chen J, Wildman RP *et al.* (2005). Major causes of death among men and women in China, *N Engl J Med* 353: 1124-1134.

Helgadottir, A., Manolescu, A., Thorleifsson, G., Gretarsdottir, S., Jonsdottir, H., Thorsteinsdottir, U., et al. (2004). The gene encoding 5-lipoxygenase activating protein confers risk of myocardial infarction and stroke, *Nat Genet* 36: 233-9.

Helgadottir, A., Gretarsdottir, S., St Clair, D., Manolescu, A., Cheung, J., Thorleifsson, G., et al. (2005). Association between the gene encoding 5-lipoxygenase-activating protein and stroke replicated in a Scottish population, *Am J Hum Genet* 76 : 505-9.

Hill, JM., Zalos, G., Halcox, JP., et al. (2003). Circulating endothelial progenitor cells, vascular function, and cardiovascular risk, *N Engl J Med* 348 :593- 600.

Hindorff, LA., Junkins, HA., Mehta, JP., Manolio, TA. (2010). A catalog of published genome-wide association studies. www.genome.gov/ gwastudies

Hivert, MF., Manning, AK., McAteer, JB., *et al.* (2009). Association of variants in RETN with plasma resistin levels and diabetes-related traits in the Framingham Offspring Study, *Diabetes* 58: 750–756.

Iizuka, K., Bruick, R. K., Liang, G., Horton, J. D., and Uyeda, K. (2004). Deficiency of carbohydrate response element binding protein (ChREBP) reduces lipogenesis as well as glycolysis*Proc, Natl. Acad. Sci. U. S. A.* 101: 7281-7286

International HapMap consortium. (2005). A haplotype map of the human genome, *Nature* 437: 1299-1320.

International HapMap comsortium. (2007). A second generation human haplotype map of over 3.1 million SNPs, *Nature* 449: 851-861.

Ishii, S., Iizuka, K., Miller, B. C., and Uyeda, K. (2004). Carbohydrate response element binding protein directly promotes lipogenic enzyme gene transcription, *Proc. Natl. Acad. Sci. U. S. A.* 101: 15597-15602

Jalkanen, S., and Salmi, M. (2001). Cell surface monoamine oxidases: enzymes in search of a function, *EMBO J.* 20:3893-3901.

JC., and Gomez Garcia, EB. (2004). Genetic variability of von Willebrand factor and risk of coronary heart disease: the Rotterdam Study, *Br J Haematol* 124: 343-347.

Jian, Wu., Yin, Wang., Yi, Zhang., Longjiang, Li. (2010). Association Between *IL-16* Polymorphisms and Risk of Coronary Artery Disease, *DNA and Cell Biology* . 00. (0) 1-1.

Johnson, R.C., Mayadas, T.N., Frenette, P.S., Mebius, R.E., Subramaniam, M., Lacasce, A., Hynes, R.O. and Wagner, D.D. (1995) Blood cell dynamics in P-selectin-deficient mice, *Blood* 86: 1106–1114.

Johnson, R.C., Chapman, S.M., Dong, Z.M., Ordovas, J.M., Mayadas, T.N., Herz, J., Hynes, R.O., Schaefer, E.J. and Wagner, D.D. (1997). Absence of P-selectin delays fatty streak formation in mice, *J. Clin. Invest.* 99: 1037–1043.

Joles, JA., Koomans, HA. (2004). Causes and consequences of increased sympathetic activity in renal disease, *Hypertension* 43: 699–706.

Kaikita, K., Ogawa, H., Yasue, H., Sakamoto, T., Suefuji, H., Sumida, H. and Okumura, K. (1995). Soluble P-selectin is released into the coronary circulation after coronary spasm, *Circulation* 92: 1726–1730.

Kariyazono, H., Ohno, T., Khajoee, V., et al. (2004). Association of vascular endothelial growth factor (VEGF) and VEGF receptor gene polymorphisms with coronary artery lesions of Kawasaki disease, Pediatr Res 56:953–9.

Kathiresan, S., Melander, O., Guiducci, C., Surti, A., Burtt, NP., Rieder, MJ., et al. (2008). Six new loci associated with blood low-density lipoprotein cholesterol, high-density lipoprotein cholesterol or triglycerides in humans, *Nat Genet* 40:189–197

Kooner, JS., Chambers, JC., Aguilar-Salinas, CA., Hinds, DA., Hyde, CL., Warnes, GR., et al. (2008). Genome-wide scan identifies variation in MLXIPL associated with plasma triglycerides, *Nat Genet* 40:149–151

Kunnari, A., Ukkola, O., Kesaniemi, YA. (2005). Resistin polymorphisms are associated with cerebrovascular disease in Finnish Type 2 diabetic patients, *Diabet Med* 22: 583–589.

Lander, ES. (1996). The new genomics: global views of biology, *Science* 274: 536-9.

Lanktree M. (2008). Genetic Basis of Coronary Artery Disease, *UWOMJ* 77(2): 55-58

Lee, TS., Lin, CY., Tsai, JY., Wu, YL., Su, KH., Lu, KY., Hsiao, SH., Pan, CC., Kou, YR., Hsu, YP., Ho, LT. (2009). Resistin increases lipid accumulationby affecting class A scavenger receptor, CD36 and ATP-binding cassette transporter-A1 in macrophages, *Life. Sci* 16: 97-104.

Li, G., Xu, J., Wang, P., Velazquez, H., Li, Y., et al. (2008). Catecholamines regulate the activity, secretion, and synthesis of renalase, Circulation 117: 1277–1282.

Libby, P. and Hansson, G.K. (1991). Involvement of the immune system in human atherosclerosis: current knowledge and unanswered questions, *Lab. Invest.* 64: 5–15.

Lusis, AJ., Mar, R., Pajukanta P. (2004). Genetics of atherosclerosis, Annu Rev *Genomics Hum Genet* 5: 189-218.

Ma, L., Tsatsos, N. G., and Towle, H. C. (2005). Direct Role of ChREBP/Mlx in Regulating Hepatic Glucose-responsive Genes, *J. Biol. Chem.* 280: 12019–12027

Mannuccio, MF., Lotta, LA., Peyvandi, F. (2010). Genome-Wide Association Studies in Myocardial Infarction and Coronary Artery Disease, *J Teh Univ Heart* Ctr 3 116-121

Matsumoto, T., Claesson-Welsh, L. (2001). VEGF receptor signal transduction. *Sci STKE* 112:RE21.

The International HapMap Consortium. (2003). The International HapMap Project. *Nature* 426: 789 -96.

McEver, R.P., Beckstead, J.H., Moore, K.L., Marshall-Carlson, L. and Bainton, D.F. (1989). GMP-140, a platelet alpha-granule membrane protein, is also synthesized by vascular endothelial cells and is localized in Weibel–Palade bodies, *J. Clin. Invest.* 84: 92–99.

Menzaghi, C., Coco, A., Salvemini, L., et al. (2006). Heritability of serum resistin and its genetic correlation with insulin resistance-related features in nondiabetic Caucasians, *J Clin Endocrinol Metab* 91: 2792–2795.

Meroni, G., Cairo, S., Merla, G., Messali, S., Brent, R., Ballabio, A., and Reymond, A. (2000). Mlx, a new Max-like bHLHZip family member: the center stage of a novel transcription factors regulatory pathway? Oncogene 19: 3266-277

Minn, A. H., Hafele, C., and Shalev, A. (2005). Thioredoxin-Interacting Protein Is Stimulated by Glucose through a Carbohydrate Response Element and Induces ß-Cell Apoptosis, *Endocrinology* 146: 2397–2405

Mohty, D., Pibarot, P., Despres, JP., *et al.* (2009). Age-related differences in the pathogenesis of calcific aortic stenosis: The potential role of resistin, *Int J Cardiol* in press.

Nehal, N,. Mehta, Mingyao, Li., Dilusha William, Amit V. Khera., Stephanie DerOhannessian., Liming Qu et al. (2011). The novel atherosclerosis locus at 10q11 regulates plasma CXCL12 levels , Eur Heart J.00. (0) 1-1

Neumann, J., Ligtenberg, G., Klein, II., Koomans, HA., Blankestijn, PJ. (2004). Sympathetic hyperactivity in chronic kidney disease: pathogenesis, clinical relevance, and treatment, *Kidney Int* 65: 1568–1576.

Norata, GD., Ongari, M., Garlaschelli, K., Tibolla, G., Grigore, L., Raselli, S., et al. (2007). Effect of the -420C/G variant of the resistin gene promoter on metabolic syndrome, obesity, myocardial infarction and kidney dysfunction, *J Intern Med* 262: 104–112.

Ohashi, K., Ouchi, N., Kihara, S., Funahashi, T., Nakamura, T., Sumitsuji, S., et al. (2004). Adiponectin I164T mutation is associated with the metabolic syndrome and coronary artery disease, *J Am Coll Cardiol* 43: 1195-1200.

Pajukanta, P., Cargill, M., Viitanen, L., Nuotio, I., Kareinen, A., Perola, M., et al. (2000). Two loci on chromosomes 2 and X for premature coronary heart disease identified in early- and late-settlement populations of Finland, Am *J Hum Genet* 67 : 1481-93.

Pan, LA., Chen, YC., Huang, H., Zhang, L., Liu, R., Li, X., Qiang, O., Zeng, Z,. (2009). G771C Polymorphism in the MLXIPL Gene Is Associated with a Risk of Coronary Artery Disease in the Chinese: A Case-Control Study, *Cardiology*. 114(3): 174-8.

Peart, WS. (1977). The kidney as an endocrine organ. Lancet 2: 543–548.of death, cardiovascular events, and hospitalization, *N Engl J Med* 351: 1296–1305.

Pritchard, JK. (2001). Are rare variants responsible for susceptibility to complex diseases? Am J Hum Genet 69 : 124-37.

Rajala, MW., Obici, S., Scherer, PE., Rossetti, L. (2003). Adipose-derived resistin and gut-derived resistinlike molecule-beta selectively impair insulin action on glucose production, *J Clin Invest* 111: 225–230.

Ramírez, M. & San Millán, JL. (2006). Adiponectin and resistin in PCOS: aclinical, biochemical and molecular genetic study, *Hum Reprod* 21: 2257–2265.

Rehman, J., Li, J., Parvathaneni, L., et al. (2004). Exercise acutely increases circulating endothelial progenitor cells and monocyte-/macrophagederived angiogenic cells, *J Am Coll Cardiol* 43: 2314–8

Reich, DE. , Lander, ES. (2001). On the allelic spectrum of human disease, *Trends Genet* 17 : 502-10

Reilly, MP., Lehrke, M., Wolfe, ML., Rohatgi, A., Lazar, MA., Rader, DJ. (2005). Resistin Is an Inflammatory Marker of Atherosclerosis in Humans, *Circulation* 111: 932-939.

Rizkalla, J., Melone, M., Zhao, A., Rashid, S. (2009). The Pathophysiological Role of resistin in Impaired Lipoprotein Metabolism in Obesity, *Circulation* 120: S529.

Samadi Rad, B., Seifi, M., Ghasemi, A., Khosravi, M., Afghan, MR. , Daghigh Azar, B. (2009). The association of ACE gene insertion/deletion polymorphism with coronary artery disease in Iranian subjects, 8th International Congress on Coronary Artery Disease - ICCAD. Czech Republic, Prague, (Octobr, 2009): 521-527

Samani, NJ., Burton, P., Mangino, M., Ball, SG., Balmforth, AJ., Barrett J., et al. (2005). A genomewide linkage study of 1,933 families affected by premature coronary artery disease: The British Heart Foundation (BHF) Family Heart Study, *Am J Hum Genet* 77 : 1011-20.

Sarwar, N., Danesh, J., Eiriksdottir, G., Sigurdsson, G., Wareham, N., Bingham S, et al. (2007). Triglycerides and the risk of coronary heart disease: 10 158 incident cases among 262 525 participants in 29 Western prospective studies, *Circulation* 115: 450–458

Salmi, M., and Jalkanen, S. (2001). VAP-1: an adhesion and an enzyme, *Trends Immunol.* 22: 211–216.

Shalaby, F., Rossant, J., Yamaguchi, TP., et al. (1995). Failure of blood-island formation and vasculogenesis in Flk-1-deficient mice, *Nature* 376: 62– 6.

Shalaby, F., Ho, J., Stanford, WL., et al. (1997). A requirement for Flk1 in primitive and definitive hematopoiesis and vasculogenesis, *Cell* 89: 981–90.

Stoeckman, A. K., Ma, L., and Towle, H. C. (2004). Mlx is the functional heteromeri partner of the carbohydrate response element-binding protein in glucose regulation of lipogenic enzyme genes, J. Biol. Chem. 279 (15) : 15662–15669.

Strehlow, K., Werner, N., Berweiler, J., et al. (2003). Estrogen increases bone marrow-derived endothelial progenitor cell production and diminishes neointima formation, *Circulation* 107:3059–65.

Towle, H. C. (2005). Glucose as a Regulator of Eukaryotic Gene Transcription, *Trends Endocrinol. Metab.* 16: 489–494

Takahashi, T., Yamaguchi, S., Chida, K., Shibuya, M. (2001). A single autophosphorylation site on KDR/Flk-1 is essential for VEGF-A-dependent activation of PLC-gamma and DNA synthesis in vascular endothelial cells, *EMBO J* 20: 2768 –78.

Ukkola, O., Kunnari, A., Kesaniemi, YA,. (2008). Genetic variants at the resistin locus are associated with the plasma resistin concentration and cardiovascular risk factors, *Regul Pept* 3: 56–59.

Vaessen, N., Heutink, P., Janssen, JA., Witteman, JCM., Testers, L., Hofman, A., Lamberts, SWJ., Oostra, BA., Pols, HAP., and Van Duijn CM. (2001). A polymorphism in the gene for IGF-I. Functional properties and risk for type 2 diabetes and myocardial infarction, *Diabetes* 637-642.

Van der Meer, IM., Brouwers, GJ., Bulk, S., Leebeek, FW., van der Kuip ,DA., Hofman, A., Witteman, JC., Gómez García EB. (2004). Genetic variability of von Willebrand factor and risk of coronary heart disease: the Rotterdam Study, Br J Haematol 124(3): 343-7.

Verma, S., Li, SH., Wang, CH., Fedak, PWM., Li, RK., Weisel, RD., Mickle, AG. (2003). Resistin promotes endothelial cell activation: further evidence of adipokine endothelial interaction, *Circulation* 108: 736–740

Vora, D.K, Fang, Z.-T., Liva, S.M., Tyner, T.R., Parhami, F., Watson, A.D., Drake, T.A., Territo, M.C. and and Berliner JA. (1997). Induction of P-Selectin by oxidized lipoproteins-separate effects on synthesis and surface Expression Circ Res 80: 810-818

Waltenberger, J., Claesson-Welsh, L., Siegbahn, A., Shibuya, M., Heldin, CH. (1994). Different signal transduction properties of KDR and Flt1, two receptors for vascular endothelial growth factor, *J Biol Chem* 269:26988 –95.

Wang, XL., McCredie, RM. and Wilcken DEL. (1996). Common DNA polymorphisms at the lipoprotein lipase gene. Association with severity of coronary artery disease and diabetes, *Circulation* 93:1339-1345.

Wang, L., Fan, C., Topol, SE., Topol, EJ., Wang, Q. (2003). Mutation of MEF2A in an inherited disorder with features of coronary artery disease. *Science* 302: 1578-81.

Watson, M.L., Kingsmore, S.F., Johnston, G.I., Siegelmann, M.H., Le Beau M.M., Lemons, R.S., Bora, N.S., Howard, T.A., Weissman, I.L., McEver, R.P. and Seldin, M.P. (1990) Genomic organization of the selectin family of leukocyte adhesion molecules on human and mouse chromsome 1, *J. Exp. Med.* 172: 263–272.

Wellcome trust case control consortium. (2007). Genome-wide association study of 14,000 cases of seven common diseases and 3,000 shared controls, *Nature* 447: 661-678.

Werner, N., Priller, J., Laufs, U., et al. (2002). Bone marrow-derived progenitor cells modulate vascular reendothelialization and neointimal formation: effect of 3-

hydroxy-3-methylglutaryl coenzyme A reductase inhibition, Arterioscler *Thromb Vasc Biol* 22: 1567–72.

Werner, N., Kosiol, S., Schiegl, T., et al. (2005). Circulating endothelial progenitor cells and cardiovascular outcomes, *N Engl J Med* 353: 999–1007.

Wolfe, RA., Ashby, VB., Milford, EL., Ojo, AO., Ettenger, RE., et al. (1999). Comparison of mortality in all patients on dialysis, patients on dialysis awaiting transplantation, and recipients of a first cadaveric transplant, *N Engl J Med* 341: 1725–1730.

Wolf G. (2004). Insulin resistance and obesity: Resistin, a hormone secreted by adipose tissue, *Nutr Rev* 62(10): 389–394.

Wright, AF. Hastie, ND. (2001). Complex genetic diseases: controversy over the Croesus code, *Genome Biol* 2 : 1-8.

Xu, J., Li, G., Wang, P., Velazquez, H., Yao, X., et al. (2005). Renalase is a novel, soluble monoamine oxidase that regulates cardiac function and blood pressure, *J Clin Invest* 115: 1275–1280.

Xu, J., Desir, GV. (2007). Renalase, a new renal hormone: its role in health and disease, *Curr Opin Nephrol Hypertens* 16: 373–378.

Yamashita, H., Takenoshita, M., Sakurai, M., Bruick, R. K., Henzel, W. J., Shillinglaw, W., Arnot, D., and Uyeda K. (2001A) glucose-responsive transcription factor that regulates carbohydrate metabolism in the live, *Proc Natl Acad Sci U S A.* 98(16): 9116-21

Yamauchi, J., Osawa, H., Takasuka, T., Ochi, M., Murakami, A., Nishida, W., et al. (2008). Serum resistin is reduced by glucose and meal loading in healthy human subjects, *Metabolism* 57: 149–156.

Zdravkovic, S., Wienke, A., Pedersen, NL., Marenberg, ME., Yashin, AI and De Faire, U,. (2002). Heritability of death from coronary heart disease: A 36-year follow-up of 20,966 Swedish twins, *J Intern Med* 252: 247-254.

Zhao, Q., Fan, Z., He, J., Chen, S., Li, H., et al. (2007). Renalase gene is a novel susceptibility gene for essential hypertension: a two-stage association study in northern Han Chinese population, *J Mol Med* 85: 877–885.

2

Multifunctional Role of TRAIL in Atherosclerosis and Cardiovascular Disease

Katsuhito Mori, Masanori Emoto and Masaaki Inaba
Department of Metabolism, Endocrinology and Molecular Medicine Osaka City University Graduate School of Medicine, Osaka Japan

1. Introduction

Tumor necrosis factor (TNF)-related apoptosis-inducing ligand (TRAIL) belongs to the TNF ligand superfamily. As the name suggests, TRAIL was identified and cloned based on its sequence homology to the extracellular domain of TNF ligand family members (Pitti et al., 1996; Wiley et al., 1995). Human TRAIL consists of 281 amino acids. TRAIL is a type II transmembrane protein with a short intracellular amino-terminal domain and an extracellular carboxy-terminal domain (Fig. 1). TRAIL is cleaved by cysteine proteases from the cell surface to form a soluble ligand, and when released soluble TRAIL is measurable in human blood. TRAIL contains cysteine residue (Cys 230) that interacts with the zinc ion, resulting in the formation of a TRAIL homotrimer (Hymowitz et al., 1999) (Fig. 1). This trimerization is necessary for TRAIL to bind to its receptors and to exert optimal biological activity, as is described below. (Hao et al., 2004; Johnstone et al., 2008; Wang, 2008; Wu et al., 2004).

TRAIL binds to five different receptors found on a variety of cells. Of these receptors, two, TRAIL-R1 (DR4) and TRAIL-R2 (DR5), contain a cytoplasmic death domain and trigger TRAIL-induced apoptosis. Two decoy receptors lacking a functional death domain, TRAIL-R3 (DcR1) and TRAIL-R4 (DcR2), compete with TRAIL-R1 and TRAIL-R2 for TRAIL binding, possibly antagonizing apoptotic signaling. In addition, osteoprotegerin (OPG) is a fifth soluble decoy receptor. Briefly, the TRAIL apoptosis pathway is initiated by the binding of a TRAIL trimer to TRAIL-R1 or TRAIL-R2, which leads to receptor trimerization. This receptor conformational change recruits the adaptor protein Fas-associated death domain (FADD) through the death domains (DD) of each protein. Subsequently, FADD interacts with caspase-8 and/or -10 through the death effector domain (DED) of each protein, resulting in the assembly of a death-inducing signaling complex (DISC). In the type I pathway, extrinsic signals proteolytically activate caspase-8 and/or -10 followed by stimulation of effector caspase-3 and -7, the key mediators of apoptosis, triggering apoptosis. In the type II intrinsic pathway, however, apoptotic commitment requires an amplification step involving the mitochondrial pathway triggered by caspase-8-dependent cleavage of the Bid protein to its active form, t-Bid (Corallini et al., 2006; Hao et al., 2004; Testa, 2010; Wang, 2008). Since TRAIL-R3, TRAIL-R4, and OPG lack intracellular functional portions, it is conceivable that they do not mediate apoptosis (Fig. 2.). However, even binding of TRAIL to death receptors such as TRAIL-R1 or TRAIL-R2 can antagonize apoptosis and induce cell proliferation under certain conditions in some cells. For example, TRAIL-R1 and TRAIL-R2 recruit receptor-interacting protein (RIP) through their DD, which can activate nuclear factor κB (NFκB). RIP-mediated NFκB activation appears to induce cell proliferation by TRAIL (Hao et al., 2004). TRAIL triggers recruitment of cellular FLICE-like inhibitory protein (cFLIP) to DISC through their DED in some instances. Some cFLIPs appear to prevent TRAIL-induced apoptosis (Hao et al., 2004; Wang, 2008). TRAIL stimulation also recruits phosphoprotein enriched in diabetes (PED) to the DISC. This process inhibits downstream caspase activation in some cases (Hao et al., 2004) (Fig. 2.). Therefore, two contradictory steps should be considered when determining the biological effects of TRAIL besides simple apoptotic signaling. First, TRAIL has death receptors (TRAIL-R1 and TRAIL-R2) and antagonized decoy receptors (TRAIL-R3, TRAIL-R4, and OPG) at the cell surface level. Second, these death receptors can counteract apoptotic signaling at the intracellular level in certain contexts. Thus, TRAIL signaling is very complicated.

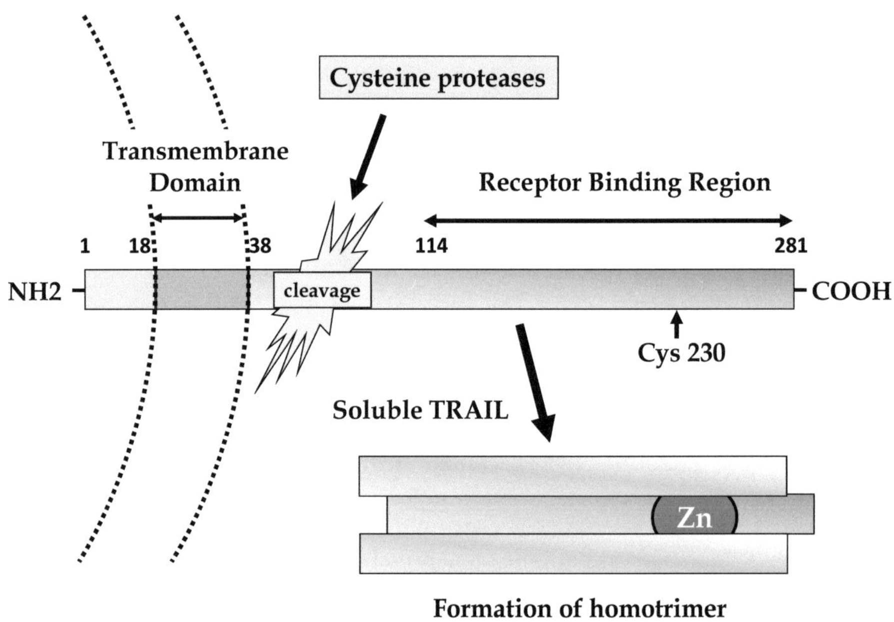

TRAIL consists of 281 amino acids with a transmembrane domain that separates the short intracellular and extracellular domains. The extracellular domain of TRAIL is cleaved and released into the bloodstream. TRAIL forms a homotrimer through interactions between zinc ions and each cysteine residue.

Fig. 1. The Structure of TRAIL.

TRAIL has attracted clinical attention as a promising agent for the treatment of cancer since it can induce apoptosis in various tumor cells without having any toxic effects on normal cells (Finnberg and El-Deiry, 2008; Wang, 2008; Wu et al., 2004). Apart from high expectations in the field of cancer, TRAIL also exhibits diverse biological effects on the immune system, hematopoiesis, and metabolic disorders, including diabetes (Afford and

Adams, 2005; Benito-Martin et al., 2009; Corallini et al., 2006; Testa, 2010; Vaccarezza et al., 2007). Recently, the involvement of TRAIL in atherosclerosis and cardiovascular diseases has been at the forefront of research efforts (Corallini et al., 2008; Kavurma and Bennett, 2008; Martin-Ventura et al., 2007). In this review, we focus on the role of TRAIL in the cardiovascular system.

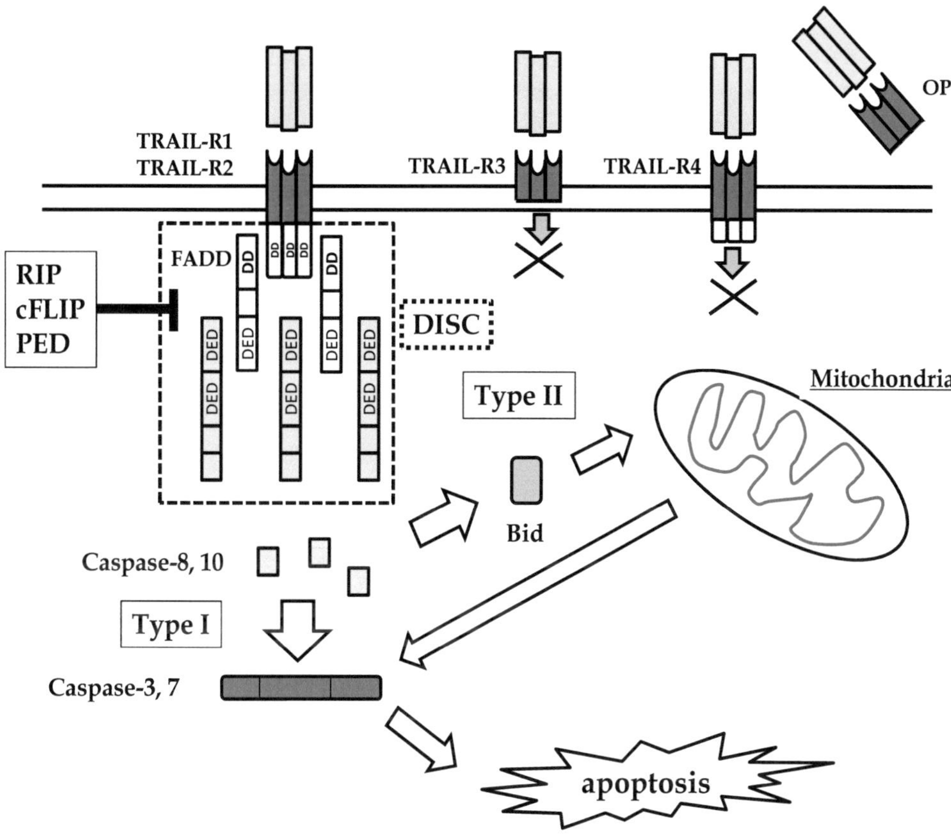

Among the five known TRAIL receptors, TRAIL-R1 and -R2 can induce intracellular apoptotic signaling. Upon binding of TRAIL to TRAIL-R1 or -R2, a death-inducing signaling complex (DISC) is formed through the recruitment of Fas-associated death domain (FADD), and subsequently results in the activation of caspase-8/10. In the type I intrinsic pathway, this activation is sufficient to conduct apoptosis through downstream effector caspases. On the other hand, activated Bid by caspase-8 amplifies apoptotic signaling through the mitochondria, which is a necessary step to induce effective downstream signaling in the type II extrinsic pathway. In addition to this activation process, it appears that at least a few other factors, such as receptor-interacting protein (RIP), cellular FLICE-like inhibitory protein (cFLIP), and phosphoprotein enriched in diabetes (PED), are antagonistic to TRAIL-induced apoptosis.

Fig. 2. TRAIL receptors and downstream apoptotic signaling.

2. TRAIL and the cardiovascular system

TRAIL and its receptors are known to be expressed in the cardiovascular system. Therefore, it is easily hypothesized that TRAIL systems may be involved in cardiovascular homeostasis and disorders. To begin with, we will summarize several *in vitro* findings that demonstrate the direct effects of TRAIL on each cellular component in the arterial wall. We will then discuss how TRAIL can act on the cardiovascular system based on evidence from animal models. Subsequently, we try to make causal inferences relating to TRAIL's role in cardiovascular diseases from cross-sectional and longitudinal clinical studies in humans. Finally, we report our recent clinical findings and debate whether TRAIL could be a common biomarker that reflects early to advanced stage atherosclerotic changes.

2.1 Effects of TRAIL on cellular components in the arterial wall (*in vitro* findings)

Endothelial cells (ECs) and vascular smooth muscle cells (VSMCs) are the principal cellular components of the normal arterial wall. Immune-inflammatory infiltrates such as activated T lymphocytes and macrophages play crucial roles in the onset and development of atherosclerosis (Libby, 2002; Weyand et al., 2008). This process is triggered and exacerbated by complicated interactions between modified lipoproteins and various cellular components. Since TRAIL and its receptors are expressed in both physiological and pathological arterial walls (Corallini et al., 2008; Kavurma and Bennett, 2008; Martin-Ventura et al., 2007; Schoppet et al., 2004), it is hypothesized that TRAIL signaling could regulate vascular wall homeostasis and morbid atherosclerosis. TRAIL is expressed in each cellular component, both in resident cells (ECs, VSMCs) and in infiltrating cells (T lymphocytes and macrophages) (Corallini et al., 2008; Kavurma and Bennett, 2008). To determine the role of TRAIL in atherosclerosis, we must first determine the effects of TRAIL on each cellular component based on results from *in vitro* studies.

ECs are located on the intima, which separates the blood stream from the vascular wall. In addition, these cells have a critical function not only as a simple barrier but also as a dynamic organ. Thus, ECs can regulate vascular tone, inflammation, thrombosis, and vascular remodeling. Balanced homeostasis in ECs protects against atherosclerosis while disruption of endothelial function results in the initiation and development of atherosclerosis (Sandoo et al., 2010). Human ECs, both human umbilical vein ECs (HUVECs) and human dermal microvascular ECs (HDMECs), express death receptors, TRAIL-R1 and TRAIL-R2. As expected, TRAIL could induce apoptosis in ECs, although this phenomenon was not observed in every cell (Li et al., 2003). This study also found that apoptosis in ECs could be reduced by treatment with caspase inhibitors and by transfection of dominant-negative FADD, suggesting the involvement of a FADD-caspase 8 pathway in this apoptotic process (Li et al., 2003). Subsequently, Secchiero et al. showed that both HUVECs and primary human aortic ECs express death TRAIL-R1, -R2 and decoy TRAIL-R3, -R4. As predicted, the removal of serum and endothelial cell growth factor (tropic withdrawal) from the cell culture system led to apoptosis. Surprisingly, TRAIL protected HUVECs from tropic withdrawal-induced apoptosis. Activation of phosphatidylinositol 3-kinase (PI3K)/Akt pathway by TRAIL appears to be involved in this anti-apoptotic action. In addition to this unexpected anti-apoptotic property, TRAIL stimulated proliferation of ECs in an ERK 1/2 dependent manner in this cell system (Secchiero et al., 2003). It has also been reported that TRAIL alone can increase HUVEC cell proliferation (Alladina et al., 2005). As reported above (Secchiero et al., 2003), inhibition of the PI3K/Akt pathway sensitizes EC cells to TRAIL-induced apoptosis (Alladina et al., 2005). More detailed investigations have found that inhibition of PI3K/Akt leads to activation of both extrinsic and intrinsic apoptotic pathways and appears to sensitize HUVECs to TRAIL-induced apoptosis by concurrent down-regulation of anti-apoptotic cFLIPs and Bcl-2 (Alladina et al.,

2005). Taken together, these results suggest that the effects of TRAIL on ECs appear to depend on cell culture conditions. Aside from cell apoptosis/proliferation, ECs have a protective role against atherosclerosis by producing nitric oxide (NO), one of the most important vasoactive factors. NO, a potent vasodilator, has antithrombotic and anti-inflammatory activity (Sandoo et al., 2010). Interestingly, TRAIL stimulates NO production through activation of endothelial NO synthase (eNOS) in HUVECs (Zauli et al., 2003). In particular, eNOS trafficking appears to be involved in TRAIL-induced eNOS activation. TRAIL can translocate eNOS from the cell membrane to the cytoplasm in HUVECs (Di Pietro et al., 2006). However, microtubule disruption with nocodazole inhibits the eNOS activity induced by TRAIL, suggesting that translocation of eNOS through cytoskeletal reorganization may be necessary for TRAIL-induced NO production (Di Pietro et al., 2006). NO synthesis with cytoskeletal alteration by TRAIL is possibly linked to the migration of HUVECs stimulated by TRAIL treatment (Zauli et al., 2003).

In terms of atherosclerosis, attachment of blood leukocytes to ECs is recognized as the first step in the initiation of this phenomenon (Libby, 2002). It is probable that TRAIL regulates this process as well. An adhesion assay using co-cultured HUVECs and HL-60 leukocytes showed that TRAIL increased the binding of leukocytes to ECs (Li et al., 2003). A later report reproduced the pro-adhesive activity of TRAIL, although its effect was much less than that of pro-inflammatory cytokines such as TNFα and interleukin-1β (Secchiero et al., 2005). When TRAIL and pro-inflammatory cytokines were evaluated at the same time, TRAIL pre-treatment showed reverse inhibition of TNFα– and IL 1β– induced HL-60 leukocyte adhesion to HUVECs. This inhibitory effect of TRAIL on cell attachment was mediated by down-regulation of the inflammatory chemokines CCL8 and CXCL10, which were stimulated by TNFα (Secchiero et al., 2005). In particular, TRAIL-R1 and TRAIL-R2 contributed to the TRAIL-induced down-regulation of chemokine release (Secchiero et al., 2005). Again, TRAIL has multiple context-dependent effects. At any rate, TRAIL may play an important role in EC function, both physiologically and pathologically.

Another physiological cellular component is the VSMCs, which are mainly localized in the media and constitute the vascular structure. Once VSMCs are transformed, however, they proliferate and migrate, contributing to the development of atherosclerosis (Ross, 1993). In advanced atheromatous plaques, apoptosis of VSMCs in the fibrous cap may be involved in plaque rupture. The former transformation exacerbates atherosclerosis (Libby, 2002), whereas the latter leads to poorer outcome (Clarke et al., 2006). TRAIL participates in the apoptosis and proliferation of VSMCs as well as ECs. For example, plaque-derived CD4 T cells expressing TRAIL induce apoptosis of VSMCs, probably through the interaction of TRAIL with TRAIL-R2 (Sato et al., 2006). On the other hand, TRAIL has been reported to act on human and rat VSMCs as an anti-apoptotic factor through TRAIL-R1 and -R2 (Secchiero et al., 2004). TRAIL promotes proliferation and migration of VSMCs through activation of ERK (Secchiero et al., 2004). Furthermore, Kavurma et al. reported that TRAIL stimulated proliferation of human VSMCs, although it induced apoptosis at high concentrations (Kavurma et al., 2008). Interestingly, they showed the importance of insulin-like growth factor-1 (IGF-1), one of the most potent growth factors, in TRAIL-induced proliferation of VSMCs. Thus, TRAIL up-regulates expression of the IGF-1 receptor in an NFκB-dependent manner (Kavurma et al., 2008). It is thus too soon to decide whether TRAIL causes apoptosis or proliferation in VSMCs, even *in vitro*.

In addition to the seemingly contradictory findings in ECs and VSMCs, a few reports have suggested that TRAIL has a pro-apoptotic effect on inflammatory lymphocytes (Janssen et al., 2005) and macrophages (Kaplan et al., 2000). In either case, TRAIL appears to have multiple functions in both physiological and pathological cells under various conditions. As described previously, the existence of five different types of TRAIL receptors and the cross-talk among multiple post-receptor signaling pathways may explain these diverse effects. On the basis of *in vitro* findings, it is very difficult to speculate the impact of TRAIL on atherosclerotic lesions *in vivo*, although the *in vitro* findings clearly indicate the involvement of the TRAIL/TRAIL receptor system in atherogenesis. In the next section, we try summarizing and discussing whether TRAIL protects against or exacerbates atherosclerosis in ways aside from its function as a mere pro-apoptotic factor.

2.2 Role of TRAIL in atherosclerosis and vascular injury (*in vivo* findings)

With regard to the role of TRAIL in the vascular wall, Secchiero et al. first demonstrated compelling *in vivo* findings using diabetic apolipoprotein E (apoE)-null mice that mimic the atherosclerotic lesions observed in humans (Secchiero et al., 2006). That is, intraperitoneal administration of recombinant human TRAIL into these mice resulted in a transient high concentration of TRAIL and subsequent protection against the development of atherosclerosis (Secchiero et al., 2006). Secchiero et al. carefully investigated the effects of TRAIL on *in vivo* atherosclerotic lesions using an adeno-associated virus containing TRAIL to ensure a low but sustained expression of TRAIL, similar to physiological conditions. TRAIL again attenuated the development of atherosclerotic plaques, even under these conditions (Secchiero et al., 2006). One of the mechanisms responsible for this effect may be selective apoptosis of infiltrating macrophages in plaque lesions. At the same time, increased VSMC levels were also observed in the fibrous caps of the atherosclerotic lesions. This increase may contribute to stabilization of the atherosclerotic plaques (Secchiero et al., 2006). Therefore, TRAIL appears to act as a protective factor against atherosclerosis *in vivo*. Subsequently, Kavurma's group showed the direct effects of TRAIL on VSMCs *in vivo*. They have already reported that TRAIL stimulates VSMC proliferation *in vitro* (Kavurma et al., 2008). To prove this using an *in vivo* model, they used a cuff-induced vascular injury method in TRAIL-null mice. In wild-type mice, this procedure can induce VSMC proliferation and intimal thickening in response to vascular injury. However, TRAIL-null mice were protected from neointimal formation and displayed reduced VSMC proliferation, suggesting a significant role for TRAIL in VSMC proliferation *in vivo* (Chan et al., 2010). Although this report showed the direct effects of TRAIL on VSMCs, the lack of atherogenic factors involved in the formation of vascular lesions should be studied further. Very recently, it has been reported that TRAIL attenuates the development of atherosclerosis using TRAIL (TRAIL −/−)/apoE (apoE −/−) double-knockout mice (Watt et al., 2011). TRAIL −/− apoE −/− mice had significantly larger atheromatous lesions compared with apoE −/− control mice at 8 weeks. The larger lesions in TRAIL −/− apoE −/− mice appeared to be due to an increase in the number of lesional VSMCs, suggesting the anti-atherogenic action of TRAIL. Intriguingly, the difference in atheromatous lesion size among these mice became smaller at 12 weeks. In contrast to Secchiero's findings, the lack of TRAIL had no effect on the macrophage content in the atheromatous lesions. There are still unsolved and controversial issues with regard to the precise mechanisms by which TRAIL acts on the arterial wall. However, TRAIL at least appears to protect against atherogenic lesions as a whole *in vivo*.

2.3 TRAIL and cardiovascular disease and prognosis (clinical findings)

Clinical studies of the relationship between TRAIL and cardiovascular diseases are also of interest. Recently, a significant relationship has been reported by a number of studies. The first study demonstrated that serum TRAIL levels were significantly lower in patients with acute coronary syndrome (ACS) compared with those with stable angina and normal coronary arteries (Michowitz et al., 2005). Subsequently, Schoppet et al. found a tendency for serum TRAIL levels to be lower in patients with coronary artery disease (CAD) compared with subjects without CAD, although this difference was not significant. To further investigate this relationship, we examined serum TRAIL levels in 285 subjects who underwent coronary angiography for suspected CAD. Interestingly, we found that serum TRAIL levels were inversely associated with the severity of CAD (Mori et al., 2010). In particular, TRAIL levels in patients with severe three-vessel disease (VD) were significantly lower than in those without CAD (Mori et al., 2010). Moreover, TRAIL was an independent and negative contributor for the presence of CAD (Mori et al., 2010). Taken together, these results suggest that lower TRAIL levels may reflect the advancement of CAD.

In addition to cross-sectional findings, recent studies have also suggested that TRAIL can be a protective predictor against cardiovascular prognosis. As previously reported (Michowitz et al., 2005), Secchiero et al. showed that serum TRAIL levels were significantly lower in patients with acute myocardial infarction (AMI) at baseline (within 24 hours from admission) compared with healthy subjects (Secchiero et al., 2009). Interestingly, serum TRAIL levels at baseline were significantly lower in patients with in-hospital adverse events compared with those who did not experience these events (Secchiero et al., 2009). Subsequently, they observed that serum TRAIL levels in AMI patients gradually recovered at discharge. Furthermore, low TRAIL levels at discharge were associated with an increased incidence of cardiac death and heart failure in the 12-month follow-up (Secchiero et al., 2009). The prognostic value of TRAIL was also examined in 351 patients with advanced heart failure (HF). Again, low serum TRAIL levels were related to a worse prognosis. The risk of mortality dropped by 70% in the highest quartile of TRAIL levels, suggesting that TRAIL is a strong inverse predictor of mortality in patients with advanced HF (Niessner et al., 2009). In addition, the role of TRAIL as a more general predictor of mortality and not limited to patients with AMI or advanced HF was investigated by a large prospective population-based study of older people (Volpato et al., 2011). Baseline TRAIL levels were inversely related to all-cause mortality over a period of six years (Volpato et al., 2011). As expected, more detailed analyses revealed that the prognostic effect of TRAIL levels was strong and highly significant in subjects with prevalent cardiovascular diseases (Volpato et al., 2011). These findings expand on the predictive ability of TRAIL at a population level with a longer follow-up period. Moreover, Secchiero et al. focused not only on TRAIL but also on OPG. As was described earlier, OPG is a soluble neutralizing receptor for TRAIL. In contrast to TRAIL, it is known that serum OPG levels are positively associated with the presence and severity of CAD and are inversely correlated with prognosis (Abedin et al., 2007; Jono et al., 2002; Kiechl et al., 2004; Omland et al., 2008; Rhee et al., 2005; Schoppet et al., 2003). In this context, both TRAIL and OPG were evaluated at the same time. The researchers found that the OPG/TRAIL ratio was significantly higher in patients with acute AMI who developed HF during the follow-up period (Secchiero et al., 2010). The increase in OPG, which is a decoy TRAIL receptor, may act against TRAIL and thus negate its protective effects on the cardiovascular system. Thus, an unbalanced OPG/TRAIL ratio may be a more accurate predictor of prognosis after AMI.

2.4 Modulating factors in TRAIL-associated biological and clinical effects

Several reports suggest that expression and/or serum levels of TRAIL are modulated by certain factors. As described above, serum TRAIL levels drop after AMI. Since proteolytic enzymes including matrix metalloproteinases (MMPs) are released following AMI, researchers have investigated whether MMPs could cleave TRAIL and thus decrease TRAIL levels, inducing AMI. In addition to MMPs, Secchiero et al. have simultaneously measured tissue inhibitors of MMPs (TIMPs) that antagonize MMPs (Secchiero et al., 2010). Among the examined MMPs and TIMPs, the circulating MMP2/TIMP2 ratio showed a significant inverse correlation with serum TRAIL levels in AMI patients (Secchiero et al., 2010). Indeed, MMP2 cleaved TRAIL and abrogated its biological activity *in vitro* (Secchiero et al., 2010). Therefore, an elevated MMP2/TIMP2 ratio following AMI may cause degradation of TRAIL, resulting in a poorer outcome. With regards to TRAIL expression, insulin has been reported to down-regulate TRAIL expression in VSMCs both *in vitro* and *in vivo* (Corallini et al., 2007). Since VSMCs are also known to release bioactive NO in response to TRAIL, it is hypothesized that chronic insulin exposure in VSMCs may induce vascular dysfunction through TRAIL suppression in diabetic patients with hyperinsulinemia or those undergoing insulin treatment. Moreover, it has been reported that activated protein C (APC), an antithrombotic and anti-inflammatory serine protease, inhibits TRAIL expression in HUVECs (O'Brien et al., 2007). In that study, intracellular signaling was thoroughly examined (O'Brien et al., 2007). However, there has been some criticism of APC-mediated decrease of TRAIL levels. It is currently unknown whether this reflects a decrease in cell-surface TRAIL expression or of TRAIL release from its intracellular pool (Secchiero and Zauli, 2008).

Statins also appear to down-regulate TRAIL expression in cytotoxic CD4 T cells in patients with ACS, resulting in protection against destabilization of plaques (Sato et al., 2010). That is, CD4 T cells are enriched in the blood of ACS patients and induce strong apoptosis of ECs, probably through TRAIL-R2 (DR5) (Sato et al., 2010). This EC apoptosis may be involved in the erosive progression of vulnerable plaques. Interestingly, statins directly block CD4 T cell-mediated EC apoptosis (Sato et al., 2010). Therefore, this protection against endothelial injury shown by statins may explain one of the pleiotropic effects of statins in cardiovascular events. On the other hand, it has been reported that statins augment TRAIL-induced apoptosis in tumor cells but not in normal cells (Jin et al., 2002), although this is not the case in vascular cells. In this regard, pioglitazone, an anti-diabetic agent, also enhances TRAIL-induced apoptosis in tumor cells (Goke et al., 2000). In clinical studies, use of various medications against diabetes, hypertension, dyslipidemia, and so on is often unavoidable. To interpret the association between TRAIL and cardiovascular lesions, it is important to pay attention to the types of interventions used.

2.5 TRAIL as a possible biomarker in early atherosclerotic lesions

As noted above, lower TRAIL levels appear to be correlated with more severe cardiovascular lesions and poorer prognosis. Thus, the next question is whether TRAIL levels also inversely reflect early atherosclerotic lesions. We therefore examined the association between TRAIL and intima-media thickness (IMT), which is a surrogate marker for atherosclerotic changes, using ultrasonography in 416 diabetic patients. We found no significant association between serum TRAIL levels and IMT (Kawano et al., 2011). Interestingly, when we focused on subjects with macrovascular diseases such as CAD, cerebrovascular diseases, and arteriosclerosis obliterans, there was a significant and reproducible association between TRAIL levels and carotid IMT. These findings suggest that TRAIL may not be a good candidate biomarker for early atherosclerotic lesions. However, TRAIL still appears to be a good biomarker of advanced atheroscletoic lesions.

In contrast to IMT, which indicates morphological wall thickening, endothelial dysfunction is recognized as reflecting earlier functional vascular damage. Flow-mediated dilatation (FMD) is a representative method of non-invasive evaluation of endothelial function. This ultrasound-based method quantifies vasodilatation in response to NO production from endothelial cells induced by shear stress (Corretti et al., 2002; Patel and Celermajer, 2006; Ter Avest et al., 2007). Since *in vitro* findings have suggested various biological effects of TRAIL on endothelial cells (as described previously), investigation of the association between TRAIL and endothelial function is of interest. In this context, we tried measuring FMD and TRAIL levels in 109 subjects (57 men and 52 women, aged 48.4 ± 16.6 years). In the trial, we focused on the following two points: First, we targeted healthy subjects to avoid various confounding biases such as metabolic disorders with concomitant drug intervention. Second, we made sure of the accuracy of FMD. It is often noted that the value of FMD is highly dependent on the technique used by various institutions (Ter Avest et al., 2007). Very recently, semi-automated equipment (Unex Co. Ltd., Nagoya, Japan) has become available for evaluating FMD that gives good reproducibility (Tomiyama et al., 2008; Tomiyama and Yamashina, 2010). We used this new equipment in this study. The serum TRAIL level was measured by an enzyme-linked immunosorbent assay kit (R&D systems, Minneapolis, USA). The mean serum TRAIL level was 75.2 ± 20.7 pg/ml, with a range of 32.4–147.4 pg/ml. The TRAIL level was not significantly correlated with FMD ($\rho = -0.128$, $p = 0.184$) (Fig. 3) (unpublished data). Again, these findings suggest that TRAIL may not be a good candidate as a biomarker of early atherosclerotic lesions.

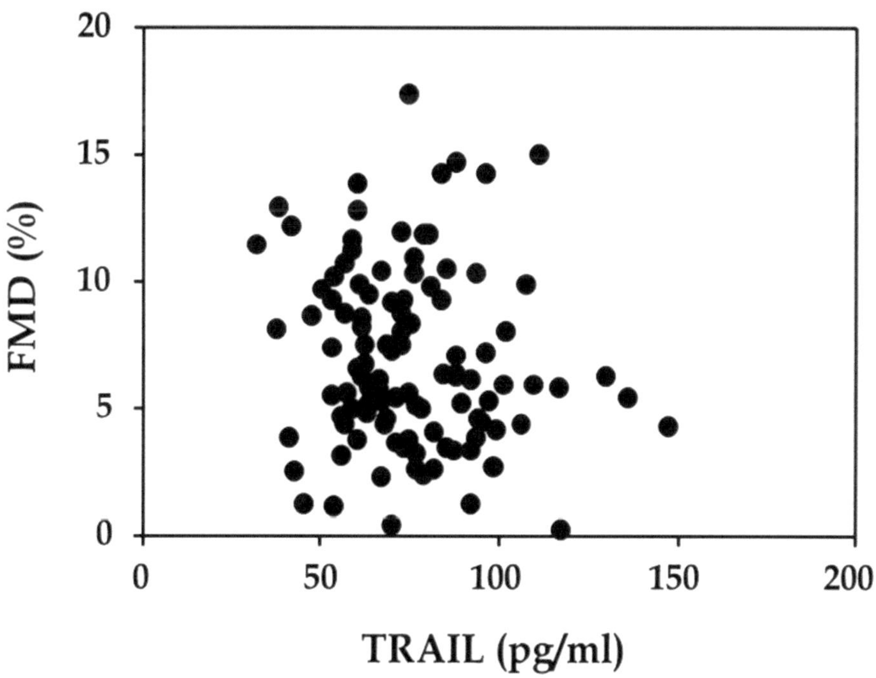

Fig. 3. The association of TRAIL with endothelial function in 109 healthy subjects.

Flow-mediated dilatation (FMD) was used to evaluate endothelial function in 109 healthy subjects. There was no correlation between serum TRAIL levels and FMD ($\rho = -0.128$, $p = 0.148$).

3. Conclusions

Recent emerging evidence has suggested the definite involvement of TRAIL in cardiovascular diseases. Taken together, these results have shown that lower serum TRAIL levels appear to be associated with worse prognosis in patients with CAD and HF. One of most important question is why TRAIL levels are lower in such conditions. It is necessary to investigate how TRAIL is produced and cleared in humans in future studies. In addition, to confirm the direct effects of TRAIL on cardiovascular diseases, administration of recombinant TRAIL may be a powerful approach. In fact, recombinant TRAIL induces apoptosis in a wide variety of tumor cells and prevents tumor progression and metastasis in the field of cancer therapy (Johnstone et al., 2008; Wang, 2008; Wu et al., 2004). Further studies are needed to address these problems.

4. Acknowledgment

This review was supported in part by a Grant-in-Aid for scientific research (No. 20591068) from the Japan Society for the Promotion of Science (to ME and KM). The authors thank Dr. Naoya Kawano, Dr. Hidenori Koyama, Ms. Yuko Kikukawa, Ms. Hisako Fujii, Dr. Sanae Fukuda, Mr. Hidekichi Tokai, Dr. Yoshinobu Hirayama, and Dr. Yasuyoshi Watanabe for their help with the study to investigate the association between TRAIL levels and FMD in healthy subjects (Fig. 3).

5. References

Abedin, M, et al. (2007). Relation of osteoprotegerin to coronary calcium and aortic plaque (from the Dallas Heart Study). *Am J Cardiol*, Vol. 99, No. 4, (February 2007) pp. 513-518, ISSN 0002-9149

Afford, SC, Adams, DH. (2005). Following the TRAIL from hepatitis C virus and alcohol to fatty liver. *Gut*, Vol. 54, No. 11, (October 2005) pp. 1518-1520, ISSN 0017-5749

Alladina, SJ, et al. (2005). TRAIL-induced apoptosis in human vascular endothelium is regulated by phosphatidylinositol 3-kinase/Akt through the short form of cellular FLIP and Bcl-2. *J Vasc Res*, Vol. 42, No. 4, (June 2005) pp. 337-47, ISSN 1018-1172

Benito-Martin, A, et al. (2009). Transcriptomics illustrate a deadly TRAIL to diabetic nephropathy. *Nefrologia*, Vol. 29, No. 1, (February 2009) pp. 13-19, ISSN 0211-6995

Chan, J, et al. (2010). TRAIL promotes VSMC proliferation and neointima formation in a FGF-2-, Sp1 phosphorylation-, and NFkappaB-dependent manner. *Circ Res*, Vol. 106, No. 6, (February 2010) pp. 1061-71, ISSN 1524-4571

Clarke, MC, et al. (2006). Apoptosis of vascular smooth muscle cells induces features of plaque vulnerability in atherosclerosis. *Nat Med*, Vol. 12, No. 9, (August 2006) pp. 1075-1080, ISSN 1078-8956

Corallini, F, et al. (2006). TRAIL, caspases and maturation of normal and leukemic myeloid precursors. *Leuk Lymphoma*, Vol. 47, No. 8, (September 2006) pp. 1459-1468, ISSN 1042-8194

Corallini, F, et al. (2007). Insulin down-regulates TRAIL expression in vascular smooth muscle cells both in vivo and in vitro. *J Cell Physiol*, Vol. 212, No. 1, (March 2007) pp. 89-95, ISSN 0021-9541

Corallini, F, et al. (2008). TRAIL and osteoprotegerin: a role in endothelial physiopathology? *Front Biosci*, Vol. 13, No. (November 2007) pp. 135-147, ISSN 1093-4715

Corretti, MC, et al. (2002). Guidelines for the ultrasound assessment of endothelial-dependent flow-mediated vasodilation of the brachial artery: a report of the International Brachial Artery Reactivity Task Force. *J Am Coll Cardiol*, Vol. 39, No. 2, (January 2002) pp. 257-265, ISSN 0735-1097

Di Pietro, R, et al. (2006). Tumor necrosis factor-related apoptosis-inducing ligand (TRAIL) regulates endothelial nitric oxide synthase (eNOS) activity and its localization within the human vein endothelial cells (HUVEC) in culture. *J Cell Biochem*, Vol. 97, No. 4, (October 2005) pp. 782-794, ISSN 0730-2312

Finnberg, N, El-Deiry, WS. (2008). TRAIL death receptors as tumor suppressors and drug targets. *Cell Cycle*, Vol. 7, No. 11, (May 2008) pp. 1525-1528, ISSN 1551-4005

Goke, R, et al. (2000). Regulation of TRAIL-induced apoptosis by transcription factors. *Cell Immunol*, Vol. 201, No. 2, (June 2000) pp. 77-82, ISSN 0008-8749

Hao, C, et al. (2004). Modulation of TRAIL signaling complex. *Vitam Horm*, Vol. 67, No. (April 2004) pp. 81-99, ISSN 0083-6729

Hymowitz, SG, et al. (1999). Triggering cell death: the crystal structure of Apo2L/TRAIL in a complex with death receptor 5. *Mol Cell*, Vol. 4, No. 4, (November 1999) pp. 563-571, ISSN 1097-2765

Janssen, EM, et al. (2005). CD4+ T-cell help controls CD8+ T-cell memory via TRAIL-mediated activation-induced cell death. *Nature*, Vol. 434, No. 7029, (March 2005) pp. 88-93, ISSN 1476-4687

Jin, Z, et al. (2002). Enhanced sensitivity of G1 arrested human cancer cells suggests a novel therapeutic strategy using a combination of simvastatin and TRAIL. *Cell Cycle*, Vol. 1, No. 1, (November 2002) pp. 82-89, ISSN 1538-4101

Johnstone, RW, et al. (2008). The TRAIL apoptotic pathway in cancer onset, progression and therapy. *Nat Rev Cancer*, Vol. 8, No. 10, (September 2008) pp. 782-798, ISSN 1474-1768

Jono, S, et al. (2002). Serum osteoprotegerin levels are associated with the presence and severity of coronary artery disease. *Circulation*, Vol. 106, No. 10, (September 2002) pp. 1192-1194, ISSN 1524-4539

Kaplan, MJ, et al. (2000). TRAIL (Apo2 ligand) and TWEAK (Apo3 ligand) mediate CD4+ T cell killing of antigen-presenting macrophages. *J Immunol*, Vol. 164, No. 6, (March 2000) pp. 2897-2904, ISSN 0022-1767

Kavurma, MM, Bennett, MR. (2008). Expression, regulation and function of trail in atherosclerosis. *Biochem Pharmacol*, Vol. 75, No. 7, (December 2007) pp. 1441-1450, ISSN 1873-2968

Kavurma, MM, et al. (2008). TRAIL stimulates proliferation of vascular smooth muscle cells via activation of NF-kappaB and induction of insulin-like growth factor-1 receptor. *J Biol Chem*, Vol. 283, No. 12, (January 2008) pp. 7754-7762, ISSN 0021-9258

Kawano, N, et al. (2011). Association of serum TRAIL levels with atherosclerosis in patients with type 2 diabetes mellitus. *Diabetes Res Clin Pract*, Vol. 91, No. 3, (January 2011) pp. 316-320, ISSN 1872-8227

Kiechl, S, et al. (2004). Osteoprotegerin is a risk factor for progressive atherosclerosis and cardiovascular disease. *Circulation*, Vol. 109, No. 18, (May 2004) pp. 2175-2180, ISSN 1524-4539

Li, JH, et al. (2003). TRAIL induces apoptosis and inflammatory gene expression in human endothelial cells. *J Immunol*, Vol. 171, No. 3, (July 2003) pp. 1526-1533, ISSN 0022-1767

Libby, P. (2002). Inflammation in atherosclerosis. *Nature*, Vol. 420, No. 6917, (December 2002) pp. 868-874, ISSN 0028-0836

Martin-Ventura, JL, et al. (2007). Trail and vascular injury. *Front Biosci*, Vol. 12, No. (May 2007) pp. 3656-3667, ISSN 1093-4715

Michowitz, Y, et al. (2005). The involvement of tumor necrosis factor-related apoptosis-inducing ligand (TRAIL) in atherosclerosis. *J Am Coll Cardiol*, Vol. 45, No. 7, (April 2005) pp. 1018-1024, ISSN 0735-1097

Mori, K, et al. (2010). Association of serum TRAIL level with coronary artery disease. *Thromb Res*, Vol. 125, No. 4, (December 2009) pp. 322-325, ISSN 1879-2472

Niessner, A, et al. (2009). Prognostic value of apoptosis markers in advanced heart failure patients. *Eur Heart J*, Vol. 30, No. 7, (February 2009) pp. 789-796, ISSN 1522-9645

O'Brien, LA, et al. (2007). Activated protein C decreases tumor necrosis factor related apoptosis-inducing ligand by an EPCR- independent mechanism involving Egr-1/Erk-1/2 activation. *Arterioscler Thromb Vasc Biol*, Vol. 27, No. 12, (October 2007) pp. 2634-2641, ISSN 1524-4636

Omland, T, et al. (2008). Circulating osteoprotegerin levels and long-term prognosis in patients with acute coronary syndromes. *J Am Coll Cardiol*, Vol. 51, No. 6, (February 2008) pp. 627-633, ISSN 1558-3597

Patel, S, Celermajer, DS. (2006). Assessment of vascular disease using arterial flow mediated dilatation. *Pharmacol Rep*, Vol. 58 Suppl, No. (March 2007) pp. 3-7, ISSN 1734-1140

Pitti, RM, et al. (1996). Induction of apoptosis by Apo-2 ligand, a new member of the tumor necrosis factor cytokine family. *J Biol Chem*, Vol. 271, No. 22, (May 1996) pp. 12687-12690, ISSN 0021-9258

Rhee, EJ, et al. (2005). Relationship of serum osteoprotegerin levels with coronary artery disease severity, left ventricular hypertrophy and C-reactive protein. *Clin Sci (Lond)*, Vol. 108, No. 3, (December 2004) pp. 237-243, ISSN 0143-5221

Ross, R. (1993). The pathogenesis of atherosclerosis: a perspective for the 1990s. *Nature*, Vol. 362, No. 6423, (April 1993) pp. 801-809, ISSN 0028-0836

Sandoo, A, et al. (2010). The endothelium and its role in regulating vascular tone. *Open Cardiovasc Med J*, Vol. 4, No. (February 2011) pp. 302-12, ISSN 1874-1924 (Electronic)

Sato, K, et al. (2006). TRAIL-expressing T cells induce apoptosis of vascular smooth muscle cells in the atherosclerotic plaque. *J Exp Med*, Vol. 203, No. 1, (January 2006) pp. 239-250, ISSN 0022-1007

Sato, K, et al. (2010). Statins reduce endothelial cell apoptosis via inhibition of TRAIL expression on activated CD4 T cells in acute coronary syndrome. *Atherosclerosis*, Vol. 213, No. 1, (May 2010) pp. 33-39, ISSN 1879-1484

Schoppet, M, et al. (2003). Increased osteoprotegerin serum levels in men with coronary artery disease. *J Clin Endocrinol Metab*, Vol. 88, No. 3, (March 2003) pp. 1024-1028, ISSN 0021-972X

Schoppet, M, et al. (2004). Localization of osteoprotegerin, tumor necrosis factor-related apoptosis-inducing ligand, and receptor activator of nuclear factor-kappaB ligand in Monckeberg's sclerosis and atherosclerosis. *J Clin Endocrinol Metab*, Vol. 89, No. 8, (August 2004) pp. 4104-4112, ISSN 0021-972X

Secchiero, P, et al. (2003). TRAIL promotes the survival and proliferation of primary human vascular endothelial cells by activating the Akt and ERK pathways. *Circulation*, Vol. 107, No. 17, (April 2003) pp. 2250-2256, ISSN 1524-4539

Secchiero, P, et al. (2004). TRAIL promotes the survival, migration and proliferation of vascular smooth muscle cells. *Cell Mol Life Sci*, Vol. 61, No. 15, (August 2004) pp. 1965-1974, ISSN 1420-682X

Secchiero, P, et al. (2005). TRAIL counteracts the proadhesive activity of inflammatory cytokines in endothelial cells by down-modulating CCL8 and CXCL10 chemokine expression and release. *Blood*, Vol. 105, No. 9, (January 2005) pp. 3413-3419, ISSN 0006-4971

Secchiero, P, et al. (2006). Systemic tumor necrosis factor-related apoptosis-inducing ligand delivery shows antiatherosclerotic activity in apolipoprotein E-null diabetic mice. *Circulation*, Vol. 114, No. 14, (September 2006) pp. 1522-1530, ISSN 1524-4539

Secchiero, P, Zauli, G. (2008). The puzzling role of TRAIL in endothelial cell biology. *Arterioscler Thromb Vasc Biol*, Vol. 28, No. 2, (January 2008) pp. e4; author reply e5-6, ISSN 1524-4636

Secchiero, P, et al. (2009). Potential prognostic significance of decreased serum levels of TRAIL after acute myocardial infarction. *PLoS One*, Vol. 4, No. 2, (February 2009) pp. e4442, ISSN 1932-6203

Secchiero, P, et al. (2010). An imbalanced OPG/TRAIL ratio is associated to severe acute myocardial infarction. *Atherosclerosis*, Vol. 210, No. 1, (December 2009) pp. 274-277, ISSN 1879-1484

Secchiero, P, et al. (2010). Metalloproteinase 2 cleaves in vitro recombinant TRAIL: potential implications for the decreased serum levels of TRAIL after acute myocardial infarction. *Atherosclerosis*, Vol. 211, No. 1, (March 2010) pp. 333-336, ISSN 1879-1484

Ter Avest, E, et al. (2007). What is the role of non-invasive measurements of atherosclerosis in individual cardiovascular risk prediction? *Clin Sci (Lond)*, Vol. 112, No. 10, (April 2007) pp. 507-516, ISSN 1470-8736

Testa, U. (2010). TRAIL/TRAIL-R in hematologic malignancies. *J Cell Biochem*, Vol. 110, No. 1, (March 2010) pp. 21-34, ISSN 1097-4644

Tomiyama, H, et al. (2008). The relationships of cardiovascular disease risk factors to flow-mediated dilatation in Japanese subjects free of cardiovascular disease. *Hypertens Res*, Vol. 31, No. 11, (December 2008) pp. 2019-2025, ISSN 0916-9636

Tomiyama, H, Yamashina, A. (2010). Non-invasive vascular function tests: their pathophysiological background and clinical application. *Circ J*, Vol. 74, No. 1, (November 2009) pp. 24-33, ISSN 1347-4820

Vaccarezza, M, et al. (2007). A role of the TRAIL-TRAIL receptor system in the pathogenesis of diabetes. *Acta Biomed*, Vol. 78 Suppl 1, No. (May 2007) pp. 262-267, ISSN 0392-4203

Venuraju, SM, et al. (2010). Osteoprotegerin as a predictor of coronary artery disease and cardiovascular mortality and morbidity. *J Am Coll Cardiol*, Vol. 55, No. 19, (May 2010) pp. 2049-2061, ISSN 1558-3597

Volpato, S, et al. (2011). Association of tumor necrosis factor-related apoptosis-inducing ligand with total and cardiovascular mortality in older adults. *Atherosclerosis*, Vol. 215, No. 2. (December 2010) pp. 452-458, ISSN 1879-1484

Wang, S. (2008). The promise of cancer therapeutics targeting the TNF-related apoptosis-inducing ligand and TRAIL receptor pathway. *Oncogene*, Vol. 27, No. 48, (October 2008) pp. 6207-6215, ISSN 1476-5594

Watt, V, et al. (2011). TRAIL attenuates the development of atherosclerosis in apolipoprotein E deficient mice. *Atherosclerosis*, Vol. No. (February 2011) pp. ISSN 1879-1484

Weyand, CM, et al. (2008). T cells in arteritis and atherosclerosis. *Curr Opin Lipidol*, Vol. 19, No. 5, (October 2008) pp. 469-477, ISSN 0957-9672

Wiley, SR, et al. (1995). Identification and characterization of a new member of the TNF family that induces apoptosis. *Immunity*, Vol. 3, No. 6, (December 1995) pp. 673-682, ISSN 1074-7613

Wu, XX, et al. (2004). TRAIL and chemotherapeutic drugs in cancer therapy. *Vitam Horm*, Vol. 67, No. (April 2004) pp. 365-383, ISSN 0083-6729

Zauli, G, et al. (2003). Tumor necrosis factor-related apoptosis-inducing ligand (TRAIL) sequentially upregulates nitric oxide and prostanoid production in primary human endothelial cells. *Circ Res*, Vol. 92, No. 7, (March 2003) pp. 732-740, ISSN 1524-4571

3

Indications for Coronary Angiography

Karl Poon and Darren Walters
The Prince Charles Hospital
Australia

1. Introduction

Since the first serendipitous selective coronary angiography was performed by pediatric cardiologist Dr. Mason Sones in 1958 during ventriculography and aortography (Sones et al., 1959), invasive coronary angiography has become well established as the diagnostic gold standard for coronary artery disease.

Coronary angiography provides definitive information of "luminology" (radiographic outline using a contrast agent) of the coronary arteries. It is the standard with which other diagnostic modalities are compared. Millions are performed annually worldwide. Whilst the risk of coronary angiography of complications is very low in experienced hands the procedure is invasive and, requires dedicated infrastructure and expense. There are certain specific indications for coronary angiography. The general indication for a coronary angiography is to define the coronary artery anatomy. More detailed guidelines for coronary angiography date back to 1999 from the American College of Cardiology (Scanlon et al., 1999). This of course predated the enormous technological advancement over the past decade, the development in computed tomography coronary angiography, the widespread adoption of coronary stenting, the improvement afforded by drug eluting stents, and the availability of new antiplatelet therapy that enhanced the safety of all coronary interventions.

This chapter examines the appropriate indications for invasive coronary angiography in the current era, assesses the role of non invasive CT coronary angiography, and incorporates the emerging adjunctive role in the management of patients undergoing percutaneous cardiac structural interventions. Case vignettes are included in this chapter to illustrate the indications and use of coronary angiography in the current era.

It must be stressed whilst guidelines do provide recommendations regarding the indications for invasive coronary angiography, many more complex clinical and non clinical factors exist for each individual patient and the clinician must exercise clinical acumen to proceed to perform an invasive diagnostic and/or therapeutic procedure.

2. Indications for coronary angiography

Coronary angiography involves the opacification of the lumen in coronary arteries and acquisition of this luminogram under fluoroscopy. Consequently the indication for coronary angiography is predominantly focused on the diagnosis of any conditions that can lead to luminal compromise. This anatomical study defines the origin, course and pattern of epicardial arteries, with a spatial resolution that is still superior to other non-invasive imaging modalities. There are however limitations to coronary angiography. Aside from the obvious invasive nature and attendant risks, it provides only a projection of the lumen outlined by contrast and hence no information on the extent of atheroma contained within the vessel wall or the functional significance of the stenosis which can only be inferred. Both of these limitations can be overcome by the use of intravascular modalities such as intravascular ultrasound, optical coherence tomography and fractional flow reserve assessment. When combined with these adjuncts, coronary angiography serves as a formidable tool in guiding revascularization strategies, with a body of scientific data that has been well validated to provide long term prognostic benefit.

The guiding principle in determining the indication behind the decision to undertake coronary angiography in a given patients is similar to that underpinning the decision to undertake any *invasive* investigations in medicine. The decision to proceed is based on that the knowledge gained from the investigation outweighs the perceived risk, that the result will benefit the patient, in that it will likely change management and the available treatment option will improve symptoms and/or prognosis. The risks and complications of coronary angiography are covered elsewhere in this book and this chapter will focus on the indications of coronary angiography. Relative and absolute contraindications are also covered briefly.

The indications for coronary angiography have been divided into the follow *clinical* categories:

1. Coronary artery disease
    1. Stable pattern
        i. suspected coronary artery disease
        ii. known coronary artery disease
    2. Unstable pattern
        i. Acute coronary syndrome with unstable haemodynamics or rhythm
        ii. Unstable angina and Non-ST elevation MI
        iii. ST elevation MI
        iv. Out of hospital cardiac arrest
    3. Special considerations
        i. Congestive cardiac failure
        ii. Preoperative assessment for non cardiac surgery
        iii. The value of non invasive computed tomography coronary angiography
    4. Relative and absolute contraindications
2. Prelude to structural cardiac disease/valvular heart disease intervention
3. Case vignettes of the use of coronary angiography in the contemporary era

3. Coronary artery disease

Coronary angiography is pivotal in the diagnostic algorithm as the gold standard for the confirmation of coronary artery stenosis. A number of well defined clinical scenarios often lead to the suspicion of coronary artery disease. This section is separated into patients who present in stable pattern, symptomatic or asymptomatic; and patients who present in an acute manner highly suggestive of coronary artery disease, i.e. acute coronary syndromes. Specifics scenarios, such as the role of coronary angiography in the investigation of congestive cardiac failure, pre-valvular surgery and the emerging role of computed tomography coronary angiography will be covered too.

3.1.1 Coronary artery disease – stable pattern – *suspected* coronary artery disease

The assessment of patients with symptoms suggestive of coronary artery disease (CAD) depends on three key factors: the clinical assessment of the quality of symptoms, the clinical risk profile, and the presence of existing abnormalities on surface electrocardiogram suggestive of CAD.

The ACC/AHA guidelines on exercise testing (Gibbons, 2002) provide classification of symptoms as typical, atypical angina and non-anginal chest pain (table 1). It is well known symptoms alone have a poor predictive value and differ between males and females (Hemingway et al, 2006, 2008). Combined with the underlying clinical risk profile however, a more reliable pre-test probability on CAD can be generated (table 2).

Chest pain	Definition
Typical/definite angina	Substernal chest pain or equivalent • Provoked by exertion or emotional stress • Relieved by rest/nitroglycerin
Atypical/probable angina	Chest pain or discomfort with two characteristics of definite or typical angina
Non-anginal chest pain	Chest pain or discomfort that meets one or none of the typical angina characteristics

Table 1. Classification of chest pain

Age	Sex	Typical/definite angina	Atypical/probable angina	Nonanginal chest pain	Asymptomatic
<39	Male	Intermediate	Intermediate	Low	Very low
	Female	Intermediate	Very low	Very low	Very low
40-49	Male	High	Intermediate	Intermediate	Low
	Female	Intermediate	Low	Very low	Very low
50-59	Male	High	Intermediate	Intermediate	Low
	Female	Intermediate	Intermediate	Low	Very low
>60	Male	High	Intermediate	Intermediate	Low
	Female	High	Intermediate	Intermediate	Low

Table 2. Pretest probability of coronary artery disease based on age, sex and symptoms (adapted from Gibbons et al, 2002)

The resting surface electrocardiogram (ECG) is important in the initial evaluation of the patient for two reasons. First, it provides a screening tool to assess for remote infarctions (Ammar et al 2004; Michael et al, 2007), with changes such as pathological Q waves, and other non-specific ST segment and T wave changes. Second, any such changes may guide the choice of the appropriate functional study. The presence of a left bundle branch block, for example, essentially renders exercise stress electrocardiography uninterpretable and confounds assessment of stress echocardiography or perfusion studies (La Canna et al, 1992).

Non-invasive tests such as exercise or pharmacological stress studies form an important pathway in the diagnostic algorithm. The value of a functional study cannot be overemphasized in patients with atypical or noncardiac chest pains. A negative functional study, such a negative treadmill test to 12 minutes on the Bruce protocol, provides sufficient prognostic information to negate any further investigations (Myers et al 2002; Marshall et al, 2010). The ischaemic burden as determined from imaging tests also provides pertinent guidance as to the appropriateness of revascularization. A substudy (Shaw et al 2008) of the COURAGE trial (Boden et al, 2007), which showed no benefit of PCI over optimized medical therapy, did show mortality and MI benefit with revascularizing patients with >10% ischaemic myocardial burden. A well executed functional study may also assist in localizing the appropriate territory for revascularization, especially in the setting of multi-vessel intermediate lesions.

Patients with positive stress tests, especially with high risk features (table three), suggestive of significant ischaemic burden, should proceed to coronary angiography for risk stratification with a view to possible percutaneous or surgical revascularization. Indeed, of the indications of coronary angiography outlined in the ACC guideline for stable angina, a positive stress test with high risk features carries the highest level of evidence (Level A) compared to all other indications (level B to C).

Noninvasive test results predicting high risk for adverse outcome (> 3% annual mortality rate)
Severe resting left ventricular dysfunction (LVEF <35%)
High-risk treadmill score (score ≤ -11)
Severe exercise induced left ventricular dysfunction (exercise LVEF <35%)
Stress-induced large perfusion defect (particularly if anterior)
Stress-induced moderate-size multiple perfusion defects
Large, fixed perfusion defect with left ventricular dilatation or increased lung uptake
Stress-induced moderate-size perfusion defect with left-ventricular dilatation or increased lung uptake
Echocardiographic wall motion abnormality (involving >2 segments) developing at low dose of dobutamine (≤ 10mg/kg/min) or at a low heart rate (<120bpm)
Stress echocardiographic evidence of extensive ischaemia

Table 3. High risk features in noninvasive tests

In some patients, however, it may be appropriate to consider coronary angiography as the initial investigation to confirm coronary artery disease. Patients who are symptomatic despite adequate or maximal antianginal therapy should proceed to coronary angiography with a view to revascularization for symptomatic benefit. As outlined in the ESC guideline on myocardial revascularization (Wijns et al, 2010), patients deemed to have a high pretest probability of coronary disease are advised against (IIIA and IIIB recommendations) non-invasive tests but to proceed to coronary angiography (IA recommendation). Patients intolerant of non-invasive testings, or with left ventricular dysfunction, could be considered for coronary angiography. Cardiac transplant patients continue to form an important group of the patients in whom coronary angiography is routinely performed for follow up for transplant vasculopathy. It continues to be a class II recommendation for patients awaiting organ transplant aged 40 years or older.

3.1.2 Coronary artery disease – stable pattern – *known* coronary artery disease

There is no role for surveillance routine coronary angiography in *stable asymptomatic* patients with known CAD, previous coronary interventions or coronary bypass surgery, unless as part of a research protocol. Patients who have documented coronary artery disease and previous interventions or CABG, who have developed recurred or worsening symptoms, coronary angiography is indicated and may be combined with percutaneous revascularization. It is reasonable to proceed to coronary angiography directly in these patients. Whilst functional non-invasive tests will still provide localizing data for inducible ischaemia, intravascular testing modalities such as intravascular ultrasound, optical coherence tomography and fractional flow reserve testing allow a robust evidence based approach to guide any revascularization (Tonino et al 2009; Pijls et al 2007).

3.2 Coronary artery disease – unstable pattern

3.2.1 Acute coronary syndromes – with haemodynamic instability or rhythm disturbance

Patients who presented with acute coronary syndromes with clinical instability (table 4) should proceed to urgent angiography with a view to possible revascularization (Hochman et al, 2006) either percutaneously or surgically if indicated.

Clinical instability in acute coronary syndromes
Cardiogenic shock
haemodynamic instability - severe hypotension on ischaemia
Recurrent/Persistent ischaemia and/or chest pain
Instability in cardiac rhythm e.g. major ventricular arrhythmia

Table 4. Clinical instability in acute coronary syndromes

3.2.2 Acute coronary syndromes – unstable angina and non ST elevation acute coronary syndromes (non STEACS)

Non STEACS is the most frequent presentation of acute coronary syndromes and carries at least as poor an outcome as STEACS (Chan et al 2009, Polonski et al, 2010). It is recommended (ESC and ACC class I recommendation) that patients who presented with non STEACS should be treated with an invasive strategy of coronary angiography. This is especially for patients with evidence of ischaemia on ECG or biomarkers, the two most powerful predictors of adverse events, as a prelude to definitive treatment for unstable coronary culprit lesions. Several meta-analyses including a Cochrane review (Hoenig et al, 2006; Fox et al, 2010; Mehta et al, 2005) of randomized controlled trials have concluded a routine invasive strategy improved ischaemic endpoints - reducing recurrent ischaemia, rehospitalisation and revascularization; and a more recent meta-analysis of three RCTs (FRISC-II, ICTUS, RITA-3) in 2010 (Fox et al, 2010) showed the benefit of a routine invasive strategy in cardiovascular death or non fatal MI was maintained at five years. Whilst the meta-analysis was conclusive, one must note the heterogeneity in the trials included. The most controversial trial, published in 2005, comparing a routine invasive vs. conservative strategy, ICTUS (de Winter et al, 2005), was the only trial to show no difference in the ischaemic end points between the two strategies. Five year follow up data from this study continued to show no long-term benefit of an early invasive strategy in reducing death or MI (Damman et al, 2010). Notably, 54% of the initially conservatively treated patients received revascularization within one year. It is likely the ability of the ICTUS trial to demonstrate difference in clinical outcomes has been significantly compromised by the cross over rate (Cannon, 2004) from medical therapy to invasive treatment.

As a result of the heterogeneity between trials (inclusion criteria, definitions of MI, intensity of pharmacological treatment and frequency of revascularization) and the confounding results, this issue of routine invasive vs. conservative treatment strategy continues to spurn passionate debate (Bittl & Maron, 2010; Thompson, 2010). The 2011 ACC guidelines (Anderson et al, 2011) acknowledge that in selective patients without high-risk features who have been stabilized, an initially conservative strategy may not be inappropriate, especially those with serious co morbidities or contraindications to angiography and intervention who have an elevated risk for clinical events, for example, patients with advanced malignancy and a history of contrast allergy who declines invasive procedures. The decision to avoid angiography in these patients may be made by considering the clinical evaluation of the physician and patient preference. It is those patients enjoying satisfactory quality of life who demonstrate the highest clinical risk profile that derive the most benefit and should receive an early invasive strategy.

When an early invasive approach has been decided for a patient, the exact timing to invasive coronary angiography is not very well established and subject to ongoing research. This of course differs from the management in STEACS where urgent reperfusion is vital. Various trials have attempted to answer the question of timing of coronary angiography in NSTEACS. The risk of adverse cardiovascular events is time dependant. These events in the unstable patient group are more common in the early phase after initial clinical presentation. An early invasive treatment may prevent impending reinfarction or ischaemia, but the counterargument is that an adequate pre procedural period of pharmacotherapy may "prepare" the lesion better to minimize complications such as no reflow. The data is not definitive. Small trials (Neumann et al, 2003), non-clinical primary endpoints (Montalescot et al, 2009), possibly underpowered studies (Mehta et al, 2009) are all factors that make definitive evidence based recommendations difficult.

Whilst the evidence differs between various trials, it is reasonable the low to intermediate risk NSTEACS patients undergo coronary angiography within 72 hours. This is reflected in the conservative arm of recent studies in whom a delayed approach is now considered a median of 24 hours after the onset of symptoms compared to 72 hours 10 years ago. Based on subgroup analysis on the TIMACS study in which patients with a GRACE score >140 benefited most from an early invasive strategy, this group of high risk patients would benefit from prompt (<24 hours) coronary angiography.

	Patients	Study design	Median early vs. Late difference (hrs)	Primary endpoint	Results	Other findings
TACTICS TIMI 18 (2001)	NSTEACS	Angiography 4-48 vs. selective invasive	22hrs vs. 79 hrs	6 month death, MI, rehospitalization for MI	15.9% vs. 19.4% (p=0.025)	
ISAR-COOL (2003)	NSTEACS	Angiography < 6 hrs vs. > 72 hrs	2.4 hrs vs. 86 hrs	30 day death or large MI	5.9% vs. 11.6% (p=0.04)	
TIMACS (2009)	NSTEACS, <24 hrs of pain	Angiography < 24 hrs vs. >36 hrs after randomization	14 hrs vs. 50 hrs	6 month death, MI, stroke	9.6% vs. 11.3% (p=0.15)	Refractory ischaemia 3.3% vs. 1.0% (p<0.001)
ABOARD (2009)	NSTEACS	Angiography "immediate" vs. delayed	70 min vs. 21 hrs	Peak troponin I during hospitalization	2.1 vs. 1.7 ng/mL	2^0 death, MI, urgent revascularization 13.7% vs. 10.2% p=0.31

Table 5. Timing of coronary angiography in NSTEACS

3.2.3 Acute coronary syndromes – ST elevation ACS

The cornerstone of management in ST elevation ACS is the timely restoration of flow in the infarct related artery. The accepted strategies for reperfusion include primary PCI and thrombolysis. If available within a timely fashion from an experienced team, urgent coronary angiography and primary PCI offers better patient outcomes than thrombolysis in STEACS. In addition, primary PCI is recommended in patients with cardiogenic shock or contraindication to thrombolysis.

In patients with failed thrombolysis, or recurrent ischaemia after initially successful thrombolysis, urgent coronary angiography should be considered, as shown in a meta-analysis in 2007 (Wijeysundera et al, 2007). Rescue PCI is associated with significant risk reduction in reinfarction and heart failure, as well as a trend towards mortality reduction. In the REACT trial (Gerschlick et al, 2005), there was a significant reduction of the primary composite end point of death, reinfarction, stroke or severe heart failure at six months for rescue PCI, compared to both conservative treatment of repeat thrombolysis. Long term data (Carver et al, 2009), median 4.4 years, from this trial reinforced the mortality reduction of rescue PCI over both conservative treatment or repeat thrombolysis (RR 0.41, p=0.004; RR 0.43, p=0.006, respectively). Repeat thrombolysis is contraindicated. It is associated with excessive bleeding and no benefit in reperfusion. In patients who presented to a non PCI-capable centre, if transfer to a PCI-capable centre can be undertaken such that the delay between first medical contact and balloon inflation is less than two hours, patient should be transferred to the PCI-capable centre. Established logistics and personnel arrangement must be in place for this to take place.

In patients with successful thrombolysis, the timing of transfer to a PCI-capable facility and the timing of angiography have been addressed in several contemporary trials and meta-analyses. Several recent meta-analyses (Borgia et al, 2010; Desch et al, 2008; Savio et al, 2010) which included studies such as CARESS-AMI (Di Mario et al, 2009), TRANSFER-AMI (Cantor et al, 2010) and NORDISTEMI (Bøhmer et al, 2009), demonstrated that early transfer to a PCI capable facility is associated with a significant reduction in the combined endpoint of 30 day mortality, re-infarction, ischaemia. The benefit appears to be driven most by a reduction of re-infarction and ischaemia. Current ESC and ACC guidelines recommend this pharmacoinvasive strategy, or "drip and ship" strategy, the prompt transfer of thrombolyzed patients to a PCI capable hospital within 24 hours.

The timing of coronary angiography deserves special mention. In stable patients successfully thrombolyzed, having been transferred to a PCI capable facility, coronary angiography and PCI should be deferred until 3 to 24 hours after thrombolysis. Whilst immediate coronary angiography appears attractive a proposition, evidence from "facilitated PCI" suggests otherwise. Facilitated PCI is a strategy of *immediate* angiography and PCI after pharmacotherapy such as upstream full or half dose thrombolytic therapy, with or without glycoprotein IIb/IIIa inhibitor. Several trials have addressed this question. ASSENT-4 (ASSENT-4 investigators, 2006), assessing tenecteplase then PCI compared to primary PCI, showed increased rates of ischaemic and bleeding complications with facilitated PCI, and FINESSE (Ellis et al, 2008, reduced reteplace and abciximab then PCI vs. abciximab then PCI vs. PCI) showed no difference in the mortality, ventricular function or cardiogenic shock but excess bleeding. A meta-analysis (Keeley et al, 2006) of 18 trials over 3 decades showed no benefit of facilitated PCI over primary PCI. There is currently no data to recommend the use of "facilitated" PCI. Pharmacoinvasive strategy is encouraged but facilitated PCI is not.

Coronary angiography should be performed prior to definitive surgical treatment for mechanical complications of any myocardial infarction (e.g. ventricular septal defect, acute mitral regurgitation or ventricular aneurysm). There are some situation however where the delays associated with angiography may outweigh the benefits of defining the coronary anatomy. For example angiography should not delay emergent surgical treatment of VSD and shock or aortic dissection.

3.2.4 Out of hospital cardiac arrest (OOHCA)

Patients who have survived an out of hospital cardiac arrest with return of spontaneous circulation (ROSC) may or may not present with diagnostic ischaemic ECG changes. In patients with definitive changes such as ST elevation, they should be treated as outlined above with an immediate invasive strategy. In haemodynamically and rhythmically stable patients after cardiac arrest, the appropriate timing (immediate vs. deferred) of coronary angiography is the subject of particular interest. Up to 80% of OOHCA patients have had an acute coronary syndrome as the precipitant (Pell et al, 2003) and ECG changes are not necessarily predictive (Aurore et al, 2011). Given this finding, it was not surprising some studies (Dumas et al, 2010; Reynolds et al, 2009; Spaulding et al, 1997; Sunde et al, 2007; Stub et al 2010) have shown an improved outcome, including cardiac ejection fraction,

	Patients	Study design	Primary endpoints	Results	Hrs to PCI in transfer group	Other findings
CARESS-in-AMI (2008)	75 y.o. or younger STEACS, ½ reteplace with abciximab, heparin, aspirin within 12 hours of pain	Immediate transfer for angiography ±PCI vs. standard treatment (with transfer for rescue if needed)	30 day death, reinfarction, refractory ischaemia	RR 0.40 (p=0.004)	<3 (median 2.2)	
TRANSFER-AMI (2009)	STEACS, tenecteplase within 12 hours of pain	Immediate transfer for angiography± PCI within 6 hours vs. standard-treatment (deferred > 24 hrs)	30 day death, reinfarction, recurrent ischaemia, new CCF, cardiogenic shock	RR 0.64 (p=0.004)	<6 (median 3.9)	
NORDISTEMI (2010)	75 y.o. or younger, STEACS, teneteplase <6 hr of pain, tenecteplase	Immediate angiography ±PCI vs. Deferred	12 month death, reinfarction, stroke, new ischaemia	RR 0.72 (NS)	As soon as possible (median 2.7)	30 day death, reinfarction, stroke or new ischaemia (RR 0.49 p=0.03)

Table 6. Timing of transfer of STEACS patients to a PCI capable facility

neurological recovery and survival, with this strategy. The largest study of this patient group is the PROCAT registry (Dumas et al, 2010) from Paris suggested that immediate angiography and successful PCI improved survival (odds ratio 2.06, p=0.013). Given the evidence leading centers have adoped a strategy of immediate coronary angiography and revascularisation as indicated after an OOHCA with ROSC. Indeed, this is the recommendation endorsed by the International Liaison Committee on Resuscitation (ILCOR, 2010) but the level of evidence is relatively low. Coma or significant neurological compromise are common in this patient group and these should not preclude consideration of angiography with full neurological recovery in initially comatose STEACS patients found in various registries (Garot et al, 2007; Hosmane et al, 2009). Further, the induction of hypothermia (Bernard et al, 2002; Wolfrum et al, 2008) should be incorporated as part of the treatment strategy for those undergoing immediate angiography.

3.3 Special considerations

3.3.1 Congestive cardiac failure

Invasive coronary angiography is useful in the investigation of left ventricular systolic dysfunction for an ischemic aetiology, especially in the presence of suggestive features such as angina, remote history of severe angina or even silent infarction, ischaemia on surface electrocardiogram, or regional wall motion abnormalities on cardiac imaging. Since the 1999 ACC guideline, the advance of non-invasive computed tomography coronary angiography (Andreini et al, 2009), with its high sensitivity and negative predictive value, may justify its use for this particular indication rather than invasive coronary angiography. The negative predictive value of a normal scan has been shown to approach 100%.

3.3.2 Preoperative assessment for noncardiac surgery

The premise of preoperative cardiac, in particular coronary, assessment for noncardiac surgery is to prevent peri operative cardiac adverse events and mortality. Surgery places significant physiological stresses that may cause cardiac ischaemia from stenosed epicardial arteries as well as inflammation and activation of the coagulation cascade possibly precipitating acute coronary syndromes.

As a general rule, the patient should be managed as would be in a non-surgical setting and testing of any type should only be undertaken if it is likely to change peri operative management. As such, in any emergency life saving operations, it is accepted any cardiac investigations should not be performed.

Coronary angiography has a limited role in the *routine* management of patients planned for non-cardiac surgery. A comprehensive discussion on the preoperative assessment of noncardiac surgery is beyond the scope of this chapter but the key determinants are: patient symptoms and clinical risk profile, surgical risk estimate (table 7) (Boersma et al, 2005), and the patient's functional capacity.

Surgical risk estimate (adapted from Boersma et al, 2005) – risk of MI and cardiac death at 30 days		
Low risk <1%	Intermediate risk 1-5%	High risk >5%
Breast	Abdominal	Aortic and major vascular surgery
Dental	Carotid	Peripheral vascular surgery
Endocrine	Peripheral arterial angioplasty	
Eye	Endovascular aneurysm repair	
Reconstructive	Head and neck surgery	
Orthopaedic - minor e.g. knee	Neurological/major orthopaedic	
Urologic - minor	Pulmonary/renal/liver transplant	
	Urologic - major	

Table 7. Risk of adverse cardiac events in different surgical scenarios

Patients who have stable angina or are asymptomatic can generally proceed with surgery. Patients who have worsening symptoms of ischaemia probably deserve further assessment, namely in the form of functional studies, prior to elective surgery. The same indications for coronary angiography and/or intervention should apply here as would be in the non-surgical setting. The cardiac risks of the particular operation should be assessed. It is a class I recommendation (Poldermans et al, 2009) that pre-operative coronary angiography be performed in acute coronary syndromes as well as in patients with angina refractory to medical therapy. Pre-operative angiography is not recommended in cardiac-stable patients undergoing low-risk and even intermediate risk surgery.

Evidence of improved outcome with revascularization prior to surgery however is lacking. There is little data pertaining to the benefit of revascularization in patients undergoing non cardiac vascular surgery, a subset of surgical patients known for high cardiac co-morbidity. One study (McFalls et al, 2004 - Coronary Artery Revascularization Prophylaxis CARP study) on stable CAD patients with preserved LV failed to demonstrate improved outcome with prophylactic revascularization compared to optimized medical therapy. Another study (Poldermans et al, 2007 - DECREASE-V pilot study), assessed the same concept on complex CAD with impaired LV systolic function, and reached the same conclusion. This was despite 75% of these cases having three vessel or left main coronary artery disease. On the currently limited available data, prophylactic revascularization cannot be recommended.

3.3.3 Non invasive computed tomography coronary angiography (CTCA)

Over the past decade the technological advances in CTCA have meant that the technology is emerging as an important investigation in a range of clinical scenarios. Aside from its non-invasive nature, CTCA provides information about both vessel lumen and important information on the composition of plaque and the vessel wall as well as other cardiac structures. However, it is important to note the spatial and temporal resolutions remain inferior to invasive coronary angiography with the current technology. Various multicentre studies (Budoff et al, 2008; Miller et al, 2008; Mowatt et al, 2008) on 64 slice CTCA have been published and confirmed its inferiority to invasive coronary angiography particularly in its specificity and the limitation on small vessel definition (table 8). The evidence for its clinical application continues to evolve.

Study author	Sensitivity per vessel	Specificity per vessel	Sensitivity per patient	Specificity per patient	Negative predictive value (per atient)	Positive predictive value (per patient)
Budoff et al 2008	84%	90%	95%	83%	99%	64%
Meijboom et al 2008	95%	77%	99%	64%	97%	86%
Miller et al 2008	75%	93%	85%	90%	83%	91%

Table 8. Meta-analyses of accuracy 64 slice CTCA compared to coronary angiography

Guidelines on the appropriateness of CTCA (Taylor et al, 2010) published in 2010 attempted to address the use of this rapidly evolving technology. The indications chosen mirrored that of invasive coronary angiography. In view of its high sensitivity, CTCA is particularly suited to low to intermediate risk patients in the setting of stable symptomatic patients, low risk acute coronary syndromes and heart failure patients. Patients with normal CTCA findings convey a very low risk of future cardiac events and cardiac mortality (Hulten et al, 2011). Patients at high risk of coronary artery disease are advised against CTCA as this represents hindrance to timely diagnosis and management of CAD with the additional risk of contrast and radiation. It has no role in the preoperative assessment of non-cardiac surgery. It is deemed appropriate in the assessment of graft patency for symptomatic patients with previous CABG. To reflect the emerging role of left main stenting, CTCA has been deemed appropriate as a means for routine follow up screening of left main stent(s) in *asymptomatic* patients.

Unless the limitations of CTCA can be sufficiently improved upon, it is likely CTCA will continue to be utilized in a complementary role to invasive coronary angiography in the assessment of CAD. Of course the major advantage of angiography remains the ability to proceed on to coronary intervention as part of the imaging procedure.

3.4 Relative and absolute contraindications

The only absolute contraindication is if a patient refuses the test fully understanding the risk and benefit of his/her decision, refuses any treatment for CAD regardless of the result of the coronary angiography, or if other medical co-morbidities rendering imaging of the coronaries and revascularization inappropriate or impossible. Subjecting the patient to even the small risks of a coronary angiogram with no foreseeable gain cannot be justified. Relative contraindications include situations which increase the likelihood of complications, e.g. bleeding diathesis, coagulopathy (iatrogenic i.e. warfarin or pathological), renal impairment, anaemia, contrast allergy, active infection and aortic valve vegetation. If these relative contraindications are reversible the patient should be appropriately prepared and coronary angiography deferred.

4. Valvular heart disease and structural heart disease intervention

The assessment of the coronary anatomy prior to cardiac valvular surgery is routine although not necessarily evidence driven. Whilst surgery for valvular heart disease has been performed for many years, percutaneous intervention for structural or valvular heart disease has been generating significant interest over the recent years. Transcatheter aortic valve implants (TAVI) have already demonstrated significant mortality benefit in patients deemed unsuitable for surgery compared to medical therapy, in the first RCT on TAVI (PARTNERS trial) (Leon et al, 2010). Several investigational percutaneous treatment options also exist for mitral regurgitation. Percutaneous coronary revascularization has been a prerequisite for the TAVI procedures and as such all patients underwent coronary angiography. The incidence of coronary disease in this patient group is high, up to 70% the PARTNERS trial. Coronary angiography is a pivotal part in the assessment for TAVI suitability. The increasing percutaneous treatment options will likely generate in the future specific college endorsed guideline to incorporate the role of coronary angiography in pre structural heart intervention..

4.1 Pre valvular surgery

It is routine to perform coronary angiography prior to valve surgery although there is no evidence to guide such practice (Bonow et al, 2006; Vahanian et al, 2007). This is especially logical in older patients with cardiac risk factors, or suggestion of CAD from symptoms, ECG, cardiac imaging or non-invasive function studies. The indication is less clear in younger patients, and special caution must be exercised in aortic valve surgery for infective endocarditis given the risk for vegetation embolization. No definitive data are available to define the clinical benefit of revascularization in the setting of corrective valve surgery. Whilst it is reasonable to expect benefit in prognostic disease, the same generalization may not apply to single vessel non prognostic lesions which would otherwise not necessarily be revascularized in a non-surgical setting. The role of CTCA is yet to be defined but its application here may reasonably mimic that outlined previously, in a low to intermediate risk group of patients undergoing valvular surgery (Meijboom et al, 2006).

4.1.1 Pre percutaneous valve implant

This is a developing area in which the role of coronary angiography appears crucial. Coronary angiography and if necessary percutaneous revascularization were a requisite for all TAVI trials so as to allow for direct comparison with the CABG + AVR subgroup. It seems nonetheless reasonable for this group of high risk patients, often with symptoms indistinguishable from ischaemia, to undergo coronary angiography. In addition, the left heart catheterization is pivotal for necessary measurement of aortic dimensions, angulation, coronary ostia position and origin, and assessment of vascular access. It should be noted the indication of revascularization in patients undergoing TAVI stems from its equivalent in surgical treatment, the exact timing and completeness of revascularization are yet to be defined.

The more difficult question relates to the need for coronary angiography in patients who may not otherwise meet the indications for coronary angiography, e.g. pulmonary valve implant in a young congenital heart disease patient, mitral valve clip in severe functional mitral regurgitation. These patients are managed the patient in a similar fashion to the conventional indications for coronary angiography.

4.1.2 Other structural cardiac interventions

There is limited evidence to support routine coronary angiography in structural cardiac interventions such as patent foramen ovale and atrial septal defect closure, coarctation stenting, patent ductus arteriosus interventions. It is often performed however based on the individual patient's clinical risk profile. The discovery of prognostically significant coronary artery disease not amenable to percutaneous coronary interventions may sway treatment towards a complete surgical treatment option. Coronary angiography does not increase the invasive nature of these procedures and add little incremental risk.

5. Case vignettes of the use of coronary angiography in the contemporary era

Case One – atrial septal defect with multi-vessel coronary artery disease

A 73 year old female presented with NYHA (New York Heart Association) class II exertional dyspnoea. Her cardiac risk factors included hypertension and hyperlipidaemia. A transthoracic echocardiogram demonstrated two small secundum atrial septal defects (ASD), with moderate right ventricular dilatation and normal systolic function. Percutaneous ASD closure was attempted. Coronary angiography was performed, especially given the uncharacteristically late presentation of her ASD, as well as her cardiac risk factors. This demonstrated prognostically significant triple vessel disease (Figure 1a, 1b, 2c), with an osital 90% left circumflex artery stenosis, 90% mid left anterior descending artery bifurcation stenosis and a 90% distal right coronary artery stenosis. Given the unfavourable percutaneous prospect for the coronary lesions, she was referred for surgical complete revascularization and ASD closure. She was discharged uneventfully one week after surgery. Coronary angiography should be considered prior to structural cardiac interventions in patients with cardiac risk factors and may alter management.

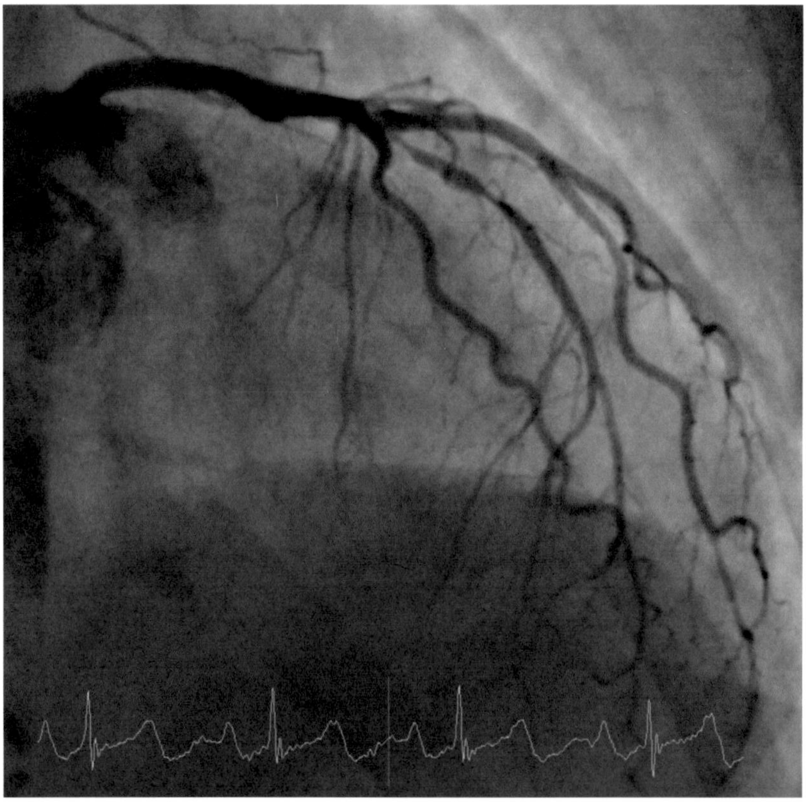

Fig. 1a. Left anterior artery stenoses

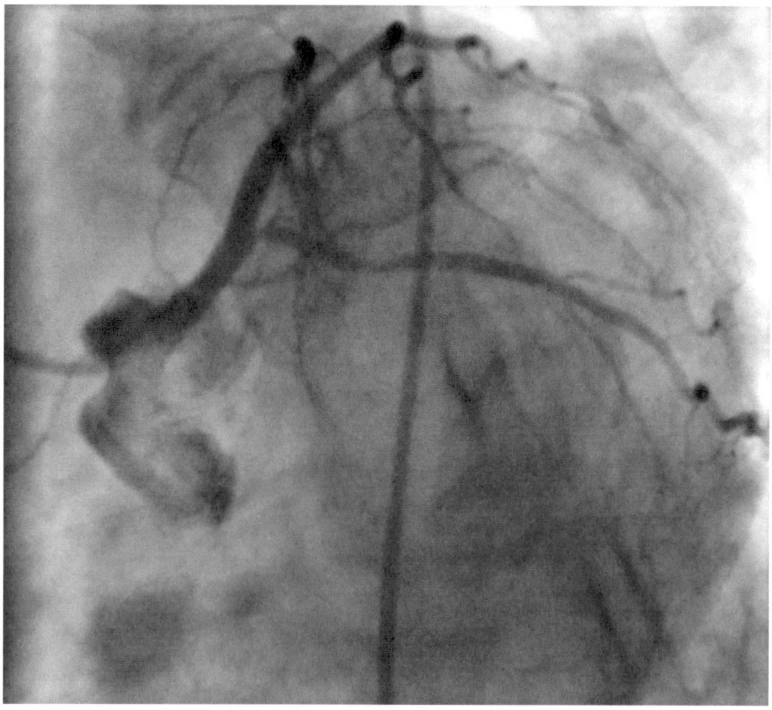

Fig. 1b. Ostial left circumflex stenosis

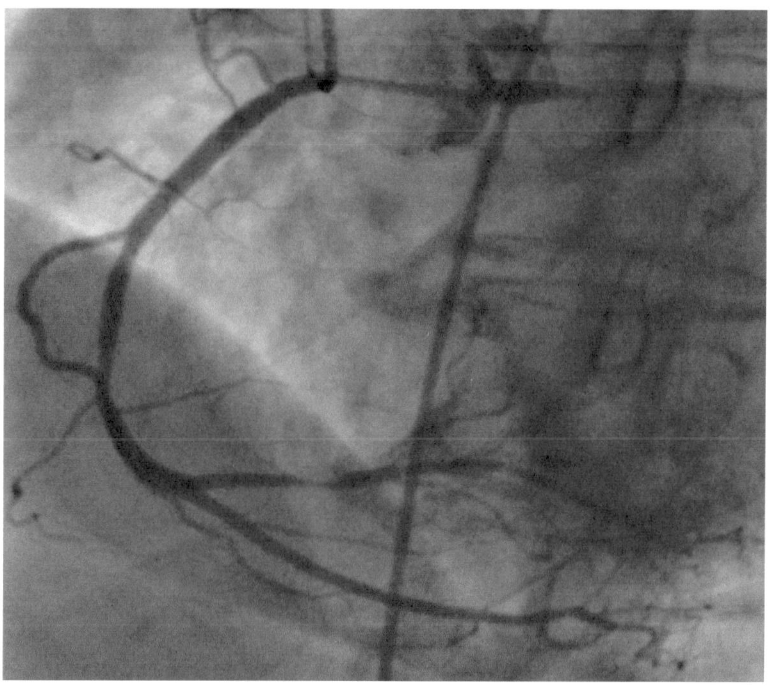

Fig. 1c. Posterolateral branch stenosis

Case Two - post TAVI angiogram

An 84 year old male represented with angina two years after a successful transcatheter aortic valve implant (TAVI) with a bioprosthetic CoreValve®. His NYHA symptomatology improved from Class IV to Class I. His coronary angiogram and graft study prior to his TAVI showed patent grafts (LIMA-LADD1-LAD; SVG-OM1; SVG-PDA) but severe native disease including a severely diseased grafted PDA with no prospect for surgical or percutaneous revascularization. A coronary angiogram and graft study was performed through his CoreValve® to assess if his underlying disease had progressed (Figure 2a).

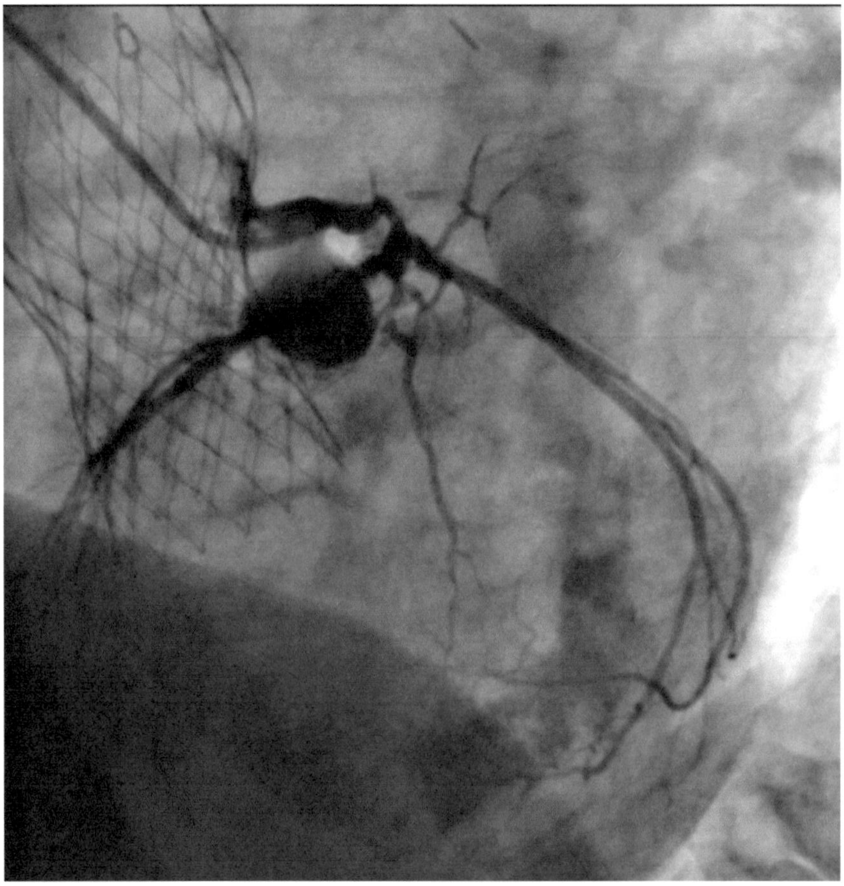

Fig. 2a. Angiography with a 5 French Judkins Left 5 catheter through a CoreValve ® bioprosthesis

This demonstrated patent grafts as previously noted but progression in his PDA disease (Figure 2b). Percutaneous, or surgical, treatment remained an unfavourable prospect and he was successfully treated with intensified medical therapy with CCS (Canadian Cardiovascular Society) I angina. Coronary angiography can be safely performed through CoreValve struts but care must be exercised with the choice and manipulation of catheters.

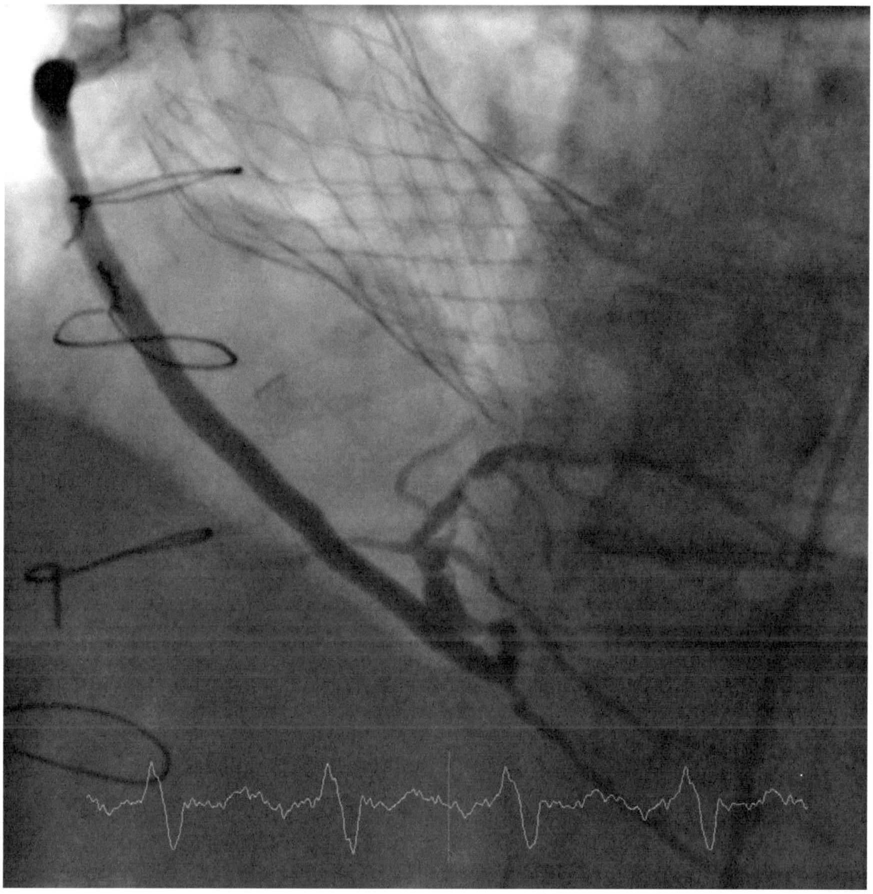

Fig. 2b. Severe native posterior descending artery disease not amenable to percutaneous treatment

Case Three - percutaneous treatment of left main stenosis and aortic stenosis

A 76 year old male with severe aortic stenosis was referred for possible percutaneous treatment due to his high surgical risk. Assessment for TAVI entailed a coronary angiogram, aortogram and an iliofemoral angiogram (Figure 3a). Coronary angiography revealed a significant left main stenosis (Figure 3b) which on intravascular ultrasound measured 5.8 mm2. A multidisciplinary heart team assessed the data and concluded surgical treatment to be prohibitively high risk. The patient then underwent left main stenting with a drug eluting stent under IVUS guidance. Satisfactory stent expansion was attained with a final diameter of 4.5mm (Figure 3c). The patient then proceeded to a successful TAVI (CoreValve®) implant and continued to enjoy excellent symptom relief at six months.

Coronary angiography, and arterial (aortic, iliac, and femoral) assessment, form an integral part of TAVI assessment. Elderly patients with severe aortic stenosis often have severe co-existing coronary artery disease as well as peripheral vascular disease as demonstrated by this case. Optimizations of the coronary status, as well as an appreciation of the peripheral vasculature, are absolutely paramount to a successful TAVI implant and to avoid vascular complications.

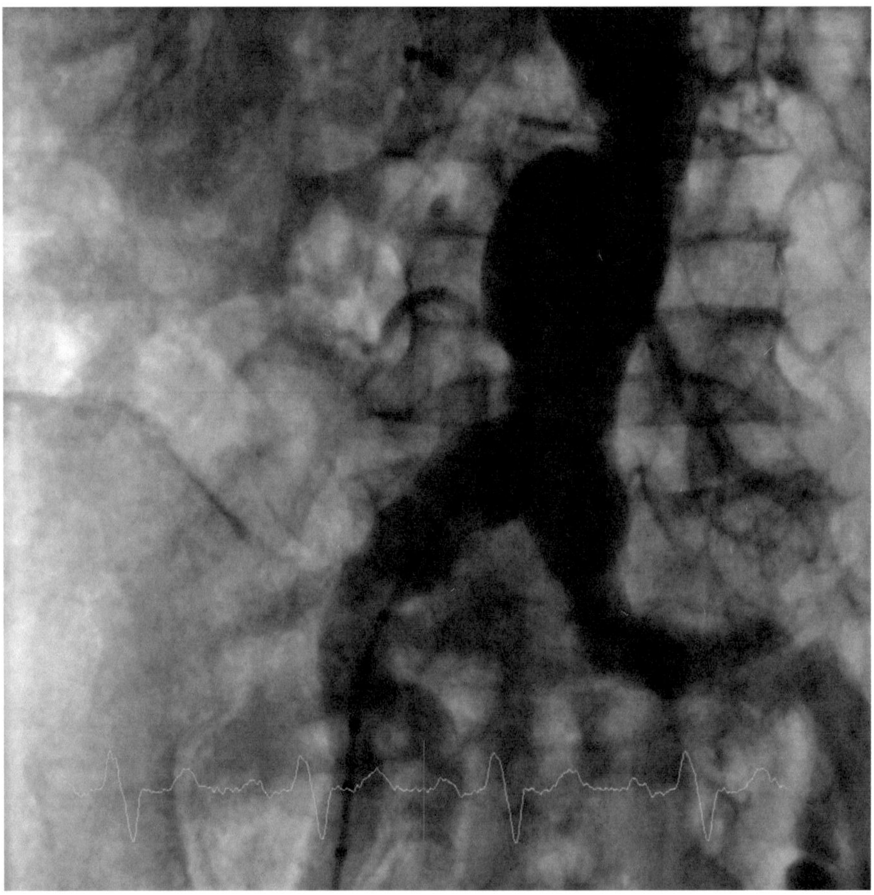

Fig. 3a. Tortuous aorta and iliac arteries, important information for TAVI transfemoral access.

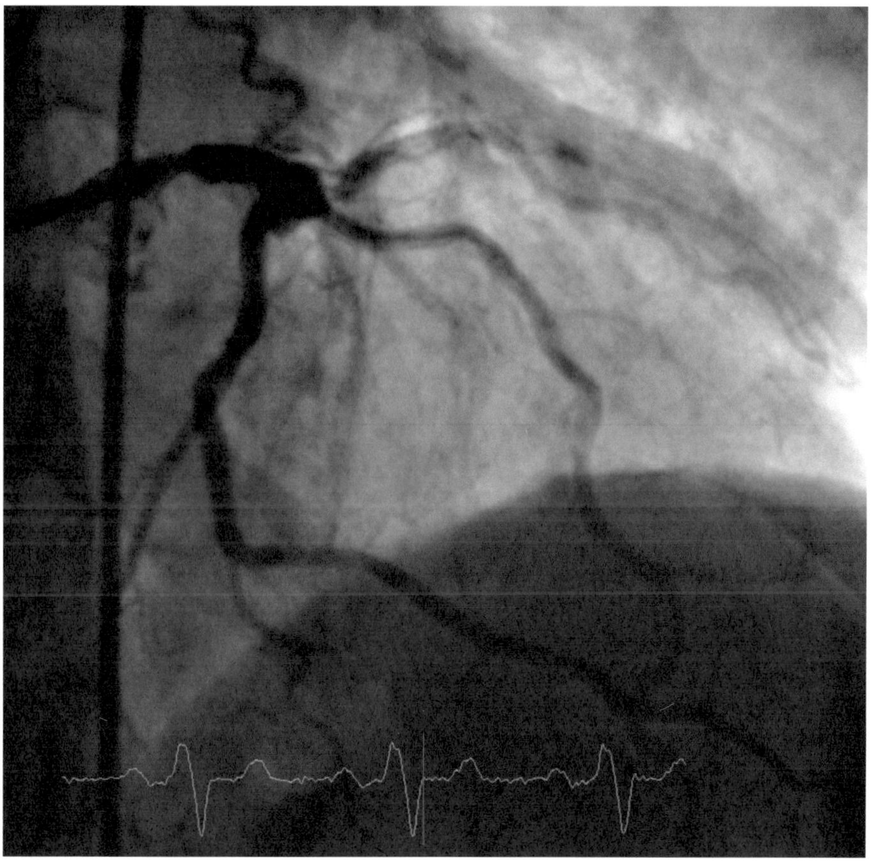

Fig. 3b. Mid shaft left main stenosis

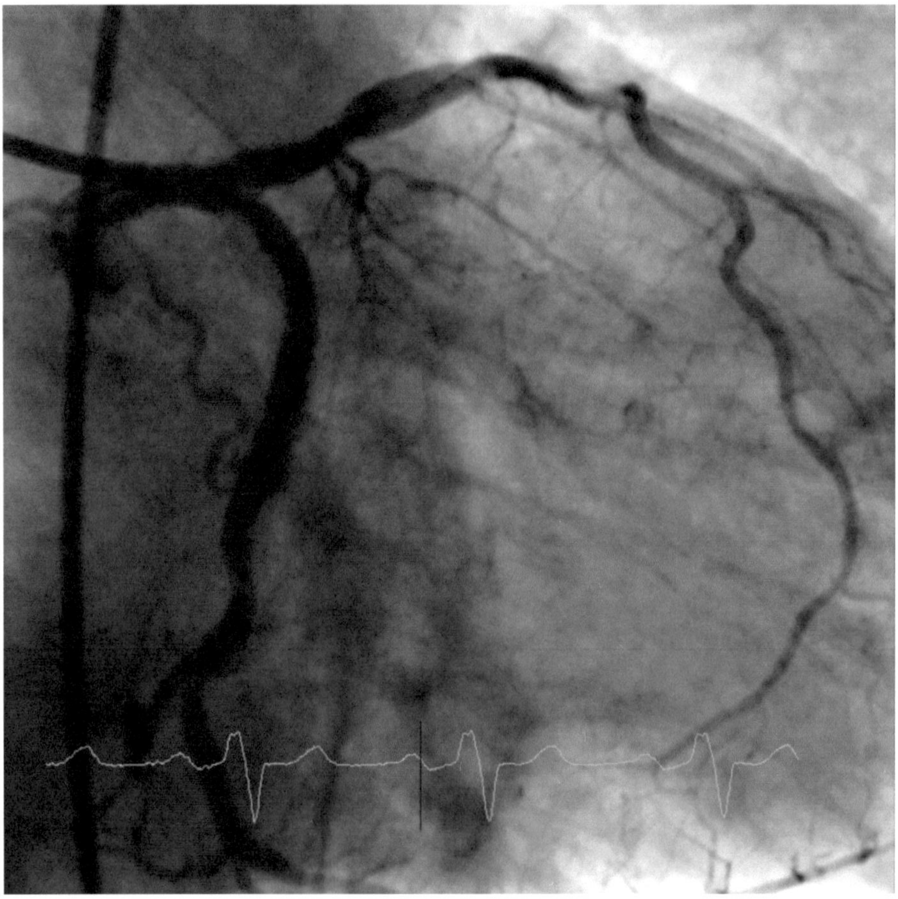

Fig. 3c. Drug eluting stent deployment in left main guided by IVUS

Case Four - anomalous coronary artery

A 63 year old male underwent coronary angiography after being successfully thrombolyzed for an inferior STEACS, 24 hours after his original pain onset. Coronary angiography via his right femoral artery showed a normal left coronary system but the origin of the right coronary artery (RCA) was not in the usual sinus. An Amplatz left catheter 2 (AL2) eventually revealed (Figure 4a) an anomalous RCA from the opposite sinus (ACAOS). A 95% stenosis in the mid RCA was found and after trying various catheters, an EBU (extra back up) 3.5 guiding catheter (Medtronic ®), traditionally a left coronary catheter, made it possible for a successful intervention and the placement of a coronary stent (Figure 4b and 4c). A CTCA (Figure 4d) was performed to ascertain the course of the RCA and confirmed ACAOS. Percutaneous coronary intervention in anomalous coronary arteries required innovative use of guiding catheters.

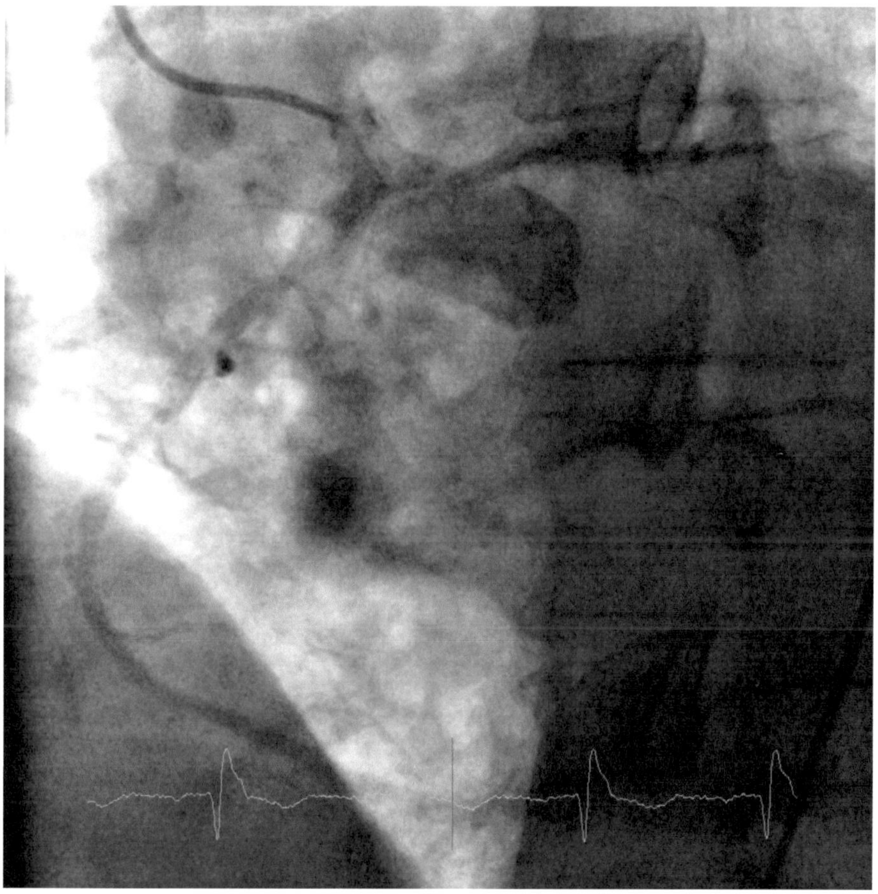

Fig. 4a. Right coronary artery injection with a 5Fr AL2 catheter showing an anomalous right coronary origin with impossible selective engagement

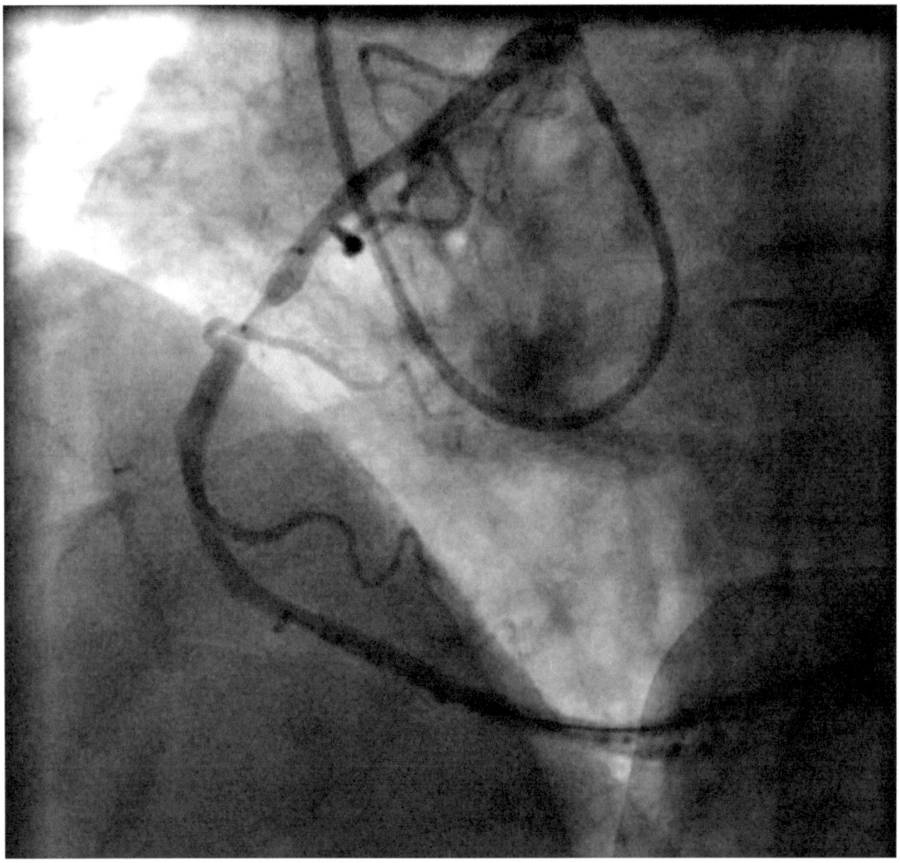

Fig. 4b. A 6Fr EBU catheter used to engage the anomalous origin. Traditional right coronary catheters would not have been useful.

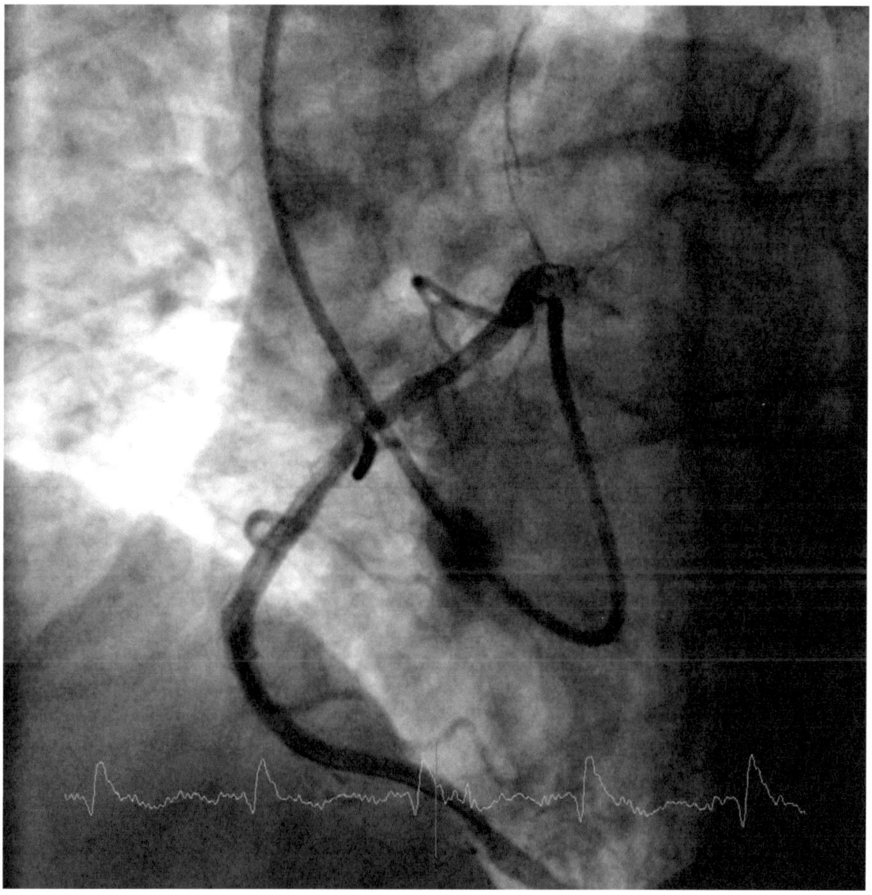

Fig. 4c. Successful placement of a drug eluting stent in the mid RCA with no residual stenosis.

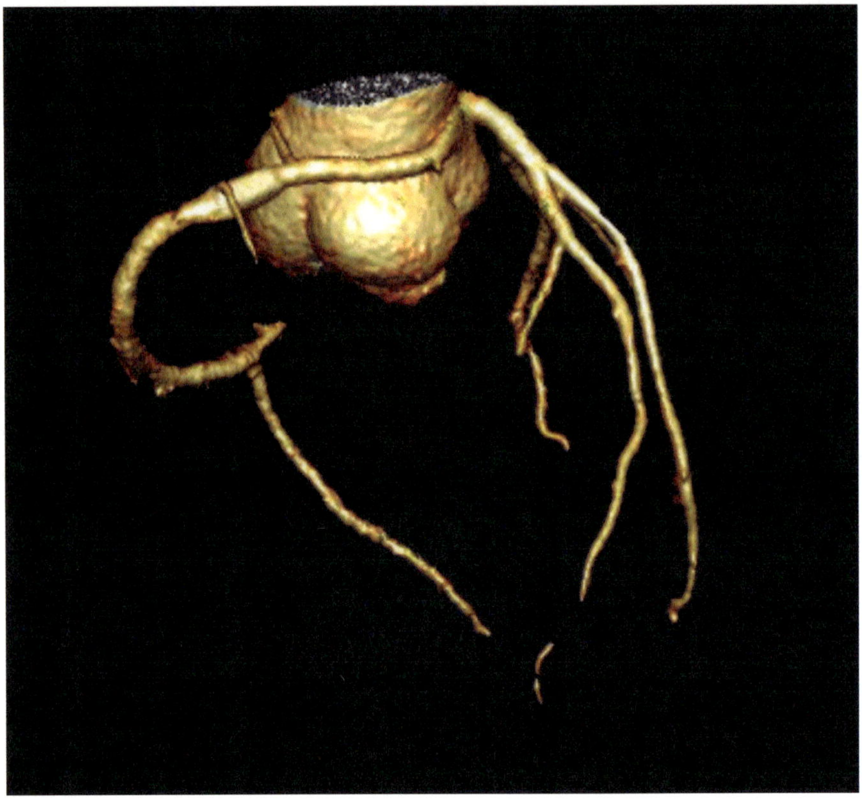

Fig. 4d. CTCA 3D reconstruction shows the origin and course of the anomalous right coronary artery clearly and defines its ante-aortic course.

Case Five - CTCA in graft assessment

A 69 year old male developed atypical chest pain 12 months after his coronary bypass graft (LIMA-LAD; RA-ramus; SVG-OM1). During the initial angiographic assessment he underwent IVUS of his left main and left anterior descending artery indeterminate lesions. IVUS showed his LM to be 5.44mm2 and LAD 3.96mm2. These were thought be suggest significant stenoses. To investigate his current atypical chest pain an MPS (Figure 5a) was performed which showed no inducible ischaemia or symptoms. A CTCA (Figure 5b) was performed which however suggested possible occluded LIMA graft. A coronary angiogram and graft study (Figure 5c and 5d) confirmed this finding that the LIMA graft had become atretic and normal coronary flow seen in the LAD. His other grafts were patent as was shown on the CTCA. This case demonstrated the value of CTCA in identifying graft patency and position, often facilitating the location of the graft anastomosis at the aorta. The atypical symptoms, patent coronary arteries and grafts, correlated well with his negative functional study. The LIMA-LAD graft probably underwent atresia as a result of no physiological implication to his intermediate LM and LAD lesions even though the diameters measured fulfilled conventional criteria for significant lesions.

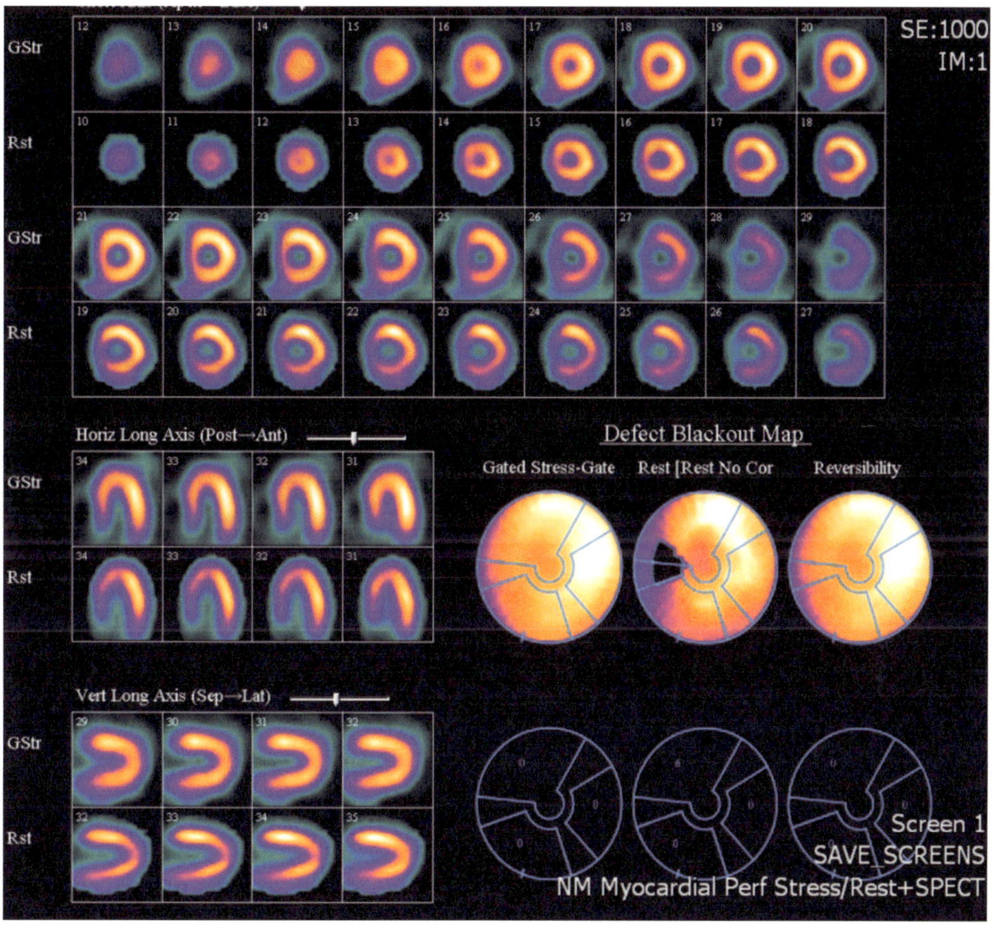

Fig. 5a. Myoperfusion study with no significant inducible ischaemia.

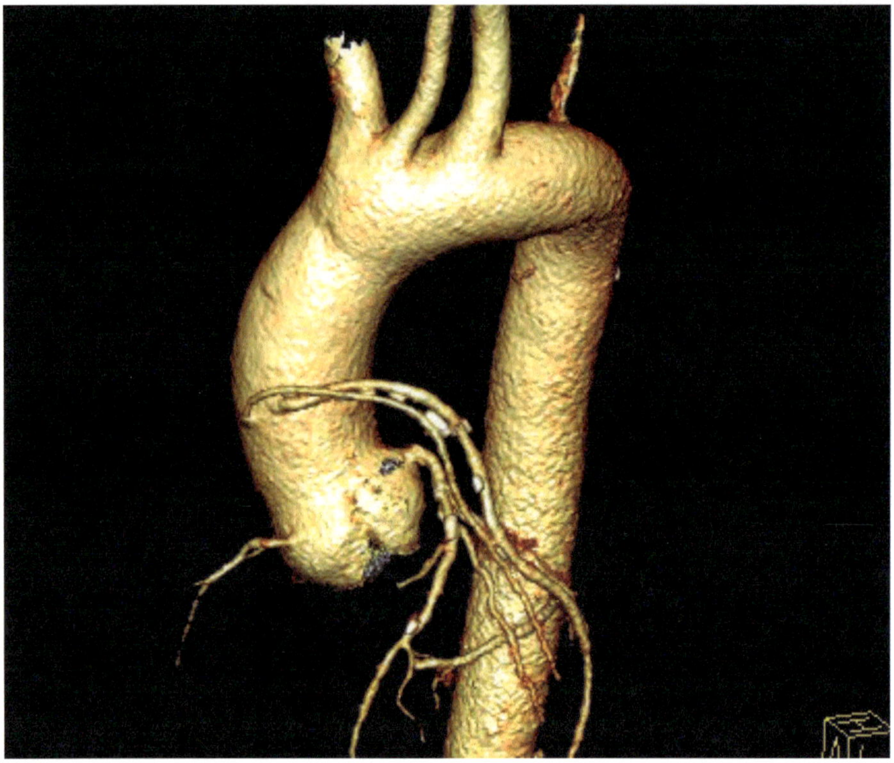

Fig. 5b. Position of two aortic grafts demonstrated clearly on CTCA. No LIMA flow demonstrated.

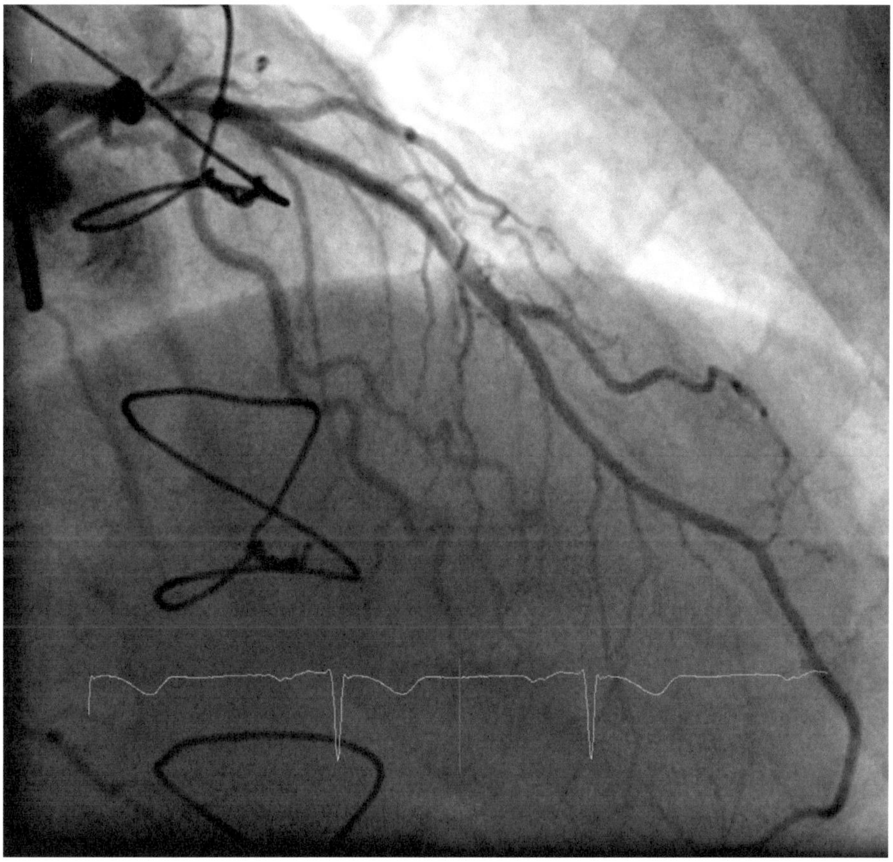

Fig. 5c. LAD artery with no obvious proximal stenosis and normal coronary flow.

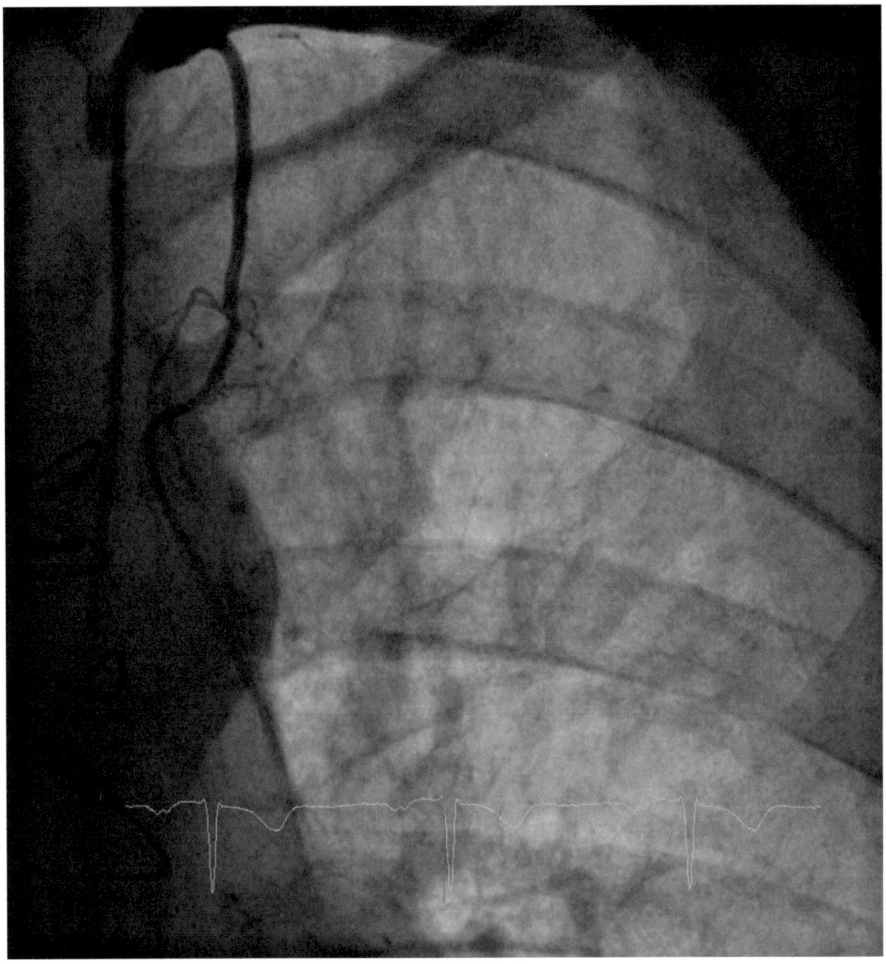

Fig. 5d. Small atretic LIMA.

Case Six - balanced ischaemia on MPS in a high risk patient

A 67 year old male with 20 years of diabetes mellitus II and 40 pack year history of smoking presented with six months of worsening exertional dyspnoea and chest pain. A myoperfusion study performed at a satisfactory level of workload demonstrated a small area of mildly reversible ischaemia in the inferolateral area. Given the abnormal findings, the patient proceeded to coronary angiography. This revealed severe distal left main artery stenosis, with a subtotally occluded left circumflex and a proximal severe RCA stenosis. Left ventricular function was normal. The extent and severity of disease was of prognostic significance. The patient underwent uneventful coronary bypass grafting and was discharged from the hospital one week after. This patient exhibited a high pretest probability based on the clinical profile. Whilst the myoperfusion study was suggestive, it underestimated the extent of disease likely due to the balanced ischaemia from the RCA and LM stenoses. Complex distal left main stenosis, especially bifurcation stenosis, is best treated with surgical revascularization.

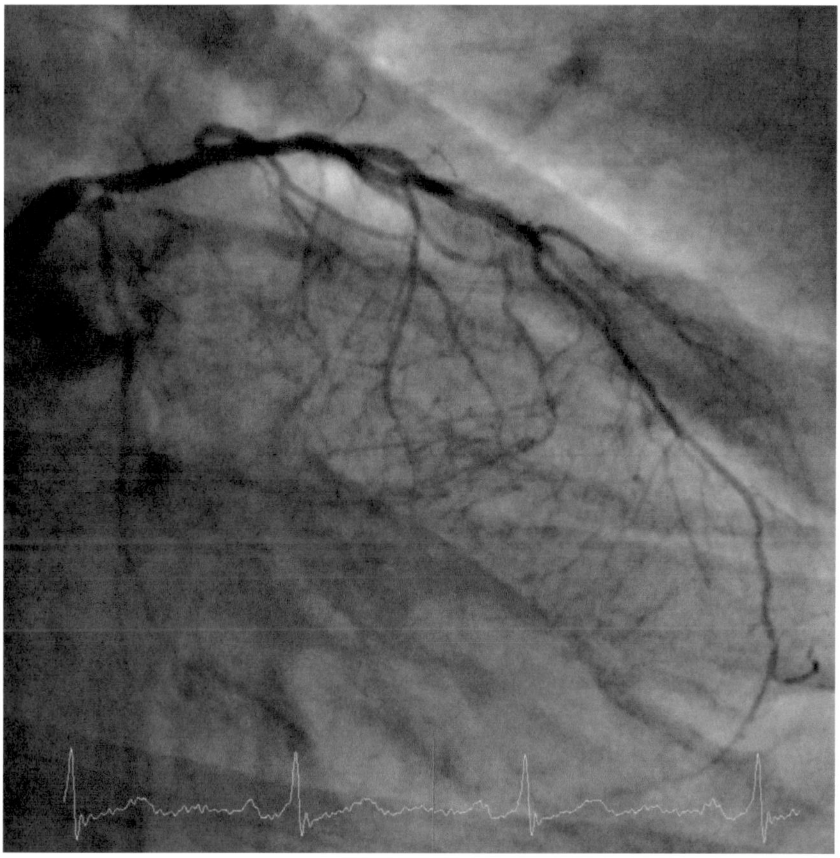

Fig. 6a. Distal left main eccentric stenosis and ostial circumflex stenosis.

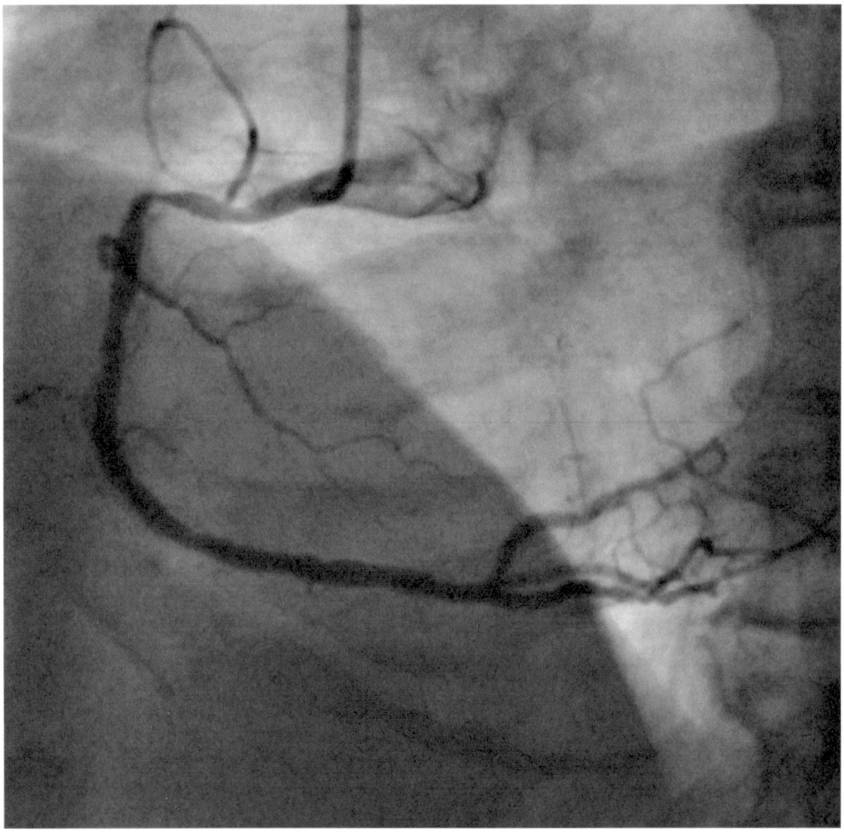

Fig. 6b. Proximal right coronary artery stenosis

6. Conclusion

Coronary angiography remains the most accurate diagnostic modality for coronary artery disease. It provides a definitive assessment of coronary artery lumen and provides an avenue to percutaneous intervention. It is pivotal in the treatment on unstable or acute coronary syndromes and life saving in cardiogenic shock and STEACSs. Indications for invasive coronary angiography have changed incrementally over the decade since ACC/AHA guidelines on the topic were published. The advent of noninvasive CTCA has changed the landscape for the diagnosis of CAD but CTCAs seem destined only for the low to intermediate risk patients. Coronary angiography also serves a pivotal role in the burgeoning field of percutaneous structural cardiac interventions, especially percutaneous valve implants.

7. References

Andreini D, Pontone G, Bartorelli AL, Agostoni P, Mushtaq S, Bertella E, Trabattoni D, Cattadori G, Cortinovis S, Annoni A, et al. (2009). Sixty-Four-Slice Multidetector Computed Tomography: An Accurate Imaging Modality for the Evaluation of Coronary Arteries in Dilated Cardiomyopathy of Unknown Etiology *Circ Cardiovasc Imaging* 2(3): 199 - 205.

Anderson JL, Adams CD, et al. (2011). 2011 ACCF/AHA Focused Update Incorporated into the ACC/AHA 2077 Guidelines for the management of patients with unstable angina/Non-ST Elevation myocardial infarction, A report of the American College of Cardiology Foundation/American Heart Association Task Force on Practice Guidelines, *Circulation*. 2011; 123 [Epub ahead of print]

ASSENT-4 investigators, (2006). Primary versus tenecteplase-facilitated percutaneous coronary intervention in patients with ST-segment elevation acute myocardial infarction (ASSENT-4 PCI): randomised trial. *Lancet* 367:569–578.

Aurore A, Jabre P, Liot P, Margenet A, Lecarpentier E, Combes X. (2011). Predictive factors for positive coronary angiography in out-of-hospital cardiac arrest patients. *Eur J Emerg Med.* 18(2):73-6.

Bernard SA, Gray TW, Buist MD, Jones BM, Silvester W, Gutteridge G, et al. (2002). Treatment of comatose survivors of out-of-hospital cardiac arrest with induced hypothermia. *N Engl J Med* 346: 557 – 563

Bittl JA, Maron DJ. (2010). Having It Both Ways *J. Am. Coll. Cardiol.*, 55(9): 865 - 866.

Boden WE, O'Rourke RA, Teo KK, et al. (2007). Optimal medical therapy with or without PCI for stable coronary disease. *N Engl J Med* 356:1503-1516

Boersma E, Kertai MD, Schouten O, Bax JJ, Noordzij P, Steyerberg EW, Schinkel AF, van Santen M, Simoons ML, Thomson IR, Klein J, van Urk H, Poldermans D. (2005). Perioperative cardiovascular mortality in noncardiac surgery: validation of the Lee cardiac risk index. *Am J Med* 118:1134–1141.

Bøhmer E, Hoffmann P, Abdelnoor M, Arnesen H, Halvorsen S. (2010). Efficacy and safety of immediate angioplasty versus ischemia-guided management after thrombolysis in acute myocardial infarction in areas with very long transfer distances: results of the NORDISTEMI (NORwegian study on DIstrict treatment of ST-Elevation Myocardial Infarction) *J Am Coll Cardiol* 55:102-110.

Bonow RO, Carabello BA, Kanu C, de Leon AC Jr, Faxon DP, Freed MD, Gaasch WH, Lytle BW, Nishimura RA, O'Gara PT, O'Rourke RA, Otto CM, Shah PM, Shanewise JS, Smith SC Jr, Jacobs AK, Adams CD, Anderson JL, Antman EM, Faxon DP, Fuster V, Halperin JL, Hiratzka LF, Hunt SA, Lytle BW, Nishimura R, Page RL, Riegel B. (2006). ACC/AHA 2006 guidelines for the management of patients with valvular heart disease: a report of the American College of Cardiology/American Heart Association Task Force on Practice Guidelines (writing Committee to Revise the 1998 guidelines for the management of patients with valvular heart disease) developed in collaboration with the Society of Cardiovascular Anesthesiologists endorsed by the Society for Cardiovascular Angiography and Interventions and the Society of Thoracic Surgeons. *J Am Coll Cardiol.* 48: e1–e148.

Borgia, F, Goodman SC, Halvorsen S, Cantor WJ, Piscione F, Le May MR, Fernandez-Aviles F, Sanchez PL, Dimopoulos K, Scheller B, Armstrong PW and Di Mario C. (2010). Early routine Percutaneous coronary intervention after fibrinolysis vs. standard therapy in ST-segment elevation myocardial infarction: a meta-analysis, *Eur Heart J* 31 (17):2156-2169

Budoff MJ, Dowe D, Jollis JG, et al. (2008). Diagnostic performance of 64-multidetector-row coronary computed tomographic angiography for evaluation of coronary artery stenosis in individuals without known coronary artery disease. *J Am Coll Cardiol* 52:1724–32.

Cannon CP. (2004). Revascularisation for everyone? *Eur Heart J* 25:1471–1472

Cantor WJ, Fitchett D, Borgundvaag B, Ducas J, Heffernan M, Cohen EA, Morrison LJ, Langer A, Dzavik V, Mehta SR, Lazzam C, Schwartz B, Casanova A, Goodman SG. (2009). Routine early angioplasty after fibrinolysis for acute myocardial infarction. *N Engl J Med* 360:2705–2718.

Carver A, Rafelt S, Gershlick AH, et al. REACT Investigators. (2009). Longer-term follow-up of patients recruited to the REACT (Rescue Angioplasty Versus Conservative Treatment or Repeat Thrombolysis) trial *J Am Coll Cardiol* 54:118-126.

Chan MY, Sun JL, Newby LK, Shaw LK, Lin M, Peterson ED, Califf RM, Kong DF, Roe MT. (2009). Long-term mortality of patients undergoing cardiac catheterization for ST-elevation and non-ST elevation myocardial infarction, *Circulation*. 19(24):3110-7

Damman P, Hirsch A, Windhausen F, Tijssen JGP, de Winter RJ, ICTUS Investigators. (2010). 5-year clinical outcomes in the ICTUS (Invasive versus Conservative Treatment in Unstable coronary Syndromes) trial: a randomized comparison of an early invasive versus selective invasive management in patients with non–ST-segment elevation acute coronary syndrome *J Am Coll Cardiol* 55:858-864.

de Winter RJ, Windhausen F, Cornel JH, et al (2005). Invasive versus Conservative Treatment in Unstable Coronary Syndromes (ICTUS) Investigators. Early invasive versus selectively invasive management for acute coronary syndromes. *N Engl J Med* 353: 1095-1104.

Desch S, Eitel I, Rahimi K, de Waha S, Schuler G, Thiele H, (2010). Timing of invasive treatment after fibrinolysis in ST elevation myocardial infarction – a meta-analysis of immediate or early routine versus deferred or ischaemia-guided randomized controlled trials, *Heart*, 96(21):1695-1702

Di Mario C, Dudek D, Piscione F, Mielecki W, Savonitto S, Murena E, Dimopoulos K, Manari A, Gaspardone A, Ochala A, Zmudka K, Bolognese L, Steg PG, Flather M. (2008). Immediate angioplasty versus standard therapy with rescue angioplasty after thrombolysis in the Combined Abciximab Reteplase Stent Study in Acute Myocardial Infarction (CARESS-in-AMI): an open, prospective, randomised, multicentre trial. *Lancet* 371:559–568

D'Souza SP, Mamas MA, Fraser DG, Fath-Ordoubadi F. (2010). Routine early coronary angioplasty versus ischaemia-guided angioplasty after thrombolysis in acute ST-elevation myocardial infarction: a meta-analysis *Eur Heart J first published online October 28, 2010*

Dumas F, Cariou A, Manzo-Silberman S, et al. (2010) Immediate percutaneous coronary intervention is associated with better survival after out-of-hospital cardiac arrest: insights from the PROCAT (Parisian Region Out of hospital Cardiac ArresT) registry. Circ Cardiovasc Interv 3:200–7

Ellis SG, Tendera M, de Belder MA, van Boven AJ, Widimsky P, Janssens L, Andersen HR, Betriu A, Savonitto S, Adamus J, Peruga JZ, Kosmider M, Katz O, Neunteufl T, Jorgova J, Dorobantu M, Grinfeld L, Armstrong P, Brodie BR, Herrmann HC, Montalescot G, Neumann FJ, Effron MB, Barnathan ES, Topol EJ. (2008). Facilitated PCI in patients with ST-elevation myocardial infarction. *N Engl J Med* 358:2205–2217.

Fernandez-Aviles F, Alonso JJ, Castro-Beiras A, Vazquez N, Blanco J, Alonso-Briales J, Lopez-Mesa J, Fernandez-Vazquez F, Calvo I, Martinez-Elbal L, San Roman JA, Ramos B. (2004). Routine invasive strategy within 24 hours of thrombolysis versus ischaemia-guided conservative approach for acute myocardial infarction with ST-segment elevation (GRACIA-1): a randomised controlled trial. *Lancet* 364:1045–1053

Fox KA, Clayton TC, Damman P, Pocock SJ, de Winter RJ, Tijssen JG, Lagerqvist B,Wallentin L. (2010). Long-term outcome of a routine versus selective invasive strategy in patients with non-ST-segment elevation acute coronary syndrome a meta-analysis of individual patient data. *J Am Coll Cardiol* 55:2435–2445.

Garot P, Lefevre T, Eltchaninoff H, Morice MC, Tamion F, Abry B, Lesault PF, Le Tarnec JY, Pouges C, Margenet A, Monchi M, Laurent I, Dumas P, Garot J, Louvard Y. (2007). Six-month outcome of emergency percutaneous coronary intervention in resuscitated patients after cardiac arrest complicating ST-elevation myocardial infarction. *Circulation*. 115: 1354–1362.

Gershlick AH, Stephens-Lloyd A, Hughes S, et al. (2005). Rescue angioplasty after failed thrombolytic therapy for acute myocardial infarction. *N Engl J Med*. 353:2758–68

Hoenig MR, Doust JA, Aroney CN, Scott IA. (2006). Early invasive versus conservative strategies for unstable angina & non-ST-elevation myocardial infarction in the stent era. *Cochrane Database Syst Rev* 3: CD004815.

Hosmane VR, Mustafa NG, Reddy VK, et al. (2009). Survival and neurologic recovery in patients with ST-segment elevation myocardial infarction resuscitated from cardiac arrest. *J Am Coll Cardiol* 53:409–15.

Hulten EA, Carbonaro S, Petrillo SP, Mitchell JD, Villines TC. (2011). Prognostic value of cardiac computed tomography, A systematic review and meta-analysis, *J. Am. Coll. Cardiol* 57:1237-1247.

ILCOR, Part 9: Acute coronary syndromes 2010 International Consensus on Cardiopulmonary Resuscitation and Emergency Cardiovascular Care Science with Treatment Recommendations_Nolan, JP, Hazinski MF, et al, Part 1: Executive summary 2010 International Consensus on Cardiopulmonary Resuscitation and Emergency Cardiovascular Care Science With Treatment Recommendations Resuscitation 81S (2010) e175–e212*Resuscitation* 81S (2010) e1–e25

Keeley EC, Boura JA, Grines CL. (2006). Comparison of primary and facilitated percutaneous coronary interventions for ST-elevation myocardial infarction: quantitative review of randomised trials *Lancet* 367:579-588

Leon MB, Smith CR, Mack M, et al. (2010). Transcatheter aortic-valve implantation for aortic stenosis in patients who cannot undergo surgery. *N Engl J Med* 2010; DOI:10.1056/NEJMoa1008232

McFalls EO, Ward HB, Moritz TE, Goldman S, Krupski WC, Littooy F, Pierpont G, Santilli S, Rapp J, Hattler B, Shunk K, Jaenicke C, Thottapurathu L, Ellis N, Reda DJ, Henderson WG. (2004). Coronary-artery revascularization before elective major vascular surgery. *N Engl J Med* 351:2795 - 2804.

Mehta SR, Cannon CP, Fox KA, Wallentin L, Boden WE, Spacek R, Widimsky P, McCullough PA, Hunt D, Braunwald E, Yusuf S. (2005). Routine vs selective invasive strategies in patients with acute coronary syndromes: a collaborative meta-analysis of randomized trials. *JAMA* 293:2908–2917.

Mehta SR, Granger CB, Boden WE, et al. (2009). Early versus delayed invasive intervention in acute coronary syndromes. *N Engl J Med.* 360: 2165–75.

Meijboom WB, Meijs MF, Schuijf JD, et al. (2008) Diagnostic accuracy of 64-slice computed tomography coronary angiography: a prospective, multicenter, multivendor study. *J Am Coll Cardiol* 52:2135-44

Meijboom WB, Mollet NR, Van Mieghem CAG, Kluin J, Weustink AC, Pugliese F, Vourvouri E, Cademartiri F, Bogers AJJC, Krestin GP, *et al.* (2006). Pre-Operative Computed Tomography Coronary Angiography to Detect Significant Coronary Artery Disease in Patients Referred for Cardiac Valve Surgery *J. Am. Coll. Cardiol.*, 48(8): 1658 - 1665.

Miller JM, Rochitte CE, Dewey M, *et al.* (2008). Diagnostic performance of coronary angiography by 64-row CT. *N Engl J Med* 359:2324–36.

Montalescot G, Cayla G, Collet JP, et al. (2009). Immediate vs delayed intervention for acute coronary syndromes: a randomized clinical trial. *JAMA*. 302:947–54.

Mowatt G, Cook JA, Hillis GS, et al. (2008). 64-Slice computed tomography angiography in the diagnosis and assessment of coronary artery disease: systematic review and meta-analysis. *Heart* 94:1386–93.

Neumann FJ, Kastrati A, Pogatsa-Murray G, et al. (2003). Evaluation of prolonged antithrombotic pretreatment ("cooling-off" strategy) before intervention in patients with unstable coronary syndromes: a randomized controlled trial. *JAMA*. 290:1593-9.

Pell JP, Sirel JM, Marsden AK, Ford I, Walker NL, Cobbe SM. (2003). Presentation, management, and outcome of out of hospital cardiopulmonary arrest: comparison by underlying aetiology. *Heart* 89:839—42

Poldermans D, Bax JJ, Boersma E, De Hert S, Eeckhout E, Fowkes G, Gorenek B, Hennerici MG, Iung B, Kelm M, Kjeldsen KP, Kristensen SD, Lopez-Sendon J, Pelosi P, Philippe F, Pierard L, Ponikowski P, Schmid JP, Sellevold OF, Sicari R, Van den Berghe G, Vermassen F, Hoeks SE, Vanhorebeek I. (2009). Guidelines for preoperative cardiac risk assessment and perioperative cardiac management in noncardiac surgery: the Task Force for Preoperative Cardiac Risk Assessment and Perioperative Cardiac Management in Non-cardiac Surgery of the European Society of Cardiology (ESC) and endorsed by the European Society of Anaesthesiology (ESA). *Eur Heart J* 30:2769-2812.

Reynolds JC, Callaway CW, El Khoudary SR, Moore CG, Alvarez RJ, Rittenberger JC. (2009). Coronary angiography predicts improved outcome following cardiac arrest: propensity-adjusted analysis. *J Intensive Care Med* 24:179-86.

Spaulding CM, Joly LM, Rosenberg A, et al. (1997). Immediate coronary angiography in survivors of out-of-hospital cardiac arrest. *N Engl J Med* 336:1629-33.

Stub D, Hengel C, Chan W, Jackson D, Sanders K, Dart AM, Hilton A, Pellegrino V, Shaw JA, Duffy SJ, Bernard S, Kaye DM. (2011). Usefulness of cooling and coronary catheterization to improve survival in out-of-hospital cardiac arrest. *Am J Cardiol.* 107(4):522-7. Epub 2010 Dec 22.

Sunde K, Pytte M, Jacobsen D, et al. (2007) Implementation of a standardised treatment protocol for post resuscitation care after out-of-hospital cardiac arrest. *Resuscitation* 73:29– 39.

Taylor AJ, Cerqueira M, Hodgson JM, et al. (2010). ACCF/SCCT/ACR/AHA/ASE/ASNC/NASCI/SCAI/SCMR 2010 appropriate use criteria for cardiac computed tomography: a report of the American College of Cardiology Foundation Appropriate Use Criteria Task Force, the Society of Cardiovascular Computed Tomography, the American College of Radiology, the American Heart Association, the American Society of Echocardiography, the American Society of Nuclear Cardiology, the North American Society for Cardiovascular Imaging, the Society for Cardiovascular Angiography and Interventions, and the Society for Cardiovascular Magnetic *Resonance J Am Coll Cardiol* 56:1864-1894.

Thompson PL. (2010). The invasive approach to acute coronary syndrome: true promise or false premise? *Med J Aust*; 192 (12): 694-695.

Vahanian A, Baumgartner H, Bax J, Butchart E, Dion R, Filippatos G, Flachskampf F, Hall R, Iung B, Kasprzak J, Nataf P, Tornos P, Torracca L, Wenink A. (2007). Grupo de Trabajo sobre el Tratamiento de las Valvulopatías de la Sociedad Europea de

Cardiología: guidelines on the management of valvular heart disease. *Eur Heart J.* 28: 230–268.

Wijeysundera HC, Vijayaraghavan R, Nallamothu BK, et al. (2007). Rescue angioplasty or repeat fibrinolysis after failed fibrinolytic therapy for ST-segment myocardial infarction: a meta-analysis of randomized trials. *J Am Coll Cardiol.* 49:422–30

Wolfrum S, Pierau C, Radke PW, Schunkert H, Kurowski V. (2008). Mild therapeutic hypothermia in patients after out-of-hospital cardiac arrest due to acute STsegment elevation myocardial infarction undergoing immediate percutaneous coronary intervention. *Crit Care Med* 36:1780–6

4

History of Coronary Angiography

Ryotaro Wake, Minoru Yoshiyama et al.*
Osaka City University Graduate School of Medicine,
Osaka City General Hospital, Tsukazaki Hospital
Japan

1. Introduction

Diagnostic cardiac catheterization is recommended whenever it is clinically important to define the presence of cardiac disease that cannot be evaluated adequately by noninvasive techniques. Because the risk of a major complication from cardiac catheterization is less than 1% with mortality of less than 0.08%, many doctors can perform the catheterization safely now. We discuss the history of coronary angiography.

2. X-ray

We must talk about X-rays, at first, when we discuss the history of coronary angiography.
In 1895, Roentgen discovered the x-rays. In 1896, X-rays of fractures had been obtained and published. Walter B. Cannon observed the movements of the opaque mass in the stomach and subsequently with mixing bismuth subnitrate described the nature and site of peristaltic activity in cats as seen on the fluoroscopic screen.
Walsh published "The Röntgen Rays in Medical Work. New York: William Wood, 1898." He reproduced a chest film that clearly showed the position and dimensions of the heart and describe a number of cardiac and aortic conditions that he visualized radiographically. The radiograph in his book required an exposure time of 20 minutes, with the tube only 30 inches (76 cm) from the radiographic plate (Figure 1).

3. Angiogram

Visualization of human blood vessels was achieved in January 1896, during the month after the announcement of Roentgen's discovery, when Haschek and Lindenthal injected Teichmann's mixture, composed mainly of calcium carbonate, into the blood vessels of an amputated hand. A published photograph of their original roentgenogram clearly showed the potential of the method for visualizing the vascular bed (Figure 2).
Morton who was a pioneer American radiologist wrote a text entitled "The X-ray, or, Photography of the Invisible and Its Value in Surgery. New York: American Technical

* Hidetaka Iida, Hiroaki Takeshita, Takanori Kusuyama, Hitoshi Kanamitsu, Hideya Mitsui, Yukio Yamada, Shinichi Shimodozono and Kazuo Haze
Osaka City University Graduate School of Medicine, Osaka City General Hospital, Tsukazaki Hospital, Japan

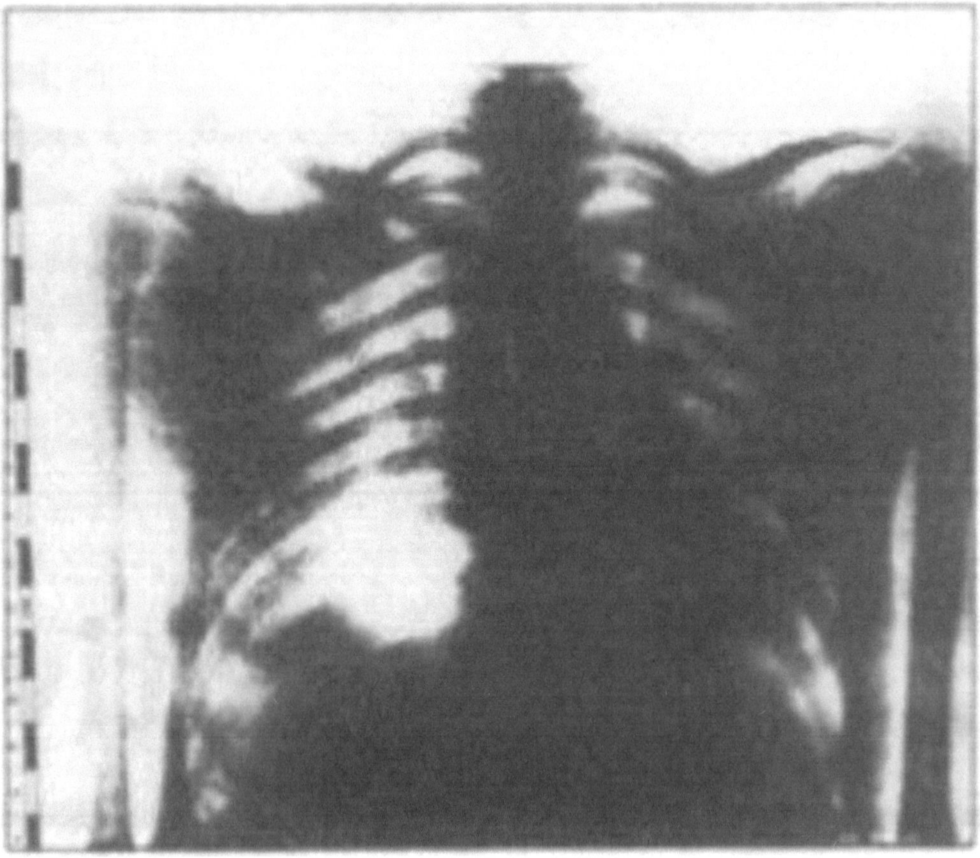

Fig. 1. The chest film from "The Röntgen Rays in Medical Work".

Book Company. 1896." In this book, his remarks concerning contrast studies are intriguing.

In teaching the anatomy of the blood vessels, the X-ray opens out a new and feasible method. The arteries and veins of dead bodies may be injected with a substance opaque to the X-ray and thus, their distribution may be more accurately followed than by any possible dissection. The feasibility of this method applies equally well to the study of the structures and organs of the dead body. To a certain extent, therefore, X-ray photography may replace both dissection and vivisection, and in the living body, the location and size of a hollow organ may be ascertained by causing the subject to drink a harmless fluid more or less opaque to the X-ray, or an effervescing mixture which will cause distention, and then taking the picture.

In 1920, a radiographic atlas devoted only to the systemic arteries of the body was published in England, "The X-ray atlas of the systemic arteries of the body. London: Balliere, Tindall, and Cox, 1920," by Orrin. The reproductions showed blood vessels in cadavers with great clarity (Figure 3).

In 1910, Franek and Alwens introduced a suspension of bismuth and oil into the hearts of dogs and rabbits directly through the large veins and observed the passage of droplets from the heart into the lungs. In 1922, the work of Sicard and Forestier represented the next major advance, when they used Lipiodol, an early oil-based contrast medium, to study the bronchial tree and then the spinal subarachnoid space. In 1923, they injected 5 ml of Lipiodol into the femoral vein of a dog and, with the aid of fluoroscopy, watched droplets move with increasing speed from the iliac vein into the heart. The Lipiodol was then pulverized by ventricular contraction, thrown with great speed into the pulmonary artery and finally spread as multiple emboli into the small vessels of the lungs, disappearing in 10-12 minutes. Nextly, they repeated the experiment with human subjects, in whom they carefully observed the course of the opaque oil from the antecubital vein to the pulmonary capillaries. They reported that the patients coughed as the oil reached the lungs but suffered no other ill effects.

In 1923, Berberich and Hirsch reported the first arteriograms and venograms obtained in human subjects, using 20% strontium bromide (Figure 4). In 1924, Brooks described the intraarterial injection of sodium iodide as a means of showing vessels of the lower extremities in humans (Figure 5).

In 1928, Moniz et al. described carotid angiography and its application to the study of cerebral lesions (Figure 6).

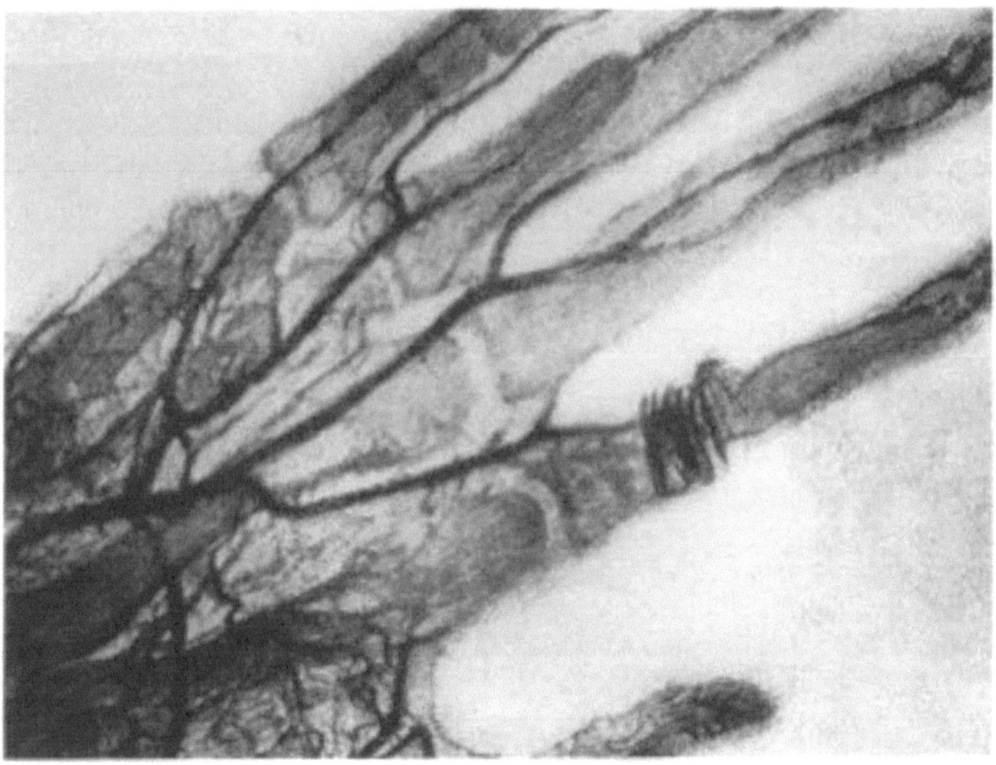

Fig. 2. A roentgenogram made by Haschek and Lindenthal after the injection of Teichman's mixture into the blood vessels of an amputated hand (Haschek E. Lindenthal O'F. A contribution to the practical use of the photography according to Röntgen. Wien Klin Wochenschr 1896:9:63.).

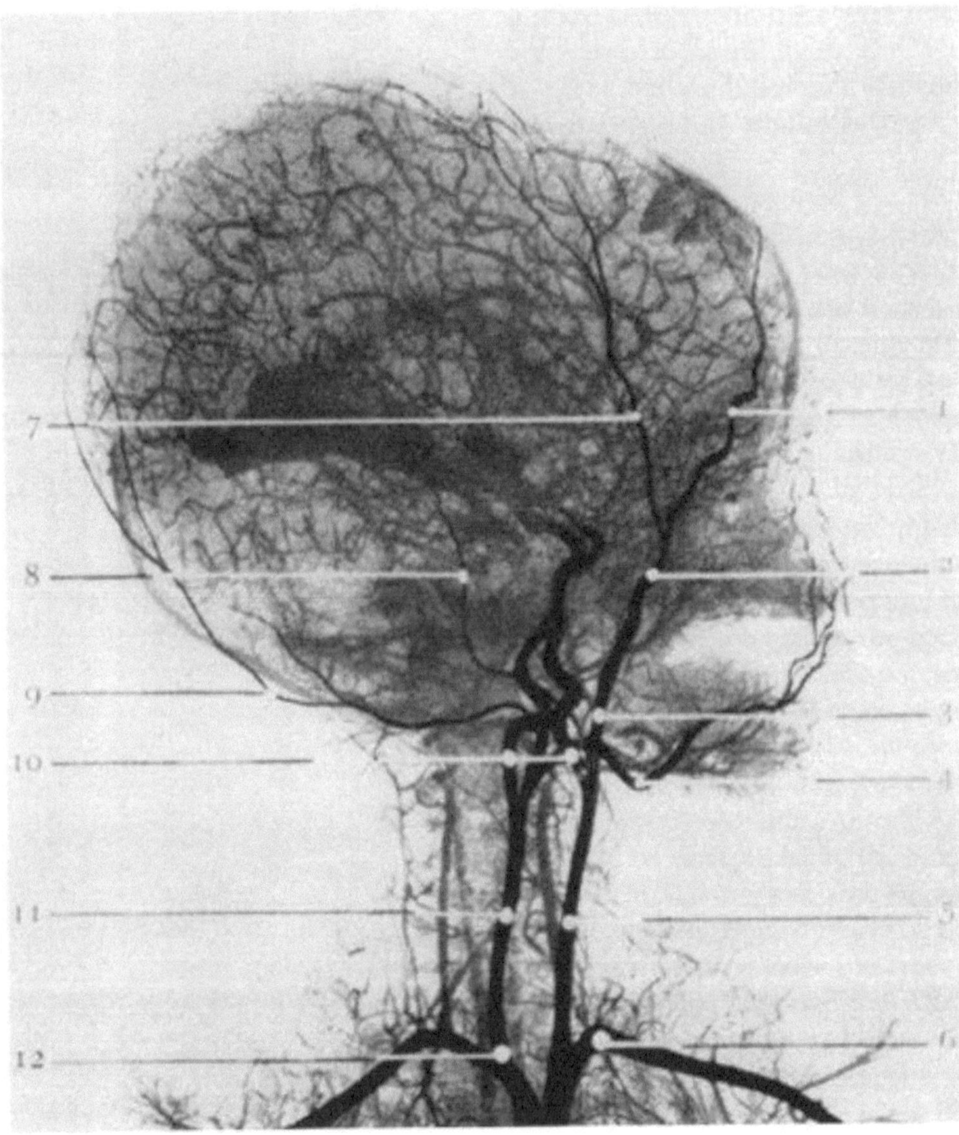

Fig. 3. Reproduction of a 1920 roentgenogram of a cadaver after the injection of opaque medium into the cerebral vessels (Orrin HC. The x-ray atlas of the systemic arteries of the body. London: Balliere, Tindall, and Cox,1920.).

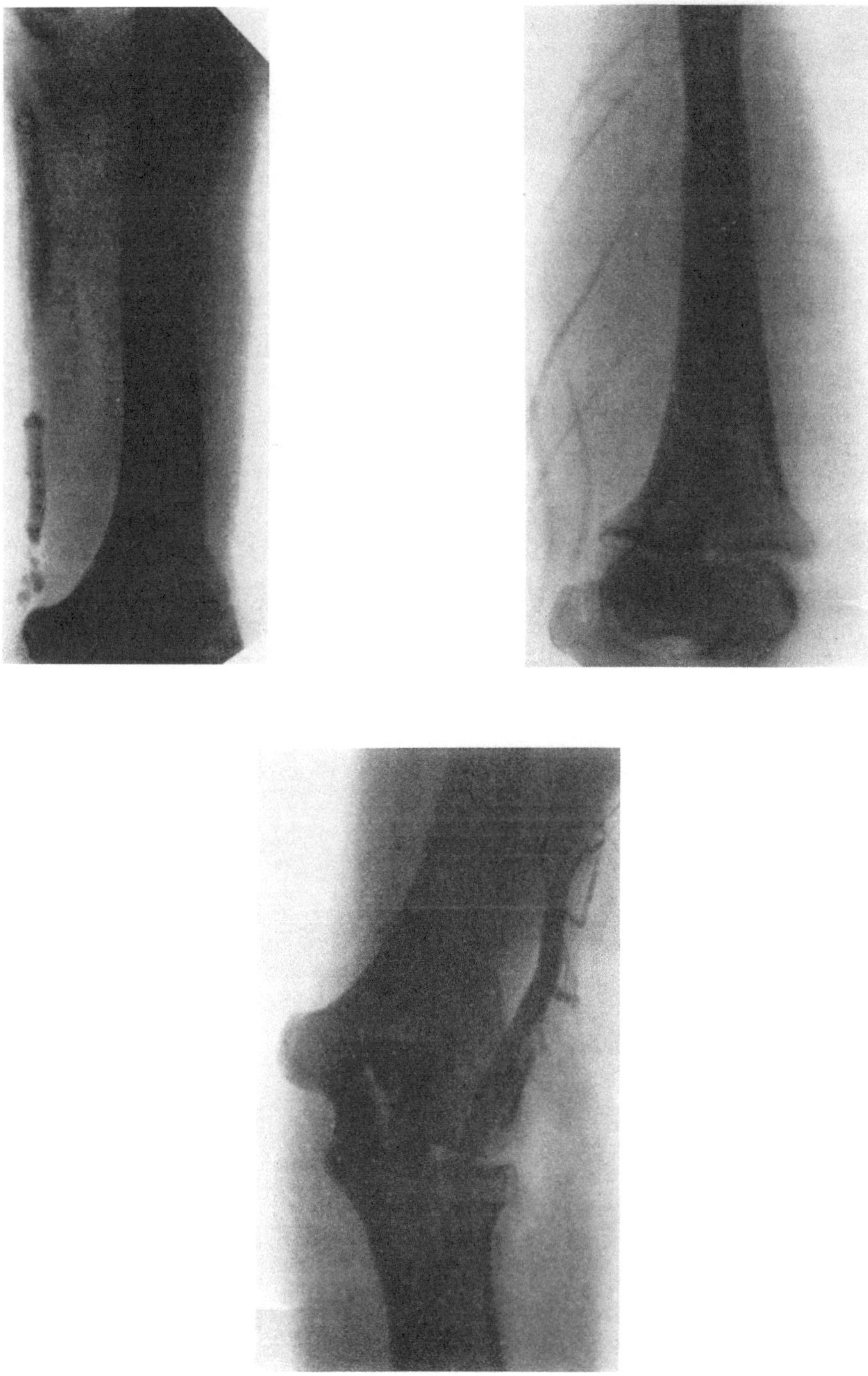

Fig. 4. Venographic studies obtained by Berberich and Hirsch in 1923. They injected 20% strontium bromide into the veins of the upper extremity (Berberich J Munchen Klin Wochenschr 1923;49:2226).

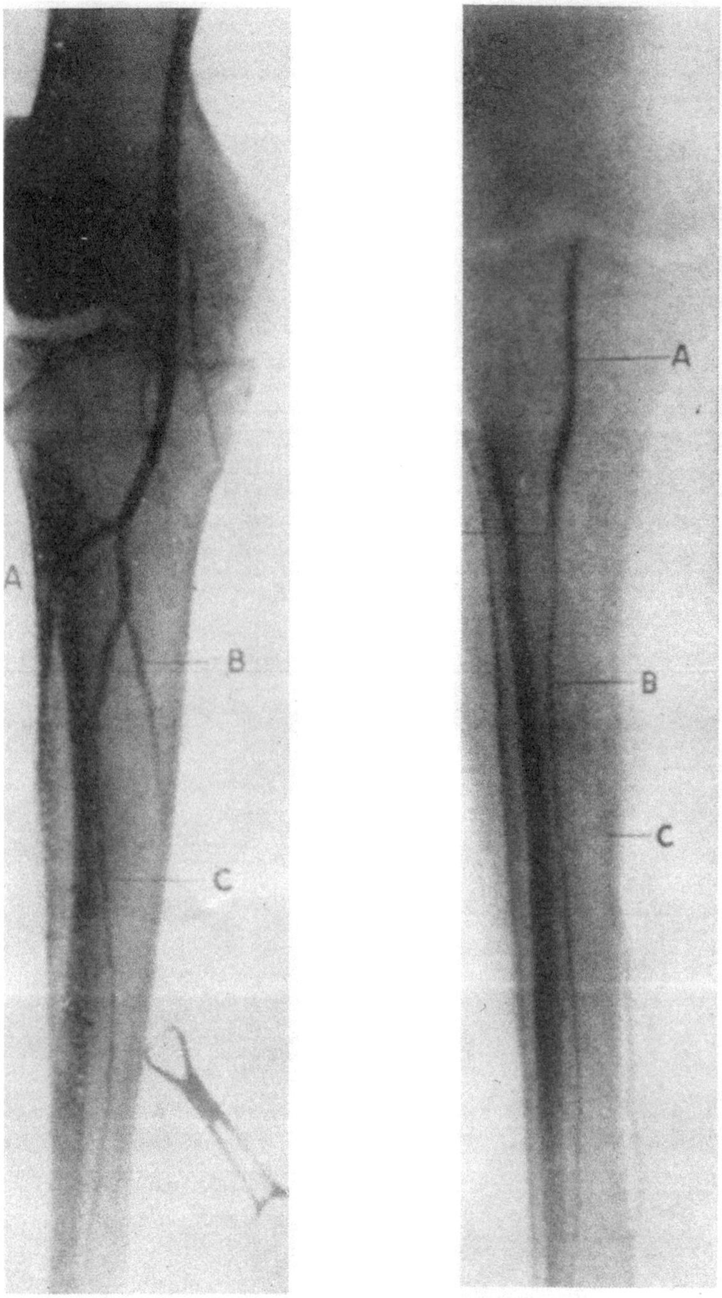

Fig. 5. The first femoral arteriogram obtained in a human subject. Brooks used sodium iodide as a means of demonstrating the vessels of the lower extremities in 1924(Brooks B. Intraarterial injection of sodium iodide. JAMA 1924; 82:1016.).

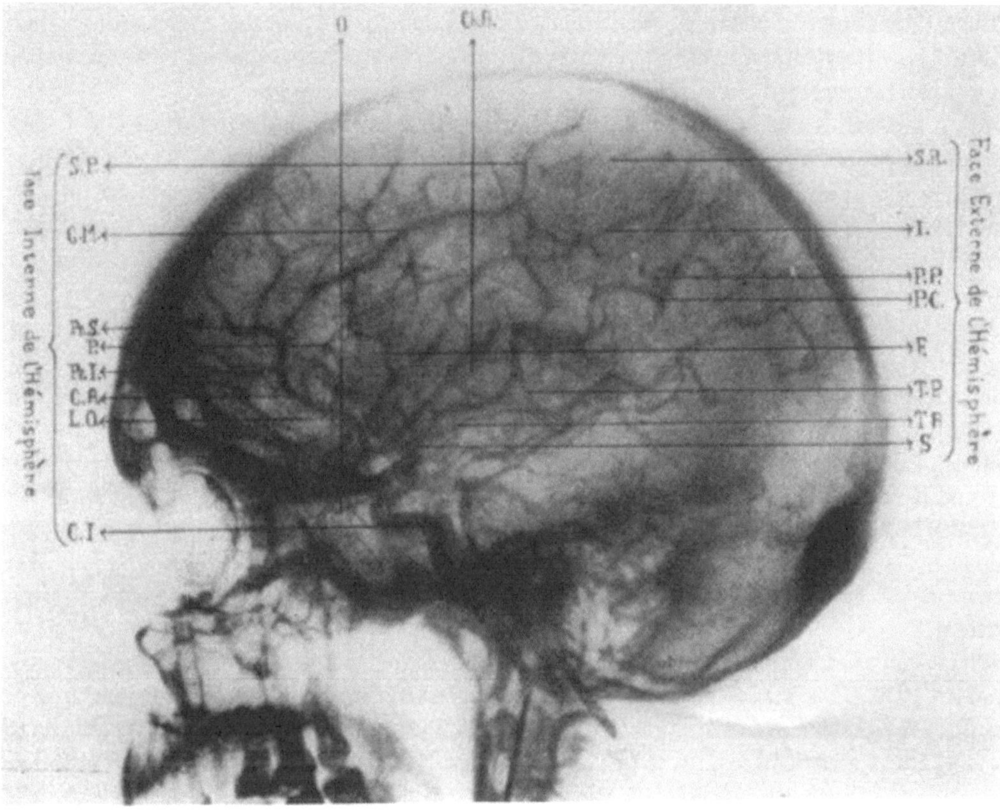

Fig. 6. Reproduction of a cerebral arteriogram (Moniz E. J Radiol Electrol Med Nucl 1928;12:72.)

4. Cardiac catheterization

As Andre Cournand remarked in his Nobel lecture of Decenber, 11th, 1956 (http://nobelprize.org/nobel_prizes/medicine/laureates/). Cournand and his colleagues led us into a new era in the understanding of cardiac function in humans. According to Cournand, cardiac catheterization was performed and so named by Claude Bernard in 1844. The subject was a horse, and both the right and left ventricles were entered by retrograde approach from the jugular vein and carotid artery.
His careful application of scientific method to the study of cardiac physiology using the cardiac catheter demonstrated the enormous value of this technical innovation. An era of investigation of cardiovascular physiology in animals then followed, resulting in the development of many important techniques and principles (pressure manometry, the Fick cardiac output method), which awaited direct application to the patient with heart disease.

In 1928, Werner Forssmann, having practiced on a cadaver, inserted a 65 cm catheter into his own antecubital vein until he felt that it had reached the right atrium [1] (Figure 7). With the catheter dangling from his arm, he walked through a hospital basement to the radiographic room. There he obtained a roentgenogram that confirmed his belief that the catheter tip had in fact reached the right atrium.

During the next 2 years, Forssmann continued to perform catheterization studies including six additional attempts to catheterize himself. Bitter criticism, based on an unsubstantiated belief in the danger of his experiments, caused Forssmann to turn his attention to other concerns, and he eventually pursed another catheter-related career as a urologist. Nevertheless, for his contribution and foresight he shared the Nobel Prize in Medicine with Andre Cournand and Dickinson Richards in 1956. Forssmann's primary goal in his catheterization studies was to develop a therapeutic technique for the direct delivery of drugs into the heart.

He wrote, "If cardiac action cases suddenly, as is seen in acute shock or in the heart disease, or during anesthesia or positioning, one is forced to deliver drugs locally. In such cases the intracardiac injection of drugs may be life saving. However, this may be a dangerous procedure because of many incidents of laceration of coronary arteries and their branches leading to cardiac tamponade, and death. Because of such incidents, one often waits until the very last moment and valuable time is wasted. Therefore I started to look for a new way to approach the heart, and I catheterized the right side of the heart through the venous system."

Others, however, appreciated the potential of using Forssmann's technique as a diagnostic tool. In 1930, Klein reported 11 right heart catheterizations, including passage to the right ventricle and measurement of cardiac output using Fick's principle. In 1932, Padillo and coworkers reported that right heart catheterization and measurement of cardiac output in two subjects. Except for these few early studies, application of cardiac catheterization to study the circulation in normal and disease states was fragmentary until the work of Andre Cournand and Dickinson Richards, who separately and in collaboration produced a remarkable series of investigations of right heart physiology in humans [2]. In 1947, Dexter reported his studies on congenital heart disease and passed the catheter to the distal pulmonary artery, describing "the oxygen saturation and source of pulmonary capillary blood" obtained from the pulmonary artery wedge position [3]. Subsequent studies from Dexter's laboratory [4] and by Werko elaborated the use of this pulmonary artery wedge position and reported that pressure measured at this position was a good estimate of pulmonary venous and left atrial pressure. During this exciting early period, catheterization was used to investigate problems in cardiovascular physiology by McMichael and Sharpey-Shafer in England. Lenegre and Maurice in Paris and Warren, Stead, Bing, Dexter, Cournand and others in the United States [5-9].

Further developments came rapidly in the 1950s and 1960s. Retrograde left heart catheterization was first reported by Zimmerman and others [10] and Limon-Lason and Bouchard in 1950. The percutaneous (rather than cut-down) technique was developed by Seldinger in 1953 and was soon applied to cardiac catheterization of both the left and right heart chambers [11]. Trans-septal catheterization was first developed by Ross [12] and Cope [13] in 1959 and quickly became accepted as a standard technique. Selective coronary angiography was reported by Sones and others in 1959 and was perfected to remarkable excellence over the ensuing years [14]. Coronary angiography was modified for a percutaneous approach by Ricketts and Abrams [15] in 1962 and Judkins [16] in 1967. In 1970, Swan and Ganz introduced a practical balloon-tipped, flow-guided catheter technique enabling the application of catheterization outside the laboratory [17]. Better radiographic imaging techniques and less toxic radiographic contrast agents have been developed progressively, as many numbers of diagnostic catheterizations has performed (Figure 8).

In 1977, Grüntzig and others introduced the technique of balloon angioplasty, known as percutaneous transluminal coronary angioplasty (PTCA) [18].

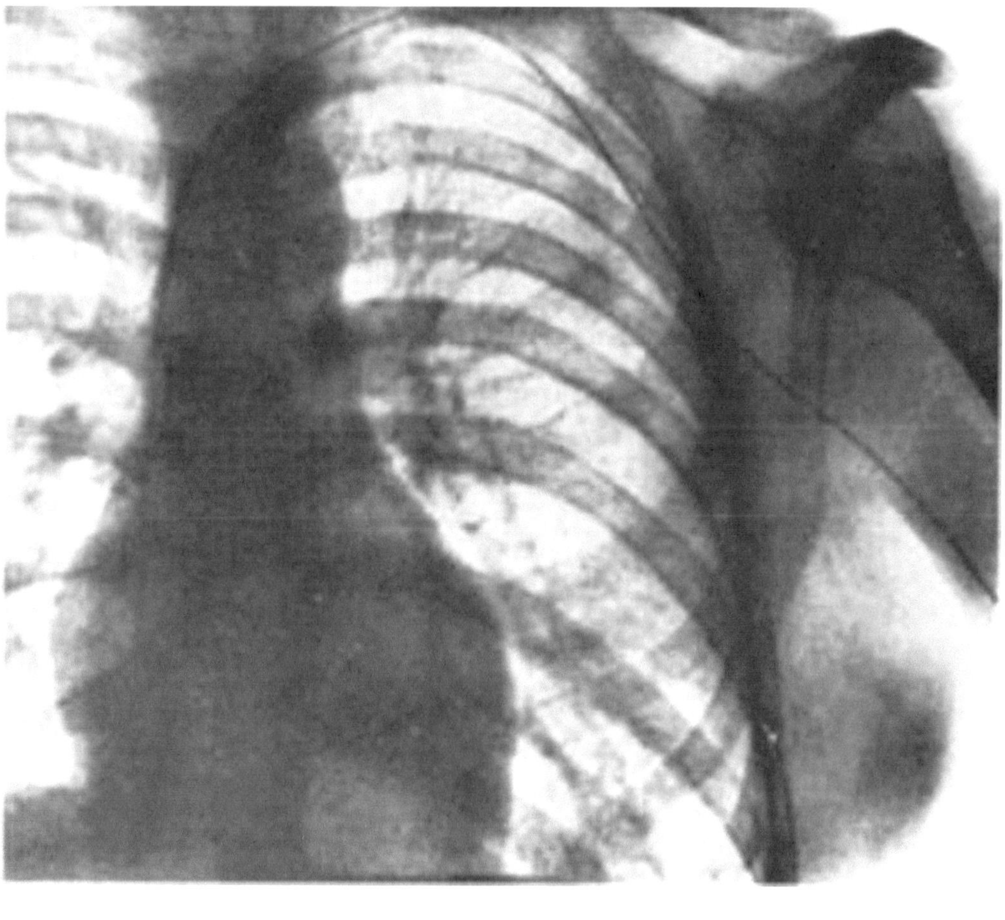

Fig. 7. The first documented cardiac catheterization. At age 25, while receiving clinical instruction in surgery at Eberswalde, Werner Forssmann passed a catheter 65 cm through one of his left antecubital veins until its tip entered the right atrium. He then walked to the radiology department where this roentgenogram was taken (Klin Wochenschr 1929;8:2085. Springer-Verlag, Berlin, Heidelberg, New York).

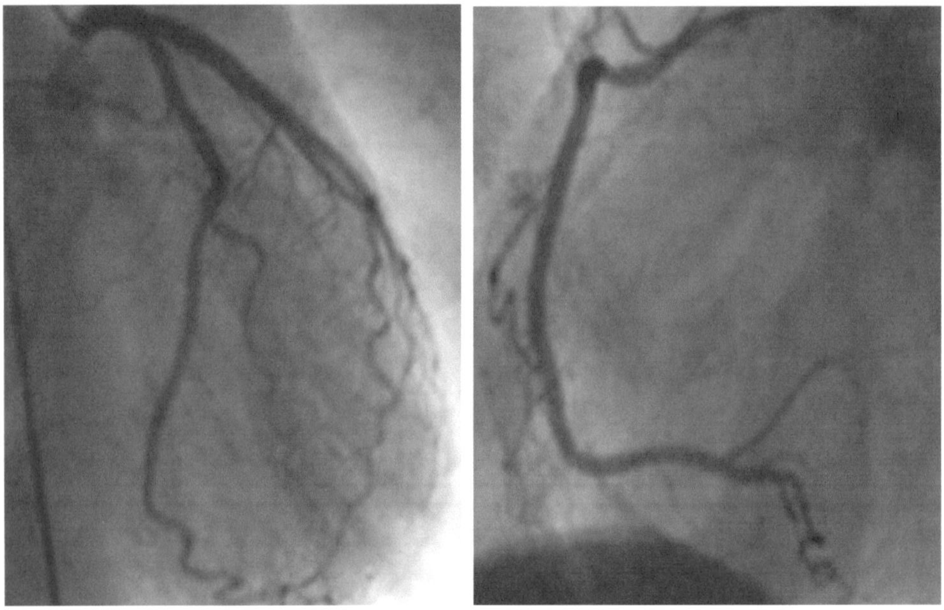

Fig. 8. Normal coronary angiogram. Left panel: left coronary artery. Right Panel: right coronary artery.

5. Equipments for coronary angiography

In the 1960s, great strides were made in the quality of image amplification, particularly with the introduction of the cesium iodide tube. Simultaneously, powerful generators capable of millisecond exposures and high contrast levels were developed. Cine cameras evolved into dependable instruments with fine-quality lenses that provide extraordinarily good resolution in modern 35-mm cine angiocardiography. Videotape recording techniques improved strikingly. Instantaneous playback of tape-recorded images has afforded great utility and safety in determining whether desired anatomic and physiologic information has been attained, thereby precluding additional unnecessary studies (Figure 8).

The introduction of angled views for the study of congenital and acquired heart disease was an important technical innovation [19]. Equipment companies responded with engineering advances that made angled views relatively simple: the C-arm, the U-arm, and the parallelogram.

Recently, the development of non-invasive angiography device is advancing. Echocardiography, scintigraphy, cardiac computed tomography and cardiac magnetic resonance imaging play increasingly important roles in the evaluation of the heart and great vessels, non-invasively. It is already an established technique for the evaluation of congenital heart disease, cardiac tumors and disorders of the aorta and pericardium. They can evaluate ventricular function and regurgitation of blood across heart valves.

6. Conclusion

Medicine moves so fast that its evolution tends to be forgotten. In particularly, techniques that have become an integral part of the standard device of diagnosis or therapy are passed

to each new generation of physicians and trainees. We perform them without their having sense of efforts involved in the initial development of those techniques.
In this one decade, we would be astonished at how far the field has come and how much information can be gathered on the structure and function of the heart from diagnostic imaging. A century is a short time in the history of medicine, but it has been an eventful lifetime.

7. References

[1] Shapiro, S.M. et al. (1997) Primary pulmonary hypertension: improved long-term effects and survival with continuous intravenous epoprostenol infusion. *J Am Coll Cardiol*, Vol.30, No.2, pp. 343-349
[2] Cournand, A. et al. (1945) Measurement Of Cardiac Output In Man Using The Technique Of Catheterization Of The Right Auricle Or Ventricle. *J Clin Invest*, Vol. 24, No.1, pp. 106-116
[3] Dexter, L. et al. (1947) Studies Of Congenital Heart Disease. Ii. The Pressure And Oxygen Content Of Blood In The Right Auricle, Right Ventricle, And Pulmonary Artery In Control Patients, With Observations On The Oxygen Saturation And Source Of Pulmonary "Capillary" Blood. *J Clin Invest*, Vol. 26, No. 3, pp. 554-560
[4] Hellems, H.K. et al. (1949) Pulmonary capillary pressure in man. *J Appl Physiol*, Vol. 2, No. 1, pp. 24-29
[5] Bing, R.J. et al. (1947) Catheterization of the coronary sinus and the middle cardiac vein in man. *Proc Soc Exp Biol Med*, Vol. 66, No. 1, pp. 239
[6] Bing, R.J. et al. (1947) Physiological studies in congenital heart disease. *Bull Johns Hopkins Hosp*, Vol. 80, No.2, pp. 107-120
[7] Burchell, H.B. et al. (1948) Cardiac catheterization in the diagnosis of various cardiac malformations and diseases. *Mayo Clin Proc*, Vol. 23, No. 22, pp. 481−487
[8] Stead, E.A., Jr. and Warren, J.V. (1947) Cardiac output in man; an analysis of the mechanisms varying the cardiac output based on recent clinical studies. *Arch Med Interna*, Vol. 80, No. 2, pp. 237-248
[9] Stead, E.A., Jr. et al. (1948) Cardiac output in congestive heart failure; an analysis of the reasons for lack of close correlation between the symptoms of heart failure and the resting cardiac output. *Am Heart J*, Vol. 35, No.4, pp. 529-541
[10] Zimmerman, H.A. et al. (1950) Catheterization of the left side of the heart in man. *Circulation*, Vol. 1, No. 3, pp. 357-359
[11] Seldinger, S.I. (1953) Catheter replacement of the needle in percutaneous arteriography; a new technique. *Acta radiol* 39 (5), 368-376
[12] Ross, J., Jr. (1959) Transeptal left heart catheterization: a new method of left atrial puncture. *Ann Surg*, Vol. 149, No. 3, pp. 395-401
[13] Cope, C. (1959) Technique for transseptal catheterization of the left atrium; preliminary report. *J Thorac Surg*, Vol. 37, No. 4, pp. 482-486
[14] Ryan, T.J. (2002) The coronary angiogram and its seminal contributions to cardiovascular medicine over five decades. *Circulation*, Vol. 106, No. 6, pp. 752-756
[15] Ricketts, H.J. and Abrams, H.L. (1962) Percutaneous selective coronary cine arteriography. *JAMA*, Vol. 181, pp. 620-624
[16] Judkins, M.P. (1967) Selective coronary arteriography. I. A percutaneous transfemoral technic. *Radiology*, Vol. 89, No.5, pp. 815-824

[17] Swan, H.J. et al. (1970) Catheterization of the heart in man with use of a flow-directed balloon-tipped catheter. *N Engl J Med*, Vol. 283, No. 9, pp. 447-451
[18] Gruntzig, A.R. et al. (1979) Nonoperative dilatation of coronary-artery stenosis: percutaneous transluminal coronary angioplasty. *N Engl J Med*, Vol. 301, No. 2, pp. 61-68
[19] Bargeron, L.M., Jr. et al. (1977) Axial cineangiography in congenital heart disease. Section I. Concept, technical and anatomic considerations. *Circulation*, Vol. 56, No. 6, pp. 1075-1083

5

Coronary Angiography - Physical and Technical Aspects

Maria Anna Staniszewska
Medical University of Lodz, Department of Medical Imaging Techniques
Poland

1. Introduction

Diseases of coronary system and heart are the main reason of deaths in highly civilized population. Then the appropriate diagnostic methods and treating of early disorders are very important for a population health care. As the imaging techniques play a great role in good diagnosis they are intensively used and developed. Among the most commonly used methods is coronary angiography, which involves coronary vessels visualization during exposure to x-rays, after filling them up with contrast agents.
There are two versions of the procedure:
CCA – conventional coronary angiography, performed under control of x-ray unit with C-arm,
CTA - CT angiography, performed under control of computerized tomography (CT scanner).

2. CCA

2.1 Description of the procedure

A patient lies in a supine position on the table which is a part of the C-arm unit. The x-ray tube moves rotationally in two perpendicular planes (horizontal and vertical); it makes possible any needed type of projection. (The most common projections are: LAO, LAO/Cranial, LAO/Caudal, RAO). The principal current-voltage parameters are chosen automatically.
Good practice rules require keeping the x-ray tube under the table. This allows avoiding an unnecessary irradiation of the staff and makes the doses to a patient lower.
To visualize coronary vessels a contrast agent is administered intravenously. intravenously: first a thin catheter is introduced the brachial artery or the femoral artery (there are two alternative access routes) and its movement is traced by fluoroscopy and observed on monitor by the operator.
(Physiological parameters of a patient of patient are permanently monitored during the procedure.)
The operating team consists of 3 to 4 persons: usually there are an operator (with assistant if necessary), instrumenting nurse and anaesthetic nurse. All the staff remind around the patient table and thus may be exposed to quite high doses of radiation. (There are mainly scattered x-rays). The most exposed member of the team is the operator: the doses registered for such persons may achieve the highest level measured for occupational exposures [1,2].

Patient exposure results mainly from the primary x-ray beam which covers a part of the back surface (the area of left shoulder) by the most time of the procedure. The remaining parts of the patient's body are exposed rather to scattered radiation.
The images created during the procedure can be registered in three ways:

a. Real-time images (fluoroscopic images) observed only by the operator,
b. Some chosen moments of the procedure recorded in radiography mode (so-called acquisition),
c. Long periods of exposure can be recorded in so-called "cine-mode" (if this mode is implemented in the x-ray system).

The results of CCA procedure are analyzed by cardiologists during its performance and also retrospectively afterwards.
Most of x-ray units used nowadays in cardiology are equipped with the digital image recording system. They are two types of them: (1) image intensifier based systems and (2) flat-panel fluoroscopy systems.
The first one uses conventional technology: the output screen of image intensifier is projected in a video camera or a CCD camera to produce an electronic information. (In the previously used conventional image intensifier analogue system the output screen had been projected on the *film* by optical lens).
In the flat-panel systems signals created by x-rays are electronic and are thus recorded simultaneously.
(The fundamental difference between "analogue" and "digital" systems concerns to way of image *archiving* (i.e. film or electronic information). The *both* systems produce the "real-time" image, although the flat-panel systems create the image by dividing the primarily detected signal. That is why the modern x-ray system has much higher output capacity and thus higher doses are possible).

2.2 Technical requirements for x-ray systems used for CCA

X-ray system used for CCA procedures should be equipped as follows:

- constant potential generator of minimum 80 kW (in possibly rectangular pulses),
- x-ray tube focuses 1.2/0.5mm,
- overcouch image detector,
- distance between x-ray tube and image detector is tracked (minimum focus skin distance 30 cm),
- concave couch top for patient comfort (made from low-attenuating materials),
- dose-area product meter (display visible for operator),
- staff protective shielding.

The system should also have the following additional tools and fulfil the following requirements:

- display of fluoroscopy time, total dose-area product (fluoroscopy and radiographic) and estimated skin entrance dose,
- minimum two dose-rate options (Low-Medium-High or Low- Standard),
- additional filtration (Cu preferred) and collimators incorporating circular shutters,
- flexibility of pulsed fluoroscopy mode,
- image hold system,
- possibility of AEC mode choice by the user by the user (IMAGE or DOSE weighted).

Additionally in some x-ray systems there are also available partially absorbent contoured filters to control the bright spots produced by the lung tissue bordering the heart.

2.3 X-ray dosimetry in CCA

The quantities used to assess radiation risk in interventional radiology are following:
Entrance air kerma (EAK), surface dose , dose-area product (DAP), absorbed organ dose, effective dose.
EAK, surface dose and DAP are available for measurements. The remaining can be evaluated experimentally or theoretically.
EAK and surface dose can be measured directly (using appropriately calibrated devices) or indirectly (by thermoluminescence (TL) dosimeters or film badges). The indirect methods need a calibration of dosimeters by the comparison to a reference meter for the standardized exposure (in a competitive laboratory). These methods are routinely applied to individual dosimetry of occupationally exposed persons, but are also used for patients in radiological procedures. (TL dosimeters are preferred for the staff in interventional procedures.)
X-ray systems used for CCA are obligatory equipped with a DAP-meter to summarize the emission in all modes of work (i.e. fluoroscopy, radiography, cine). (Dose Area Product= DAP [$mGy.cm^2$]). Measurements are performed by the transmission chamber placed on the x-ray tube output.
Absorbed organ doses are necessary for evaluation of a possible effect for an exposed human. They can be estimated theoretically or experimentally. Theoretical evaluation relies on Monte Carlo simulation performed for mathematical human phantom at assumed exposure conditions. In the experimental method the physical anthropomorphic phantom is used which is exposed at assumed exposure conditions while the dosimeters are placed inside. (TL dosimeters are used usually for this purpose.)
On the basis of the absorbed organ doses the evaluation of the equivalent dose and the effective dose are possible [3,4].

Equivalent dose (in an organ or body part)

$T_i=w_R.D_i$ [Sv] where w_R-the radiation weighting factor ($w_R=1$ for x-rays, γ-rays and electrons), D_i- the dose absorbed in "i" organ (or body part).

Effective dose (whole body)

$E_{ff}= \sum w_i.D_i$ [Sv] had been implemented to evaluate overall risk for health resulted from exposure to ionizing radiation. This value is fully justified if irradiation of the body is uniform enough: if opposite deterministic effects can appear despite the very low value of the E_{ff} .
Both quantities (T_i and E_{ff}) are used for the dose limits applied for occupational exposure.

2.4 Doses to patients

The doses obtained by the patients undergoing CCA procedures are dependent on:
- patient architecture (BMI-body mass index),
- emission effectiveness of the x-ray system,
- applied dose-rate mode,
- total exposure time,
- mode of work (number of acquisitions -radiographic or cine).

The entrance surface dose to patient dramatically increased when the focus-to-skin distance becomes too short.
The patient doses are significantly higher when the high dose-rate mode is activated or if pulsed fluoroscopy of high number of pulses per second is chosen. These doses are also

inversely proportional to the diameter of the image intensifier. The entrance dose to skin may locally achieved values exceeding the threshold of deterministic effects and the skin injuries of patients undergoing interventional procedures are reported [5].
Generally, exposure of the patients during CCA procedures is extremely non-uniform:high doses are received on a small are of the back while the remaining parts of the body practically stay out of the primary beam. Although effective dose is not a good measure of radiation risk for that, this quantity is used after all. The measurable quantities, i.e. entrance surface dose (or air kerma) and DAP, have more practical meaning. These quantities are proportional to each other:

$$DAP = EAK_c . S$$

where EAK_c -the entrance air kerma in the centre of the beam, S - mean value of incident x-ray beam are (on patient's skin).
(Both values are averaged over the total exposure time, because their varies from one projection to another.)
DAP (and EAK_c) values have to be displayed on the monitors of x-ray system and should be registered in the patient record. (Especially when EAK_c>1Gy and exceeds the threshold of deterministic skin effects.)
As the doses to patients in CCA are affected by a number of factors the range of their values is very wide. The examples are presented in Table 1 and Table 2.
To keep the radiation risk to patients on an acceptable level and control it the reference levels are introduced also for interventional cardiology procedures (like for another radiological procedures).

Number of patients	DAP [Gy.cm^2]	Time of fluoroscopy [min]	Number of frames	Reference
130	72 +/-55	0.35+/-0.25	1550+/-775	[7]
78	73	9.9	1079	[8]
100	60.6	-	412	[9]
117	1.1 - 11.3	0.3 - 22	-	[10]
8	22 - 93	2 - 21	Doctor 1	[11]
3	14 - 44	1 – 4	Doctor 2	
106	35 - 160	4.8+/-3.5	39+/-11	[12]
62	37-190	4.2+/-3.0	30+/-10	
90	3.1-57.2	1.5-5.1	639	[13]
76	44.5	6	10	[14]
194	64 - 281	0.4 - 33	200-1911	[6]

Table 1. The doses to patients in CCA procedures (according to [6])

Effect of pulsed fluoroscopy on the patient dose in CCA were investigated by [16]:
X-ray systems with pulsed fluoroscopy (5 vendors): 10 units; average surface dose rate: 22.52+/-4.5 mGy/min, (25, 30 and 50 pulses/sec);
X-ray systems with conventional fluoroscopy (3 vendors): 3 units; average surface dose rate: 23.93+/-2.77 mGy/min.

X-ray system	DAP [Gy.cm^2]		Time of fluoroscopy [min]	
	median	range	median	range
CCD	30.0	1.1-135.2	3.8	1.1 - 57.0
FP	31.0	14.7-75.9	4.0	0.8- 39.4

Table 2. Median and range of DAP and fluoroscopy time in CCA for different x-ray systems [15]

2.5 Doses to staff

The main inconvenience of CCA procedures (generally - interventional radiology) is the necessity to work standing near the patient during exposure, i.e. in the radiation field. Thus the staff is also exposed mainly to scattered radiation, but primary x-rays are also possible. The factors affecting staff dose are as follows:

- relative position with respect to patient,
- patient body typ (BMI),
- irradiated patient volume,
- x-ray tube position,
- time of exposure,
- effective use of protection shielding.

Thus, staff and patient doses are partially linked: higher exposure for patient means higher irradiation to staff. This is especially true for an operator and the person standing nearby him (an assistant or instrumenting nurse). Additional factor determining the doses to staff is an professional experience and good training in the procedure performance: good manual skills make the exposure time shorter.

Patients with high BMI need a high dose-rate to produce the diagnostic image and then the scattered x-rays also achieve high intensity (especially near the patient).

X-ray tube in undercouch position allows to reduce the doses (mainly for eyes and thyroid of the operator) and also allows avoiding the contact with primary x-rays. (The old x-ray systems had the tube in overcouch position which caused very high doses to operator's hands).

The problem of radiation risk to staff in interventional cardiology had been widely discussed many times. The resulting essential conclusions are the recommendations concerning performance of the interventional procedures and elaboration of the methodology for evaluation radiation risk for the staff [1,17].

The main recommendations concerning the proceeding of the staff during CCA can be summarized in the three points:

- time of exposure possibly short,
- distance to patient possibly long,
- protection shield used effectively.

The recommendations concerning radiation risk rely upon evaluation of the doses to the staff.

Because of the spatial distribution of x-rays affecting staff exposure the special dosimetric requirements are introduced for this group of workers: they should have been equipped with minimum two dosimeters, one under the protective apron (at the chest level) and the second over the apron at the collar level. The first dosimeter is used to evaluate the effective dose and the second can be used to evaluate the equivalent dose to the eyes. (Also for the thyroid if it is not shielded.) Additional dosemeter(s) can be use to evaluate the equivalent

dose(s) to the hands. The protective aprons used by the staff in interventional procedures should have Pb-equivalent of 0.35mm.
As the doses to staff in CCA are affected by a number of factors the range of their values is very wide (the same concerns patients) and many studies were performed to evaluate them. The range of the doses shows the results given in the paper from the USA [18], where on the basis of the rich collection of published data the exposure for operators in cardiovascular procedures from the early 1970's through the present was analyzed. The range of effective doses from 0.02μSv to 38 μSv per one cardiac diagnostic catheterization procedure was found.
Another survey had been performed by European research group SENTINEL in a sample of European cardiac centres and the results have been published recently [19]. According to this study the results for the first operator are as follows:

a. annual effective dose: median 1.3mSv, third quartile 1.4mSv,
b. equivalent dose over the apron: median 11.1mSv, third quartile 14mSv.

Although the above values are rather low it should be underlined that they may be many times higher (even up the annual limits) , especially for inexperienced staff or in a case of clinically difficult patient.

3. CTA

A very dynamic development computerized tomography (CT) Which occurred during last decade creates quite new possibilities for this imaging method. The rotation time below one second together with a rich software allow applying CT to diagnostics of dynamic physiological processes and quickly moving objects (organs). On the other hand, increasing frequency of heart diseases in population linked the health needs With technological achievements in the CT technique to implement this imaging method to cardiology.
Although traditional (conventional) coronary x-ray diagnostics remain a gold standard these procedures are invasive and resulted in high radiation doses both to patients and to staff. Therefore CT procedures became an alternative and comfortable method for heart diagnosis.
For technological reasons the possibilities of CT are limited to diagnostics, without further therapeutic activity (i.e. angioplasty). However, cardiovascular CT plays an increasingly important role in planning for cardiovascular interventions (those are performed under C-arm x-ray units).
Improvements in spatial and temporal resolution, scan time, scan range and advanced image postprocessing (very important in clinical practice) have made *CT angiography* (CTA) an excellent tool for identifying patients in need of invasive therapy and for mapping out the best percutaneous or surgical approach. In some cases CTA provides complementary information to conventional angiography (CCA).
As coronary disease is jointed with calcification of coronary arteries evaluation of this process is a good indicator of pathology. CTA gives possibility to display calcifications (3D) and to assess them quantitatively: it is so-called "calcium scoring".
Although history of CTA had begun with four-slice scanners, the real development came with 64-slice scanners with appropriate combination of spatial and temporal resolution.
Generally, the heart can be imaged well if its structures do not move significantly during the scanning time. This condition is fulfilled during the diastolic phase of cardiac cycle. For

selection of the proper phase for CT images recording ECG gating (triggering) is applied. Additionally, to collect sufficient image data the table speed should not exceed $v = SC \cdot f_H$ and pitch should not exceed $p = f_H \cdot t_{rot}$,
where SC- total collimation width (CT primary beam), f_H- frequency of heart, t_{rot}- rot1ation time. (For example: if t_{rot}=0.5sec and f_H=60bpm then $p \le 0.5$)
The main benefit from CTA is the evaluation of cardiac structure and function. That concerns coronary anomalies, right and left ventricular function, left ventricular ejection fraction and myocardial viability assessment, when the results of other modalities are inadequate [1,2].
According the American College of Cardiology Foundation (ACCF) the principal indications to cardiac CT are as follows [3]:

- low and intermediate pretest probability of obstructive coronary artery disease (CAD),
- noncontrast CT calcium scoring for patients at intermediate risk of coronary heart disease, and for low-risk patients with a family history of disease,
- coronary CT is especially recommended for patients with reduced left ventricular ejection fraction at low or intermediate pretest probability of disease,
- preoperative CT angiography for both heart surgery and noncoronary indications in the setting of risk of CAD.

3.1 Description of the procedure

General rules for exposure parameters:
Slice thickness <1mm, pitch<1, $t_{rot} \le 0.5$sec, kilovoltage U≥100kV, mAs and physical filtration are dependent on the CT scanner, ECG-gating.
The main stages of CT study protocol are as follows:

- The heart rate control and regulation (if necessary: should have been lower than 65bpm),
- Calcium scoring,
- i.v. injection of contrast agents,
- CT angiography.

Ad.1. The required heart rate is dependent on the scanner software: at the high cardiac rate the registered imaging data also have to be reconstructed very quickly (practically immediately). This is possible only with the newest scanners. Lowering the heart rate is achieved pharmacologically.
Ad.2. Calcium scoring is performed on the basis of pre-contrast images. The high attenuation of x-ray in calcified structure allows to differentiate them from the soft tissues.
Ad.3. Contrast agent (iodine compound) is injected automatically in the rate adapted to data acquisition.
Ad.4. CT coronary angiogram: the data acquisition starts automatically when the signal in the descending aorta reaches a predefined threshold (usually 100 HU). The entire volume of the heart is scanned during a few seconds: the newest versions of CT scanners (≥64-slice) do it during one breath-hold (<10sec) under ECG control. The tube voltage, anode current and gantry rotation time are dependent on the scanner type and model and version of software.
After completing acquisition of primary data, elaboration of them (post-processing) begins. The software dedicated to coronary procedures is necessary for that. Such software is offered by the vendors on user's requirement.

It should be underlined that imaging possibilities of each CT scanner are determined by its technical configuration (number of detectors, generator, etc.) but even more by the installed version of software.
The principal algorithms for image post-processing are [4]:
- curved and multiplanar reformats (MPR),
- shaded-surface display (SSD),
- maximum intensity projection (MIP),
- volume rendering (VR).

The axial images produced by hardware (so-called row data) are essential and should be used but reformatted images may improve lesion detection and classification (particularly coronal and oblique views). The axial images and MPRs are used for diagnosis and the SSD and MIPs are for display purposes.
The results of CTA are evaluated or consulted by a cardiologist.

3.2 Dosimetry in CT

Because of special exposure system CT needs the special dosimetry quantities, i.e.: dose-length-product (DLP) and computed-tomography-dose- index (CTDI).
CTDI is treated as an estimation of mean absorbed dose to the whole scanned volume. This quantity also evaluates the level of radiation risk for given procedure at assumed exposure parameters.
CTDI is calculated *automatically by scanner* software on the basis the selected exposure parameters and is displayed on CT monitor. The DLP is then computed as a product of CTDI (averaged over the whole scan length) and the scan length: such value is displayed on CT monitor after the examination is completed.
Independently, *CTDI can be computed* on the basis of measurements performed for particular dosimetric phantoms. For that purpose DLP is measured using special pencil-shaped chamber (external probe) to summarize the dose from incident photons during the tube rotation on the whole length of scanned object. (This is also performed during the acceptance or constancy Quality Control (QC) tests for CT scanner.)
Final evaluation of risk to patient in CT procedures is based on the effective dose. As in the other radiological techniques this quantity can be estimated theoretically (Monte Carlo simulation) or experimentally (TL dosimeters inside the anthropomorphic phantom). Additionally - the effective dose obtained in the particular procedure can be estimated indirectly:

$$E_{ff} = k \, . \, DLP$$

where DLP - value for the procedure, k - transition coefficient for the examined body part (computed theoretically). The above evaluation is applied for adult patients only.
For coronary examinations the transition coefficient $k=0.014\ mSv.mGy^{-1}.cm^{-1}$ is used which corresponds to the chest as the examined region [5].
The problem of doses in CTA is considered only for patients as the staff is out of radiation area.

3.3 Doses to patients and radiation protection in CTA

Because of exposure conditions in CTA (thin slices and low pitch) the doses to patients are relatively high, especially at 64-slice scanners. It was an inspiration to implement the methods of dose reduction without loss of image quality.

The doses can be reduced by lowering of current-voltage parameters, implementation of x-rays intensity modulation (for three axis) and shortening of scanned body length.
The special solution for dose reduction being dedicated to cardiac CT examinations is change of image acquisition technique from RGH to PGA [6].
RGH = Retrospectively Gated Helical: the patient and table move through the gantry at a steady speed. A low pitch (0.2 to 0.4) is needed to cover the entire cardiac volume, especially to compensate for any ectopic beats, which can result in misregistration and gaps in coverage. Thus, the same anatomy can be exposed to the x-ray beam many time (up to five) to ensure enough coverage, causing the high absorbed doses.
PGA= Prospectively Gated Axial: the table is stationary during PGA image acquisition, then moves to the next location for another scan that is initiated by the next normal cardiac cycle. The x-rays emission is then dynamically predicted on the basis of ECG signal.
Diagnostic values of images obtained for PGA protocol were not found to be lower for RGH while the doses where substantially lower [6]. In the same study including 203 CTA exams (82 with routine RGH and 121 with the PGA) the doses were evaluated for protocol including scout images, low-dose calcium scoring scans, test-bolus scan and CT coronary angiogram. The exams were performed by using 64-slice CT scanner (LightSpeed VCT XT, GE). The effective doses were as follows:
RGH: (8.7-23.2) mSv, mean: 18.4 mSv;
PGA: (0.75-6.67) mSv; mean: 2.84 mSv.
For comparison, the results of the big study involved nearly 2000 patients examined (CTA) in 50 hospitals in 2007 in Germany and US show the range of effective dose (8-18) mSv with median 12 mSv. The reduced 100 kV tube voltage was used in 5% of patients, with sequential scanning in 6%. ECG gating was applied in 73% exams [7].
The influence of lower tube voltage is illustrated also by the results CTA performed using 320-MDCT for anthropomorphic phantom (ECG gating was simulated) [8].
The results are given in Table 3.

Heart rate= 60bpm	100kV	120kV	135kV
Midbreast	13.4±3.6	21.7±4.1	29.3±5.2
Breast	11.8±0.6	18.9±1.1	24.8±1.5
Lung	12.2±2.6	19.1±3.2	26.5±5.0
Thyroid	0.4±0.1	0.7±0.1	0.9±0.2
Heart rate=75bpm	100kV	120kV	135kV
Midbreast	38.3±2.0	59.7±3.1	77.8±3.7
Breast	26.2±1.7	44±1.1	52.8±4.1
Lung	38.0±1.6	58.9±1.7	78±2.9
Thyroid	0.8±0.2	1.0±0.2	2.2±0.5

Table 3. The effect of tube voltage and heart rate on absorbed doses [mGy] in CTA (according to [8]).

4. Comparing CCA and CTA

Primary x-ray beam in the CCA is focused on nearly the same area of a patient's body by most time of the procedure, and then very high local doses are possible. (Skin injuries and even of x-ray burn cases were reported in the paper [9]).

Moreover, a possibility to destroying the vessel wall during catheter operations also exists.

Patient entrance doses change with body thickness, required image quality and distance to x-ray tube focus. Because medical staff have to work in direct neighbourhood of x-ray source and x-rays scattered on a patient's body, the doses to the staff are related to the patient doses.

Thus, the procedures are still treated as invasive and risky for both patients and the staff despite the benefit from "traditional" angiographies.

Good spatial and temporal resolution of modern CT scanners is the reason of positive features of CTA in comparison to conventional angiography [10,11,12], i.e.:

- better detection of stenosed lesions,
- possibility to delineate a cross-sectional cut of the artery,
- non-invasive procedure contrary to the conventional angiography or intravascular ultrasound.

All of the above reasons have made CTA an excellent technique for quick (emergency) cardiac diagnosis and for qualification patients for angioplasty. Moreover, coronary CTA includes a complete evaluation of the lungs and chest. Contrary to to conventional cardiac angiography (CCA) the staff are completely unexposed in CTA.

The only deficiency of CTA in comparison to CCA is its exclusive diagnostic character: any further intervention as angioplasty is not possible in CTA technique. That needs continuing of treatment action in more "traditional" way – at C-arm unit control.

For comparison of doses to patients in both imaging techniques techniques the measurements were performed using multislice CT scanners (MSCT) and C-arm units.

The measurements were performed for

- two sixteen-slice CT scanners (made by two manufacturers),
- one sixty-four-slice CT scanner,
- three C-arm units of different manufacturers.

For each controlled C-arm unit the organ doses in "traditional" coronary angiography were distributed extremely non-uniformly: from up to 100 mGy in the area of the primary x-ray beam interaction to about zero in quite near vicinity of that. For that in all the phantom examinations doses for both lungs and doses for elements of skeleton differed significantly in dependence on the composition of projections.

That was not observed for CTA procedures, when the magnitude of doses inside the scanned volume was similar.

The detailed results were published [13]. Below the most important values of are presented in the Tables 4 to 6.

To summarize of the presented results:

1. In coronary angiography carried out by C-arm units patient organ doses are distributed non-uniformly inside patient body (from up to 100 mGy in area of primary x-ray beam to about zero in quite near vicinity). Therefore, a low effective dose does not mean the low absorbed doses at all.

2. Doses to patients in CTA procedures covering the chest are distributed more uniformly and are dependent on the scanner configuration and protocol of the procedure.

CCA	CTA
1st manufacturer: 0.9 – 1.4	16-slice scanner: 5.4
2nd manufacturer: 1.3 - 3.2	64-slice scanner: 23.1
3rd manufacturer: 6.2 - 18.8	(The both scanners made by 1st manufacturer.)

Table 4. Effective doses to patients in coronary procedures [mSv]

Organ	Eight exposures carried out by C-arm units designed by three manufacturers.	Four exposures carried out by C-arm units the same type (made by the1st manufacturer)
Lungs	2.95 - 23.68	2.95 - 5.64
Stomach	0.07 - 59.76	0.22 - 0.75
Upper Large Intestine	<0.1 - 10.73	0.10 - 0.37
Red Bone Marrow	1.75 - 23.90	1.75 - 3.30
Thyroid	0.13 - 2.03	0.13 - 2.03
Heart	0.52 - 27.15	1.39 - 3.75

Table 5. Range of absorbed doses [mGy] in CCA

Organ	Sixteen-slice CT	Sixty-four-slice CT
Lungs	25.8	64.5
Stomach	5.7	44.2
Upper Large Intestine	1.5	8.1
Red Bone Marrow	10.9	31.4
Thyroid	6.8	11.7
Heart	29.0	77.7

Table 6. Absorbed doses [mGy] to patients in CTA (both CT scanners made by 1st manufacturer)

5. References

5.1 References for CCA

[1] International Commission on Radiological Protection, Publication 85, Avoidance of Radiation Injuries from Medical Interventional Procedures, 2001.

[2] Vano E, Gonzales L, Guibelalde E, et al:Radiation exposure to medical staff in interventional and cardiac radiology. Br.J.Radio., 71,954-960,1998.

[3] International Commission on Radiological Protection, Publication 60, Recommendations of the International Commission on Radiological Protection, 1991.

[4] International Commission on Radiological Protection, Publication 103, The 2007 Recommendations of the International Commission on Radiological Protection, 2007.

[5] Vano E, Arranz L, Sastre JM, et al: Dosimetric and radiation protection considerations based on some cases of patient skin injuries in interventional cardiology. Br.J.Radiol., 71, 510-516, 1998.

[6] Bor D, Olgar T, Toklu T, et al.: Patient doses and dosimetric evaluations in interventional cardiology. Physica Medica, 25,31-42, 2009.

[7] Maccia C: An optimization study of cardiac interventional radiology procedures: an experience in France. ERPET in Madrid, p.113-119, 1997.

[8] Hansson B, Karambatsakidou A: Relagtionships between entrance skin dose, effective dose and dose area product for patients in diagnostic and interventional cardiac procedures. Radia.Prot.Dosimetry. 90: 141-144, 2000.

[9] Van de Putte S, Verhaegen F, Taeymans Y, et al.: Correlation of patient skin doses in cardiac interventional radiology with dose-are product. Br.J.Radiol. 73: 504-513, 2000.

[10] Clark AL, Brennan AG, Robertson LJ, et al.:Factors affecting patient radiation exposure during routine coronary angiography in a tertiary referral centre. Br.J.Radiol. 73: 184-189, 2000.

[11] McFadden SL, Money RB, Shepherd PH: X-ray dose and associated risks from radiofrequency catheter ablation procedures. Br.J.Radio. 75: 253-265, 2002.

[12] Delichas MG, Psarrakos K, Molyvda Athanassopoulou E, et al.:Radiation doses to patients undergoing coronary angiography and percutaneuos transluminal coronary angioplasty. Radiat.Prot.Dosimetry.103(2):149-154, 2003.

[13] Sandborg M, Fransson SG, PetterssonH: Evaluation of patient and staff absorbed doses during coronary angiography and intervention by femoral and radial artery access routes. Eur.Radiol. 14(4):653-658, 2004.

[14] Leung KC, Martin CJ: Effective doses for coronary angiography. Br.J.Radiol. 69:426-431, 1996.

[15] Tsapaki V, Kottou S, Kollaros N, et al.: Dose performance evaluation of a charge coupled device and a flat-panel digital fluoroscopy system recently installed in an interventional cardiology laboratory. Radiat.Prot.Dosimetry. 111(3): 297-304,2004.

[16] Chida K, Fuda K, Saito H, et al.: Patient skin dose in cardiac interventional procedures: conventional fluoroscopy versus pulsed fluoroscopy. Catheter Cardiovasc Interv.69(1):115-121, 2007.

[17] International Commission on Radiological Protection, Publication 75, General Principles of Monitoring for Radiation Protection of Workers, 1997.

Kim KP, Miller DL, Balter S, et al.: Occupational radiation doses to operators performing cardiac catheterization procedures. Health Phys. 94(3):211-227,2008.

[18] Padovani R: Optimisation of patient and staff exposure in interventional radiology. In: Radiation Protection in Medical Physics, edited by Y.Lemoigne and A.Caner, Springer in Cooperation with NATO Public Diplomacy Division, The Netherlands, 2011.

5.2 References to CTA

[1] Korosoglou G, Mueller D, Lehrke S, et al.: Quantitative assessment of stenosis severity and atherosclerotic plaque composition using 256-slice computed tomography. Eur.Radiol 20:1841-1850,2010.

[2] Rutten A, Meijs MFL, de Vos A, et al.: Biphasic contrast medium injection in cardiac CT: moderate versus high concentration contrast material at identical iodine flux and iodine dose. Eur.Radiol. 20: 1917-1925, 2010.

[3] Taylor A, Cerquiera M in Journal of the American College of Cardiology, October 2010: according to AuntMinnie.com (November 1,2010): New cardiac CT guidelines expand use for low-risk patients.

[4] W.A.Kalender: Computed Tomography. Publicis MCD Verlag, Munich 2000.

[5] Bischoff B, Hein Fm Meyer T, et al.: Impact of a reduced tube voltage on CT angiography and radiation dose: results of the PROTECTION I study.JACC Cardiovasc Imaging 2:940-946, 2009.

[6] AuntMinnie.com February 15, 2007: Radiation dose slashed in 64-slice coronary CTA (by Eric Barnes)

[7] AuntMinnie.com February 3, 2009: JAMA study finds wide variation in cardiac CTA dose (by Eric Barnes)

[8] Nikoito D, Khosa P, Lin PJ, et al.:Absorbed radiation dose in radiosensitive organs during coronary CT angiography using 320-MDCT: effect of maximum tube voltage and heart rate variations. AJR.195(6):1347-1354, 2010.

[9] Vano E, Gelcolea J., Galvan C et.al. Skin radiation injuries in patients following repeated coronary angioplasty procedures. The British Journal of Radiology 2001; 74: 1023-1031.

[10] De Backer G, Ambrosioni E, Borch-Johnson K, et al. European quidelines on cardiovascular disease prevention in clinical practice. Eur.J.Cardiovasc.Prev. Rehabil. (2003), 10(4):S1-10.

[11] Nieman K, Cademartiri F, Lemos PA, et al.Reliable non-invasive coronary angiography with fast submillimeter multislice spiral computed tomography. Circulation 2002, 106: 2051-2054.

[12] Ropers D, Baum U, Polite K, et.al. Detection of coronary artery stenoses with thin-slice multi-detector row spiral computed tomography and multiplanar reconstruction. Circulation 2003. 107:664-666.

[13] Staniszewska MA, Jazwinski J: MSCT and C-arm units: doses to patients in the chest angiography procedures. Pol.J.Radiol. 73(1):43-49, 2008.

6

Procedural Techniques of Coronary Angiography

Jasmin Čaluk
BH Heart Center Tuzla
Bosnia-Herzegovina

1. Introduction

Coronary angiography is an invasive diagnostic procedure in which radiocontrast is injected into the coronary arteries under X-ray guidance in order to display the coronary anatomy and possible luminal obstruction. Despite the advances in other diagnostic methods, it remains to be "the golden standard" of coronary disease diagnostics. Although today the complication rate is far lower than previously, the possibility of complication still exists, and an invasive cardiologist must be able to complete the procedure flawlessly, and to competently deal with complications, should they occur. In order to be able to do that, he/she must master the proper techniques in performing the coronary angiography procedure, and be comfortable with all the available access-sites.

2. Cath lab

The procedure is performed in a specifically designed room, very much resembling the operating room, called the catheterization laboratory, or cath lab (Fig.1). Recordings are made using a special X-ray machine, called cardioangiograph (Fig.1). Today, these machines are completely digitalized, enabling superb picture quality, with the lowest possible radiation doses, and some additional features, such as precise measurements and quantifications of the recorded angiograms, connections to additional devices, such as intravascular ultrasound, easy and large-capacity data storage etc. It is convenient to have a wide choice of spare catheters, multi-packs, guidewires, coronary angioplasty ballons, coronary stents, and other equipment in the cath lab itself, so it can be used without time-delay. The space should be intuitively organized, and the spare devices, sterile gowns, gloves, drapes etc. must be easily accesible. Defibrillator, endotracheal tubes, temporary pacemakers and leads, oxygen supply, and other cardiopulmonary resuscitation equipment must be held in the cath lab at all times. Just outside of the cath lab is the control-station with monitors for angiogram, patient data, electrocardiogram (ECG), haemodynamics etc (Fig.2). Modern cardioangiographs allow for data analysis both from the control station outside the cath lab, as well as from within the cath lab, using specifically designed control-commands at the table.

3. Coronary angiography: Preparation

Coronary angiography is performed under local anesthesia. The procedure is sterile, and all potential access sites must be disinfected, shaved, and sterilized. At the beginning of the procedure, the patient lays down in supine position on the cardioangiograph table, and is prepared for the procedure in sterile conditions (Fig.3).

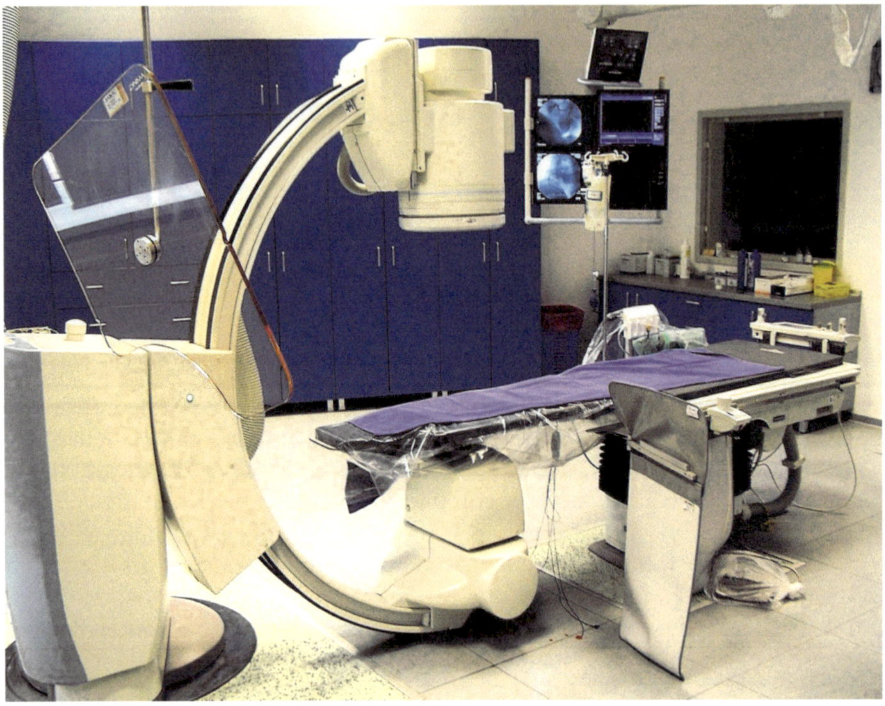

Fig. 1. Catheterization laboratory

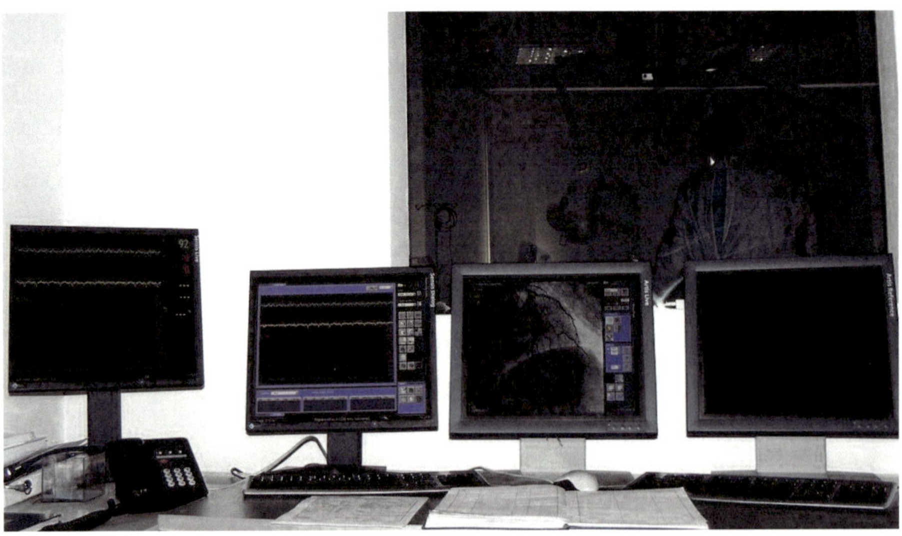

Fig. 2. Control-station with monitors outside the catheterization laboratory

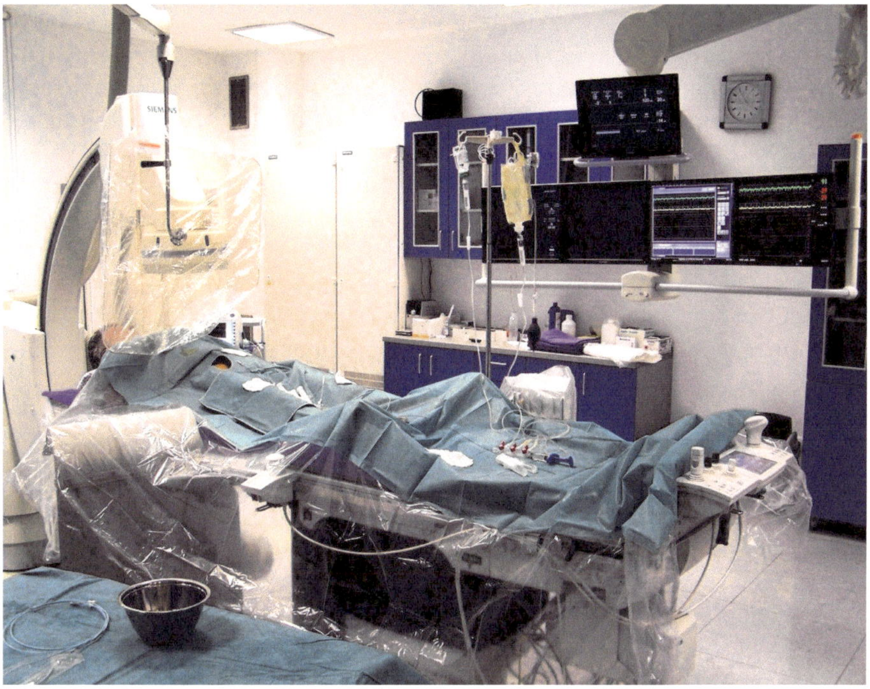

Fig. 3. The patient in supine position on the cardioangiograph table

Coronary angiography is performed with the patient in the fasting state, except in emergency cases, e.g. acute myocardial infarction, in which the degree of urgency prevails over the risks of aspiration incidents, which are generally very rare. In many institutions today, it is common not to administer pre-medication prior to coronary angiography, except in certain specific conditions. In other institutions, the patients are given 10 mg diazepam p.o. and 25 mg diphenhydramine p.o. 30-60 min before the procedure. If the patient has a known allergy to radiocontrast, prednisone can be administered at 60 mg p.o. every 8 hours for two days prior to the procedure. Other institutions have the policy to administer hydrocortisone 80-120 mg IV some 30 min before the procedure, along with 50 mg diphenhydramine p.o. The patients with a history of radiocontrast allergy must be monitored after coronary angiography for signs of acute allergy: urticas on skin or itchy skin, swelling of tongue, stuffy nose or signs of respiratory distress.

The table set for coronary angiography (Fig. 4) can differ from one institution to another, but generally it has the following list of items and equipment:

- sterile drapes to cover the patient and radiation-protection screens,
- sterile swabs for cleaning the arterial access site,
- a bowl of Betadine solution for cleaning the arterial access site,
- lidocaine for local anesthesia, 15-20 ml of 2% solution (in some cases, for more sensitive patients, more may be needed)
- punction neelde for arterial cannulation,
- an 11-mm or 15-mm blade,
- syringes and needles,
- two containers, one with 500 ml of saline solution with 5,000 U of heparin added,
- arterial sheath with a dilator,

- a J-shaped guidewire,
- diagnostic catheters for coronary angiography; start with the most common JL4 and JR4 with angulated pigtail if left ventriculography and/or aortography is planned,
- a three-outlet manifold which is to be connected to pressure transducer, saline solution container, and radiocontrast container on side-outlets, to the syringe for radiocontrast application on the proximal end, and with its distal end to diagnostic/therapeutic catheters during the procedure.

During the procedure, the patient must be monitored by several systems, and the ECG is absolutely essential. The patient also must have an ECG recording done just before the procedure actually starts. For practical reasons, during the angiography itself, there is really no need to apply the precordial leads, since the basic four electrodes can provide enough information for ECG monitoring during coronary angiography and percutaneous coronary interventions (PCI). Four electrodes should be placed on the calf or thigh and on the shoulders or upper arms (Watson & Hunter, 2011).

The area of the puncture site must be shaved, disinfected, then anesthetized, and only then punctured. The center of the field for shaving and disinfection is the puncture site. The disinfection is performed starting at the center, and spiraling outwards, at least twice, using Betadine. Thereafter, the site is wiped off with a third swab. If the procedure is planned to be performed via the femoral artery, than both right and left groins must be shaved and disinfected, in case that the operator must switch to contralateral artery. Only after the disinfection of the puncture site, the patient is covered with a sterile drape. Most centers today use single-use pre-packed sterile drapes. These drapes have openings conveniently placed at the location of patient's left and right inguinal area (Fig.5, Fig. 6).

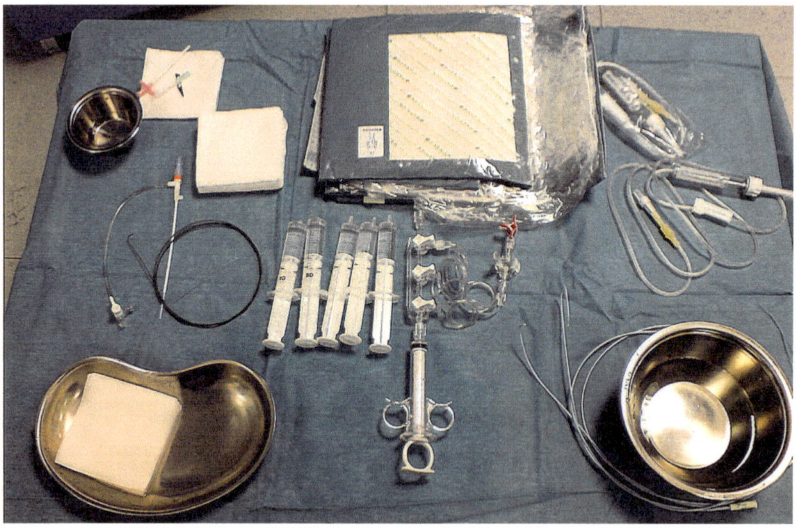

Fig. 4. The table set for coronary angiography

The patient must be warned not to move his/her hands downward, towards the disinfected areas of planned vascular access. The radiation shield and image intensifier/digital flat panel detector are also covered with sterile covers. The manifold is connected and flushed, and then zeroed for pressure monitoring.

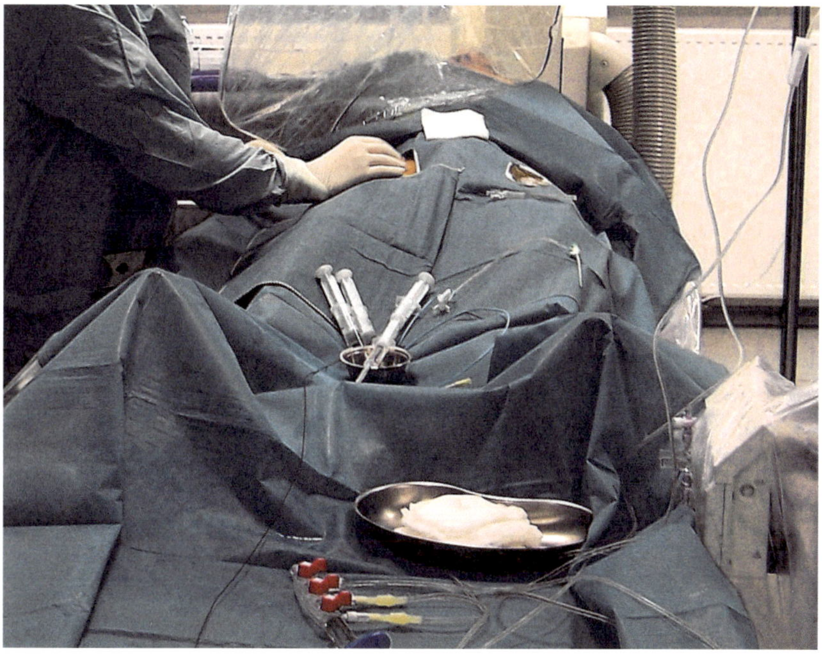

Fig. 5. Sterile drape openings in patient's inguinal area, femoral pulse palpation

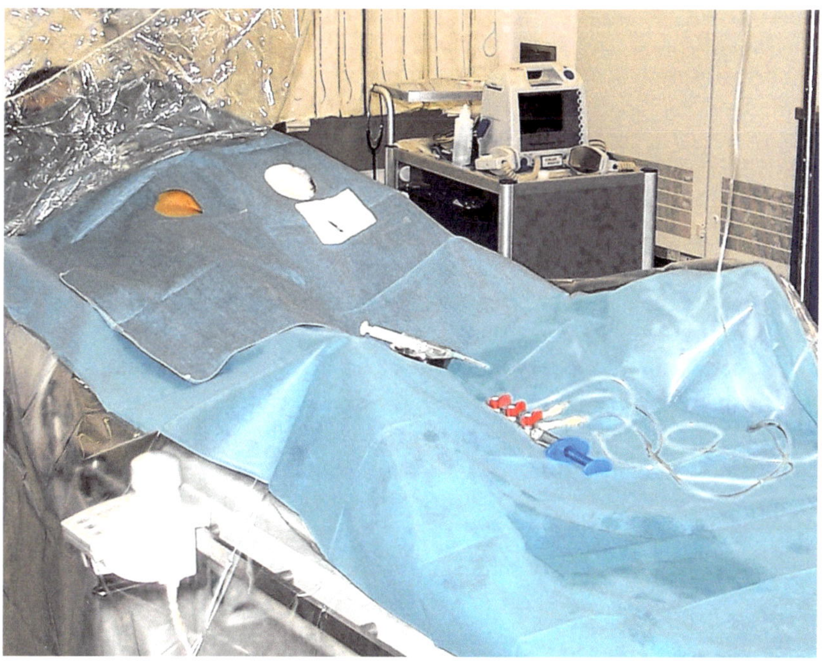

Fig. 6. Sterile drape openings in patient's inguinal area

4. Catheter menu

Coronary angiography is performed with the use of specifically designed diagnostic catheters. More than 95% of all procedures can be completed using catheters Judkins left 4 (JL4), and Judkins right 4 (JR4). Also, a pigtail catheter is used for obtaining left ventriculogram, if it is recorded. Usually the catheters come pre-packed in a sterile envelope, in which JL4, JR4 and pigtail catheters are present. Diagnostic catheters are more elastic than the catheters used for PCI, and can be manipulated into the coronary ostium. However, sometimes the anatomy of the aortic arch and coronary ostia requires the use of different types of catheters. Today, the catheter menu is abundant with different versions, and at least one of the available catheters will be able to adequately cannulate even the most difficult and distorted coronary ostia (Fig.7). It is necessary to know the shapes of those catheters in order to choose the appropriate-ones for certain anatomical variants. Therapeutic (guiding) catheters are somewhat stiffer and do not forgive an imperfect position, because the insertion of interventional equipment (coronary guidewires, angioplasty balloons, stents etc.) creates much more backforce than does the radiocontrast injection. Therefore, an unstable catheter with inadequate backup will be frequently displaced out of the coronary ostium. This is why coronary stenting, even more than diagnostic coronary angiography, requires the use of dedicated guiding catheters.

5. Arterial puncture

The standard technique of arterial puncture used today is Seldinger technique (Powell & Moxey, 2011), cleverly developped by Sven-Ivar Seldinger, a Swedish radiologist, in 1953. The procedure of arterial puncture is performed as follows: firstly, at the site of arterial puncture, an appropriate pulse has to be palpated in order to locate the artery (Fig.5). A local anesthesia is applied, usually with 10-15 ml of 1% or 2% lidocaine for local infiltration of the skin and subcutaneous tissues. Then, a percutaneous puncture of the desired vessel with a hollow beveled tapered-tip needle is made. The pointy tip at the distal end of the needle is the first one in contact with the skin, and subsequently with the artery, while the distal needle opening faces upwards. The needle is held in the operator's hand like a pencil, at an angle of 30°-45° against the surface of the skin. Arterial puncture is made by advancing the needle to the site of the arterial pulse. An experienced operator will usually feel when the needle has punctured the arterial wall. A correct arterial puncure is confirmed by the pulsatile back-flow of the bright-red blood from the proximal end of the needle (Fig.8).

It is not necessary to have a syringe attached to the needle during arterial puncture, because the arterial pressure will produce a pulsatile jet of blood when the needle tip reaches the arterial lumen. If the backflow is slow and barely pulsatile (or seems to be continuous, without pulsations), and the blood is dark-red, the needle tip has punctured the vein. In certain circumstances, however, even correct arterial puncture may resemble venous puncture: shock, hypotension, severe bradycardia, very low oxygen saturation, cardiac arrest and/or resuscitation etc.

After the arterial puncture, an atraumatic, curved-tipped guide wire (J-wire with moveable inner core) is passed through the needle and advanced into the artery (Fig.9). The needle is then removed, leaving the guide wire in the vessel. The site of puncture at the skin level is usually widened by a couple of milimetres using a small and shallow cut by a surgical scalpel, an 11-mm or 15-mm blade to facilitate the passage of the arterial sheath. The sheath with a plastic dilator inside of it is advanced over the guide wire, and into the artery. The dilator is removed, leaving the sheath in the vessel, and a haemostatic valve prevents bleeding through the sheath. It also provides access for the passage of catheters and other devices into the vessels, with no blood loss. The side arm of the sheath is aspirated and injected with heparinized saline before the advancement of catheters. During arterial puncture and sheath placement, the patient may develop a vasovagal reaction due to puncture and vessel manipulation, which will manifest as hypotension and bradycardia. Atropine IV usually swiftly reverts the condition, and sometimes elevation of patient's legs and high-rate saline infusion with oxygen supplementation should be implemented additionally. The technique of direct arterial approach, with the preparation and direct visualization of the artery at the puncture site is today very rarely used, and therefore discussed elsewhere.

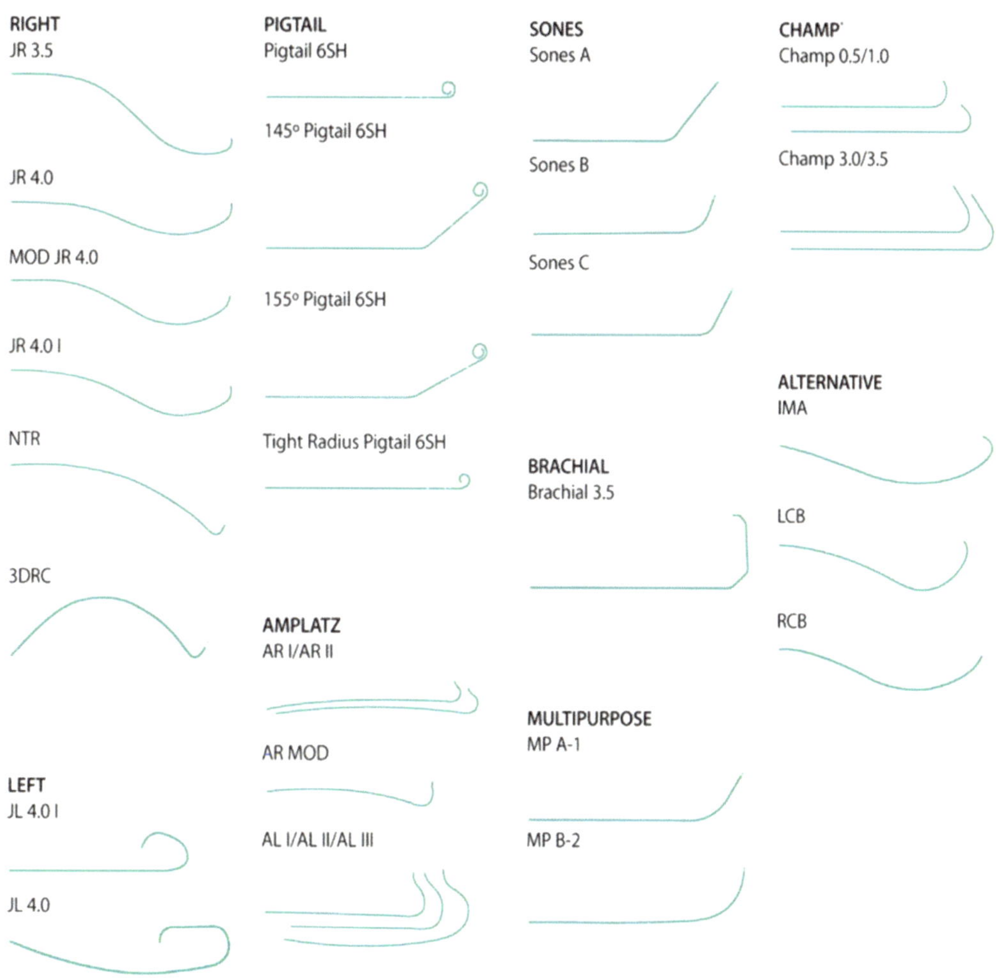

Fig. 7. Diagnostic catheter curves, picture courtesy of Medtronic

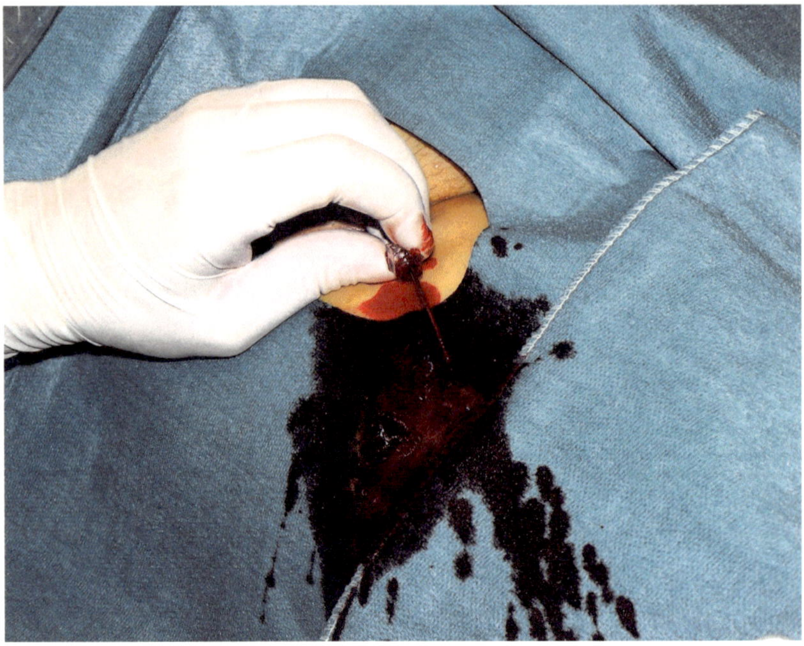

Fig. 8. Pulsatile back-flow of the bright-red blood from the proximal end of the needle

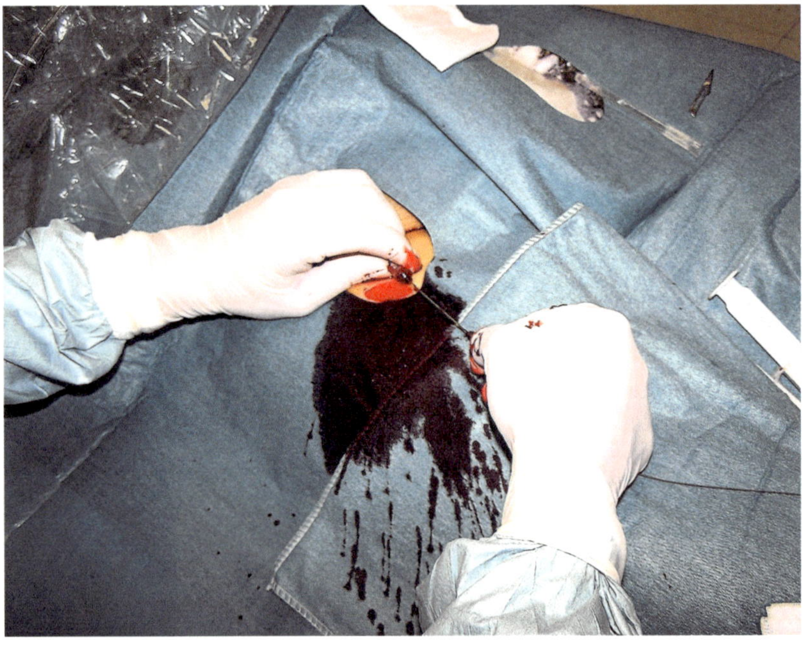

Fig. 9. J-wire is passed through the needle and advanced into the artery

6. Vascular access

6.1 Femoral approach

Preferences of particular access sites vary in different centers, but the most commonly used are right femoral and right radial artery. The percutaneous transfemoral approach has been routinely used for cardiac catheterization and coronary angioplasty (Kwac et al, 2010). Right transfemoral approach is favoured because of the larger artery diameter, and therefore the possibility to insert larger arterial sheaths, catheters and bulkier devices, in comparison with the transradial approach. If there is a peripheral vascular problem, the left femoral, or right or left radial or brachial approaches can be used. The femoral approach is the most comfortable access for the operator. Its main disadvantage is the time-delay after the angiography and before mobilizing the patient. After the femoral pulse is palpated (Fig.5) and local anesthesia applied, the puncture of the femoral artery is performed some 2 cm below the inguinal ligament (Fig.10), at the *punctum maximum* of the pulse. The inguinal ligament is attached to *spina illiaca anterior superior* on one end, and with the pubic bone on the other (Fig.10). This makes determining of its anatomical location easier, because overlapping skin crease in obese patients can be located more distally, thus deceptively making the less experienced operators prone to puncturing too distally. Puncture through the ligament itself will make the haemostasis very difficult, because the ligament is a firm structure which precludes adequate pressure application against the artery after angiography.

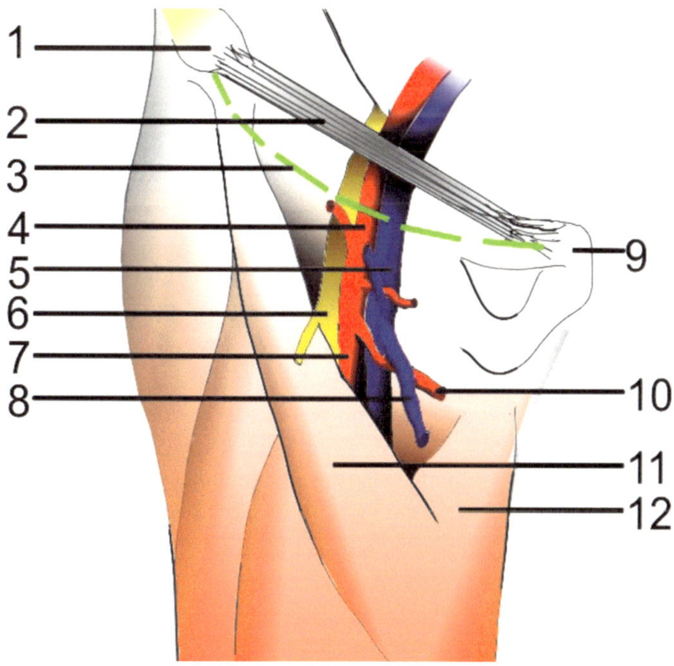

Fig. 10. Inguinal area anatomy; 1 - spina iliaca anterior superior, 2 - inguinal ligament, 3 - skin crease, 4 - common femoral artery, 5 - common femoral vein, 6 - femoral nerve, 7 - deep femoral artery, 8 - saphenous vein, 9 - pubic bone, 10 - superficial femoral artery, 11 - sartorius muscle, 12 - abductor longus muscle

6.2 Radial approach

Alternative access when femoral puncture is unavailable or cannot be used, is radial or brachial approach. While the femoral access is still most widely used in the USA and the most of Europe, Asia and Americas, radial access is becoming more and more popular in Europe, thanks to its advantage of avoiding prolonged periods of patients' bed-rest after the procedure. The transradial approach has gained popularity in recent years mainly because of the significantly decreased access-site complications and the greater patient comfort it offers (Tomassini et al, 2011). However, the prevalence of transradial approach for coronary procedures worldwide is still quite low and nowadays, in the United States, for example, the favourite strategy for bleeding prevention is mostly based on the adoption of new antithrombotic drugs (such as bivalirudin and fondaparinux) rather than on the selection of an alternative, safer vascular access route (Rigattieri et al, 2010). Also, radial approach is somewhat more difficult to master, and requires more training than the femoral one. The main setback is the small diameter of the vessel, and the fact that the radial artery is prone to spasm. Allen's test is also mandatory to determine the ability of the ulnar artery to take over the circulation to the hand in case of an irreversible damage to the radial artery. Another disadvantage of right radial approach is the considerable technical difficulty in evaluating left interior mammary arterial graft. Instead, the left radial approach can be used. The third reason because of which radial artery might not be used is the inability to use that particular artery as a potential free arterial bypass-graft, should the bypass-surgery be indicated. Also, there has been some controversy in radiation dose to the operator when using radial approach. There were reports of significantly higher radiation doses for the operator in comparison to femoral approach, especially during the learning phase. Before proceeding with transradial coronary angiography, it is wise to administer premedication in order to reduce the probability of radial artery spasm or thrombosis. Premedication cocktail containing nitroglycerin and verapamil has been documented to be effective in preventing radial spasms. However, verapamil is relatively contraindicated for some patients with left ventricular dysfunction, hypotension and bradycardia. Intra-arterial premedication with 100 µg of nitroglycerin and 3,000 units of heparin is effective in preventing radial spasms during transradial cardiac catheterization, according to Chen et al (2006). Some authors recommend an intra-arterial cocktail consisting of 5 mg of verapamil plus 200 µg nitroglycerine in 10 ml of normal saline, and others (Pancholy et al, 2006) use 200 µg/ml of nitroglycerin solution injected on the lateral and medial aspect of the previous location of the radial artery pulsation, should the arterial spasm occur after administration of lidocaine for local anesthesia, and before radial cannulation. During transradial coronary angiography, the wire should always go smoothly. If the operator feels some resistance, a peripheral radial angiogram should be taken. There is a possibility that a radial loop with recurrent radial artery exists, and the operator will be forced to change the access site. Left radial approach can be used comfortably: it is possible to bend the patient's arm over the abdomen and perform the procedure. Left radial approach is also favoured when re-evaluating left interior mammary artery (LIMA) to left anterior descending coronary artery (LAD) bypass grafts. The transradial approach can be safely proposed for all patients, with a low conversion rate to transfemoral approach when an attempt on both radial arteries is considered first (Guédès et al, 2010). Instead of JL4 used in transfemoral approach, for an average sized patient, a JL3.5 can be used. The catheters should always be exchanged over a long wire, so that renegotiating the wire through this spasm-prone and often tortuous vessel can be avoided. Some population studies have shown that patients prefer radial access because of early ambulation (Cooper et al, 1999) and some cardiologists also strongly prefer it. However, one should bear in mind that the most important indication for PCI today is acute myocardial infarction. This important setting must be considered when discussing the preffered vascular access, because this is the primary circumstance in which PCI improves survival. It can be expected that difficulties with radial approach and conversion to femoral approach may delay time to reperfusion, jeoppardizing the lives of critically ill patients, especially those in cardiogenic shock, requiring intra-aortic balloon pump, for example. So the question is: with the increased use of radial approach, should it become the new standard of care, especially regarding emergency interventions for acute myocardial infarction, and can primary PCI (pPCI) be routinely performed through radial approach?And the answer is: No. As for the setting of acute myocardial infarction (AMI), Vorobcsuk et al (2009) performed a systematic review and meta-analysis of 12 trials comparing the radial versus the femoral approach. They found no significant difference in the time to reperfusion between the two groups but found access site failure when transradial approach was used, which contributed to longer procedure times (Jolly et al, 2009). Recent systematic reviews and meta-analyses of trials in the acute setting of ST-elevation AMI, where time is of the essence, have shown radial access to be associated with a 10% crossover rate increasing "time to reperfusion" in the individual case (Vorobcsuk et al, 2009). Those trials usually excluded unstable patients in cardiogenic shock requiring additional treatment options, such as intra-aortic balloon pumps, central venous access or temporary pacing. These patients are automatically treated using femoral access as it is more convenient and appropriate to use one access site. In some circumstances these patients arrest on the table necessitating cardiopulmonary resuscitation, and femoral access is simply easier and less fiddly under difficult circumstances (Patterson & Foale, 2011). Radial artery puncture can only be attempted once. If that attempt fails, the morbidity associated with access site crossover occurs, including the risk of radial artery occlusion, but also the need for double site post-procedural care (Stella et al, 1997). The radial approach therefore increases procedure times, not only because of the steep learning curve to this technically more challenging approach. Radial artery anomalies are also relatively common and are a cause of transradial procedure failure even for experienced radial operators (Lo et al, 2009). Even when operators achieve equal procedural times using radial and femoral approach, there is still significantly greater fluoroscopy time with radial approach PCI. Inevitably an increase in the irradiation of staff and patient follows (Brasselet et al, 2008). Femoral access is easier for training, not limited by anomalous radial artery anatomy, and allows for both left and right mammary arterial bypass graft evaluation. It is also convenient if a venous puncture is necessary for obtaining haemodynamic measurements. In these circumstances, an adjecent femoral vein puncture requires "same-site" postprocedural management. Surely this does not mean that the transradial technique should be dismissed as a cardiology fashion. It should be learned because it has certain advantages in diagnostic coronary angiography and *elective* PCI, it is associated with an earlier patient discharge, and can be applied in circumstances of severe aortoiliac disease which precludes the use of femoral approach. However, in primary PCI, the current enthusiasm for using transradial approach is not sufficiently justified in evidence, and especially not justified enough to dismiss the femoral route from current training programmes.

6.3 Brachial approach

Brachial approach remains an option too, most commonly the right brachial approach. The brachial artery is the distal continuation of the axillary artery, and itself separates distally into ulnar and radial arteries. Percutaneous transbrachial approach is useful and safe alternative for performing coronary angiography as well as PCI. The advantage of the brachial approach as an alternative to the radial one is that brachial approach needs no special premedication, and can be performed using the exactly same equipment (arterial sheath and catheters), often even the larger-ones, including 7 Fr size, although most operators usually use the shorter brachial sheaths. For brachial approach it is necessary that an arm-board be placed for the patient's arm and hand during the preparation of the patient for the procedure. The antecubital fossa should be prepped and draped, and the technique of local anesthesia, arterial puncture, sheath placement etc. is generally similar to the one used for femoral access. When puncturing the brachial artery, care must be taken not to puncture the posterior arterial wall too. The complication rate is relatively low, and in the large series has not exceeded 2% (Gonzalez et al, 1991). Complications of this site of arterial access include: brachial artery thrombosis, hemmorhage, pseudoaneurysm formation, cellulitis, phlebitis, and median nerve traction with possible irreversible damage.

6.4 Axillar approach

Axillary artery cannulation is a useful technique for obtaining central arterial access in patients with severe peripheral vascular disease in the lower and upper extremities, although it is very rarely used today. The axillary artery, which is the direct continuation of the subclavian artery, courses from the outer margin of the first rib to the tendon of *musculus teres major*, where it becomes brachial artery. The lateral portion of the axillary artery is cannulated, just lateral to the head of *musculus pectoralis minor*. The patient's underarm must be shaved and prepped in sterile fashion. The arm is hyperabducted and externally rotated in order to access the artery (Gonzalez et al, 1991). After applying local anesthesia, a skin incision is made using a no. 11 blade, and through that incision, an 18-gauge needle is advanced until pulsatile backflow is obtained. Care must be taken to only perform a single-wall puncture. Then, a J-wire and thereafter a side-arm sheath-dilator are placed into the artery as with other accesses, and angiography can be conducted. After the procedure, the patient is advised not to use the arm for at least one day to avoid bleeding. Complications of axillary arterial cannulation include arterial thrombosis, brachial plexus injury, hemorrhage, and pseudoaneurysm formation.

7. Performing the coronary angiography

Through the sheath placed into peripheral artery through which the vascular access is enabled, and over the guidewire, the first coronary diagnostic catheter is introduced through the peripheral artery (Fig.11), and farther into the aorta. Care must be taken that the atraumatic J-tip of the guidewire precedes the catheter, as to avoid injury to the vascular endothelium. The J-wire is 0.035 or 0.038 inch in diameter. There are many different types of guidewires, different in length, structure, coatings, diameter, tip structure and shape, and materials, available for different diagnostic and interventional vascular procedures. The usual choice is the 0.035 inch wire with a 3 mm J-tip. For tortuous vessels, a hydrophilic wire, such as Terumo Glidewire, or Wholey Wire with soft, floppy tip may be used. Glidewire should not be used through the needle, because of the possibility to damage the hydrophilic coating. Also, when advancing the catheter, the proximal part of the J-wire has to be visible on the outside of the catheter and secured by the operator's hand (Fig.11), as to avoid embolization of the J-wire into the patient's circulation. That would require an emergency vascular surgical procedure to remove the J-wire from the patient's aorta. Under the X-ray guidance, the guidewire tip is advanced up to the ascending aorta, and into the aortic root. Holding it in place, the coronary diagnostic catheter is advanced over the guidewire until it reaches the ascending aorta.

After the catheter reaches the Valsalva sinus in the aorta, the guidewire is withdrawn leaving the catheter in place. The outside portion of the catheter is connected to a manifold (Fig.12). The manifold is on the other side connected to the syringe (or an automated injection-device) for radiocontrast application, and on its side arms to the saline infusion, to the transducer for invasive blood-pressure monitoring, and to a radiocontrast container from which radiocontrast is taken into the syringe. Through the manifold, the operator controls the contrast injection, blood pressure, injections of heparinized saline if necessary, etc. To ensure that there is no air or clot within the coronary catheter, a syringe is connected to the catheter to aspirate and discard at least some 5 ml of blood. This is the approximate volume of the catheter lumen. Some operators instead just allow a small "bleed back" from the catheter, after which the catheter is connected to the three-port manifold.

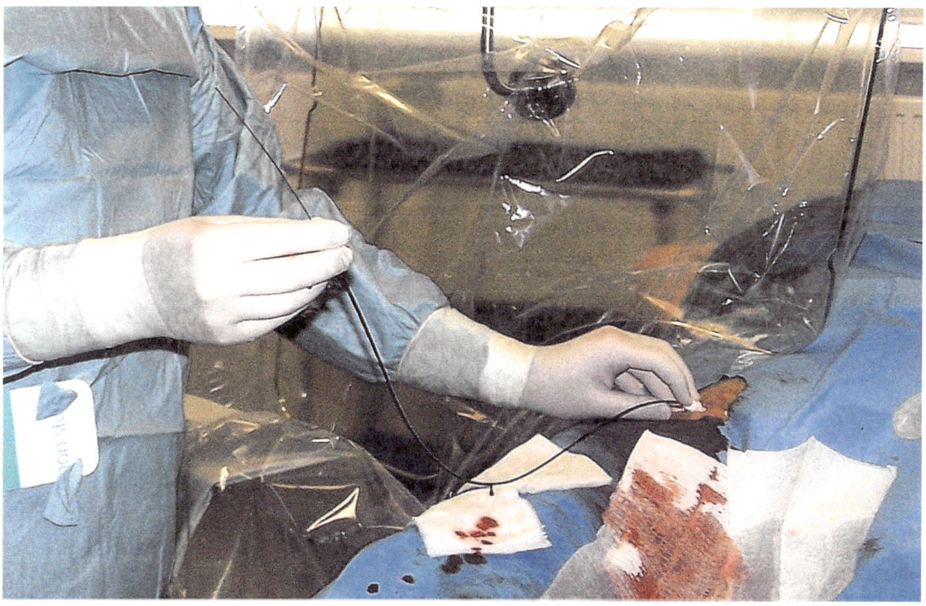

Fig. 11. Through the arterial sheath and over the guidewire, the first coronary diagnostic catheter is introduced into the artery; note the proximal end of the wire outside of the catheter

When connecting the catheter to the manifold, it is important to connect using the fluid-against-fluid method, i.e. to let the blood back-bleed from the catheter, and at the same time to allow saline flush from the manifold. This manner of connecting the catheter to the manifold prevents air embolism from air bubbles from within the catheter, or from within the manifold.

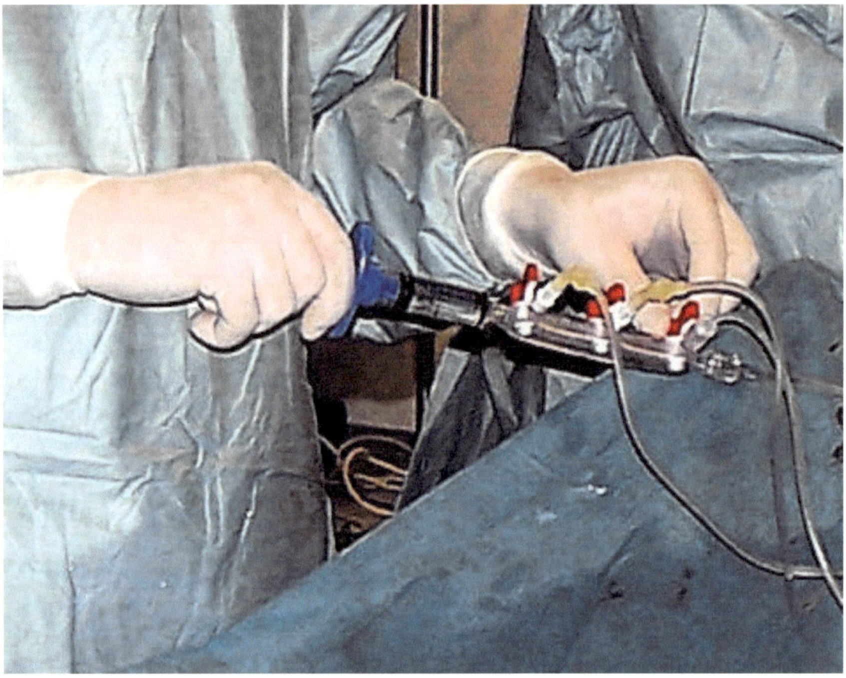

Fig. 12. Manifold with connections

7.1 Left coronary artery engagement

Under fluoroscopic guidance, the catheter is advanced into the coronary ostium, and several recordings of the left coronary artery are taken. The most commonly used catheter diameters are 6 Fr, but diameters from 4 Fr to 8 Fr can also be used. Diagnostic and therapeutic coronary catheters are pre-shaped to suite specific aortic and coronary anatomy. The most commonly used diagnostic catheters for coronary angiography are JL4 (Judkins left 4 cm curve) for the left, and JR4 for the right coronary artery. Both types of catheters were ingeniously designed by Judkins, and are easy to use, because they can engage the coronary ostia with very little manipulation. In fact, Judkins himself said that "no points are earned for coronary catheterization - the catheters know where to go if not thwarted by the operator" (Judkins, 1968). When cannulating the left coronary artery, the catheter is supposed to be unfolded in *en face* position in the ascending aorta. The best view to see the coronary ostia (both left and right) and to perform the ostial coronary cannulation is left anterior oblique (LAO) 50°, because sinus of Valsalva and aortic root are not superimposed on either of the coronary ostia. Cannulating the left coronary artery (LCA) in antero-posterior (AP) position is not recommended because it is difficult to appreciate the ostium, and ostial Left Main Coronary Artery (LMCA) stenoses can be easily missed.

For engagement of the LCA, the J-wire is advanced to the level of aortic valve. Then, the JL4 catheter is placed as low as possible facing the left coronary ostium. The guidewire is slowly withdrawn, and the catheter tip is already in the LMCA or just below it. If it is below the ostium, than it should be withdrawn ever so slightly, and it will fall into the LMCA ostium. Some operators fear that this method might be a bit risky, so they prefer to leave the catheter tip above the level of the left sinus of Valsalva, then withdraw the guidewire from the catheter, and thereafter advance the catheter tip downwards and into the LMCA ostium. This, on the other hand, carries some risk of scratching the surface of the aortic endothelium and embolizing atheromas if they are located in catheter's path. If the catheter tip is at the level of the ostium, but not within the ostium itself, it is usually easily inserted into the ostium by a clockwise or counter-clockwise torque. An injection of 5-10 ml of contrast close to the expected location of the coronary ostium reveals the position of the catheter tip within the aortic root and facilitates a precise cannulation. If the aorta is dilated, a JL5 or JL6 catheters may be required, while in small individuals, or with small aortic arches, a JL3.5 or even JL3 catheters may be used to cannulate the left coronary artery. Multiple recordings are taken from diffrerent perspectives. The optimal positions for recording the left coronary artery are discussed later in the chapter.

7.2 Right coronary artery engagement

After recording the luminograms of the left coronary artery, the catheter is removed over the J-wire, and another catheter, the one for the right coronary artery (RCA) is inserted through the sheath and into the aorta, up to the right coronary ostium, also in the LAO position. After reaching the ascending aorta with the tip of the right coronary catheter and removing the guidewire from inside of it, the catheter is aspirated and connected to manifold. The JR4 catheter is advanced into the aortic root, some 2 cm above the valve level. Then, the operator applies a clockwise rotation with some traction to the catheter. The catheter is slowly rotated using the rotation swivel at the distal portion of the manifold, where the coronary catheter is attached. As the catheter rotates, the torque should be reduced, so that there is no overshoot of the catheter over the right coronary ostium. The catheter rotates and descends somewhat, thereafter cannulating the right coronary ostium. If the first rotation is unsuccessful in cannulating the artery, the catheter should be rotated counter-clockwise to the initial position as to avoid the kinking of the catheter. The problem to find the coronary artery is most commonly due to the origin of the RCA superiorly and more leftwards than usual. It may even arise from the left coronary sinus, close to the LMCA. Using an Amplatz left (AL) 1 or 2 coronary catheter can be helpful to perform selective cannulation of such an RCA. Usually two, but sometimes more right coronary artery luminograms from different projections are recorded, and the catheter is removed. If the right coronary artery ostium is oriented straight downwards, a multipurpose (MP) catheter may be required. In contrast, if the ostium is oriented upwards, a "shepherd's crook" (SC) catheter or internal mammary (IM) catheter may be required. The optimal positions for recording the right coronary artery are discussed later in the chapter.

7.3 Contrast injection technique

The syringe with radiocontrast is held with the handle elevated, so that any air-bubbles inside of the syringe can rise to plunger, and are less likely to be injected into the patient's coronaries. A significant air-embolism into a coronary artery may result in asystole, and cardiac massage should be initiated. This usually reverts pretty quickly, as the air components of the bubble (nitrogen, oxygen, carbon-dioxide etc) are dissolved in the blood. Of course, the operator must previously make sure that there are no air-bubbles inside of the syringe. The radiocontrast must be injected vigorously enough to ensure that it temporarily replaces the blood in the coronaries, with a continuous back-flow into the aortic root. A weak injection may appear as a pulsatile contrast flow with filling-defects, and fail to display the coronary lumen adequately. It sometimes causes the operator to declare a coronary stenosis existence in a place where only a simple contrast filling defect exists. On the contrary, a too-forceful injection can, in extreme cases, cause a coronary dissection, although this event is extremely rare today. If there is no contrast back-flow to the aortic root, or if the back-flow is inadequate, there may be an ostial lesion present.

7.4 Pressure damping

During the cannulation of the coronary artery ostia, a special care must be taken to monitor the blood pressure. A sudden fall in blood pressure may lead to ventricular fibrillation and cardiac arrest. An immediate defibrillation usually restores the normal heart rhythm, although sometimes a full spectre of cardiopulmonary resuscitation has to take place, along with the cardiac massage, endotracheal intubation, artificial ventilation etc. This usually occurs if there is a severe ostial stenosis in the LMCA or the RCA, or if the artery is very prone to severe spasms, or if the conus branch is superselectively cannulated during the RCA engagement. It is a sign of a total coronary obstruction. Pressure damping or "ventricularization", called so because the pressure waveform resembles that of the ventricle, especially with very low diastolic pressure, can also be the result of placement of the catheter tip with the end-hole against the vessel wall, or presence of a thrombus, or an air bubble inside the catheter lumen, and sometimes also occurs after kinking the catheter body.

Whenever blood-pressure damping occurs during the coronary artery engagement, it is best to remove the catheter immediately (Conti et al, 1980). A repeated, careful cannulation may be attempted, best preceded by administration of nitroglycerin. If pressure damping occurs again, the angiogram can be swiftly recorded, and the operator must remove the catheter immediately. Sometimes, a non-selective or semi-selective opacification from the aortic root, with the catheter just in front of the coronary ostium may be sufficient to delineate the ostial coronary disease. There is also an option to use the side-hole catheters, which enable coronary perfusion through the sideholes located just proximally to the catheter tip.

8. Coronary anatomy and the purposeful angiographic projections

Since the coronary arteries are three-dimensional structures, and the X-ray image is two-dimensional, several different perspectives of observing the coronary luminograms are necessary in order to adequately depict the coronary artery anatomy, the location, the extent, and the degree of coronary obstruction. The projections are defined according to the position of the digital flat panel detector, or image intensifier, depending on what kind of cardioangiograph is used. The X-ray tube is under the cardioangiograph table (Fig.1), i.e. under the patient. The positions can be defined as a combination of antero-posterior (AP), cranial, caudal, left or right lateral, and left or right anterior oblique (LAO and RAO, respectively). Extremely rarely, practically almost never, are posterior oblique positions used in diagnostic coronary angiography. The eleven regularly used positions at varying angles are: AP, AP-cranial, AP-caudal, left lateral, right lateral, RAO (right anterior oblique),

RAO-cranial, RAO-caudal, LAO (left anterior oblique), LAO-cranial, and LAO-caudal. These positions are also defined by angles to cranial or caudal, and angles to the left or to the right. These angles may vary depending on patients' anatomy, coronary anatomy, position of the heart etc.

8.1 Radiological coronary anatomy

Left coronary artery is a complex structure, and demands usually at least 4-5 projections. In those, the Left Main (LM, or LMCA) coronary artery has to be clearly visible, along with its bifurcation and branches. The LMCA is a short artery, with variable length, usually bifurcating into the left anterior descending and left circumflex coronary artery. Sometimes LMCA can be very short, almost non-existant as such, in which case there is a "shotgun-ostium" of the left anterior descending (LAD) and the left circumflex (CX) coronary artery. The LMCA is rarely longer than 2 cm.

The LAD passes down the anterior interventricular sulcus and usually extends around the heart's apex. It usually gives rise to two diagonal branches (D-1 and D-2), although they may also vary in number. Diagonal branches are positioned on the left anterolateral part of the heart's surface. The LAD also gives rise to septal perforators. The first one (1st septal) is usually the largest of all the perforators. It marks the border between the proximal and the mid portion of the LAD. The distal portion of the LAD is the distal 1/3 of the vessel, and has no specific landmark as to define it against the mid part. It is important to note the largest septal branch if the patient is to be subjected to alcohol septal ablation for hypertrophic obstructive cardiomyopathy.

The circumflex artery is positioned in the atrio-ventricular (AV) groove and is located on the left side of the heart. It gives rise to several atrial branches, but also to very important marginal branches. As they are positioned on the *margo obtusus cordis*, they are called the obtuse marginal (OM) branches. There are usually three of them (OM-1, OM-2, and OM-3), but their number can also vary individually. Marginal branches are important to define, because they are an available target for coronary bypassing if surgical revascularization is planned. The CX artery is usually anatomically non-dominant, meaning that it does not give rise to posterior lateral (PLA), nor posterior-descending (PDA) artery, which in that case originate from the right coronary artery (RCA). If the CX continues through the AV-groove and gives rise to PLA, while the PDA originates from RCA, than CX and RCA are co-dominant. If the CX gives rise to both PLA and PDA, while the RCA is small and terminates before bifurcating to PLA and PDA, than the CX is anatomically dominant. In this case, it is usually the largest artery in coronary circulation. If it is non-dominant, than the territories of blood supply of both LAD and RCA are larger and more significant than the CX one.

The right coronary artery (RCA) can vary in the position of its ostium. It gives rise to conus-branch, which supplies the right ventricular infundibulum. The second most proximal branch of the RCA is the sinoatrial node artery. The RCA continues on along the right-side AV-sulcus giving rise to a few right-atrial branches. It also gives rise to one or two acute marginal branches, called so because they are positioned on the *margo acutus cordis*. They supply the right ventricular myocardium. Before reaching the crux cordis, the RCA also gives off a few posterior right ventricular branches on the right-diaphragmatic surface of the heart. Finally, at the crux cordis, on the heart's posterior wall, the RCA is bifurcating into the PLA and the PDA. This RCA dominance is the most common situation, present in some 85%

of all human hearts. The PLA and the PDA have several smaller branches, e.g. the posterior septal perforators originating from the PDA. In the crux region, the atrioventricular node artery origins from the RCA, and passes vertically upward towards the AV-node. This is why ischemia in the region of RCA at the time of an acute inferior-wall myocardial infarction can be associated with different degrees of heart block.

8.2 The best projections for evaluating the left coronary artery

Left caudal view (LAO-caudal, or "spider" view) is excellent for evaluation of the LMCA and its bifurcation into the LAD and CX, or trifurcation into the LAD, CX and intermediate branch if it exists (Di Mario and Sutaria, 2005). Interventionalists use it in many cases for wiring the LAD or the CX. It forshortens the mid and the distal segment of the LAD, and should not be used to evaluate these segments, although it can pretty nicely separate LAD from diagonals and septals. Also, it can be very useful in viewing ostia of high marginal branches, and therefore is used for wiring these branches too. It is usually done in 25-40° caudal and 30-50° to the left.

Left cranial (LAO-cranial) view is very good for showing the ostium of the LMCA, but considerably forshortens the proximal half of the LAD. It is convenient for separating the diagonals and the septals from the LAD, though, and can be used to guide the guidewire into and from these branches during interventions. The CX and its high-originating branches are not appreciated well in this projection, but if the CX is dominant, this projection can be useful to depict the very distal parts of the CX.

Cranial (AP-cranial) projection displays the ostium of the LMCA (Di Mario and Sutaria, 2005), similarly to the LAO-cranial view. Although some operators use it to intervene on the proximal LAD, the aouthor's opinion is that the overlap of the CX is too distracting, and that there are better projections for interventions and evaluation of the proximal LAD than the AP-cranial. This projection can be useful for evaluating the mid and distal segments of the LAD and diagonals' take-off, although the diagonal ostia can be overlapped with the main-course LAD. The CX in this view often looks confusing for the inexperienced operator, especially in its proximal and mid segments, but if it is dominant, this can be a very useful projection for evaluating the very distal portions of the CX.

Caudal (AP-caudal) is a very good projection for evaluation of the LMCA, its bifurcation (or in some cases trifurcation), ostial LAD, and the intire CX if it is not dominant. This is the author's favourite projection for interventions on the CX. It can be useful for ostial stent placement in the LAD, similarly to LAO-caudal. Some operators prefere wiring of the marginal branches in RAO-caudal, but in that projection, the marginal ostia are often overlapped with the main course CX. The author feels that AP-caudal is the best projection for evaluating the CX in its entirety, including the marginal ostia, meaning that this projection is also probably the best for wiring those too. It is especially good for treating bifurcational lesions on CX + marginals, but in author's experience also good for treating bifurcation lesions on LMCA + LAD + CX, along with the spider-view. However, if the CX is anatomically dominant, the distal portions of the artery will usually overlap with 3rd marginal branch, PLA and/or PDA. For these, in the case of CX dominance, the cranial projections should be used.

Right cranial (RAO-cranial) projection is the most useful if it is performed with increased cranial angulation of 30°, or in some cases even more. This projection shows nicely the mid part of the LAD with the take-offs of diagonal branches and can in most instances be very useful for treating bifurcation lesions within the LAD + diagonals. Sometimes, the diagonal ostia will overlap, and LAO-cranial, LAO-caudal or AP-cranial will be better for that purpose. If the LMCA is very short, even proximal and ostial LAD can be nicely appreciated in steep RAO-cranial. The CX can be appreciated in this view only if it is dominant, and that goes only for its most distal parts. The proximal and the mid segment of the CX cannot be adequately evaluated in this view.

Right caudal (RAO-caudal) view is very good for evaluating the distal LAD. The proximal and the mid part of the LAD are overlapped with diagonals in most cases, so this should be taken into consideration when evaluating LAD in RAO-caudal. Still, some stenoses of the LAD can only be seen here, so it requires operator's attention. The LMCA is displayed in this view, although the bifurcation itself is being overlapped in most patients by the ostial segments of the LAD and the CX. The CX artery can be nicely evaluated in RAO-caudal, but to be sure, the AP-caudal should always be taken.

Left lateral is rarely used today. It can be useful to display LIMA-LAD anastomosis, the mid and the distal portions of the LAD, and to separate the LAD from the diagonals, LAD being the closest to the sternum. Pure RAO is rarely used today, since it does not display any of the LCA segments ideally, except it can be useful for evaluating the distal LAD. Pure LAO is very useful for cannulation of both LCA and RCA, but is not very useful in evaluating LCA or its branches, so it is not being routinely used for LCA today. Straight AP is also not an ideal projection for evaluation of the LCA, and for any of the segments, there are many more useful projections.

8.3 The best projections for evaluating the right coronary artery

Many operators believe that two projections can be quite enough for evaluation of the RCA since it has less complex anatomy in comparison to the LCA. The RCA can be viewed nicely in LAO, but even better in LAO-caudal, which is better than the former one in displaying the crux. The crux with the bifurcation of the RCA into the PLA and the PDA is also very nicely displayed in AP-cranial, and in some cases in RAO-cranial projection. Some operators use only simple LAO and RAO to evaluate the RCA. Left cranial (LAO-cranial) displays best the proximal and the distal RCA and is very good for displaying the crux. It can also be pretty good for displaying the PLA and the PDA (Di Mario and Sutaria, 2005). Cranial (AP-cranial), sometimes with just a small angulation to the right (5-10°) is very good for displaying the crux, the PLA and the PDA. The mid-RCA is best displayed in lateral and the RAO-view, but in most cases, LAO can be sufficient for this segment also.

8.4 Angiographic studies and engagement of coronary bypass grafts

When a previously operated patient, who had undergone a bypass-coronary revascularization, is subjected to coronary angiography, beside evaluating the native coronary arteries, a study of bypass-grafts is also necessary. The operator should read the surgical report in order to find out how many, and which bypass grafts there are. The venous, or free arterial bypass grafts, i.e. the bypass grafts for aorto-coronary bypassing are best cannulated from RAO 40°, but some operators cannulate them from LAO 50°, just as they do for native coronaries. Still, from RAO 40° there is the best depiction of the grafts' origin from the aorta. The bypass graft for the RCA can usually be cannulated using the standard JR4, or JR3.5, sometimes JR3 catheter. The origin of the graft to the RCA is usually in the ascending aorta, just above the sinotubular junction. The cannulation is performed by placing the catheter high in the ascending aorta, applying clockwise-rotation, and, at the same time, pushing the catheter a bit downwards. If Judkins catheters are inadequate, RCB (right coronary bypass) catheter can also be used for cannulating the SVG (saphenous vein graft) to RCA.

The JR4 or JR3.5 catheters can also be used to cannulate all the other bypass grafts. Those grafts' origins are usually located higher in the ascending aorta, just beneath the arch. If the grafts for LAD, diagonals, intermediate, and obtuse marginals are unreachable with JR catheter, an LCB (left coronary bypass), or an AL catheter can be used. If grafts cannot be found selectively, an aortography in LAO position can be used to determine their origin, position, or stumps if they are occluded. For obtaining a proper evaluation, after aortography, a selective cannulation of the grafts should be reattempted.

Left internal mammary arterial graft can be cannulated using the IMA (internal mammary artery) catheter, but JR4, JR3.5, JR3, or short tip JR can also be used in certain situations. The ostium of the left internal mammary artery (LIMA) is engaged in 50° LAO position, although sometimes it can be viewed better from AP or RAO 40° position. First in 50° LAO, a J-wire is passed into the left subclavian artery, beyond LIMA. Than the IMA catheter is passed over the wire, also beyond the LIMA origin. Then, from the position best suited for the operator (AP, LAO 50°, or RAO 40°), the catheter is slowly withdrawn, rotating the tip counterclockwise. Small test-injections are needed to display the ostium of the LIMA. The angiography should be performed from several positions, especially paying attention to the distal anastomosis with the LAD, since this position is the one most prone to iatrogenic injury from manipulation during the grafting procedure, thus being the most prone to developing a significant stenosis. A 90° left-lateral position is almost mandatory in displaying LIMA-LAD graft, since it is very good to depict the distal anastomosis.

For cannulating the right interior mammary artery (RIMA), the brachicephalic artery is engaged, J-wire is advanced distally to the RIMA origin, from the right subclavian to the right axillary artery. The IMA catheter is advanced also distally over the wire. In the LAO 50° projection, after removing the J-wire, the catheter is slowly withdrawn, and with occasional test-injections engaged into the RIMA ostium.

The right gastroepiploic artery has been used for coronary bypass, although very rarely. Surgeons sometimes use it when mammary arteries and saphenous vein grafts are unavailable. It is cannulated by first entering the hepatic artery using the cobra catheter. The operator must then advance a hidrophylic guidewire into the gastroduodenal artery, and then into the right gastroepiploic artery. Selective angiography of the letter will be enabled by switching the catheter, usually to right Judkins (Di Mario and Sutaria, 2005). The procedure is performed very rarely, and because of the unusual anatomy for the invasive cardiolgist, can be time-consuming.

9. After the procedure

The operator should always review his/her angiographic recordings before withdrawing the catheter, because standard projections used may not adequately reveal the condition of the coronary circulation, and additional shots may be necessary. The further therapeutic strategy should be considered (medical, surgical or interventional treatment). After the catheter is removed, and the procedure is finished, the patient is transfered out of the catheterization laboratory. Arterial sheath is removed, and manual pressure is applied onto the site of arterial puncture in order to stop the bleeding. That is followed by mechanical compression of that site in order to definitely stop the bleeding. The patient is later mobilized, and if there is no indication for the patient to stay in the hospital further, he/she is discharged on the next day, or sometimes on the same day after the procedure.

9.1 Haemostasis

Haemostasis is an important practical matter. Complications from diagnostic cardiac catheterization are rare, but if they happen, those related to haemostasis are the most common ones. When a patient comes out of the hospital after coronary angiography or coronary stenting, and gets a groin haematoma, he/she will most likely quickly forget the top-notch, several million euros costing equipment used during the procedure, as well as the skills of the operator who performed sometimes very difficult intervention, but will remember a large haematoma, and often complain about it to his family, neighbours, and friends. Therefore, it is very important to adequately perform haemostasis, not only for obvious medical, but also for "public-relation" reasons. The details of haemostasis and its possible complications are discussed elsewhere. However, there are a few points that need to be noted. Haemostasis may be difficult if the patient is obese, if there is high blood pressure (always try to regulate the blood pressure prior to sheath removal), or if clotting time is prolonged. If there is no vital indication, coronary angiography should be avoided if INR is >1.6, otherwise, the sheath should be sutured and removed upon achieving a more appropriate INR value. A significant aortic regurgitation with *pulsus celer et altus* can also make the post-sheath-removal hold difficult.

Large sheaths create bigger holes in the arterial wall, so the bigger the sheath diameter, the more difficult haemostasis will be. The patients who frequently elevate intra-abdominal pressure by sneezing, coughing or performing Valsalva maneuvers can prolong bleeding from the vascular access site. Same is true for restless patients, so those sometimes need to be sedated and observed by a nurse. In order to facilitate the haemostasis process, haemostatic devices have been developed, such as: collagen plugs, external pressure devices, vascular clips, external C clamps, topical haemostatic accelerators etc.

10. Non-coronary left heart catheterization

Sometimes, an additional catheter, called pigtail-catheter (because of its shape) is inserted into ascending aorta to perform aortography, and/or into the left ventricle to perform left ventriculography. Today, with skilled echocardiographers and top-notch cardiac ultrasound devices, these additional procedures are rarely used, but will be described too, so as to give the readers the necesary technical information about the value of these procedures, as well as how they should be performed.

10.1 Left ventriculography

Today, with skilled echocardiographers and excellent cardiac ultrasound equipment, there is far less need to perform left ventriculoghaphy than previously. With reliable echocardiograms, avoiding left ventriculography spares the patient from additional contrast administration, which is especially important if the patient already has impaired renal function. Also, without left ventriculography there is less radiation both for the patient and for the operator. If the patient is in heart failure or cardiogenic shock, every additional volume intake can prove to be risky for his/her condition. However, some operators and some centers prefer to perform the left ventriculography, especially if there is doubt about echocardiography findings, or if there is no echocardiography finding available.

In order to perform the left ventriculoghaphy, the operator advances the pigtail catheter over a J-wire to the aortic root. The author's choice is usually the angled version of the pigtail catheter. The J-wire is withdrawn into the catheter, with the J-wire tip just inside the catheter tip to add to the catheter stiffness in order to successfully pass over the aortic valve. The position of the digital flat-panel detector or the image intensifier is in RAO 30°. The catheter with the wire inside of it is advanced farther, so that the body of the catheter "bounces off" the aortic valve, and the distal curve faces upwards. Then the catheter is rotated in a clockwise fashion, being at the same time slowly withdrawn. This causes the catheter to rotate, and when the aortic valve opens, slip through the aortic ostium and into the left ventricle. If there are difficulties to pass the catheter into the left ventricle this way, the catheter tip is withdrawn into the ascending aorta, and the valve is probed with the J-wire. When the wire passes into the ventricular cavity, the catheter is advanced into the ventricle over the wire. Sometimes, a Glidewire with hydrophyllic coating must be used to pass the aortic valve, especially if there is a tight aortic stenosis. Also, sometimes it might be easier to pass the valve with a Judkins right coronary catheter.

The catheter is then held with the tip in the middle of the ventricle. The proximal end of the catheter is connected to the injector after it has been adequately aspirated and flushed. Through the automated injector, some 35–50 ml of contrast is injected into the ventricle at the rate of 12-15 ml/s, delineating the left ventricular cavity and displaying the left ventricle contractility. Intracavitary thrombi can be seen as hypodensities or filling-defects of contrast within the left ventricle. Mitral regurgitation, if exists, can be seen and semi-quantified, using degrees from 1 to 4, with 4 being the most severe. Care must be taken when advancing the pigtail catheter into the left ventricle, because the mechanical contact with endocardium can provoke premature ventricular beats, even ventricular tachicardia. It can also provoke a complete heart block if the patient already has a right bundle-branch block, and the catheter irritates the left bundle-branch upon contact with left ventricular endocardium. If there are foreign masses within the left ventricle, such as thrombi or vegetations, those can be fragmented and embolized into systemic circulation, causing potentially catastrophic outcomes. A combination of a fragile myocardium and too vigorous catheter manipulation can cause myocardial rupture with fatal cardiac tamponade and refractory shock. Entanglement of the catheter into the chordae tendineae of the mitral valve or hooking the catheter tip on a mitral cusp can result in seemingly severe mitral regurgitation, so care must be taken to avoid this. In exceptional circumstances, catheter tip can theoretically rip a mitral cusp or break up a chorda or two, causing acute mitral regurgitation of various degree, thus complicating the left ventriculography.

After the ventriculography, the catheter is connected to manifold to record pressures in the left ventricle. Upon withdrawal of the catheter over the aortic valve, pressure curves in the aorta are also noted, and pressure values recorded. The systolic pressures in the aorta and the left ventricle are noted for transvalvular aortic pressure gradient. Care must be taken not to declare aortic stenosis in patients with previously unrecognized hypertrophic obstructive cardiomyopathy with high pressure-gradients across the left ventricular outflow tract, which may mimic the haemodynamics of aortic stenosis, with pressure gradients between the middle of the left ventricle and the ascending aorta.

Calculation of the left ventricular ejection fraction (LVEF) is usually performed using the software already incorporated into the imaging review station. Some operators use the semi-quantitative eye-ball method in LVEF estimation, which has, when used by experienced operators, shown a surprisingly good correlation with the actual value of LVEF measured invasively in several studies. The software calculates LVEF by subtracting left ventricular end-systolic volume from the left ventricular end-diastolic volume.

Mastering the left ventriculography is important as the transfemoral - transcatheter aortic valve implantation is being performed increasingly. For severely stenosed aortic valves, it may be easier to pass the valve using an AL catheter and a Glidewire.

10.2 Aortography

Aortography is defined as a radiographic recording of injection of a large volume of radiocontrast into the aortic root. Most commonly, some 50 ml of radiocontrast, at a rate of 15-25 ml/sec with a 0.5 sec linear rise is used. The catheter of choice is a sidehole catheter, usually the pigtail shape. The best projection for estimation of aortic regurgitation is LAO 45°. Aortic regurgitation is semi-quantified and described in degrees from 1 to 4, much like mitral regurgitation. If the patient is subjected to invasive diagnostics because of suspected coarctation of aorta, the coarctation will be best visible if aortography is performed in LAO 20° position. Using the pressure monitoring, the gradient across the coarctation can also be measured. For evaluation of a suspected patent ductus arteriosus, the shot is usually taken at a very steep LAO projection. Aortography is usually done for evaluating the ascending aorta for dilation or aneurysm, and/or aortic regurgitation. The J-wire and the catheter are positioned in the ascending aorta, inside the root or at the level of sinotubular junction. Anatomy and dimensions of the ascending aorta and aortic arch are noted, as well as aortic regurgitation (if such a disorder exists), and/or aorto-coronary bypass grafts, also if they exist. Care must be taken that the catheter does not protrude back into the left ventricle during injection, which can make quantification of the aortic regurgitation difficult.

11. Conclusion

Invasive cardiologists today generally continue their education and become interventionalists. Anyone who wants to become a good interventionalist must be able to routinely perform diagnostic coronary angiography and to be able to solve the problems that might occur during the procedure. Therefore, the techniques of performing coronary angiography must be mastered by an invasive cardiologist. That creates the conditions for swift procedures, informative findings, purposefull conclusions and further recommendations, and last, but not least, the maximum safety for the patient. However, even with most carefully conducted coronary angiograms, there can be false readings. This is especially true for less experienced operators, who can sometimes misinterprete the finding, thus affecting the final recommendation for further treatment. These pitfalls may be: inadequate number of projections, ostial coronary occlusions without visible stumps, superselective injection, e.g. especially if LAD and CX have (almost) separate ostia, catheter induced coronary spasm, congenital coronary anomalies, pulsatile injection of radiocontrast with filling defects mimicking coronary atherosclerotic obstruction, myocardial bridging - the key to recognize it is the fact that the lumen normalizes upon muscle relaxation, i.e. during diastole. Today, coronary angiogram projections must be observed by the operator in the context of future percutaneous coronary intervention. The lesions are not assessed only as significant or non-significant, but are evaluated regarding their length, their position regarding side-branches and other caracteristics important for the possible intervention. Therefore, it is of paramount importance to adequately display the coronary arteries and their lesions, in appropriate projections, with an adequate number of different views, still remaining rational regarding radiation and contrast medium consumption. Interventional procedures in cardiology today have expanded beyond the treatment of coronary artery disease. We are witnessing a technopharmacological improvement which enabled the interventional, catheter-based treatment of valvular heart disease, closure of interatrial and interventricular septal defects, relief of aortic coarctations, interventional treatment of hypertrophic obstructive cardiomyopathies, paravalvular leak closure, left atrial appendage closure, peripheral vascular disease treatment etc, and the basis for performing any of the interventional procedures, especially percutaneous coronary interventions, is mastering coronary angiography first.

12. References

Brasselet C, Blanpain T, Tassan-Mangina S, Deschildre A, Duval S, Vitry F, Gaillot-Petit N, Clément JP, Metz D. (2008) Comparison of operator radiation exposure with optimized radiation protection devices during coronary angiograms and ad hoc percutaneous coronary interventions by radial and femoral routes. *Eur Heart J* 2008 Jan;29(1), pp. 63-70, ISSN 0195-668x

Chen CW, Lin CL, Lin TK, Lin CD. (2006) A simple and effective regimen for prevention of radial artery spasm during coronary catheterization. *Cardiology.* 2006;105(1): pp. 43-7, ISSN 1878-5409

Conti CR, Levin DC, Grossman W. (1980). Coronary Angiography, In: *Cardiac catheterization and angiography*, Grossman W, pp. 147-169, Lea & Febiger, ISBN 0-8121-0712-4, Philadelphia, Pa, USA

Cooper CJ, El-Shiekh RA, Cohen DJ, Blaesing L, Burket MW, Basu A, Moore JA. (1999). Effect of transradial access on quality of life and cost of cardiac catheterization: a randomized comparison. *Am Heart J* 1999 Sep;138(3 Pt 1): pp. 430-6, ISSN 0002-8703

Di Mario C & Sutaria N. (2995). Coronary angiography in the angioplasty era: projections with a meaning. *Heart* 20052005;91: pp. 968-976, ISSN 1355-6037

Gonzalez A, Rahimtoola SH, Kulick DL. (1991). Technique of Vascular Access, In: *Techniques and Applications in Interventional Cardiology*, Kulick DL and Rahimtoola SH, pp. 1-18, MosbyYear Book, ISBN 0-8151-7048-3, St. Louis, MO, USA

Guédès A, Dangoisse V, Gabriel L, Jamart J, Chenu P, Marchandise B, Schroeder E. (2010) Low rate of conversion to transfemoral approach when attempting both radial arteries for coronary angiography and percutaneous coronary intervention: a study of 1,826 consecutive procedures. *J Invasive Cardiol.* 2010 Sep;22(9): pp. 391-7, ISSN 1042-3931

Jolly SS, Amlani S, Hamon M, Yusuf S, Mehta SR. (2009). Radial versus femoral access for coronary angiography or intervention and the impact on major bleeding and ischemic events: a systematic review and meta-analysis of randomized trials. *Am Heart J* 2009 Jan;157(1): pp. 132-40, ISSN 0002-8703

Judkins MP: Percutaneous transfemoral selective coronary angiography. *Radiol Clin North Am* 6 1968 Dec;6(3): pp. 467-92, ISSN 0033-8389

Kwac MS, Yoon SJ, Oh SJ, Jeon DW, Kim DH, Yang JY. (2010). A rare case of radial arteriovenous fistula after coronary angiography. *Korean Circ J.* 2010 Dec;40(12): pp. 677-9, ISSN 1738-5520

Lo TS, Nolan J, Fountzopoulos E, Behan M, Butler R, Hetherington SL, Vijayalakshmi K, Rajagopal R, Fraser D, Zaman A, Hildick-Smith D. (2009). Radial artery anomaly and its influence on transradial coronary procedural outcome. *Heart* 2009;95: pp. 410-415, ISSN 1355-6037

Pancholy SB, Coppola J, Patel T. (2006). Subcutaneous administration of nitroglycerin to facilitate radial artery cannulation. *Catheter Cardiovasc Interv.* 2006 Sep;68(3): pp. 389-91, ISSN 1522-1946

Patterson T, Foale RA. (2011) If the radial artery is the new standard of care in primary percutaneous coronary intervention, why is most intervention done by the femoral approach? *Heart* 2011;97: pp. 521-522, ISSN 1355-6037

Powell D & Moxey CF. (2011). Diagnostic Catheterization, In: *Invasive Cardiology: a manual for cath lab personnel, 3rd Edition*, Watson S & Gorski KA, pp. 143-162, Jones & Bartlett Learning, ISBN 978-0-7637-6468-5, Sudbury, MA, USA.

Rigattieri S, Di Russo C, Silvestri P, Fedele S, Loschiavo P. (2010). Our technique for transradial coronary angiography and interventions. *Indian Heart J.* 2010 May-Jun;62(3): pp. 258-61. ISSN 0019-4832

Stella PR, Kiemeneij F, Laarman GJ, Odekerken D, Slagboom T, van der Wieken R. (1997). Incidence and outcome of radial artery occlusion following transradial artery coronary angioplasty. *Cathet Cardiovasc Diagn* 1997 Feb;40(2): pp. 156–8, ISSN 0098-6569

Tomassini F, Gagnor A, Varbella F. (2011). Successful use of an extra-long hydrophilic-coated sheath in enlarged aorta to overcome extreme tortuosity of right subclavian artery via transradial approach during coronary angiography. *J Invasive Cardiol.* 2011 Mar;23(3): pp. 56-7, ISSN 1042-3931

Vorobcsuk A, Konyi A, Aradi D, Horváth IG, Ungi I, Louvard Y, Komócsi A. (2009) Transradial versus transfemoral percutaneous coronary intervention in acute myocardial infarction: systematic overview and meta-analysis. *Am Heart J* 2009 Nov;158(5): pp. 814-21, ISSN 0002-8703

Watson S & Hunter J. (2011) Cath Lab Staff Duties, In: *Invasive Cardiology: a manual for cath lab personnel, 3rd Edition*, Watson S & Gorski KA, pp. 119-129, Jones & Bartlett Learning, ISBN 978-0-7637-6468-5, Sudbury, MA, USA.

7

Risks and Complications of Coronary Angiography: Contrast Related Complications

S. Mohammad Reza Khatami
Nephrology Research Center, Tehran University of Medical Sciences
Iran

1. Introduction

Since Wilhelm Röntgen reported his novel discovery of the X- Ray in 1895(Röntgen, 1898 as cited in Weinmann etal., 2005), the Diagnostic imaging has been an integral part of medicine. He was decorated by the second class of Prussian crown medal and he was also awarded the first physic Nobel Prize at 1901. Levy- Dorn was another pioneer in radiology who understood the potential importance of X-ray in medicine and opened a daily private office for medical examination with X-ray in 1896 just one year after innovation of X-ray by Röntgen. He pointed to the danger of this method to the living organism very early (Hierholzer K & Hierholzer J 1997; Nitze, 1895; as cited in Hierholzer K & Hierholzer J, 2002) Since X-rays are not sufficiently absorbed by soft tissue, contrast media (CM) is used to highlight organs or pathologies. Osborne etal reported that inorganic Iodine enhanced the urinary tracts X-ray images (Osborn etal., 1923). But the most important contributor to the field of urological imaging came from the field of agriculture when A Binz and C Räth, two scientists from the Berlin agricultural college synthesized a new organic iodinated molecule "Selectan"(Binz & Räth 1928 as cited in Hierholzer K & Hierholzer J, 2002), and a research fellow used this agent in clinical investigations. (Swick 1929a, 1929b as cited in Hierholzer K & Hierholzer J, 2002; Weinmann etal., 2005).

In 1928 an urologist, Forssmann, used one of these agents in his own coronary arteries (Hricak & Barbarive 1984).This was an unexpected methodological contribution of urological research to cardiology.

From 1929 on, serial production of Uroselectan was established. This agent was a big step forward in safety, because ionic iodide (Sodium Iodide and Lithium Iodide) cannot be used in a clinical setting. In the early 1950s, a new generation of iodinated agents was launched, which were derivatives of triiodinated benzoic acid, e.g. diatrizoate (Urografin etc.). These agents became standard in diagnostic imaging for the next 30 years and are still widely used in many countries. Almen suggested that non-ionic molecules could reduce osmolality (Almen, 1969, as cited in Weinmann etal., 2005), an idea that was the basis of safer compounds that entered routine clinical use in the 1980s. Water-soluble, non-ionic iodinated contrast agents are now the workhorses in contrast based imagings. More than 90% of contrasts media are used in western countries are non-ionic CM.

There are two main complications of contrast media. The aim of this chapter is to discuss these two major side effects of CM. the most important of these two complication is contrast induced nephropathy (CIN) which will be described in details and the other is anaphylaxis reactions to the CM which will be mentioned briefly at the end of the chapter.

2. Contrast induced nephropathy

According to the report of American Heart Association statistics committee and stroke statistics subcommittee updated at 2007, from 1979 to 2004 the number of cardiac catheterization has been increased 334%. Meanwhile from 1987 to 2004 the number of percutaneous coronary intervention (PCI) has also increased 326%.IN 2004 more than 1,297.000 cardiac catheterization and in 2006 at least 1,313,000 PCI were performed in U.S (American Heart Association statistics committee and stroke subcommittee, 2007). In 2003, about 80 million doses of CM were used worldwide (Persson, 2005). Now in U.S more tha 10 millions radiological examinations with CM are performed annually which 4 millions of these procedures are cardiac catheterizations. In western countries 6000 diagnostic cardiac catheterization and 2000 therapeutical procedure are done per 1million habitants (Costa, 2004; Ultramari etal., 2006). On the other hand the physicians are dealing with a significant increase in the prevalence and incidence of cardiovascular diseases, chronic kidney diseases and diabetes which are considered as risk factors of CIN development. All these patients are in increased need to such a diagnostic and the therapeutical maneuver.

CIN is a very interesting Issue for researchers. It is a type of acute kidney injury (AKI) which in contrast to all other causes of AKI, the exact time of injurious insult is known. Accordingly, it may help the investigators to find a more preciously diagnostic tool beside to develop more effective prophylactic and therapeutical interventions.

CIN is a matter of health conflicts. It is an important causes of increased resource utilization, prolonged hospital stay, increased in hospital and long term mortality and provoke the progression of CKD (Bartholomew etal., 2004; Goldenberg etal., 2009; Gruberg etal., 2000; James etal., 2010; McCullough etal., 1997; Solomon etal., 2009; Subramanian etal., 2007).

2.1 Physicochemical properties and classification of Contrast Media (table1)

CM is derivatives of tri-Iodinated benzene and is classified according to their Ionization, osmolality and structural properties. The ionized media are dissociated in water, while the nonionic agents are not dissociated although they are soluble in water. The ratio of iodine to dissolved particles, describes an important relationship between opacification and osmotoxicity of a contrast agent, higher this ratio, more desirable. In high osmolal CM this ratio is 1.5, which in low-osmolal and iso-osmolal CM this ratio is 3 and 6 respectively. With lowering the osmolality, the viscosity will increase. Viscosity has some deleterious effect on renal blood flow and urinary flow in tubules. Contrast agents are completely filtered. With reabsorption of water in tubules the concentration of CM reaches 50-100 times of plasma concentration.

The first generation CM was Ionic. They had 3 atoms of Iodine, one atom of sodium and 2 active osmotic particles in each molecule,therefore their osmolality was very high (1200-1800 mosm/kgH2o), so they called hyper-osmolal contrast media (HOCM). From late 80s, the next generation of these agents has been marketed. They are non-Ionic. They have only one somatically active particle. They have been known as Low-osmolal Contrast Media (LOCM) because their osmolality is lower than first generation but yet significantly higher than plasma osmolality (600—900 mosm/kgH2o). The third generation of CM is Iso-osmolal Contrast Media (IOCM) (≈300 mosm/kgH2o). They are non-ionic dimers. They have two benzene rings rather than one ring of previous generations. This structure allows 6 Iodine atoms to attach to the one cosmetically active particle.

Type	Name	osmolality (mosm/kg water)	ionicity	mono/dimer	amount of iodine iodine mg/mL	iodine ratio	viscosity mPa.sec at 37^{0c}
HOCM	Iothalamat	1695	Ionic	monomer	400	3:2	2.8
LOCM	Iomeprol	720	nonionic	monomer	350	3:1	4.8
LOCM	Iopentol	683	nonionic	monomer	310	3:1	6.5
LOCM	Iopromide	586	nonionic	monomer	350	3:1	4.7
LOCM	Iopamidol	653	nonionic	monomer	300	3:1	4.6
LOCM	Ioversol	719	nonionic	monomer	320	3:1	6
LOCM	Iohexol	667	nonionic	monomer	300	3:1	5.7
LOCM	Ioxaglate	584	ionic	dimer	320	3:2	7.8
IOCM	Iodixanol	290	nonionic	dimer	320	6:1	11.4

Table 1. Types of contrast media and their physicochemical properties

2.2 Definition & diagnosis

Definition of CIN is a matter of controversy and there is no a unique accepted definition. CIN is a rapid decline in renal function after CM administration while there is obviously no other causes of acute kidney injury (AKI).

Serum creatinine is the standard marker for detecting CIN. Small changes in serum creatinine after CM exposure are seen but it is not considered clinically relevant.

In last two decade, different criteria of renal function deterioration were defined in clinical trials. But the two most popular are: 1- A 25% relative increase of serum creatinine from baseline and 2- An absolute increase of 0.5 mg/dl of serum creatinine from the base. It will happen within 2 days to one week after contrast exposure. None of these two criteria are accurate. The most common method for the assessment of kidney function consists of using the Glomerular Filtration Rate (GFR) which usually measured by creatinine clearance. But serum creatinine is not a real-time marker of change in kidney function. It is neither a specific nor a sensitive marker of GFR evaluation. In the case of rapid changes in kidney function serum creatinine has a 48-72 hours delay related to GFR changes. It cannot show the small changes of GFR too, and other factors rather than GFR may affect the blood level of serum creatinine. Even in patients with stable serum creatinine the GFR may significantly be declined. So many investigators are trying to redefine the cutoff point level of serum creatinine increment. For instance the recent definition of AKI, considers a 0.3 mg/dl increase of serum creatinine as an evidence of AKI development rather than a 0.5 mg/dl increase (Shah & Mehta, 2006). Weisbord etal showed that only a 0.25-0.3 mg/dl increase in serum creatinine after coronary angiography was accompanied with significant increase of mortality within 30 days of procedure (Weisbord etal., 2006). In another study only a 5% increases of serum creatinine within 12 hours after the contrast exposure had 75% sensitivity and 72% specificity for detecting CIN. It also had a strong correlation with the development of renal failure during next 30 days (Ribichini etal., 2010).

Recently more sensitive markers of GFR have been developed and validated. The most promising markers are Cystatin-C and Neutrophilic Gelatinase Associated Lipocaline (NGAL). Cystatin-C may be more accurate than serum creatinine in predicting renal function. In patients with GFR lower than 60ml/min, Cystatin-C may be a better marker of both early detection of CIN and prediction of major side effects like death and chronic dialysis. But it is not known whether the increased level of Cystatin-C is due to the decreased GFR or it is released from atherosclerotic plaques during angiography .If Cystatin-C increases by more than 10% within 24 hours, then it is a good marker of CIN occurrence and further events. But an increase of less than 10% from baseline will rule out the diagnosis of CIN and the patient can be discharged without any caution (Briguori etal., 2010).There is no study to evaluate the validity of Cystatin-C in earlier time. Cystatin-C has to be better validated in different situations.

NGAL is also an early diagnostic biomarker of acute kidney injury, but studies for validating this biomarker in CIN are limited. It's specificity and sensitivity in diagnosis of CIN in children has been identified (Hirsch etal., 2007).

The most accurate method for measuring GFR is radionuclide techniques which are expensive and labor-intensive. The Cockcroft-Gault or MDRD equations are useful for the calculation of GFR in clinic.

The problem with Studies, regarding CIN is that nearly in all these studies contrast nephropathy is defined by serum creatinine increment which is a soft outcomes value. If hard outcomes like the need for dialysis, readmission, other clinical complications and death are considered, it may cause better understanding the nature of AKI including CIN and therefore its better management. It may also be more useful if RIFLE classification is taken into account rather than Acute Kidney Injury Network criteria for better definition of CIN. Further studies should be done to validate this classification for CIN diagnosis.

The differential diagnosis of CIN is cholesterol atheroemboli, volume depletion and interstitial nephritis.

2.3 Incidence

CIN is the third cause of AKI in hospitalized patients. The cumulative incidence of CIN is 10% of all AKI (Tepel etal., 2006). The incidence of CIN in patients without any risk factor is 0.6-2.3%, but in high risk patients it will be raised up to 90% (McCullough etal., 2006A ; Toprak & Cirit 2002). In two studies in 1979 and 2002, CIN was the third cause of in-hospital AKI (Nash etal., 2002). These studies showed no change in the incidence of CIN in this period (12% in 1979 and 11% in 2002).

Three factors increase the incidence of CIN in future: 1) increase in burden of CKD, 2) Increase in incidence of diabetes, and 3) increase in diagnostic and therapeutically measures requiring CM.

The incidence of CIN is dependent on the renal function. With serum creatinine more than 1.3mg/dl and more than 1 mg/dl in men and women respectively the risk of CIN will significantly increase (Lamiere etal., 2006). It has been shown that by increasing serum creatinine from 1.2 to 2.9mg/dl the risk of CIN increases from 4% to 20% (Barrett etal., 1992;). The incidence of CIN in patients with serum creatinine of 3 mg/dl with or without diabetes is more than 30%.In another study the risk of CIN in patients with serum creatinine equal to1.5mg/dl was 8%, but with serum creatinine of 6.8mg/dl the risk of CIN has been increased to 92% (McCullough etal.,1997). In patients with normal renal function, even in the presence of diabetes or other risk factors the incidence of CIN is less than 2% (Lamiere etal., 2006). The incidence of CIN in diabetic patients with normal serum creatinine is 3.7% (Rihal etal., 2002).In patient with severe renal failure and diabetes the need to dialysis will be increase to 12% if CIN develops after CM exposure (Manske etal.,1990).

With regards to coronary angiography the incidence of CIN after this procedure has been reported to be 3-14%. Only 2% of patients without diabetes and with serum creatinine of 1.1 mg/dl will develop CIN after coronary angiography (McCullough etal.,1997; Rihal etal., 2002).

2.4 Natural course

The natural history of CIN includes an increase of serum creatinine mostly after 24 hours of CM exposure, which picks in 3-7 days and return to normal within 2 weeks. Most patients are non-oliguric but the urine output is usually declined (Rudnick etal., 1995).

CIN is generally and potentially a reversible acute renal failure, but it should not be considered as a benign disorder, because in 30% of patients, renal function would not be fully recovered (Maydoon etal., 2001). The patients with CIN rarely need dialysis. According to a study among 0.8% of patients who needed dialysis after PCI, 13% remained on dialysis for lifetime (McCullough etal., 1997). Another study reported that 13-50% of CIN patients who had needed renal replacement therapy, they may remain on dialysis for the rest of life (Toprak, 2007). If even CIN recovered completely, it will cause more morbidities including bleeding, infection, prolonged hospital stay, increased resource utilization, increase in the risk of CKD and increased in-hospital and long term mortality rate (Gruberg etal., 2000; Perazella, 2009; Rihal etal., 2002). CIN also causes increase in cardiovascular morbidities. The rate of both in-hospital and long term mortality will also significantly be increased due to CIN (Gruberg etal., 2000; Liss etal., 2006; Marenzi etal., 2004; McCullough etal., 1997; Rihal etal., 2002, Weisbord etal., 2006). The overall mortality rate of patients with CIN is 1.1-34%, but it is not obvious that CIN perse is the cause of mortality or CIN is more prevalent in patients who are sicker and their co-morbidities are more than control patients (McCullough etal., 1997 Rudnick & Feldman, 2008).

The in-hospital mortality rate of CIN is estimated to be 22-25%. Meanwhile the rate of death within 5 years is significantly higher in this group of patients in comparison with control group (McCullough etal., 1997; Rihal etal., 2002). Odds of in-hospital death are related to rate of serum creatinine increment (Weisbord etal., 2006). CIN is a cause of CKD in the coming months (Liss etal., 2006). Although it is not known that whether the direct nephrotoxic effect of contrast agents is the cause of CKD or the background renal disease will be unmasked by CIN.

2.5 Risk factors

The risk factors of CIN are shown in table 2. Previous chronic kidney disease (CKD) is the leading and the single most important risk factor of CIN (McCullough etal., 2006B; Rihal etal., 2002; Rudnick etal., 1995). The most important cause of delaying or cancelling angiography is renal failure. In a recent cohort, the Glomerular Filtration Rate (GFR) of 60 ml/min considered as a cutoff point (Bartholomew etal., 2004; Mehran etal., 2004). Diabetes is the second most important risk factor of CIN (McCullough etal., 1997,2006; Rudnick etal., 2006; Weisberg etal., 1994). It remains unclear whether diabetes is a risk factor of CIN perse or it makes the patient prone to this complication because nearly all diabetic patient have overt or covert renal disease (Manske etal., 1990). So the diabetic patients with CKD are the highest risk group (McCullough etal., 2006aTepel etal., 2006; Toprak & Cirit, 2006).

Class IV heart failure is another risk factor of CIN (McCullough etal., 2006B). Many of these patients also have several other risk factors like renal disease (atherosclerotic renal disease) or decreased effective circulating volume and low GFR. Acute myocardial infarction (AMI) is another independent risk factor of CIN if the CM is given within 24hours after the AMI (Rihal etal., 2002; Marenzi etal., 2006a). S-T elevation myocardial infarction (STEMI) also increases the risk of CIN in the time of PCI. The mortality rate of these patients is high too. There is a positive correlation between the mortality rate of these patients and the volume of contrast that is being used for coronary angiography (Marenzi etal., 2006b). Old age (Iokavou etal., 2003), hypovolemia (McCullough etal., 2006B) and hypotension are other risk factors of CIN. Hypovolemia is among few risk factors which are preventable and should be corrected promptly before starting the procedure. The medications that cause extra-cellular contraction like diuretics or cause vascular tonicity changes like non-steroidal anti-inflammatory drugs (NSAIDS) may be involved in development of CIN or at least may increase the severity of the disease. The use of angiotensin converting enzyme inhibitors (ACIs) or angiotensin receptor blockers (ARBs), while the blood pressure is in normal range are not considered contraindicated and could be continued.

Patient related factors	**Procedure related factors**
CKD	*hyper-osmolal CM*
Diabetes mellitus	*high volume of CM*
Age	*repeated exposure to CM within 24 hours*
Hypovolemia	*intra-arterial injection of CM*
Hypotension	
Low ejection fraction	
Class IV CHF	
Concomitant use of other nephrotoxics	
Hypoalbumenimeia (<3.5g/dL)	
Renal transplantation	
Recent AMI (24 hours before angiography)	
Anemia	

Table 2. Risk factors for CIN

Low hematocrite is associated with increased risk of CIN (Nikolsky etal., 2005), but there is no study to show that correction of anemia will decrease the incidence of CIN.
There are few retrospective studies showing high incidence of CIN in renal transplanted patients (up to 21%), but these patients had other risk factors like diabetes, renal failure, concomitant use of nephrotoxic agents and volume depletion (Ahuja etal., 2000). The coronary artery bypass graft (CABG) at the day of angiography will also increase the risk of CIN (Ranucci etal., 2008). Nowadays in contrast to what is mentioned in the literature multiple myeloma is not considered as a risk factor for CIN.

2.6 Type of CM

The safety of a contrast agent depends in large part on the amount of CM that must be administered. The body's ability to tolerate any substance depends on the amount given. Even isotonic saline is toxic at very large doses. High dosages that disturb the ionic and osmotic balance in the body will elicit adverse reactions without exhibiting a direct interaction with other molecules (chemotoxicity). This kind of toxicity is based on the osmotic activity of the agent or, more precisely, on the osmotic load (mosmol/kg body weight). The important properties of a CM that determine its nephrotoxicity are: osmolality, volume, and repeated use, route of use, viscosity and Ionicity.
Here we briefly review the role of each of the properties of a CM in the development of CIN.

2.7 Osmolality / viscosity (Table2)

Now the HOCM is completely replaced by LOCM or IOCM. There is no doubt that osmolality is a main factor in nephrotoxicity of a CM (Barrett & Carlisle, 1993; Rudnick & Goldfarb, 2003). Although in patients with normal renal function this factor is not important (Barrett & Carlisle, 1993). But in chronic renal failure patients, particularly in diabetic patients, use of HOCM is contraindicated (Solomon, 2005, Solomon & Dumouchel, 2006).The incidence of CIN with HOCM in patients with risk factors is two times in comparison with LOCM (Barrett & Carlisle, 1993).

All studies showed that nephrotoxicity of low osmolal media is lower than hyperosmolal one (Barrett & Carlisle, 1993; Rudnick etal., 1995), but there are many controversies about the difference of LOCM and IOCM in terms of CIN (Aspelin etal., 2003; Barrett etal., 2006; Carraro etal., 1998; Liss etal., 2006; McCullough etal., 2006C; Rudnick etal.,2006; Solomon etal.,2007; Thomsen etal., 2008).The viscosity of IOCM is higher than LOCM and this property of IOCM may offset the benefit of lower osmolality of newer developed agents (Aspelin etal., 2003; Barrett & Carlisle, 1993; Rudnick & Goldfarb, 2003, Seeliger etal., 2007). Systematic reviews were not also able to solve the contradictory results concerning the difference between low and iso-osmolal CM (Heinrich etal., 2009, Reed etal., 2009,McCullough etal., 2006C., Solomon & Dumouchel, 2006). NEPHRIC study showed that with IOCM the risk of CIN in high risk diabetic patients is significantly lower than LOCM (Aspelin etal., 2003). This study is criticized by few numbers of patients. In a meta-analysis it was also shown that IOCM are less nephrotoxic than LOCM (McCullough etal,. 2006C), but in another larger meta-analysis there was no significant difference between LOCM and ICOM in term of nephrotoxicity (Heinrich etal., 2009). In a retrospective study, LOCM was less nephrotoxic than IOCM (Liss etal., 2006). This study showed that the risk of renal failure in future is increased by IOCM whether they had CIN or not.

According to the published studies, the American college of cardiology/American Heart association (ACC/AHA) recommended that there is no difference between low and iso-osmolal agents in CKD patients. The exception is Iohexol and Ioxaglate. The IOCM has lower probability of CIN than these two LOCM (Kushner etal., 2009).

The exact role of Ionicity in development of CIN is not known. The only meta-analysis in this regard showed that Ionic IOCM is similar to nonionic LOCM (Barrett & Carlisle, 1993).

2.8 Contrast Media volume

There is a direct relation between dose of CM and CIN development (Manske etal., 1990; McCullough etal., 1997; Rudnick et al., 1995). The probability of CIN is increased with higher volume of CM. On average, in coronary angiography, PCI and CT scan 130cc, 190cc and 100 to150cc CM is used. Although it has been shown that no patient with less than 100cc CM has developed CIN (Gruberg etal., 2001; McCullough etal., 1997), but unfortunately wide range of the volume of CM defined as cut off value (30-200cc). The relation between the dose of CM and CIN is particularly evident in moderate to severe renal failure patients (CKD3-5) which they should be received ultra-low dose of CM. Unfortunately, the need for CM for interventional purposes is much higher than this safe volume (250-300cc). In the study of Rihal etal it has been shown that with each 100cc CM, the risk of CIN will be increased 12% (Rihal etal., 2002). In another study the risk of CIN is serious when the volume of CM exceeds more than 3.7 fold of creatinine clearance (Laskey etal., 2007).Repeated use of CM within 72 hours increases the risk of CIN

3. Pathogenesis

The primary mechanism of CIN is Ischemia and direct tubular toxicity of CM to epithelial tubular cells.In experimental studies, after contrast infusion there is an early brief vasodilatation of renal vasculature, followed by a long term vasoconstriction (Arakawa etal., 1996; Seeliger etal., 2007). This biphasic response has not been evident in human and mostly increase of renal blood flow has been shown (Weisberg etal.,1992). These studies carried out the direct measurement of blood flow by hemodilution techniques. Nevertheless, if renal blood flow is measured directly by an intra-renal artery guide-wire, no difference of blood flow could be detected at the time of ventriculography, while subsequently by further CM infusion, the blood flow is decreased by3.7-39.5% from base (Mockel etal., 2008).Although these studies showed mild to moderate decrease of renal blood flow after exposure to CM, these findings nevertheless cannot describe the longitudinal decrement of GFR in CIN patients.

3.1 Medullary Hypoxemia

To overcome the discrepancy between renal blood flow rate and GFR decrement, medullary Hypoxemia due to regional blood flow changes is in the focus of attention in describing the pathophysiology of CIN. According to this hypothesis, the pathogenetic axel of CIN is medullary hypoxemia (Agmon etal., 1994; Heyman etal, 2008).

Physiologically, blood flow in outer medulla is low and this part of nephron works in relatively hypoxic state. The cause of this condition is the unique structure of vasa recta which is vital for countercurrent solute exchange. Low blood flow of medulla is also important to maintain the gradient in distal nephron. Meanwhile the thick ascending Limb of Henle as a hard worker of nephron needs a high level of oxygen. Due to this contradictory status, this part of nephron is more vulnerable to ischemic injuries. The decrease of blood flow in outer medulla is critical. In normal physiological conditions, the mechanisms responsible for blood flow and tubular transport are tubule-glomerular feedback, autoregulation and glomerulo-tubular balance which operate hand in hand to maintain the integrity of nephron and the system to work properly. The vasodilators (nitric oxide, prostaglandins, adenosin, dopamin, urodilantin) and vasoconstrictors (local endothelin, AngiotensinII, vasopressin) and transport inhibitors (PDF2, Adenosin, dopamine) together balance the supply and demand of oxygen in this part of nephron. Release of vasoconstrictor mediators or blockade of vasodilator mediators may play a role in the pathogenesis of CIN (Heyman etal., 1994). CM makes imbalance of these mediators. They cause decrease of oxygen tension both in cortex and medulla. It may be due to increased work of active transport in medullary tick ascending limb of Henle in response to osmotic diuresis of hyperosmolal agents.

Proximal tubules reabsorb a scant amount of CM. The osmotic property of CM causes less water reabsorption and increased intra-tubular pressure. The distal delivery of salt and water will be increased in this state which in turn activates tubule glomerular feedback and decreased GFR.

Increased pressure of intrestitium is also a factor for decreasing GFR. It also causes medullary hypoxia. CM may decrease renal blood flow by direct vasoconstriction of renal vasculature. This effect may be due to the change of calcium metabolism (Bakris & Burnett, 1985), or local increase of adenosin (Pflueger etal., 2000) and endothelin (Bagnis etal., 1997).

By CM infusion, the oxygen tension in outer medulla is decreased, nevertheless the sodium delivery to thick ascending Limb of Henle is increased due to osmotic diuresis of CM but the low oxygen pressure in this part of nephron is not related to the osmolality of CM (Liss etal., 1998). Administration of A1 adenosin receptor antagonists could not humiliate the decreased oxygen tension (Liss etal., 2004), but it seems that prostaglandins and nitric oxide could counteract vasoconstrictor effect of CM (Agmon etal., 1994). In animals, nitric oxide depletion has an effective role in vasoconstriction (Agmon etal., 1994; Ribeiro etal., 2004).

3.2 Reactive oxygen species

The role of oxidative stress in pathogenesis of Ischemia/reperfusion injuries is well known. Activation of oxidative stress processes in ischemia produce reactive oxygen species (ROS) which have a known role in AKI. The diseases which are considered as risk factors of CIN (CKD, CHF, and Diabetes) are associated with high oxidative stress state.
Experimental studies demonstrated that therapeutical strategies reduce the production of ROS and/or increase the nitric oxide activity and by these mechanisms halt the renal injuries due to Ischemia in different models of AKI including CIN. The rational use of antioxidants such as acetylcystein or allopurinol in preventing CIN is to lower or inhibit the oxidative stress processes.

3.3 Direct cytotoxicity

It is not known how much physicochemical properties of Iodinated CM are responsible for CIN and whether direct cytotoxicity of CM play any role in pathogenesis of CIN or not. In vitro studies showed that CM particularly HOCM is cytotoxic to mesangial and tubular cells (Itoh etal., 2006; Peer etal., 2003). The mechanism of such cytotoxicity is not known, but possibly cellular energy failure, disintegration of calcium homeostasis, apoptosis mechanisms and oxidative stress play a role (Beeri etal., 1995; Haller & Hizoh, 2004; Humes etal., 1987;). Internalization of non-ionic agents are seen in proximal tubules, (nephrosis osmotic), but these pathologic findings are also seen in patients who take CM without renal function deterioration (Persson & Tepel, 2006).CM may cause vasoconstriction by direct action on smooth muscles of arteries. More studies, should be run to show the relation of these changes with iso-osmolal contrast agents.

3.4 Others

In experimental studies CM can decrease capillary blood flow by decreasing the velocity of erythrocytes and increasing the red blood cells aggregation. HOCM also decreases erythrocyte volume and alters its membrane deformability. Recently hemeoxygenase activator is introduced as a pathomechanism of CIN development. Hemeoxygenase inhibits ROS production, suppresses pro-apoptotic proteins, activate anti-apoptotic proteins and has anti-inflammatory and vasodilatory effects. In future this enzyme may play an important role in CIN prophylaxis in human.

4. Prophylaxis

If CIN happens, the management is supportive, and because the time of insult is known the best measure is prophylaxis. Although in many studies, meta-analysis and systematic reviews have focused on prophylactic measures of CIN, nevertheless there is no an evidence-based guideline for clinical use.

No general consensus is present about the prophylactic measures of CIN other than stopping nephrotoxic agents, hydration and use of the lowest possible volume of CM and not using HOCM. Published guidelines are according to limited studies on very heterogenic patients. So they cause more confusion rather than better understanding and enlightment of the issue of CIN to provide the best reliable prophylactic measures. Probably the European Society of Urogenital Radiology (ESUR) guideline is yet valid (Morcos etal.,1999) and further studies within last 13 years have not been demoted its validity.

4.1 Volume expansion

Theoretically, volume expansion suppresses renin-angiotensin system activity, decreases vasoconstrictor hormones like endothelin, increases sodium diuresis, inhibits tubulo-glomerular feedback, prevents tubular obstruction, protects cells against ROS and finally dilutes the CM in tubules. Overall the toxicity of CM is decreased on tubules by hydration.

Large numbers of studies are about the role of volume expansion in preventing CIN. No controversy is present about the effectiveness of volume expansion. Up to now the volume expansion is known as the most effective measure in nephroprotection of CIN (Thomsen, 2006).This benefit has been shown in many randomized controlled trials (Bader etal.,2004; Dussol etal., 2006; Merten etal., 2004; Mueller etal., 2002; Taylor etal, 1998; Trivedi etal., 2003). But it is difficult to show that which type of fluid in how much dose and at which time is more suitable (McCullough & Soman, 2005). This obscurant is due to the heterogeneity of the studies and different definitions for CIN are used. Unfortunately these studies rarely reported the hard clinical endpoints.

Solomon et al has done the first randomized controlled trials (RCT) in this regard (Solomon etal., 1994). They showed that forced diuresis with diuretic or manitol is worse than hydration with isotonic salin or 0.45% salin. This Study did also very clearly show that volume expansion is highly effective in prevention of CIN in high risk patients and since then this prophylactic measure is the key stone of CIN prevention. Intravenous fluid therapy is also superior to oral hydration (Weisbord & Pavelsky, 2008) as it was shown in the study of Solomon etal .They reported that the control group had had 10 times more CIN than case controls. Because of such significant difference, this study was stopped early. Mueller etal also showed superiority of isotonic saline to 0.45% salin in patients with normal renal function, but if renal failure is present, there is no difference between two types of fluids (Mueller etal., 2002). The study of Merten etal compared sodium bicarbonate with isotonic saline in preventing CIN. Although this study showed better results with bicarbonate, but the study is criticized in different aspects (Merten etal., 2004).

In some studies intravenous bolus of isotonic saline just before procedure, or oral hydration from the night before the procedure, or use of NaCl tablets from 2 days before contrast exposure were examined with different results. (Bader etal.,2004; Dussol etal., 2006; Taylor etal, 1998; Trivedi etal., 2003) Volume expansion with isotonic saline is safe, simple and cheap, but not all patients taking CM will unfortunately suffer it. We showed that in patients that use of isotonic salin may be associated with the hazard of overload, use of 0.45% salin may be as effective as isotonic salin (Vasheghani-Farahani etal., 2010). It has been demonstrated that 26% of high risk patients have not been received any kind of intravenous fluid, and there was no standard about the volume and the type of fluid that were being used in the remaining patients. Urine volume more than 150^{cc} / hour is shown to be a good sign of decreased risk of CIN (Stevens etal., 1999). Cardiologists are the main target group who should know and use the strategies of volume expansion.

4.2 Sodium bicarbonate

The mechanism of sodium bicarbonate in preventing CIN is not clearly understood. Theoretically Sodium bicarbonate can expand the extracellular volume.

Alternatively it has been suggested that sodium bicarbonate will decreased the amount of ROS by increasing the PH of medulla. So the kidney will be protected from oxidant injuries (Atkins, 1986; Bakris etal., 1990; Merten etal., 2004; Morcos etal., 2005; Weisbord etal., 2008). Through this line of explanation, the main protective effect of sodium bicarbonate is not through volume expansion.

There are many concerns about the role of bicarbonate in prevention of CIN (Briguori etal., 2007; From etal., 2008; Masuda etal., 2007; Ozcan etal., 2007, Recio-Mayoral etal., 2007).Most studies compared isotonic saline and sodium bicarbonate have reported contradictory results. Masuda etal., showed Bicarbonate is more effective than saline in prevention of CIN (1.7% Vs 13%) (Masuda etal.,2007). In a meta-analysis, comparing saline and bicarbonate, it was shown that rise of serum creatinine in bicarbonate group is less than salin group, but in term of need to dialysis and death there was no difference between the two groups(Hogan etal., 2008).In the largest RCT comparing salin and bicarbonate, No differences between two groups was shown (Maioli etal., 2008). In another retrospective study including 7977 patients it was shown that the risk of CIN in sodium bicarbonate is significantly higher than salin group (From etal., 2008).We showed that addition of sodium bicarbonate to isotonic salin added no benefit to isotonic salin alone in preventing CIN (Vasheghani-Farahani etal., 2009).These controversial results and heterogeneity of studies make it difficult to be able to extract a conclusion that bicarbonate is even equal to salin in preventing CIN.

4.3 N-Acetyl Cysteine (NAC)

The main mechanism of NAC may be due to its known antioxidant peculiarity. It may diminish the oxidative stress markers ((Drager etal., 2004; Efrati etal., 2003) and / or its vasodilatory effect (Fishbane etal., 2004; Stenstorm etal., 2008).CM decrease urinary nitric oxide and NAC may inhibit this effect of CM. But it has been shown that NAC has no effect on F2- isoprostane a known marker of oxidative stress (Efrati etal., 2003).

NAC has wide first-pass metabolism, so its bioavailability will be very low if it is administered orally. Meanwhile many centers use oral NAC without any evidence-based guidelines (Marenzi etal., 2006b). The drug has also wide intra-patient variation. Its half-life after intravenous injection is 40 minutes. It has wide plasma and tissue protein binding. After oral or intravenous administration of NAC the drug cannot be detected in systemic circulation. So its effectiveness may be due to secondary effects like induction of glutathione synthesis rather than its direct effect. Because there are no tool to measure these secondary effects, no optimal dose of NAC can be defined and the dose of drug for prevention of CIN is empirical.

Clinically the use of NAC was controversial from the early time. Positive and negative results about NAC have created confusions about the role of this agent in CIN prophylaxis protocols. When the first report of NAC was published by Tepel and his coworkers (Tepel etal., 2000), it caused a universal trend to use NAC in all patients have been taking CM. They showed significant decrease in the rate of CIN in patients on NAC (2% Vs 12%). Since then many studies have been conducted with contradictory results. Now After 12 years of use of NAC in prevention of CIN, there is no general consensus about this pharmacological agent. In last decade many RCTs, non-randomized studies and meta-analyses were performed with NAC (Alonso etal., 2004; Bagshaw etal., 2006, Bagshaw & Ghali, 2004; Birck etal., 2003; Duong etal., 2005; Dzgoeva etal., 1995, Isenbarger etal., 2003; Kshirsagar etal., 2004; Liu etal., 2005; Nallamothu etal., 2004; Onbasili etal., 2007; Pannu etal., 2004; Spargias et al., 2004; Zagler etal., 2006). Some of these studies showed that there is no positive effect for NAC in prevention of CIN (Onbasili etal., 2007; Spargias et al., 2004). On the other hand some meta-analyses showed effectiveness of NAC but the most of these meta- analyses had inconclusive results (Bagshaw etal., 2006; Nallamothu, 2004). In conclusion although huge data is available, the role of NAC in preventing CIN is moot yet. This discrepancy may be due to bias in the publishing of studies with positive results, so these studies should be considered with skepticism (Fishbane etal., 2008).

In a study on patients with myocardial infarction high dose intravenous NAC (1200mg) was effective in prevention of CIN (Marenzi etal., 2006b). Surprisingly no patient in this study had received fluid for volume expansion. An interesting but confusing issue in studies about NAC is the decrement of serum creatinine after CM exposure (Baker etal., 2003; Drager etal., 2004; Kay etal., 2003; Marenzi etal., 2006b). Probably NAC can decrease serum creatinine directly without affecting renal function (Drager etal., 2004). In this study the GFR of patients who were taken NAC four days before CM exposure was significantly higher than those patients were taken NAC only for two days. Interestingly this study and study of Hoffmann and coworkers showed that NAC may decrease serum creatinine in patients that had not received CM (Hoffmann etal., 2004). There are concerns that NAC with increasing tubular secretion of creatinine decreases the serum creatinine without any change in GFR. A recent meta-analysis found that NAC was more protective than saline infusion and the authors recommended the use of NAC because of its low cost, availability and paucity of side effects (Cigarroa etal., 1989). In contrast to this recommendation which is based on safety of the NAC, there is a report of anaphylactic reaction in 3-6% of patients receiving intra-venous NAC (Kanter, 2006).

Briefly, NAC may increase GFR in normal patients and restore GFR in high risk patients for CIN. But it is not known whether these effects are due to direct protective effect of NAC on kidney or it is due to alteration in creatinine metabolism. Some studies reported good effect of NAC while others did not find such positive effects.

In conclusion, there is no agreement about the NAC. Otherwise there is no guideline about the route of administration of NAC or the dose or the time of its administration. There is an important question whether its effect on serum creatinine is real or spurious. It is obvious that we need more good designed RCTs to solve these controversies.

4.4 Type and dose of Contrast Media

It is obvious that HOCM is associated with higher risk of CIN. So for prophylactic purposes it is recommended not to use this type of CM in any patients particularly in the patients with moderate or high risk of CIN. In analysis of present studies about the type of contrast, it is possible that different monomer CM have different toxic effects (Bettmann, 2005; Solomon etal., 2005). Up to now there is no evidence that CIN is more prevalent with LOCM than IOCM. There is a trend to use Iodixanol which is a dimeric IOCM (Barrett & Carlisle, 1993). But different studies showed no superiority of this agent over the other IOCM or LOCM (Baker etal., 2003; Boccolandro etal., 2003; Briguori etal., 2005). Over all, it seems that there is no difference between LOCM and IOCM in regard of CIN.

The other issue in preventing measures for CIN in the term of CM is the dose of the agent. So it is advised that the lowest possible dose of the CM should be administered in patients at risk of CIN. It is obvious that the higher the volume of the CM is associated with the higher incidence of CIN (Cigarroa etal., 1989; Manske etal., 1990), but there is no magical dose of contrast to believe that below that dose, the CIN will not occur. The renal function is an important limiting factor for dose of CM. In study of Laskey etal. it was reported that if the volume of CM exceeded 3.7 times of creatinine clearance, the risk of CIN will be higher (Laskey eal., 2002). So the absolute value of contrast volume may be too low. There are 2 formulas for calculating relatively the safe volume of CM according to renal function.

$$\text{dose of CM} = \frac{5\,\frac{ml}{kg}\ contrast\,media}{serum\,creatinine\ (\frac{mg}{dl})} \qquad (1)$$

Or,

$$= \frac{300\,ml\,contrast\,media}{serum\,creatinine} \qquad (2)$$

In any case the dose of contrast should not be exceeded by 300 ml. For IOCM and LOCM the dose may increase by 1.5 times.

4.5 Other preventive strategies

Several studies examined different pharmacologic agents to prevent CIN. Studies about fenoldopam, dopamin, calcium channel blockers, atrial natriuretic peptide, L-arginine and statines are inconclusive. Use of ATP-MgCl2 also failed to show beneficial effect. Mesna is another pharmacologic agent that can inhibit ROS related renal injury.

4.5.1 Theophylin

High level of adenosin is a possible mechanism for occurrence of CIN. It causes afferent arteriole vasoconstriction (Haller etal., 2004; Pflueger etal., 2000). Theophylin is a non specific antagonist of adenosin receptor, so it may theoretically be beneficial. Studies about the theophylin like studies of NAC are not conclusive. Few studies showed effectiveness of theophylin or aminophylin in prevention of CIN , but in a meta-analysis no positive effect of this drug was shown (Bagshaw & Ghali, 2005). So the routine use of theophylin is not recommended. In a study on patients in ICU, infusion of 200mg theophylin half an hour before contrast exposure was superior to NAC (Huber etal., 2006) but arythmogenesity of theophylin is a problem in coronary artery disease. It is possible that in the future, theophylin is replaced by a selective adenosin receptor antagonist with less toxicity and more effectiveness than theophylin in CIN prophylaxis protocols (Pflueger etal., 2000).

4.5.2 Prostaglandin analogues

Prostaglandin I1 and E1 may have some protective effects , but it is associated with severe hypotension. So their routine use is not suggested. Prostacyclin may also have such a role.

4.5.3 Ascorbic acid

Studies about the ascorbic acid are inconclusive (Briguori etal., Spargias etal., 2004). 3 grams of ascorbic acid 2 hours before contrast exposure and 2 grams at night and in the morning after procedure may decrease the risk of CIN (Spargias etal., 2004).

4.5.4 Trimetazidine

This novel pharmacologic agent interferes with different metabolic pathways. It can prevent Ischemia-reperfusion injuries. In a RCT it was effective in preventing CIN (Onbasili etal., 2007).

4.5.5 Erythropoietin

Erythropoietin may have some role in CIN prophylaxis. Its effect has been shown in some studies (Yokomaku etal., 2008).

4.6 Renal replacement therapy

The rationality for use of renal replacement therapy after contrast exposure is to remove the CM rapidly to prevent CIN (Frank etal., 2003; Marenzi etal 2003,2006b; Vogt, 2001).Each session of dialysis can remove 60-90% of administered CM (Deray etal., 2006). CM are totally eliminated by the kidneys. They are handled by the kidneys like Inulin. Different extracorporeal techniques can efficiently remove CM. So it is rational to use these techniques just after contrast exposure to prevent or reduce the risk of CIN. Recent study on severe CKD patients not on dialysis(GFR less than 15ml/min) comparing isotonic salin and prophylactic hemodialysis showed that patients on hemodialysis were discharged from the hospital while 5% of them need hemodialysis. Meanwhile, the rate of chronic dialysis at the time of discharge in salin group was 45% (Solomon etal., 2004). Nevertheless, other studies demonstrated that hemodialysis in patients with previous history of renal failure was not beneficial and the incidence of CIN will not be changed by this modality (Deray, 2006; Vogt, 2001).One meta-analysis has supported this result (Cruz etal., 2006). Patients on dialysis do not also need dialysis after contrast exposure (Hamani etal., 1998; Morcos etal., 2002).

Only few study reported the prophylactic usefulness of hemodialysis (Lee etal., 2007; McCullough & Soman, 2005). But repeatedly it has been shown that hemodialysis has no role in preventing CIN (Cruz etal., 2006; deray, 2006; Marenzi etal., 2006b). In contrast to positive studies one RCT showed that prophylactic dialysis caused more reduction of renal function and these patients need more dialysis after exposure to contrast (Vogt etal., 2001). In one meta-analysis (Cruz etal., 2008), the beneficial effect of pre-procedural extracorporeal blood purification was obscure.

It has been shown that serum creatinine four days after contrast exposure is less in dialysis group, but this difference was not significant.

CRRT, hemodiafiltration (CVVHD) and hemofiltration are also evaluated in this regard (Gabutti etal., 2003, Marenzi etal., 2003). The only technique with enthusiasm was CVVH. But this procedure is very complex and expensive and even if further studies prove its efficacy in large clinical trials, it cannot be ordinarily used in clinic (Klarenbach etal., 2006).

Overall, given the cost and logistic necessity of extra corporeal modalities, it is difficult to suggest routine use of these techniques in prophylactic protocols of CIN and further studies may show its advantage or disadvantage.

4.7 Drugs which should be stopped before procedure

At the time of planning for procedures with CM, all drugs which are taken by patients should carefully be reviewed. There is no RCT about the harmfulness of drugs, but generally speaking the following drugs may be associated with increased risk of CIN.

4.7.1 Non-Steroid Anti-Inflammatory Drugs (NSAIDs)

Case reports and clinical experiences have shown that NSAIDs may increase the incidence of CIN. There is no difference between selective or non selective cycloxygenase inhibitors. They should be stopped several days before procedure.

4.7.2 Antihypertensive agents

No antihypertensive drug is contraindicated for patients that undergo for imaging with CM. But if they cause hypotension, the risk of CIN may be increased. The use of angiotensin converting enzyme inhibitors (ACEIs) and angiotensin receptor blockers (ARBs) should not be stopped (Erley, 2006). Although In patients with serum creatinine 2 mg/dl or higher it may increase the rate of CIN. Cirit etal. have reported an increased risk of CIN with ACEIs (Cirit etal., 2006), nonetheless another study showed its preventive effect (Dangas etal., 2005).There is also a report that Captopril may cause decrease in incidence of CIN in diabetic patients(Gupta etal., 1999).
There is no study about ARBs.

4.7.3 Metformin

Metformin causes lactic acidosis in patients with renal failure. Otherwise uncontrolled diabetes is a risk factor of CIN. There is no RCT about metformin and CIN. It is recommended to continue the use of the drug until the night before the procedure (Bailey etal., 1996). Others have suggested the continuation of metformin in patients with normal renal function. If metformin is stopped, it is better to start it again when the physician is sure that CIN has not been happened.

4.7.4 Diuretics

Use of furosemide, manitol and endothelial receptor antagonists were associated with increased risk of CIN (Anto etal., 1981; Solomon etal., 1994; Weisberg etal., 1994).Forced diuresis increases the risk of CIN. Although there is no RCT about diuretics, nevertheless it is not theoretically rational to expand the volume from one hand and to contract it from the other hand. So it is recommended to discontinue diuretics 12 hours before the procedure and to restart it 24 hours after that.

4.7.5 Manitol

Like diuretics it may increase the risk of CIN in patients with forced diuresis (Solomon etal., 1994). The problem is raised in neurosurgical patients on manitol. It is suggested to stop the drugs several hours before CM administration and to monitor the hydration status of the patients very carefully (Erley, 2006)

5. Tools for assessment of patients at risk of CIN

In published study there is no controversy about the risk factors of CIN. But nearly all patients undergoing imaging with CM have more than one risk factor, so the investigators are looking for an innovative risk stratification model to detect the patients who are at a higher risk of CIN. There are different scoring tools that could detect the patients at risk of CIN before the procedure and accordingly the physicians can provide and modify the different preventive measures for these patients to decrease the risk of CIN.

Up to the present time there are two popular scoring models. Both of which have been introduced at 2004 and provide good tools for estimating the odds of the CIN. They are more or less similar with few differences in the terms of risk factors and scoring. According to the data of 8357 PCI patients, Mehran et al. determined the independent predictive factors of CIN and provided a scoring model for estimating potential risk of patients (Mehran etal., 2004). Bartholomew et al. also suggested another risk stratification model at the same year (Bartholomew etal., 2004). They evaluated the data of 2047 patients and determined the risk factors and their risk scoring. Table 3 shows these two models comparatively.
According to Mehran's model the risk score of less than 5 is associated with 7.2% risk of CIN and nearly no patients need dialysis (0.04%) but risk score more than 16 will increase the risk of CIN up to 57.7% and need to dialysis to 12.6%.
Bartholomew et al. reported no patients with risk score of less than 1 developed CIN and CIN had occurred in 25% of patients with risk score more than 9.
In regards to risk stratification models, some factors are not predictable before the procedure (like need to balloon pump or volume of contrast), so according to these models it is impossible to estimate the exact reliable and accurate risk of CIN in every patient.

Mehran model		*Bartholomew model*	
Risk factor	*Point*	*Risk factor*	*point*
Hypotension(BP<80 mmHg)	*5*	*Hypotension*	*1*
CHF	*4*	*CHF*	*1*
Intra-aorta balloon pump	*5*	*Intra-aorta balloon pump*	*2*
Diabetes	*3*	*Diabetes*	*1*
Volume of contrast	*1(/ each100cc)*	*Volume of contrast(>260cc/)*	*1*
Previous CKD: *Serum Creatinine> 132 mmol/L* *Or:* *GFR 40-60 ml/min* *GFR 20-40 ml/min* *GFR <20 ml/min*	 *4* *2* *4* *6*	*Creatinine clearance<60ml/min*	*2*
Anemia	*3*	*Peripheral vascular disease*	*1*
Age > 75 years	*4*	*Emergent PCI*	*2*

Table 3. Two most popular risk starfication models of cin

6. Recommendations

Until more accurate and universally accepted guidelines are developed, following recommendations which are based on different studies are useful in preventing CIN.The important issue is how to find the patients at risk before imaging procedures. There are some recommendations in this regard.
The American Radiology College (ARC) has suggested the measurement of serum creatinine in all patients who are suspected of having renal disease or those at risk of nephrotoxicity before the procedure (The committee on drugs and contrast media of the American College of Radiology, 2010). The patients at risk are those with a positive answer to any of the following statements: history of renal disease (including tumor or transplantation), familial history of renal disease, on diabetes therapy, having paraproteinemia disorders, having

collagen vascular disease, taking specific drugs such as metformin or NSAIDs or Nephrotoxic antibiotics. The ESUR has also recommended to measure serum creatinine in some specific patients (Thomsen & Morcos, 2005). Accordingly, the patients with a history of renal disease, renal surgery, proteinuria, hypertension, diabetes, gout, recent use of nephrotoxic drugs are considered high risk patients. The Urogenital Radiology Association also suggests that serum creatinine should be measured in all patients with history of chronic renal failure or those who are candidates for intra-arterial angiography or patients with at least one positive answer to the questioner (Thomsen & Morcos, 2006). 99% of patients with negative answers to all questions had serum creatinine less than 1.7 mg/dl (Thomsen, 2005).A good alternative surrogate marker to the serum creatinine is to measure GFR according to one of the MDRD formulas in all patients with any risk factors of CIN, because the serum creatinine has limitation to find CKD patients.
After finding the high risk patients there are some different preventive measures for people at different risks. But some general recommendations should be taken into account for all patients whether they have risk factor(s) or not.

6.1 General recommendations for all patients taking CM

1. Evaluation of risks in all patients planned to take CM.
2. Measurement of serum creatinine in all high risk patients before and after procedure.
3. List the risk factors according to present risk score models.
4. Encouraging all patients to drink water before procedure.
5. All patients should be taken LOCM or IOCM.
6. The dose of CM should be as low as possible.
7. Continuing use of angiotensin converting enzyme inhibitors and angiotensin receptor blockers is not contraindicated
8. NSAIDS should be stopped several days before procedure.
9. Use of furosemide and manitol should be stopped 12-24 hours before CM administration.
10. Stop metformin the night before procedure until ensure of not happening CIN.
11. No repetition of procedure until to be sure that CIN has not been developed.

6.2 Recommendations for low risk patients

(Normal renal function and risk score≤5 according to Mehran's score)

1. All recommendations for no risk patients
2. Oral hydration (at least 500cc pre-procedure and 2500cc within 24 hours post procedure)
3. Intravenous isotonic salin in patients who are not taking oral intake at rate of 1 ml/kg/hour starting 4 hours before procedure and continuing at least for 6 hours post procedure . It is best to continue the hydration for 24 hours after procedure.
4. No repetition of procedure until serum creatinine returns to base value.

6.3 Recommendation for moderate risk patients

(Patients with CKD1-3 and/or risk score 5-15 according to Mehran's score)

1. All recommendations for low risk patients

2. Delaying the procedure in volume depleted patients or those who have blood circulation collapse or patients with CHF until stability of hemodynamic is achieved.
3. Infusion of 0.45% salin in patients at risk of volume overload.
4. If the time to procedure is less than 6 hours (in emergent angiography) a simultaneous administration of oral and IV Fluid with the dose of 3 ml/kg/hour and maximum 300cc fluid/hour is recommended. The fluid administration should be started one hour before procedure. After procedure the fluid is continued with the rate of 1 ml/kg/hr for 12 hours.
5. Use of NAC 1200mg twice daily in the day and day after the procedure. In emergency situations use of 1200mg intravenous bolus of NAC instead of first oral dose is appropriate.
6. Measurement of serum creatinine 24-48 hours after procedure in patients with moderate and severe risk factors

6.4 Recommendations for high risk patients

(CKD4-5 and/or risk score >15 according to Mehran's score)

1. All recommendations in moderate risk patients
2. Nephrology consultation
3. Use of hydration should be individualized according to volume status of each patient with considering overload hazards.
4. In ICU patients use of 200mg theophylin 30minutes before procedure, particularly if hydration protocol could not completely be follow. But remember the side effects of this drug.

7. Anaphylactic reactions

Anaphylactic reactions to CM are well known from the early use of these agents. These reactions are dermal allergic type reactions, edema, pulmonary edema, angina pectoris, arrhythmia and hypertension crisis. Mostly these side effects are mild and there is no need to treatment. The occurrence of the serious side-effects is within 20 minutes of CM administration. They are exhibited by nausea and vomiting, urticaria, pulmonary edema, bronchospasm, laryngospasm, hypotension, tachycardia, vaso-vagal responses and seizure.

In last decade the reactions to CM have significantly decreased from 5-12% to 0.2-0.7% (Sayol & Bush, 2011). It may be due to shift from HOCM to LOCM and IOCM. Anaphylactic reaction to HOCM is more than LOCM. Ionicity is also a cause of reaction to these agents and nonionic monomers are less anaphylactic. These reactions are either chemotoxic or Anaphylactic (Idio or nonidiosynchratic).The chemotoxic reaction is related to physicochemical property of CM and its severity is dependent on the dose and concentration of the agent.

The mechanisms of anaphylactic reaction are not well understood. Histamine, Leukotriens, Basophiles and prostaglandins may be mediators of this type reaction. It is unlike that antigen- antibody interaction plays any role.

Aging, history of allergy and asthma and previous history of reaction to CM, are the risk factors of anaphylactic reactions. The patients with CKD, cardiovascular disease and epilepsy are also at increased risk. Beta blockers may increase the threshold and severity of anaphylactic reactions (Kadivar & McClennan, 2010).

Treatment of anaphylactic reactions is mostly supportive. In mild reactions anti histaminic drugs are effective, but in more severe cases use of short acting steroids is mandatory and even some critical care facilities may be necessary.

8. Alternatives to Contrast Media

Very high risk patients may be in need for other imaging techniques rather than using contras media. One of these agents is Carbone dioxide which may be a good alternative to iodinated CM. It may be used solely or in conjunction with low dose of iodinated CM. The procedure is simple and the quality of images is good. With using modern technologies such as digital subtract angiography the nephrotoxicity of this method is neglectable (Kessel etal., 2002; Liss etal., 2005; Shaw & Kessel, 2006).

The other alternative is magnetic resonance angiography (MRA). Its main complication in renal failure is nephrogenic systemic fibrosis (NSF). SO in patients with moderate to severe renal failure it is contraindicated and in patients with mild renal failure its use is cautiously recommended.

9. Conclusion

Contrast agents are associated with many complications. There are two more prevalent and important complications related to contrast media: allergic reactions and CIN. The allergic reactions are preventable by knowing the high risk patients and premedication with steroids and antihistamines.

The most important complication of contrast agents is CIN, which is usually a mild to moderate AKI that is rapidly recovered. But it could be associated with increased significant morbidity and mortality. There is no treatment for developed CIN, so it should be prevented by some measures. The proved modalities for prevention of CIN are saline administration, the lowest possible dose of CM, and use of IOCM or LOCM.

All patients at risk should be evaluated carefully before the procedures with CM and the risk factors should be stratified according to available risk stratification models.

10. References

Agmon Y, Peleg H, Greenfeld Z, etal. (1994) Nitric oxide and prostanoids protect the renal outer medulla from radiocontrast toxicity in the rat. *J Clin Invest*; 94: 1069–1075.

Alonso A, Lau J, Jaber BL, et al. (2004) Prevention of radiocontrast nephropathy with N-acetylcysteine in patients with chronic kidney disease: a meta-analysis of randomized, controlled trials. *Am J Kidney Dis*; 43:1–9.

American Heart Association statistics committee and stroke subcommittee -2007 update: A report from the AHA statistics committee and stroke subcommittee. *Circulation* 115:e69-e171.

Anto HR, Chou SY, Porush JG, Shapiro WB. (1981) Infusion intravenous pyelography and renal function. Effect of hypertonic mannitol in patients with chronic renal insufficiency. *Arch Intern Med*;141:1652–1656

Arakawa K, Suzuki H, Naitoh M, etal. (1996)Role of adenosine in the renal responses to contrast medium. *Kidney Int*; 49:1199–1206.

Araujo M, Welch WJ. (2006) Oxidative stress and nitric oxide in kidney function. *Curr Opin Nephrol Hypertens*; 15:72–77.

Aspelin P, Aubry P, Fransson SG, etal. (2003)Nephrotoxic effects in high-risk patients undergoing angiography. *N Engl J Med*;348:491–499.

Atkin JL. Effect of sodium bicarbonate preloading on ischemic renal failure. *Nephron* 1986;44:70–76.

Bader BD, Berger ED, Heede MB, et al. (2004) What is the best hydration regimen to prevent contrast media-induced nephrotoxicity? *Clin Nephrol*; 62:1–7.

Bagnis C, Idee JM, Dubois M, et al. (1997) Role of endothelium-derived nitric oxide endothelin balance in contrast medium-induced acute renal vasoconstriction in dogs. *Acad Radiol*; 4: 343–348.

Bagshaw SM, Ghali WA. (2004) Acetylcysteine for prevention of contrast-induced nephropathy after intravascular angiography: a systematic review and meta-analysis. *BMC Med*; 2:38–49.

Bagshaw SM, Ghali WA. (2005) Theophylline for prevention of contrast-induced nephropathy: a systematic review and meta analysis. *Arch Intern Med*; 165: 1087–1093.

Bagshaw SM, McAlister FA, Manns BJ, Ghali WA. (2006)Acetylcysteine in the prevention of contrast-induced nephropathy:A case study of the pitfalls in the evolution of evidence. *ArchIntern Med*;166:161–166.

Bailey CJ, Turner RC. Metformin. *N Engl J Med*; 334:574–579.

Baker CS, Wragg A, Kumar S, etal. (2003) A rapid protocol for the prevention of contrastinduced renal dysfunction: the RAPPID study. *J Am Coll Cardiol*; 41:2114–2118.

Bakris GL, Burnett JC Jr. (1985) A role for calcium in radiocontrast induced reductions in renal hemodynamics. *Kidney Int*; 27:465–468.

Bakris GL, Lass N, Gabaer AO, etal. (1990) Radiocontrast medium-induced declines in renal function. A role for oxygen free radicals. *Am J Physiol*; 175:57–60.

Barrett BJ, Parfrey PS, Vavasour HM, et al. (1992) Contrast nephropathy in patients with impaired renal function: high versus low osmolar media. *Kidney Int*;41: 1274– 1279.

Barrett B J,Carlisle E J. (1993) Meta-analysis of the relative nephrotoxicity of high- and low osmolality iodinated contrast media . *Radiology*;188:171-178.

Barrett BJ, Katzberg RW, Thomsen HS, et al.(2006) Contrast-induced nephropathy in patients with chronic kidney disease undergoing computed tomography: A double blind comparison of iodixanol and iopamidol. *Invest Radiol*;41:815–821.

Bartholomew BA, Harjai KJ, Dukkipati S, et al.(2004). Impact of nephropathy after percutaneous coronary intervention and a method for risk stratification. *Am J Cardiol*; 93:1515–1519.

Beeri R, Symon Z, Brezis M, et al. (1995) Rapid DNA fragmentation from hypoxia along the thick ascending limb of rat kidneys. *Kidney Int*; 47: 1806–1810.

Bettmann MA. (2005)Contrast medium-induced nephropathy: critical review of the existing clinical evidence. *Nephrol Dial Transplant*;20(suppl 1): i2–i7.

Birck R, Krzossok S, Markowetz F, et al. (2003) Acetylcysteine for prevention of contrast nephropathy: meta-analysis. *Lancet*; 362:598–603.

Boccolandro F, Amhad M, Smalling RW, Sdringola S. (2003) Oral acetylcysteine does not protect renal function from moderate to high doses of intravenous radiographic contrast. *Cathet Cardiovasc Interv*; 58:336–341.

Briguori C, Airoldi F, D'Andrea D, et al. (2007) Renal insufficiency following contrast media administration trial (REMEDIAL): a randomized comparison of 3 preventive strategies. *Circulation*; 115:1211–1217.

Briguori C, Colombo A, Airoldi F et al. (2005) Nephrotoxicity of low-osmolality versus iso-osmolality contrast agents: impact of N-acetylcysteine. *Kidney Int*; 68:2250–2255.

Briguori C, Visconti G, Rivera N V, etal.(2010) Cystatin C and contrast-induced acute kidney injury. *Circulation*;121:2117-2122.

Carraro M, Malalan F, Antoinione R, et al.(1998) Effects of a dimeric vs. a monomeric nonionic contrast medium of renal function in patients with mild to moderate renal insufficiency: a double-blind randomized clinical trial. *Eur Radiol*; 8:144– 147.

Cigarroa R G, Lange R A, Williams R H, Hillis L D. (1989) Dosing of contrast material to prevent contrast nephropathy in patients with renal disease. *Am J Med* ;86: 649-652.

Cirit M, Toprak O, Yesil M, et al. (2006) Angiotensin-converting enzyme inhibitors as a risk factor for contrast-induced nephropathy. *Nephron Clin Pract*; 104: c20- c27.

Costa N. (2004) Understanding contrast media. *J Infus Nurs*; 27:302–12.

Cruz D N, Perazella M A, Bellomo R, etal. (2006) Extracorporeal blood purification therapies for prevention of radiocontrast-induced nephropathy: A systematic review. *Am J Kidney Dis*; 48:361-371.

Dangas G, Iakovou I, Nikolsky E, et al. (2005) Contrast-induced nephropathy after percutaneous coronary interventions in relation to chronic kidney disease and hemodynamic variables. *Am J Cardiol*; 95:13–19.

Deray G. (2006) Dialysis and iodinated contrast media. *Kidney Int Suppl*;100:S25–S29.

Drager LF, Andrade L, Barros de Toledo JF, etal. (2004) Renal effects of N- acetylcysteine in atients at risk for contrast nephropathy: decrease in oxidant stress-mediated renaltubular injury. *Nephrol Dial Transplant*; 19:1803–1807.

Duong MH, MacKenzie TA, Malenka DJ. (2005) N-acetylcysteine prophylaxis significantlyreduces the risk of radiocontrast-induced nephropathy: comprehensive meta-analysis. *Catheter Cardiovasc Interv*; 64:471–479.

Dussol B, Morange S, Loundoun A, et al. (2006) A randomized trial of saline hydration to prevent contrast nephropathy in chronic renal failure patients. *Nephrol Dial Transplant*; 21:2120–2126.

Dzgoeva FU, Milovanov Iu S, Kutyrina IM. (1995) Acute kidney failure related to the use of x-ray contrast agents and indomethacin: the risk factors and mechanisms of its development. (Abstract)*Ter Arkh*; 67:36–39.

Efrati S, Dishy V, Averbukh M, etal. (2003) The effect of N-acetylcystein on renal function, nitric oxide, and oxidative stress after angiography. *Kidney Int*; 64:2182–2187.

Erley C. (2006) Concomitant drugs with exposure to contrast media. *Kidney Int*; 69 Suppl 100:S20–S24.

Fishbane S. (2008) N-acetylcysteine in prevention of contrast-induced nephropathy. *Clin J Am Soc Nephrol*; 3:281–287.

Frank H, Werner D, Lorusso V, et al. (2003) Simultaneous hemodialysis during coronary angiography fails to prevent radiocontrast-induced nephropathy in chronic renal failure. *Clin Nephrol*; 60:176–182.

From AM, Bartholmai BJ, Williams AW, etal. (2008) Sodium bicarbonate is associated with an increased incidence of contrast nephropathy: a retrospective cohort study of 7977 patients at mayo clinic. *Clin J Am Soc Nephrol*;3:10–18.

Gabutti L, Marone C, Monti M, etal. (2003) Does continuous veno-venous hemodiafiltration concomitant with radiological procedures provide a significant and safe removal of the iodinated contrast ioversol? *Blood Purif*; 21: 152–157.

Goldenberg I, Chonchol M, Guetta V.(2009)Reversible acute kidney injury followin contrast exposure and the risk of long-term mortality. *Am J Nephrol*; 29:136–144.

Gruberg L, Mintz GGS, Mehran R, et al. (2000)The prognostic implications of further renal function deterioration within 48 h of interventional coronary Procedur in patients with preexistent chronic renal insufficiency. *J Am Coll Cardiol*; 36: 1542-1548.

Gruberg L,Mehran R,Dangas G, etal.(2001) Acute renal failure requiring dialysis after percutaneous coronary interventions. *Catheter Cardiovasc Interv*; 52:409- 416.

Gupta RK, Kapoor A, Tewari S, et al. (1996) Captopril for prevention of contrast induced nephropathy in diabetic patients: a randomised study. *Indian Heart J* 1999; 51:521–526.

Haller C, Hizoh I. (2004)The cytotoxicity of iodinated radiocontrast agents on renal cells in vitro. *Invest Radiol*;39:149–154.

Hamani A, Petitclerc T, Jacobs C, Deray G. (1998) Is dialysis indicated immediately after administration of iodinated contrast agents in patients on haemodialysis? *Nephrol Dial Transplant* ;13:1051–1052.

Heinrich MC, Haberle L, Muller V, et al.(2009) Nephrotoxicity of iso-osmolar Iodixanol compared with nonionic low-osmolar contrast media: meta-analysis of randomized controlled trials. Radiology; 250:68–86.

Heyman SN, Rosen S, Brezis M. (1994) Radiocontrast nephropathy: a paradigm for the synergism between toxic and hypoxic insults in the kidney. *Exp Nephrol*; 2:153–157.

Heyman SN, Rosen S, Rosenberger C. (2008) Renal parenchymal hypoxia, hypoxi adaptation, and the pathogenesis of radiocontrast nephropathy. *Clin J Am Soc Nephrol*;3:288–296.

Hierholzer K, Hierholzer J: The discovery of renal contrast media in berlin. *Am J Nephrol* 2002;22:295-299.

Hirsch R, Dent C, Pfriem H, etal.(2007) NGAL is an early predictive biomarker of contrast-induced nephropathy in children. *Pediatr Nephrol*;22:2089–2095.

Hoffmann U, Fischereder M, Kruger B, etal. (2004) The value of N-acetylcysteine in the prevention of radiocontrast agent-induced nephropathy seems questionable. J *Am Soc Nephrol*;15:407–410.

Hogan SE, L'Allier P, Chetcuti S, etal. (2008) Current role of sodium bicarbonate- based preprocedural hydration for the prevention of contrast-induced acute kidney injury: Am eta-analysis. *Am Heart J*; 156:414–421.

Hricak H, Barbariv Z L(1984).Newer imaging techniques:Workshop; in *Robinson I (ed): Proc 9th Int Cong Nephrol*, , 1430-1436.

Huber W, Eckel F, Hennig M,etal. (2006) Prophylaxis of contrast material-induced nephropathy in patients in intensive care: acetylcysteine, theophylline, or both? A randomized study. *Radiology* ;239:793–804.

Humes HD, Hunt DA, White MD. (1987) Direct toxic effect of the radiocontrast agent diatrizoate on renal proximal tubule cells. *Am J Physiol*; 252: F246–255.Isenbarger

DW, Kent SM, O'Malley PG. (2003) Meta-analysis of randomized clinical trials on the usefulness of acetylcysteine for prevention of contrast nephropathy. *Am J Cardiol*; 92:1454–1458.

Itoh Y, Yano T, Sendo T, etal. (2006) Involvement of de novo ceramide synthesis in radiocontrast-induced renal tubular cell injury. *Kidney Int*; 69:288–297.

James MT, Ghali WA, Tonelli M, et al. (2010) Acute kidney injury following coronary angiography associated with a long-term decline in kidney function. *Kidney Int*; 78:803-809.

Kadivar Kh, McClennan BL. (2010) Intravenous Iodinated Contrast Media Reactions: Recognition and Response. Contemporary Diag Radiol ; 33:1-6.

Kanter M Z. (2006) Comparison of oral and i.v acetylcysteine in the treatment of acetaminophen poisoning. *Am J Health Syst Pharm*; 63:1821–1827.

Kay J, Chow WH, Chan TM, etal. (2003) Acetylcysteine for prevention of acute deterioration of renal function following elective coronary angiography and intervention: a randomized controlled trial. *JAMA*; 289:553–558.

Kessel DO, Robertson I, Patel J etal. (2002) Carbon-dioxide-guided vascular interventions: technique and pitfalls.*Cardiovasc Intervent Radiol*.;25(6):476.

Klarenbach SW, Pannu N, Tonelli MA, Manns BJ. (2006) Cost-effectiveness of hemofiltration to prevent contrast nephropathy in patients with chronic kidney disease. *Crit Care Med*;34:1044–1051.

Kshirsagar AV, Poole C, Mottl A, et al. (2004) N-acetylcysteine for the prevention of radiocontrast induced nephropathy: a meta-analysis of prospective controlled trials. *J Am Soc Nephrol*; 15:761–769.

Kushner FG, Hand M, Smith SC Jr, et al. (2009) focused updates: ACC/AHA guidelines for the management of patients with ST-elevation myocardial infarction (updating the 2004 guideline and 2007 focused update) and ACC/AHA/SCAI guidelines on percutaneous coronary intervention (updating the 2005 guideline and 2007 focused update). A report of the American College of Cardiology Foundation/American Heart Association Task Force on Practice Guidelines. *J Am Coll Cardiol*; 54:2205–2241.

Laskey WK, Jenkins C, Selzer F, et al. (2007)Volume-to-creatinine clearance ratio. *J Am Coll Cardiol*; 50:584–590.

Lee PT, Chou KJ, Liu CP, etal. (2007) Renal protection for coronary angiography in advanced renal failure patients by prophylactic hemodialysis. A randomized controlled trial. *J Am Coll Cardiol*;50:1015–1020.

Liss P, Nygren A, Erikson U, Ulfendahl HR. (1998) Injection of low and iso-osmolar contrast medium decreases oxygen tension in the renal medulla. *Kidney Int*;53:698–702.

Liss P, Carlsson PO, Palm F, Hansell P. (2004) Adenosine A1 receptors in contrast media-induced renal dysfunction in the normal rat. *Eur Radiol*;14:1297–1302.

Liss P, Eklöf H, Hellberg O, etal. (2005) Renal effects of CO2 and iodinated contrast media in patients undergoing renovascular intervention: a prospective, randomized study. *J Vasc Interv Radiol*.;16(1):57.

Liss P, Persson PB, Hansell P, Lagerqvist B. (2006) Renal failure in 57 925 patients undergoing coronary procedures using isosmolar or low-osmolar contrast media. *Kidney Int* ;70:1811–1817.

Liu R, Nair D, Ix J, et al. (2005) N-acetylcysteine for the prevention of contrast- induced nephropathy: a systematic review and meta-analysis. *J Gen Intern Med*;20:193–200.
Manske CL, Sprafka JM, Strony JT, Wang Y. (1990) Contrast nephropathy in azotemic diabetic patients undergoing coronary angiography. *Am J Med*; 89:615–620.
Maioli M, Toso A, Leoncini M, etal. (2008) Sodium bicarbonate versus Saline for the prevention of contrast-induced nephropathy in Patients with renal dysfunction undergoing coronary angiography or intervention. *J Am Coll Cardiol*;52:599–604.
Marenzi G, Marana I, Lauri G, et al. (2003) The prevention of radio contrast- agent induced nephropathy by hemofiltration. *N Engl J Med*; 349:1333–1340.
Marenzi G, Lauri G, Assanelli E, et al. (2004) Contrast-induced nephropathy in patients undergoing primary angioplasty for acute myocardial infarction. *J Am Coll Cardiol*; 44:1780–1785.
Marenzi G, Lauri G, Campodonico J, et al. (2006b) Comparison of two hemofiltration protocols for prevention of contrast-induced nephropathy in high –risk patients. *Am J Med*; 119:155-162
Marenzi G, Assanelli E, Marana I, etal. (2006a) N-acetylcysteine and contrast-induced nephropathy in primary angioplasty. *N Engl J Med*;354:2773–2782.
Marenzi G, Assanelli E, Campodonico J, etal. (2009) Contrast volume during primary percutaneous coronary intervention and subsequent contrast-induced nephropathy and mortality. *Ann Intern Med*; 150:170–177.
Masuda M, Yamada T, Mine T, et al. (2007) Comparison of usefulness of sodium bicarbonate versus sodium chloride to prevent contrast-induce nephropathy in patients undergoing emergent coronary procedure. *Am J Cardiol*; 100:781–786.
McCullough PA, Wolyn R, Rocher LL, et al. (1997) Acute renal failure after coronary intervention: incidence, risk factors, and relationship to mortality. *Am J Med*; 103:368–375.
McCullough P A, Soman S S. (2005) Contrast-induced nephropathy. *Crit Care Clin*; 21:261–280.
McCullough PA, Adam A, Becker CR, etal. (2006a) Epidemiology and prognostic implications of contrast-induced nephropathy. *Am J Cardiol*;98:5K–13K.
McCullough PA, Adam A, Becker CR, et al. (2006b) Risk prediction of contras induced nephropathy. *Am J Cardiol*; 98:27K–36K.
McCullough PA, Bertrand ME, Brinker JA, Stacul F. (2006c) A meta-analysis of the renal safety of isosmolar iodixanol compared with low-osmolar contrast media. *J Am Coll Cardiol*; 48:692–699.
Mehran R, Aymong ED, Nikolsky E, et al. (2004) A simple risk score for prediction of contrast-induced nephropathy after percutaneous coronary intervention: development and initial validation. *J Am Coll Cardiol*; 44:1393–1399.
Merten GJ, Burgess WP, Gray LV, et al. (2004) Prevention of contrast-induced nephropathy with sodium bicarbonate: a randomized controlled trial. *JAMA*; 291:2328–2334.
Mockel M, Radovic M, Kuhnle Y, etal. (2008) Acute renal haemodynamic effects of radiocontrast media in patients undergoing left ventricular and coronary angiography. *Nephrol Dial Transplant*;23:1588–1594
Morcos S K, Thomsen H S, Webb J A W and members of contrast media safety committee of the European Society of Urogenital Radiology (ESUR). (1999) Contrast media induced nephropathy: a consensus report. *Eur Radiol*;9:1602-1613.

Morcos SK, Thomsen HS, Webb JA. (2002) Dialysis and contrast media. *Eur Radiol*; 12: 3026–3030.

Morcos SK. (2005) Prevention of contrast media-induced nephrotoxicity after angiographic procedures. *J Vasc Interv Radiol*;16:13–23.

Mueller C, Buerkle G, Buettner HJ, et al. (2002) Prevention of contrast media associated nephropathy: randomized comparison of 2 hydration regimens in 1620 patients undergoing coronary angioplasty. *Arch Intern Med*; 162:329–336.

Nallamothu BK, Shojania KG, Saint S, et al. (2004) Is acetylcysteine effective in preventing contrast-related nephropathy? A meta-analysis. Am J Med; 117:938–947.

Nash K, Hafeez A, Hou S. (2002) Hospital-acquired renal insufficiency. *Am J Kidney Dis*; 39:930–936.

Nikolsky E, Mehran R, Lasic Z, etal. (2005) Low hematocrit predicts contrast-induced nephropathy after percutaneous coronary interventions. *Kidney Int*;67:706–713.

Onbasili AO, Yenicerioglu Y, Agaoglu P, et al. (2007) Trimetazidine in the prevention of contrast-induced nephropathy after coronary procedures. *Heart*;93:654-655.

Ozcan EA, Guneri S, Akdeniz B, et al. (2007) Sodium bicarbonate, N acetylcysteine, and saline for prevention of radio-contrast-induced nephropathy. A comparison of 3 regimens for protecting contrast-induced nephropathy in patients undergoing coronary procedures. A single-center prospective controlled trial. *Am Heart J*; 154:539–544.

Pannu N, Manns B, Lee H, Tonelli M. (2004) Systematic review of the impact of N-acetylcysteine on contrast nephropathy. *Kidney Int*; 65:1366–1374

Peer A, Averbukh Z, Berman S, etal.(2003) Contrast media augmented apoptosis of cultured renal mesangial, tubular, epithelial, endothelial, and hepatic cells. *Invest Radiol*; 38:177–182

PerazellaMA.(2009)Radiocontrast-induced nephropathy: an update. *Minerva Urol Nefrol* ; 61:215-233.

Persson PB (2005).Contrast medium-induced nephropathy. *Nephrol Dial Transplant*; 20 Suppl 1:i1

Persson PB, Tepel M.(2006) Contrast medium-induced nephropathy: the pathophysiology. *Kidney Int Suppl*; 100:S8–10.

Pflueger A, Larson TS, Nath KA, et al. (2000) Role of adenosine in contrast media induced acute renal failure in diabetes mellitus. *Mayo Clin Proc*; 75:1275–1283.

Ranucci M, Ballotta A, Kunkl A, et al.(2008)Influence of the timing of cardiac catheterization and the amount of contrast media on acute renal failure after cardiac surgery. *Am J Cardiol*; 101:1112–1118.

Recio-Mayoral A, Chaparro M, Prado B, et al. (2007) The reno-protective effect of hydration with sodium bicarbonate plus N-acetylcysteine in patients undergoing emergency percutaneous coronary intervention: the RENO study. *J Am Coll Cardiol*; 49:1283–1288.

Reed M, Meier P, Tamhane U U, etal.(2009)The relative safety of Iodixanol compared with low-osmolar contrast media: a meta-analysis of randomized controlled trials. *J Am Coll Cardiol*;2:645-654.

Ribeiro L, de Assuncao e Silva F, Kurihara RS, etal. (2004) Evaluation of the nitric oxide production in rat renal artery smooth muscle cells culture exposed to radiocontrast agents. *Kidney Int*; 65: 589–96.

Ribichini F, Graziani M, Gambaro G, etal. (2010) Early Creatinine shifts Predict Contrast-induced Nephropathy and persistent renal damage after angiography. *Am J Med;* 123:755-763.

Rihal CS, Textor SC, Grill DE, et al. (2002) Incidence and prognostic importance of acute renal failure after percutaneous coronary intervention. *Circulation;* 105:2259–2264.

Rudnick M R,Goldfarb S,Wexler L,etal. (1995)Nephrotoxicity of ionic and nonionic contrast media in 1196 patients: A randomized trial: the Iohexol Cooperative Study. *KidneyInt;*47:254-261.

Rudnick M, Kesselheim A, Goldfarb S. (2006) Contrast-induced nephropathy: how it develops, how to prevent it. *Cleveland Clin J Med;* 73:75–87.

Rudnick M, Goldfarb S. (2003) Pathogenesis of contrast-induced nephropathy: Experimental and clinical observations with an emphasis on the role of osmolality. *Rev Cardiovasc ed;* 4 (Suppl 5):S28–S33.

Rudnick MR, Davidson C, Laskey W, et al.(2008) Nephrotoxicity of iodixanol versus ioversol in patients with chronic renal disease. The visipaque angiography /interventions with laboratory outcomes in renal insufficiency (VALOR) trial. *Am Heart J;*156:776-782.

Rudnick M, Feldman H. (2008) Contrast-induced nephropathy: what are the true clinical consequences? *Clin J Am Soc Nephrol;* 3:263–272.

Sayol A J, Bush W H. (2011) Avoidable errors in dealing with anaphylactoid reactions to iodinated contrast media. *Invest Radiol;*46: 147–151.

Seeliger E, Flemming B, Wronski T, et al.(2007) Viscosity of contrast media perturbs renal hemodynamics. *J Am Soc Nephrol;* 18:2912–2920.

Shah SH, Mehta RL. Acute kidney injury in critical care:time for a paradigm shift? *Curr Opin Nephrol Hypertens* 2006;15:561- 565.

Shaw DR, Kessel DO. (2006) The current status of the use of carbon dioxide in diagnostic and interventional angiographic procedures. *Cardiovasc Intervent Radiol.* ;29(3):323.

Solomon R, Werner C, Mann D, et al. (1994) Effects of saline, mannitol, and furosemide to prevent acute decreases in renal function induced by radiocontrast agents. *N Engl J Med;* 331:1416–1420.

Solomon R. (2005)The role of osmolality in the incidence of contrast induced nephropathy: A systematic review of angiographic contrast media in high risk patients. *Kidney Int;*68:2256–2263.

Solomon R, Dumouchel W. (2006) Contrast media and nephropathy: findings from systematic analysis and Food and Drug Administration reports of adverse effects. *Invest Radiol;* 41:651-660.

Solomon R , Natarajan MK, Doucet S, et al. (2007) Cardiac angiography in renally impaired patients (CARE) study: A randomized double-blind trial of contrast induced nephropathy in patients with chronic kidney disease. *Circulation;* 115:3189–3196.

Solomon RJ, Mehran R, Natarajan MK, et al. (2009) Contrast-induced nephropathy and long-term adverse events: cause and effect? *Clin J Am Soc Nephrol;* 4:1162–1169.

Spargias K, Alexopoulos E, Kyrzopoulos S, et al. (2004) Ascorbic acid prevents contrast-mediated nephropathy in patients with renal dysfunction undergoing coronary angiography or intervention. *Circulation;* 110:2837–2842.

Stevens MA, McCullough PA, Tobin KJ, et al. (1999) A prospective randomized trial of prevention measures in patients at high risk for contrast nephropathy: results of the

P.R.I.N.C.E. study. Prevention of radiocontrast induced nephropathy clinical evaluation. *J Am Coll Cardiol*; 33:403–411.

Subramanian S, Tumlin J, Bapat B, Zyczynski T. (2007) Economic burden of contrast-induced nephropathy: implications for prevention strategies. *J Med Econ*; 10:119–134.

Taylor AJ, Hotchkiss D, Morse RW, McCabe J. (1998) PREPARED: Preparation for angiography in Renal Dysfunction: a randomized trial of inpatient vs. outpatient hydration protocols for cardiac catheterization in mild-to-moderate renal dysfunction. *Chest*; 114:1570–1574.

Tepel M, van der Giet M, Schwarzfeld C, et al. (2000) Prevention of radiographic contrast-agent-induced reductions in renal function by acetylcysteine. *N EnglJ Med*; 343:180–184.

Tepel M, Aspelin P, Lameire N. (2006) Contrast-induced nephropathy: a clinical and evidence-based approach. *Circulation*;113:1799–806.

The Committee on Drugs and Contrast Media of the American College of Radiology (2010). Contrast nephropathy. In: *ACR manual oncontrast media,Version 7*.28 American College of Radiology, Retrieved from: http://www.acr.org/ secondarymainmenucategories/quality_safety/contrast_manual/fullmanual.aspx

Thomsen H S. (2005)How to avoid CIN: guidelines from the European Society of Urogenital Radiology. *Nephrol Dial Transplant*; 20 (Suppl 1):i18- i22.

Thomsen H S, Morcos S K, Members of Contrast Media Safety Committee of European Society of Urogenital Radiology (ESUR). (2005) In which patients should serum creatinine be measured before contrast medium administration? *Eur Radiol*, 15: 749–756.

Thomsen H S, Morcos SK. (2006) ESUR guidelines on contrast media. *Abdom Imaging*; 31: 131–140.

Thomsen HS. (2006) Reducing the risk of contrast media induced nephrotoxicity. In: *Contrast media: safety issues and ESUR Guidelines*. Thomsen HS (ed) 53–55 Springer, 978-3-540-72783-5 Heidelberg Berlin New York,; pp.

Thomsen HS, Morcos SK, Erley CM, et al. (2008)The ACTIVE trial: comparison of the effects on renal function of iomeprol-400 and iodixanol-320 in patients with chronic kidney disease undergoing abdominal computed tomography. *Invest Radiol*; 43:170–178.

Toprak O, Cirit M, Bayata S, etal. (2003) The effect of preprocedural captopril on contrast-induced nephropathy in patients who underwent coronary angiography. (abstract) *Anadolu Kardiyol Derg*;3:98-103.

Toprak O, Cirit M.(2006) Risk factors and therapy strategies for contrast-inducednephropathy. *Renal Fail*;28:365–381.

Trivedi HS, Moore H, Nasr S, et al. (2003) A randomized prospective trial to assess the role of saline hydration on the development of contrast nephrotoxicity. *Nephron Clin Pract*; 93:c29–c34.

Ultramari FT, Bueno Rda R, da Cunha CL, et al.(2006)Contrast media-induced nephropathy following diagnostic and therapeutic cardiac catheterization. *Arq bras Cardiol*; 87:378–90.

Vasheghani -Farahani A, Sadigh G, Kassaian S E etal. (2009)Sodium Bicarbonate Plus Isotonic Saline Versus Saline for Prevention of contrast-induced nephropathy in patients undergoing coronary angiography: A randomized controlled trial; *Am J Kidney Dis* 54:610-618.

Vasheghani-Farahani A ,Sadigh G ,Kassaian S, etal. (2010) Sodium bicarbonate in preventing contrast nephropathy in patients at risk for volume overload: a randomized controlled trial. *J Nephrol*; 23:216–223.

Vogt B, Ferrari P, Schonholzer C, et al. (2001) Prophylactic hemodialysis after radiocontrast media in patients with renal insufficiency is potentially harmful. *Am J Med*; 111: 692–698.

Weinmann H J, Platzec J, Schirmer H etal.(2005) Contrast media: future aspects. *Eur Radiol*15 (Suppl4):D70-D73

Weisberg LS, Kurnik PB, Kurnik BR (1992) Radiocontrastinduced nephropathy in humans: role of renal vasoconstriction. *Kidney Int* 41:1408–1415.

Weisberg LS, Kurnik PB, Kurnik BR. (1994) Risk of radiocontrast nephropathy in patients with and without diabetes mellitus. *Kidney Int*;45:259–265.

Weisbord SD, Chen H, Stone RA, etal.(2006)Associations of increases in serum Creatinine with mortality and length of hospital stay after coronary angiography. *J Am Soc Nephrol* ; 17:2871–2877.

Weisbord SD, Pavelsky PM. (2008) Prevention of contrast-induced nephropathy with volume expansion. *Clin J Am Soc Nephrol*; 3:273–280.

Yokomaku Y, Sugimoto T, Kume S, et al. (2008) Asialoerythropoietin prevents contrast-induced nephropathy. *J Am Soc Nephrol*; 19:321–328.

Zagler A, Azadpour M, Mercado C, Hennekens CH. (2006) N-acetylcysteine and contrast-induced nephropathy: a meta-analysis of 13 randomized trials. *Am Heart J*; 151:140–145.

8

Complications of Cardiac Catetherization

Mariano García-Borbolla[1], Rafael García-Borbolla[2] and Begoña Balboa[3]
[1]Hospital Virgen Macarena
[2]Hospital de Jerez
[3]Hospital Virgen del Rocio
Spain

1. Introduction

Cardiac catheterization was primarily a diagnostic procedure that was used to evaluate hemodynamics, ventricular function, and coronary anatomy. However, the introduction of improved angioplasty equipment and new interventional devices in the 1980s made catheterization an important tool in the treatment of cardiovascular disease.

Although diagnostic catheterization and percutaneous coronary intervention are done by skin puncture rather than incision, and under local rather than general anesthesia, they can cause a variety of adverse events, ranging from minor problems without long-term sequelae to major complications requiring immediate corrective action. Furthermore, newer interventional procedures may be associated with different and, in some cases, more frequent complications.

2. Major complications

The risk of producing a major complication (death, myocardial infarction, or major embolization) during diagnostic cardiac catheterization is generally well below 1 percent. As a result, the risk-to-benefit ratio still favors performing this procedure as a part of the evaluation of potentially fatal or lifestyle limiting cardiac disease.

The risk of an adverse event, for the individual patient, is dependent upon demographics, cardiovascular anatomy, clinical circumstances including comorbidities, the experience of the operator, and the type of procedure being performed (**table 1 A-C**) [1]. Severe peripheral artery disease is a risk factor for all of the major complications.

2.1 Death

Death following diagnostic cardiac catheterization is now rare. Compared with the 1 percent mortality rate seen in the 1960s, the second registry of the Society for Cardiac Angiography revealed that the procedural mortality had fallen to 0.1 percent in the more than 200,000 patients catheterized between 1984 and 1987 [2].

High-risk subgroups have been identified in multiple large series [1-9]:

	Percent
Mortality	0.11
Myocardial infarction	0.05
Cerebrovascular accident	0.07
Arrhythmia	0.38
Vascular complications	0.43
Contrast reaction	0.37
Hemodynamic complications	0.26
Perforation of heart chamber	0.28
Other complications	0.28
Total of major complications	1.70

Noto, TJ Jr, Johnson, LW, Krone, R, et al. Cardiac catheterization 1990: A report of the Registry of the Society for Cardiac Angiography and Interventions (SCA&I). Cathet Cardiovasc Diagn 1991; 24:75.

Table 1. (A): Risk of cardiac catheterization and coronary angiography (based on 59,792 patients)

Variable	Odds ratio
Moribund	10.22
Shock	6.52
Acute MI <24 h	4.03
Renal insufficiency	3.30
Cardiomyopathy	3.29
Aortic valve disease	2.72
Mitral valve disease	2.33
Heart failure	2.33
New York Heart Association Functional	
Class I	1.00
Class II	1.15
Class III	1.32
Class IV	1.52
Hypertension	1.45
Unstable angina	1.42
Outpatient/inpatient	0.63

Moribund indicates a patient who responds poorly due to a life threatening condition.
MI: myocardial infarction.
Scanlon, PJ, Faxon, DP, Audet, AM, et al, J Am Coll Cardiol 1999; 33:1756.

Table 1. (B): Multivariate predictors of major complications of coronary angiography (based on 58,332 procedures)

Acute renal failure
Chronic renal failure secondary to diabetes
Active gastrointestinal bleeding
Unexplained fever, which may be due to infection
Untreated active infection
Acute stroke
Severe anemia
Severe uncontrolled hypertension
Severe symptomatic electrolyte imbalance
Severe lack of cooperation by patient due to psychological or severe systemic illness
Severe concomitant illness that drastically shortens life expectancy or increases risk of therapeutic interventions
Refusal of patient to consider definitive therapy such as PTCA, CABG, or valve replacement
Digitalis intoxication
Documented anaphylactoid reaction to angiographic contrast media
Severe peripheral vascular disease limiting vascular access
Decompensated heart failure or acute pulmonary edema
Severe coagulopathy
Aortic valve endocarditis

PTCA: percutaneoas transluminal coronary angioplasty; CABG: coronary artety bypass graft.
Scanlon, PJ, Faxon, DP, Audet, AM, et al, J Am Coll Cardiol 1999; 33:1756.

Table 1. (C): Relative contraindications to coronary angiography

- Patients with valvular heart disease, chronic kidney disease, diabetes mellitus requiring insulin therapy, peripheral artery disease, cerebrovascular disease, and pulmonary insufficiency all appear to have an increased incidence of death and major complications from cardiac catheterization. Mortality is especially high in those with preexisting renal insufficiency who have further deterioration of renal function within 48 hours after the procedure, particularly when dialysis is required [10].
- A similar increase in risk is seen with severe disease of the left main coronary artery (compared to single vessel disease) and with a left ventricular ejection fraction (LVEF) below 30 percent (compared to an LVEF above 50 percent).
- Age above 60 years and below one year and women have an increased mortality rate after catheterization.
- New York Heart Association functional class IV is associated with an almost tenfold increase in mortality compared with classes I and II (**table 2**).

Class	New York Heart Association functional classification	Canadian Cardiovascular Society functional classification	Specific activity scale
I	Patients with cardiac disease but without resulting limitations of physical activity. Ordinary physical activity does not cause undue fatigue, palpitation, dyspnea, or anginal pain.	Ordinary physical activity, such as walking and climbing stairs, does not cause angina. Angina with strenuous or rapid prolonged exertion at work or recreation.	Patients can perform to completion any activity requiring ≥7 metabolic equivalents, eg, can carry 24 lb up eight steps; do outdoor work (shovel snow, spade soil); do recreational activities (skiing, basketball, squash, handball, jog/walk 5 mph).
II	Patients with cardiac disease resulting in slight limitation of physical activity. They are comfortable at rest. Ordinary physical activity results in fatigue, palpitation, dyspnea, or anginal pain.	Slight limitation of ordinary activity. Walking or climbing stairs rapidly, walking uphill, walking or stair climbing after meals, in cold, in wind, or when under emotional stress, or only during the few hours after awakening. Walking more than two blocks on the level and climbing more than one flight of ordinary stairs at a normal pace and in normal conditions.	Patients can perform to completion any activity requiring ≤ 5 metabolic equivalents, eg, have sexual intercourse without stopping, garden, rake, weed, roller skate, dance fox trot, walk at 4 mph on level ground, but cannot and do not perform to completion activities requiring ≥ 7 metabolic equivalents.
III	Patients with cardiac disease resulting in marked limitation of physical activity. They are comfortable at rest. Less than ordinary physical activity causes fatigue, palpitation, dyspnea, or anginal pain.	Marked limitation of ordinary physical activity. Walking one to two blocks on the level and climbing more than one flight in normal conditions.	Patients can perform to completion any activity requiring ≤ 2 metabolic equivalents, eg, shower without stopping, strip and make bed, clean windows, walk 2.5 mph, bowl, play golf, dress without stopping, but cannot and do not perform to completion any activities requiring > 5 metabolic equivalents.
IV	Patient with cardiac disease resulting in inability to carry on any physical activity without discomfort. Symptoms of cardiac insufficiency or of the anginal syndrome may be present even at rest. If any physical activity is undertaken, discomfort is increased.	Inability to carry on any physical activity without discomfort - anginal syndrome may be present at rest.	Patients cannot or do not perform to completion activities requiring > 2 metabolic equivalents. Cannot carry out activities listed above (Specific activity scale III).

Table 2. Comparison of three methods of assessing cardiovascular disability

2.2 Myocardial infarction

Although periprocedural myocardial ischemia is fairly common, infarction is rare. The general risk of myocardial infarction (MI) in most series is less than 0.1 percent [2-7]. However, the risk of precipitating an MI in an individual patient is influenced by patient-related and technique-related factors. Risk factors that predispose patients to MI during the procedure include:

- Recent non-ST elevation acute coronary syndrome.
- Extension of disease (0.17 percent with left main coronary disease versus 0.06 percent in single vessel disease) [2].
- Diabetes mellitus requiring insulin therapy [1].

2.3 Stroke and transient ischemic attack

A stroke is a rare but potentially devastating complication of cardiac catheterization. The incidence of stroke was 0.07 to 0.10 percent in an analysis of two large databases [2,11] and has more recently been reported to be as high as 0.2 to 0.4 percent [12]. Risk factors for stroke include the severity of coronary artery disease, the length of fluoroscopy time, diabetes, hypertension, prior stroke, or renal failure [11,12]

Stroke and transient ischemic attacks are thought to be caused by disruption of atheromatous plaques on the walls of the aorta. The risk of intracerebral hemorrhage is increased in those receiving anticoagulation or thrombolytic therapy as well as with any of the following: age ≥75 years; female sex; systolic blood pressure ≥160 mmHg; black race; and low body weight (**table 3**). Based on the number of the risk factors present, the rate of intracerebral hemorrhage varies from less than 1 percent to more than 4 percent.

Risk Factors*	
Age ≥75 years	
Black race	
Female sex	
Prior history of stroke	
Systolic blood pressure ≥160 mmHg	
Weight ≤65 kg for women or ≤80 kg for men	
INR >4 or PT >24•	
Use of alteplase (versus other thrombolytic agent)	
Risk score	**Rate of intracranial hemorrhage, percent**
0 or 1	0.69
2	1.02
3	1.63
4	2.49
≥5	4.11

* Each risk factor is worth 1 point if present, 0 points if absent. Points are added to determine the risk score.

• INR: international normalized ratio; PT: prothrombin time.

Brass, LM, Lichtman, JH, Wang, Y, et al. Intracranial hemorrhage associated with thrombolytic therapy for elderly patients with acute myocardial infarction: results from the cooperative cardiovascular project. Stroke 2000; 31:1802.

Table 3. Cooperative cardiovascular project risk model for intracranial hemorrhage with thrombolytic therapy

Meticulous attention to technical factors such as wire and catheter exchanges is mandatory in all patients, regardless of risk. Transient neurologic deficits may also result from the injection of high osmolar contrast agents into the carotid or vertebral arteries. The majority of patients with a periprocedural stroke have an unfavorable neurologic outcome and, in one study, the in-hospital mortality was 32 percent [11].

2.4 Role of valvular aortic stenosis

The risk of stroke may be particularly high in patients with valvular aortic stenosis (AS) who undergo retrograde catheterization of the aortic valve [13,14]. This was demonstrated in a study of 152 patients with severe AS (mean age 71 years) who were randomly assigned to cardiac catheterization with or without catheter passage through the valve [13]. The following findings were noted:

- Detailed neurologic examination done before and after the catheterization demonstrated clinically apparent deficits in 3 percent of those who underwent retrograde catheterization, but in none of the other patients.
- Cranial MRI done before and after the catheterization demonstrated focal lesions consistent with cerebral emboli in 22 percent of those who underwent retrograde catheterization of the aortic valve, but in none of the patients who did not.

As a result, retrograde catheterization should be performed with caution in patients with severe calcific AS and only when the information sought cannot be reliably obtained noninvasively [14].

2.5 Asymptomatic embolic events

The incidence of stroke after cardiac catheterization was 0.07 to 0.10 percent in an analysis of two large databases [2,11]. However, asymptomatic embolic events are much more common [13,15,16].

This was illustrated in a prospective study of 48 patients (mean age 62 years) who underwent cardiac catheterization and angiography and, in some patients, percutaneous coronary intervention; magnetic resonance imaging (MRI) was performed before and about 24 hours after the procedure [15]. There were no embolic lesions on diffusionweighted imaging at baseline, but seven patients (15 percent) had nine cerebral infarcts after the procedure; all were asymptomatic.

Similar findings were noted in a report of 47 unselected patients in whom transcranial Doppler was used to detect microemboli and MRI to detect new lesions [16]. The median number of solid (ie, not gaseous) microemboli was significantly higher with a transradial compared to a transfemoral access (57 versus 36). New MRI lesions occurred in 5 of 33 patients (15 percent) after transradial catheterization, compared to none of nine after transfemoral catheterization. Most of the patients with new lesions remained asymptomatic.

These observations suggest that catheter manipulation in the diseased aortic root releases small pieces of atherosclerotic debris more commonly than suspected, based upon the fortunately low incidence of clinically apparent stroke. The same principles presumably apply to peripheral embolism.

3. Local vascular complications

Local complications at the site of catheter insertion are among the most common problems seen after cardiac catheterization.

These problems may include acute thrombosis, distal embolization, dissection or poorly controlled bleeding (which may be manifested as free hemorrhage or contained hematoma in the femoral or retroperitoneal areas), pseudoaneurysm, or arteriovenous fistula. Hemorrhage and hematoma are usually evident within 12 hours after the procedure by virtue of local discomfort, hypotension, or falling hematocrit, which lead to confirmatory noninvasive testing (ultrasound or CT). In contrast, other complications such as pseudoaneurysm and arteriovenous fistula may not become apparent for days to weeks afterward.

3.1 Hemostasis at the access site

The traditional approach to catheter removal at the conclusion of cardiac catheterization was local hand-applied pressure for 15 to 30 minutes.

Two alternative approaches are available: mechanical clamp compression and more importantly, arterial puncture closing devices:

3.1.1 Mechanical clamp

Mechanical clamp compression reduces the amount of staff time and effort required to assure hemostasis, and may reduce the rate of vascular complications. One trial randomly assigned 778 patients to hand applied pressure or mechanical clamp pressure; the latter reduced the frequency of ultrasound-defined femoral vascular complications (femoral artery thrombosis, echogenic hematoma, pseudoaneurysm, or arteriovenous fistulae formation) by 63 percent [17]. However, clamping does not decrease the importance of having staff in attendance to ensure that the device is placed and remains in the correct position.

The circumstances which may make mechanical clamps the preferred method of achieving hemostasis include procedures where longer hemostasis time is anticipated: larger sheaths, excessively anticoagulated patients, recognized hematoma, and dual antiplatelet therapy

3.1.2 Closure devices

Arterial puncture closing devices (APCDs) eliminate the need for prolonged arterial compression and reduce the subsequent interval of bed rest that is otherwise required. Two types of APCDs in clinical use include collagen hemostatic puncture closure devices [18-21] and suture-mediated devices [22].

APCDs may increase the risk of local vascular complications. In a meta-analysis of 30 trials including 4000 patients who underwent coronary angiography or PCI, nonsignificant increases in the incidence of groin hematoma, bleeding, and pseudoaneurysm formation were associated with use of these devices compared to manual compression [23]. When only those trials with an intention-to-treat analysis were included, the relative risks of groin hematoma and pseudoaneurysm formation were significantly increased (1.89 and 5.40, respectively).

A larger meta-analysis that included 30 studies involving 37,066 patients concluded that the risk of complications depended upon the specific device used and whether the procedure was a diagnostic catheterization or a PCI [24]. In the overall analysis, there was a significant increase in risk with an APCD (odds ratio [OR] 1.34, 95% CI 1.01- 1.79). For reports limited to diagnostic studies, there were no significant differences between APCDs and mechanical compression, although there were trends toward fewer complications with the AngioSeal

device (OR 0.71) and toward more complications with the VasoSeal and Perclose devices (OR 1.85 and 1.51, respectively).
For reports limited to PCI, there were no significant differences between APCDs and mechanical compression overall. However, there was a significant increase in vascular complications with the VasoSeal device (OR 2.52).
Closure devices also increase the risk of local infection or endarteritis [25,26]. Although this complication is infrequent (0.3 percent in one series) [26], it can be serious when it occurs. Consideration should be given to periprocedural antibiotics in immunocompromised patients following prolonged arterial access or when sterility has been breached when a closure device is used. It may also be prudent for the operator to change gloves prior to using an arterial closure device. (See 'Infection' below.) An angiogram of the femoral artery should be performed prior to use of an APCD. Use ofclosure devices should be avoided if a hematoma has formed during the procedure, or in the presence of severe iliofemoral vascular disease, and when the access site is below the bifurcation of the superficial and profunda femoral arteries.

3.1.3 Prior warfarin therapy

Among patients who are being treated with warfarin, the optimal approach is to withhold warfarin and wait until the INR reaches 1.5 before proceeding with catheterization. When the procedure cannot be delayed, it has been suggested that, in patients with an INR of 2.0 to 3.0, manual pressure hemostasis may be sufficient to prevent excess bleeding [27]. In patients with an INR >3.0, administration of fresh frozen plasma prior to arterial sheath removal may be warranted. The transradial approach may also be useful in such cases. The risk of local bleeding in warfarin-treated patients is likely to be greater in those undergoing PCI who are often treated with heparin, clopidogrel, and a glycoprotein IIb/IIIa inhibitor. These patients typically have longer intraarterial times and more manipulation of the arterial access site.increase in risk is seen with severe disease of the left main coronary artery (compared to single vessel disease) and with a left ventricular ejection fraction (LVEF) below 30 percent (compared to an LVEF above 50 percent).

3.2 Hematoma formation

Hematoma formation is not uncommon in the soft tissue of the upper thigh and the patient should be advised that the development of a large area of ecchymosis is likely. Although most resolve over a period of days, femoral nerve compression can occur, which may take weeks to months to resolve. Patients should be advised to avoid strenuous activity or lifting heavy objects within the first week following arterial catheterization. Surgical repair for a hematoma is generally not required.

3.2.1 Retroperitoneal extension

If the arterial puncture occurs above the inguinal ligament, hematoma may extend into the retroperitoneal space, causing hypotension and ipsilateral flank pain. CT scanning or abdominal ultrasonography can help to establish the diagnosis. Treatment is usually conservative, consisting of bed rest and blood transfusion rather than surgical correction. Reversal of systemic anticoagulation may be indicated if bleeding persists or is associated with hemodynamic compromise.

3.3 Arteriovenous fistula

Ongoing bleeding from the arterial puncture site may decompress into the adjacent venous puncture site, leading to the formation of an arteriovenous fistula. This complication may be recognized by the presence of a thrill or continuous bruit at the site of catheter insertion. Surgical repair is usually necessary, since fistulae tend to enlarge over time. The most common finding at surgery is a puncture site below the common femoral artery, which illustrates the importance of careful technique in avoiding this complication [1].

3.4 Prior pseudoaneurysm

If a hematoma remains in continuity with the arterial lumen, a pseudoaneurysm may develop with blood flow into and out of the hematoma cavity during systole and diastole. A pseudoaneurysm is most often recognized by the presence of a pulsatile mass with a systolic bruit over the catheter insertion site; it can be confirmed by duplex ultrasonography. Almost all pseudoaneurysms occur within the first three days after removal of the arterial sheath, and most of the remaining cases by seven days after sheath removal [28].

The main risk factor for pseudoaneurysm formation is an inadequate period of manual compression. This was illustrated in a series of 581 angiographic procedures involving transfemoral arterial catheterization [29]. A pseudoaneurysm occurred in 14 percent of the first 300 procedures in which standard manual compression was performed, compared to 1.1 percent of the next 281 procedures when manual compression was continued for at least five minutes after local bleeding had stopped.

Other risk factors include large bore sheaths, postprocedural anticoagulation, antiplatelet therapy during the intervention, age >65 years, obesity, hypertension, peripheral artery disease, hemodialysis, cannulation of the superficial rather than common femoral artery, and complex interventions [28-30].

Surgical management should be performed when a pseudoaneurysm occurs at the site of a vascular anastomosis, becomes very large and threatens or causes skin necrosis, is expanding rapidly, occurs spontaneously, as it may be infected, or there is a failure of a minimally invasive procedure [30]. Expanding hematomas have a propensity towards eventual rupture, especially if the patient is maintained on anticoagulation [1,7,31,32].

Treatment of smaller pseudoaneurysms may be accomplished with either direct ultrasound-guided compression or with ultrasound-guided local injection of thrombin or collagen into the pseudoaneurysm cavity, which has a higher success rate [28,33-35]. Although an effective approach, ultrasound-guided compression is uncomfortable for both the patient and the person applying compression.

The success rate of ultrasound-guided injection of bovine thrombin was illustrated in a series of 240 patients with simple or complex pseudoaneurysms [28]. The primary success rate was 96 percent with simple pseudoaneurysms and 89 percent with complex pseudoaneurysms. The secondary success rate was 99.6 percent (all but one patient). The authors also reviewed 34 studies with 1388 patients; the overall success rate was 97.2 percent.

The high success rate of ultrasound-guided injection has made it the treatment of choice for most postcatheterization pseudoaneurysms [30]. However, the procedure should not be performed when, as defined above, there is an indication for surgical management.

In rare cases, pseudoaneurysms less than 2 cm can be managed conservatively and monitored by serial imaging to confirm spontaneous resolution.

3.5 Arterial thrombosis

Arterial thrombosis is rare and occurs slightly more often when the brachial approach is used [3,4]. Predisposing factors to femoral artery thrombosis include small vessel lumen, peripheral artery disease, diabetes mellitus, female sex, placement of a large diameter catheter or sheath (eg, intraaortic balloon pump), or a long catheter dwell time [2-7,31,32].
Patients with lower extremity pain or paresthesia, plus reduced or absent distal pulses not responding to catheter removal, should be evaluated for possible flow obstructing thrombus or dissection. Urgent vascular surgery or thrombectomy may be required for preservation of the limb.

3.6 Radial artery access

Local vascular complications appear to occur less frequently with radial artery access. This issue was best addressed in a meta-analysis that evaluated 12 randomized trials including 3224 patients comparing radial with femoral access [36]. The risk of major adverse cardiac events was similar for the two approaches. Radial access was associated with a significantly lower incidence of access site complications (odds ratio 0.20, 95% CI 0.09-0.42), but a significantly higher rate of procedural failure (odds ratio 3.30. 95% CI 1.63-6.71), probably due to the specific technical skills required for this method.

3.6.1 Integrity of the palmar arch

Radial artery cannulation is associated with a 5 to 19 percent chance of radial artery occlusion [37]. This complication is not clinically important in most patients because the hand is perfused by both the radial and ulnar arteries with extensive collateral flow between the two. However, some patients have incomplete palmar arches, which may diminish collateral perfusion, possibly leading to hand ischemia in the presence of radial artery occlusion.
The modified Allen test has traditionally been used to identify patients at increased risk from radial artery catheterization. However, many centers now use pulse oximetry and plethysmography.
The modified Allen test, originally developed to evaluate patients with thromboangiitis obliterans, assesses the adequacy of collateral blood supply from the ulnar artery to the hand via the palmar arches. The test consists of the following steps:

- The patient's hand is initially held high while the fist is clenched and both radial and ulnar arteries are compressed; this allows the blood to drain from the hand.
- The hand is then lowered and the fist is opened.
- After pressure is released over the ulnar artery, color should return to the hand within six seconds, indicating a patent ulnar artery and an intact superficial palmar arch. The test is considered abnormal if 10 seconds or more is required for color to return.

In two large series of patients undergoing cardiac catheterization, an abnormal Allen test result was obtained in 6 and 27 percent [38,39]. The importance of an abnormal test was evaluated in a study of 55 patients undergoing coronary angiography, 20 of whom had an abnormal test [37]. After 30 minutes of subsequent radial artery occlusion, the patients with an abnormal test had significantly reduced blood flow to the thumb and an elevated thumb capillary lactate.
Based upon such observations, radial artery catheterization is usually not performed in patients with an abnormal modified Allen test. A possible exception occurs in patients with

an excessive estimated risk from a femoral approach (eg, severe peripheral artery disease, large abdominal aortic aneurysm, morbid obesity) [37].

The results of the modified Allen test can be altered by a number of factors, including overextension of the wrist, skin tension over the ulnar artery, and operator error. As a result, an appreciable number of false positive and false negative results have been reported [38]. As an alternative, many centers use a more direct assessment of blood flow to the thumb during radial artery occlusion, which can be accomplished with pulse oximetry and plethysmography [38,40].

The traditional modified Allen test was compared to pulse oximetry and plethysmography in a consecutive series of 1010 patients referred for diagnostic cardiac catheterization [38]. The modified Allen test was considered abnormal if palmar blanching persisted for ≥10 seconds after release of ulnar compression. Plethysmography was observed for two minutes during radial artery compression. Plethysmography was characterized as follows:

- **A:** no change in the amplitude of the pulse tracing during compression
- **B:** reduction in amplitude with compression
- **C:** loss of pulse tracing with initial compression, but recovery of flow during two minutes of compression (signifying development of collateral flow)
- **D:** loss of pulse tracing with no recovery

Patients in categories A, B and C were considered to have a patent ulnopalmar arch, and therefore eligible for radial catheterization.

The modified Allen test was abnormal in significantly more patients than plethysmography (6.3 versus 1.5 percent). The authors concluded that plethysmography more accurately demonstrates the adequacy of the ulnopalmar arch, and that the modified Allen test may unnecessarily exclude some patients from radial artery catheterization. However, the number of patients who underwent radial artery catheterization was not reported, and the value of either test for predicting ischemic complications following radial artery catheterization was not assessed.

4. Arrhythmias

A variety of arrhythmias and conduction disturbances can occur during catheterization. The most common, ventricular premature beats, may be induced by catheter introduction into the right or left ventricle, and are generally without clinical importance or impact.

4.1 Ventricular tachycardia or fibrillation

Ventricular tachycardia or fibrillation is rare complications of catheterization, occurring in 0.4 percent of cases in the second registry of the Society for Cardiac Angiography [2]. These arrhythmias may result from excess catheter manipulation or, more commonly, from intracoronary contrast injection. This complication occurs more commonly when ionic and hyperosmolar contrast agents are used.

4.2 Atrial arrhythmias

Atrial arrhythmias can be induced by cardiac catheterization, especially in response to catheter placement into or out of the right atrium during right heart catheterization. These arrhythmias usually do not require immediate treatment unless they produce ischemia or hemodynamic instability.

Atrial flutter is generally well tolerated and can be treated with burst atrial pacing, or electrical or pharmacologic cardioversion. Atrial fibrillation, on the other hand, can cause clinical sequelae in the setting of a rapid ventricular response or if the loss of atrial systole results in hypotension, as in a patient with mitral stenosis or diastolic ventricular dysfunction. Synchronized cardioversion should be performed immediately in patients who are hemodynamically unstable.

4.3 Bradycardia

Bradycardia commonly occurs during coronary angiography, most often at the end of the injection of ionic contrast into the right coronary artery. Forceful coughing helps to clear the contrast, support perfusion, and restore normal cardiac rhythmtachycardia or fibrillation is rare complications of catheterization, occurring in 0.4 percent of cases in the second registry of the Society for Cardiac Angiography [2]. These arrhythmias may result from excess catheter manipulation or, more commonly, from intracoronary contrast injection. This complication occurs more commonly when ionic and hyperosmolar contrast agents are used.

Vasovagal reactions, which can include bradycardia, hypotension, yawning, and/or sweating, are seen in up to 3 percent of patients, particularly if they have pain or are anxious [2]. These reactions may occur with palpation or compression of the artery prior to needle access.

Treatment usually consists of volume administration, atropine (0.5 to 1.0 mg intravenously), and removal of the painful stimulus. Patients with critical coronary or valvular disease may undergo irreversible decompensation from vagally-mediated hypotension. As a result, rapid reversal of hypotension is crucial in this setting.

4.4 Conduction disturbances

Conduction disturbances are a rare cause of bradycardia in the catheterization laboratory. Patients with pre-existing left bundle branch block may develop asystole with right heart catheterization. Patients with pre-existing right bundle branch block may develop asystole during left heart catheterization. Atropine is rarely helpful in patients who develop complete heart block, but its administration is still recommended. Coughing may help support the circulation while the right heart catheter is exchanged for a temporary pacing wire. Prophylactic placement of a temporary pacemaker is not necessary, even in patients with bundle branch block or intervention in the right coronary artery.

Frank asystole is rare and there is generally sufficient time for insertion of a pacing wire through a venous sheath [41].

5. Perforation of the heart or great vessels

Perforation is an extremely rare complication of cardiac catheterization. Higher risk procedures are those that involve stiffer catheters, including transseptal catheterization, endomyocardial biopsy, balloon valvuloplasty, needle pericardiocentesis, and placement of a pacing catheter. Older adult women appear to be at particular risk.

Cardiac perforation is generally heralded by bradycardia and hypotension due to vagal stimulation induced by blood in the pericardium. If the patient is hemodynamically stable, echocardiography is suggested to document the presence of blood in the pericardial space. However, emergent pericardiocentesis should be performed via the subxiphoid approach in the presence of hemodynamic instability.

Since pericardiocentesis is itself associated with complications, it is best performed under echocardiographic guidance or with pressure monitoring. In a study of 91 cases of acute tamponade during catheterization, pericardiocentesis was the only therapy necessary in 82 percent [42].

Reversal of anticoagulation may cause blood in the pericardial space to "gel." As a result, we generally try to aspirate the majority of the blood in the pericardial space prior to the administration of protamine [1].

6. Allergic reactions

Allergic reactions during catheterization may be precipitated by three agents: the local anesthetic, the contrast agent, or protamine sulfate.

6.1 Local anesthetic

In patients claiming previous reaction to a local anesthetic, the use of a preservative-free agent (such as bupivacaine or mepivacaine) may be a safe alternative [1].

6.2 Iodinated contrast agents

Reaction to the contrast agent occurs in up to 1 percent of patients [2-7]. The risk of such a reaction is highest in patients with a history of prior contrast reactions. Other conditions, such as asthma and other atopic diseases, also confer some risk.

There are several steps that can reduce the incidence of a reaction in a high-risk patient:

- Premedication with corticosteroids and H1 antihistamines can reduce the incidence of a severe reaction (eg, bronchospasm or shock) to below 1 percent (**table 4**).
- The patient should receive a nonionic contrast agent. The incidence of crossreactivity in patients who have had previous reactions to older agents is low, although all patients with previous reactions should be premedicated [1]. In the past, nonionic contrast agents were used selectively, given their higher cost.

Prednisone 50 mg orally 13,7, and 1 h prior to procedure [In children: 0.5 to 0.7 mg/kg orally, up to 50 mg]
Diphenhydramine 50 mg PO/IM/ or IV 1 h prior to procedure [In children: 1.25 mg/kg orally, up to 50 mg]
Lower / iso-osmolar RCM should be recommended
Emergency therapy should be available

Table 4. Pretreatment for patients with previous adverse reactions to RCM

However, the cost of nonionic contrast has fallen significantly. Thus, we recommend using nonionic contrast in all patients undergoing coronary angiography.

If a severe reaction does occur, it should be treated in the same manner as anaphylaxis, and can be sometimes be reversed by using boluses of intravenous epinephrine (1:10,000 epinephrine so that 1 mL = 0.1 mg). One mL of this solution should be administered approximately every minute until the arterial pressure is restored.

However, the rapidity of dosing must be adjusted by the degree of hypotension and the level of assessed hypoperfusion. It is rare for a patient to require a total dose of more than 1.0 mg (10 mL).

Contrast-induced acute renal failure represents another complication that is discussed below.

6.3 Protamine

Allergic reactions to protamine sulfate occur occasionally, more often in insulin-dependent diabetic patients who have received NPH insulin (which contains protamine) in the past [1]. The rapid administration of protamine sulfate can also provoke back pain of unknown etiology.

In current practice, protamine is rarely administered. Most diagnostic catheterizations are done without heparin anticoagulation and in most interventional procedures the heparin is either allowed to wear off over the next two to three hours prior to sheath removal, or the sheath is removed in the fully anticoagulated state using an arterial closure device.

7. Atheroembolism

During the process of cardiac catheterization, atheromatous debris is often scraped from the aortic wall. This debris can cause systemic embolization, including cutaneous, renal, retinal, cerebral, and gastrointestinal emboli (**photo 1** and **photo 2** and **photo 3**). To minimize the risk of stroke or visual impairment, arterial catheter exchanges are best performed over a wire in the descending aorta at the level of the diaphragm (for closed loop catheters) and in the ascending aorta for angiographic catheters. Once arterial access has been obtained, the practice of readvancing the guidewire through the infrarenal aorta rather than exchanging it through a catheter should be avoided.

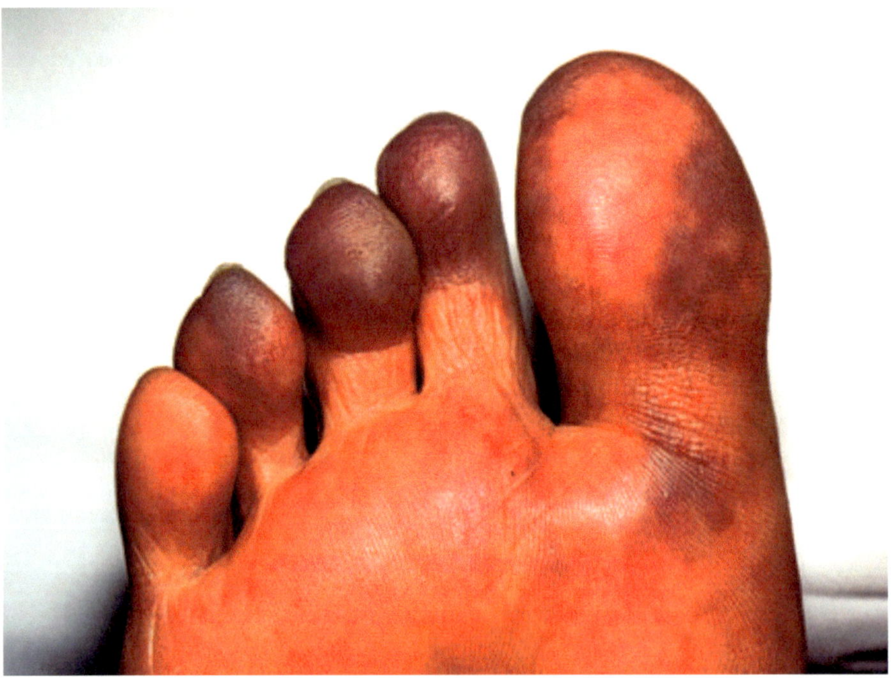

Blue toes are a classic manifestation of peripheral embolization of atheromatous material from proximal arterial sources (eg, aorta); the pedal pulses are often normal. This patient, who has a 30-year history of type 1 diabetes and severe peripheral vascular disease, presented with foot pain and discoloration. Cholesterol microemboli from the aorta were suspected to be the cause.

Photo 1. Blue toe syndrome

The high rate of release of atheromatous debris was illustrated in a series of 1000 patients undergoing percutaneous coronary intervention: 51 percent had aortic atheromatous material retrieved from the catheter after back flow of blood [43]. There were no associated in-hospital ischemic complications, probably due to sufficient withdrawal of blood containing the debris prior to the injection of contrast.

The reported incidence of atheroembolic events varies from 0.6 to 0.9 percent in retrospective studies to 1.4 to 1.9 percent in prospective series [44].

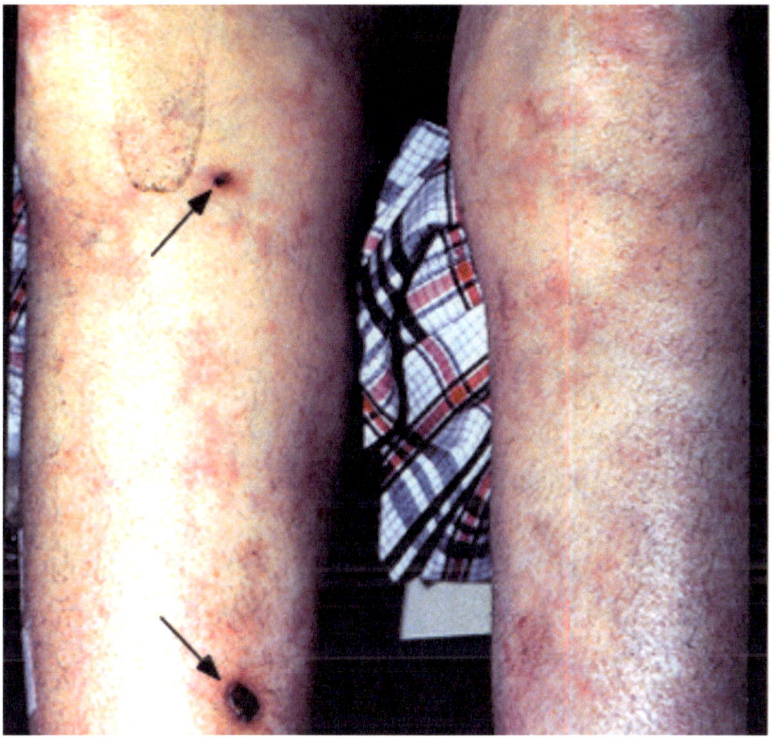

Patient with lupus and anti-phospholipid antibodies with livedo reticularis (manifested by a reddish-cyanotic, reticular pattern of the skin) which has resulted in ulcer formation (arrows).

Photo 2. Livedo reticularis

The clinical features of atheroembolism after diagnostic cardiac catheterization were examined in a prospective evaluation of 1786 patients ≥40 years of age [45]. The following observations were made:

- 25 patients (1.4 percent) were diagnosed with atheroembolism; 12 had cutaneous signs (eg, "blue toes" syndrome, livedo reticularis) (**photo 1** and **photo 2**) and 16 had acute renal failure that was considered to be atheroembolic in origin because it persisted for at least two weeks (while contrast nephropathy typically reverses within the first week).
- Eosinophil counts were significantly higher in patients suffering from atheroembolism both before and after catheterization.
- Four patients with atheroembolism died in hospital (16 percent); all had progressive renal dysfunction. The mortality rate was much lower (0.5 percent) in the patients without atheroembolism.

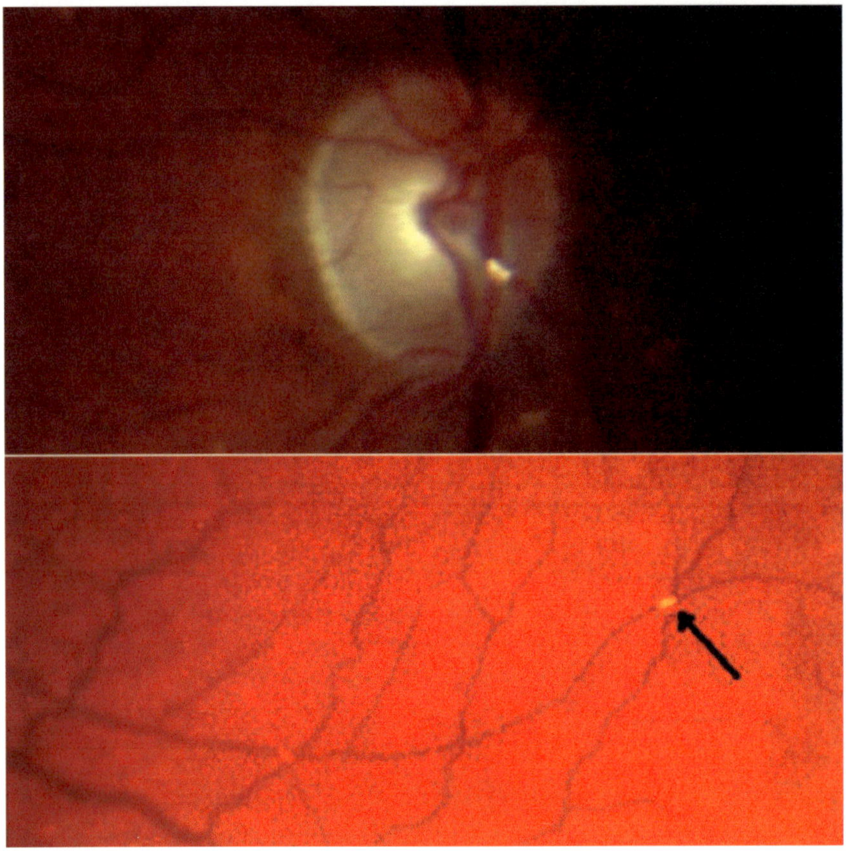

Photo 3. Hollenhorst plaque (cholesterol crystal, arrow) in retinal artery

8. Acute renal failure

There are three major causes of renal dysfunction related to cardiac catheterization: contrast-induced acute renal failure, renal atheroemboli, and hemodynamic instability with renal hypoperfusion.

8.1 Contrast nephropathy

At least 5 percent of patients who undergo cardiac catheterization experience a transient rise in the plasma creatinine concentration of more than 1.0 mg/dL (88 micromol/L) due to contrast-induced renal dysfunction [46].

However, there is substantial variability in risk among patients, some of whom have a risk that exceeds 50 percent. The risk is greatest in patients with moderate to severe renal insufficiency and diabetes.

The plasma creatinine concentration usually returns to baseline within seven days, and less than 1 percent of patients, usually diabetic patients with underlying severe chronic kidney disease, go on to require chronic hemodialysis.

Nonionic low osmolal contrast agents are now administered for the majority of radiologic procedures using intravascular contrast media, as a result of increased patient tolerability and decreased hypersensitivity reactions. However, in patients at risk for contrast nephropathy, we

prefer the use of iso-osmolal agents (approximately 290 mosmol/kg) rather than low osmolal agents (500 to 850 mosmol/kg) because of a lower risk of contrast nephropathy.
The 2007 focused update of the ACC/AHA/SCAI 2005 PCI guidelines recommended the use of iso-osmolal in preference to low osmolal agents in patients with chronic kidney disease [47].

8.2 Renal atheroemboli

The kidney is one of the principal end organs that may be affected by atheroembolic events. (See 'Atheroembolism' above.) There are three main findings that suggest that atheroemboli rather than contrast nephropathy is responsible for the development of acute renal failure after catheterization:

- The presence of other signs of embolization such as blue toes (**photo 1**), livedo reticularis (**photo 2**), Hollenhorst plaques in the retina (**photo 3**), and/or abdominal pain.
- Transient eosinophilia and hypocomplementemia.
- Persistent renal failure after seven days.

In a review of 1786 consecutive patients undergoing cardiac catheterization, acute renal failure developed in 0.9 percent overall and in 64 percent of those with evidence of any atheroembolism [45]. In this report, acute renal failure was considered to be due to renal atheroembolism if it had persisted for at least two weeks, well beyond the time at which contrast nephropathy should have resolved.

9. Infection

Cardiac catheterization procedures are performed using sterile technique. Thus, both local infection and bacteremia are rare and endocarditis prophylaxis during cardiac catheterization is not recommended for patients with valvular disease. Infection is approximately 10 times more common with the brachial approach compared to the femoral approach (0.6 versus 0.06 percent) [2-7].
Infection control guidelines for the cardiac catheterization laboratory were updated in 2006 by the Society for Cardiovascular Angiography and Interventions [48]. These guidelines emphasize the importance of handwashing caps, gowns, gloves, and masks to protect the patient against bacterial infection, and measures such as eye wear and vaccination for hepatitis B to protect laboratory personnel.

10. Radiation exposure

Patients undergoing diagnostic and interventional cardiac catheterization receive substantial radiation exposure.

11. Endomyocardial biopsy

Endomyocardial biopsy of right ventricular tissue is made using a relatively stiff catheter. Complications such as perforation of the heart or great vessels, life threatening arrhythmias, or heart block requiring permanent pacing occur uncommonly.

12. Conclusions

Cardiac catheterization is a common proceduce with very low incidence of complications nowadays. We can consider different kind of adverse events. On the one hand, the events related with the artery access, that are the most common, like haematoma, pseudoaneurysm or dissection. On the other hand, we can observe complications more severe like embolizations, renal failure or allergic reactions. Death is an uncommon complication, with a is generally well below 1 percent. It is very important to know the potential adverse events of these procedures in order to be aware to prevent it as better as possible.

13. References

[1] Baim, DS, Grossman, W. Complications of cardiac catheterization. In: Cardiac Catheterization, Angiography and Intervention, Baim, DS, Grossman, W (Eds), Williams & Wilkins, Baltimore 1996. p.17.
[2] Johnson LW, Lozner EC, Johnson S, et al. Coronary arteriography 1984-1987: a report of the Registry of the Society for Cardiac Angiography and Interventions. I. Results and complications. Cathet Cardiovasc Diagn 1989; 17:5.
[3] Dorros G, Cowley MJ, Simpson J, et al. Percutaneous transluminal coronary angioplasty: report of complications from the National Heart, Lung, and Blood Institute PTCA Registry. Circulation 1983; 67:723.
[4] Kennedy JW. Complications associated with cardiac catheterization and angiography. Cathet Cardiovasc Diagn 1982; 8:5.
[5] Noto TJ Jr, Johnson LW, Krone R, et al. Cardiac catheterization 1990: a report of the Registry of the Society for Cardiac Angiography and Interventions (SCA&I). Cathet Cardiovasc Diagn 1991; 24:75.
[6] Laskey W, Boyle J, Johnson LW. Multivariable model for prediction of risk of significant complication during diagnostic cardiac catheterization. The Registry Committee of the Society for Cardiac Angiography & Interventions. Cathet Cardiovasc Diagn 1993; 30:185.
[7] Wyman RM, Safian RD, Portway V, et al. Current complications of diagnostic and therapeutic cardiac catheterization. J Am Coll Cardiol 1988; 12:1400.
[8] King KM, Ghali WA, Faris PD, et al. Sex differences in outcomes after cardiac catheterization: effect modification by treatment strategy and time. JAMA 2004; 291:1220.
[9] Hemmelgarn BR, Southern DA, Humphries KH, et al. Refined characterization of the association between kidney function and mortality in patients undergoing cardiac catheterization. Eur Heart J 2006; 27:1191.
[10] Gruberg L, Mintz GS, Mehran R, et al. The prognostic implications of further renal function deterioration within 48 h of interventional coronary procedures in patients with pre-existent chronic renal insufficiency. J Am Coll Cardiol 2000; 36:1542.
[11] Segal AZ, Abernethy WB, Palacios IF, et al. Stroke as a complication of cardiac catheterization: risk factors and clinical features. Neurology 2001; 56:975.
[12] Hamon M, Baron JC, Viader F, Hamon M. Periprocedural stroke and cardiac catheterization. Circulation 2008; 118:678.
[13] Omran H, Schmidt H, Hackenbroch M, et al. Silent and apparent cerebral embolism after retrograde catheterisation of the aortic valve in valvular stenosis: a prospective, randomised study. Lancet 2003; 361:1241.
[14] Chambers J, Bach D, Dumesnil J, et al. Crossing the aortic valve in severe aortic stenosis: no longer acceptable? J Heart Valve Dis 2004; 13:344.

[15] Büsing KA, Schulte-Sasse C, Flüchter S, et al. Cerebral infarction: incidence and risk factors after diagnostic and interventional cardiac catheterization--prospective evaluation at diffusion-weighted MR imaging. Radiology 2005; 235:177.
[16] Lund C, Nes RB, Ugelstad TP, et al. Cerebral emboli during left heart catheterization may cause acute brain injury. Eur Heart J 2005; 26:1269.
[17] Pracyk JB, Wall TC, Longabaugh JP, et al. A randomized trial of vascular hemostasis techniques to reduce femoral vascular complications after coronary intervention. Am J Cardiol 1998; 81:970.
[18] Ward SR, Casale P, Raymond R, et al. Efficacy and safety of a hemostatic puncture closure device with early ambulation after coronary angiography. Angio-Seal Investigators. Am J Cardiol 1998; 81:569.
[19] Kapadia SR, Raymond R, Knopf W, et al. The 6Fr Angio-Seal arterial closure device: results from a multimember prospective registry. Am J Cardiol 2001; 87:789.
[20] Silber S, Gershony G, Schön B, et al. A novel vascular sealing device for closure of percutaneous arterial access sites. Am J Cardiol 1999; 83:1248.
[21] Silber S, Tofte AJ, Kjellevand TO, et al. Final report of the European multi-center registry using the Duett vascular sealing device. Herz 1999; 24:620.
[22] Baim DS, Knopf WD, Hinohara T, et al. Suture-mediated closure of the femoral access site after cardiac catheterization: results of the suture to ambulate aNd discharge (STAND I and STAND II) trials. Am J Cardiol 2000; 85:864.
[23] Koreny M, Riedmüller E, Nikfardjam M, et al. Arterial puncture closing devices compared with standard manual compression after cardiac catheterization: systematic review and meta-analysis. JAMA 2004; 291:350.
[24] Nikolsky E, Mehran R, Halkin A, et al. Vascular complications associated with arteriotomy closure devices in patients undergoing percutaneous coronary procedures: a meta-analysis. J Am Coll Cardiol 2004; 44:1200.
[25] Geary K, Landers JT, Fiore W, Riggs P. Management of infected femoral closure devices. Cardiovasc Surg 2002; 10:161.
[26] Cherr GS, Travis JA, Ligush J Jr, et al. Infection is an unusual but serious complication of a femoral artery catheterization site closure device. Ann Vasc Surg 2001; 15:567.
[27] El-Jack SS, Ruygrok PN, Webster MW, et al. Effectiveness of manual pressure hemostasis following transfemoral coronary angiography in patients on therapeutic warfarin anticoagulation. Am J Cardiol 2006; 97:485.
[28] Krueger K, Zaehringer M, Strohe D, et al. Postcatheterization pseudoaneurysm: results of US-guided percutaneous thrombin injection in 240 patients. Radiology 2005; 236:1104.
[29] Katzenschlager R, Ugurluoglu A, Ahmadi A, et al. Incidence of pseudoaneurysm after diagnostic and therapeutic angiography. Radiology 1995; 195:463.
[30] Webber GW, Jang J, Gustavson S, Olin JW. Contemporary management of postcatheterization pseudoaneurysms. Circulation 2007; 115:2666.
[31] Muller DW, Shamir KJ, Ellis SG, Topol EJ. Peripheral vascular complications after conventional and complex percutaneous coronary interventional procedures. Am J Cardiol 1992; 69:63.
[32] Popma JJ, Satler LF, Pichard AD, et al. Vascular complications after balloon and new device angioplasty. Circulation 1993; 88:1569.

[33] Paulson EK, Sheafor DH, Kliewer MA, et al. Treatment of iatrogenic femoral arterial pseudoaneurysms: comparison of US-guided thrombin injection with compression repair. Radiology 2000; 215:403.

[34] La Perna L, Olin JW, Goines D, et al. Ultrasound-guided thrombin injection for the treatment of postcatheterization pseudoaneurysms. Circulation 2000; 102:2391.

[35] Hamraoui K, Ernst SM, van Dessel PF, et al. Efficacy and safety of percutaneous treatment of iatrogenic femoral artery pseudoaneurysm by biodegradable collagen injection. J Am Coll Cardiol 2002; 39:1297.

[36] Agostoni P, Biondi-Zoccai GG, de Benedictis ML, et al. Radial versus femoral approach for percutaneous coronary diagnostic and interventional procedures; Systematic overview and meta-analysis of randomized trials. J Am Coll Cardiol 2004; 44:349.

[37] Greenwood MJ, Della-Siega AJ, Fretz EB, et al. Vascular communications of the hand in patients being considered for transradial coronary angiography: is the Allen's test accurate? J Am Coll Cardiol 2005; 46:2013.

[38] Barbeau GR, Arsenault F, Dugas L, et al. Evaluation of the ulnopalmar arterial arches with pulse oximetry and plethysmography: comparison with the Allen's test in 1010 patients. Am Heart J 2004; 147:489.

[39] Benit E, Vranckx P, Jaspers L, et al. Frequency of a positive modified Allen's test in 1,000 consecutive patients undergoing cardiac catheterization. Cathet Cardiovasc Diagn 1996; 38:352.

[40] Hovagim AR, Katz RI, Poppers PJ. Pulse oximetry for evaluation of radial and ulnar arterial blood flow. J Cardiothorac Anesth 1989; 3:27.

[41] Harvey JR, Wyman RM, McKay RG, Baim DS. Use of balloon flotation pacing catheters for prophylactic temporary pacing during diagnostic and therapeutic catheterization procedures. Am J Cardiol 1988; 62:941.

[42] Tsang TS, Freeman WK, Barnes ME, et al. Rescue echocardiographically guided pericardiocentesis for cardiac perforation complicating catheter-based procedures. The Mayo Clinic experience. J Am Coll Cardiol 1998; 32:1345.

[43] Keeley EC, Grines CL. Scraping of aortic debris by coronary guiding catheters: a prospective evaluation of 1,000 cases. J Am Coll Cardiol 1998; 32:1861.

[44] Bashore TM, Gehrig T. Cholesterol emboli after invasive cardiac procedures. J Am Coll Cardiol 2003; 42:217.

[45] Fukumoto Y, Tsutsui H, Tsuchihashi M, et al. The incidence and risk factors of cholesterol embolization syndrome, a complication of cardiac catheterization: a prospective study. J Am Coll Cardiol 2003; 42:211.

[46] Tommaso CL. Contrast-induced nephrotoxicity in patients undergoing cardiac catheterization. Cathet Cardiovasc Diagn 1994; 31:316.

[47] King SB, 3rd, Smith, SC Jr, Hirshfeld, JW Jr, et al. 2007 Focused Update of the ACC/AHA/SCAI 2005 Guideline Update for Percutaneous Coronary Intervention: a report of the American College of Cardiology/American Heart Association Task Force on Practice Guidelines: 2007 Writing Group to Review New Evidence and Update the ACC/AHA/SCAI 2005 Guideline Update for Percutaneous Coronary Intervention, Writing on Behalf of the 2005 Writing Committee. Circulation 2008; 117:261.

[48] Chambers CE, Eisenhauer MD, McNicol LB, et al. Infection control guidelines for the cardiac catheterization laboratory: society guidelines revisited. Catheter Cardiovasc Interv 2006; 67:78.

9

Diagnosis and Management of Complications of Invasive Coronary Angiography

Jong-Seon Park and Young-Jo Kim
Yeungnam University Hospital
Korea

1. Introduction

Since its introduction several decades ago, coronary angiography and intervention has become a widely and ever increasingly popular diagnostic and therapeutic modality. However, it is not devoid of occasional systemic and local complications, and their immediate detection and management are crucial to achieving a favourable clinical course. This chapter focuses on the mechanism, diagnosis and treatment of the inherent risks of coronary angiography and intervention.

2. Systemic complications

Coronary angiography and intervention comprise local procedures performed via a percutaneous vascular approach. Untoward hemodynamic and systemic hormonal changes and toxic effects of the contrast agents used might occur during and after procedures. Patient's general status, comorbid conditions and degree of systemic atherosclerosis are the most important factors predisposing to the development of systemic complications. Effective pre-procedural preparation and immediate proper treatment help prevent event occurrence and its subsequent deterioration to permanent sequelae.

2.1 Side effects of contrast agent

Use of contrast agents has a long history since the introduction of X-ray technology in 1895, and progressive changes after Douglas Cameron of Minnesota recommended the use of sodium iodide for retrograde phelography reduced toxicity leading to current angiography practices. The side effects of contrast agents are related to their osmolarity, hydrophilicity and viscosity, and there currently are different kinds of contrast media available which can be classified according to their chemical characteristics (Table 1).

Osmolarity is the most important characteristic of contrast agents, which thereby are classified into high-osmolar (~2,000 mOsm/kg), low-osmolar (600~800 mOsm/kg) and iso-osmolar (290 mOsm/kg) contrast media. Commonly, high osmolar contrast agents induce fluid shift into vessels, which can cause a febrile sensation and pain. Also, high osmolar contrast media take cellular fluid from cells including red blood cells and therefore lead to dehydration and morphological changes. Hemodilution and hypervolemia can further aggravate heart failure when present. In the past 60 years, high–osmolar contrast media with osmolarity 5~8 times higher than that of plasma have been replaced by low-osmolar contrast media having osmolarity 2~3 times higher than that of plasma.

Osmolarity	Molecular structure	Component	Iodine concentration (mg/mL)	Osmolarity (mOsmol/kg)	Viscosity at 37°C (cps)
High-osmolar	Ionic monomer	Sodium iothalamate Meglumine diatrizoate	320-370	1,500~2,100	2.75-5.0
Low-osmolar	Ionic dimer	Meglumine ioxaglate	320	580	6
		Iopamidol Iohexol Loversol Iopromide	300	520-672	4.5-6.3
Iso-osmolar	Nonionic dimer	Iotrolan	240	320	8.1
		Iodixanol	320	290	11.4

Table 1. Characteristics of contrast media

Cell membranes consist of phospholipid bilayers which are resistant to hydrophilic molecules. Therefore hydrophilic contrast agents are safer than hydrophobic ones.
Viscosity increases as iodine concentration increases and temperature decreases; therefore, contrast agents should be heated from room temperature to body temperature before use.
Early ionic contrast agents were associated with high incidence of early systemic side effects such as nausea, urticaria, pain, and heat sensation by comparison to non-ionic agents. Therefore, ionic agents have been replaced with non-ionic agents. However, the incidence of late skin reaction, i.e., 24 hours after injection of non-ionic dimeric agents is relatively high as compared to monomeric agents (Sutton et al 2001).
The side effects of contrast media are divided into anaphylactoid and non-anaphylactoid reactions. Most of the adverse effects occur within 20 minutes after administration of contrast agents. Therefore, the patient's systemic symptoms, blood pressure, heart rate and rhythm, and respiratory status should be carefully monitored early after contrast injection. Furthermore, the catheterization laboratory always should be ready for cardiopulmonary resuscitation.

2.1.1 Anaphylactoid reactions

Anaphylactoid reaction is a life-threatening side-effect of contrast media which occurs within 20 minutes and requires immediate, intensive therapy; the incidence of use of high osmolar contrast agent is approximately 1~3 % and a fatal reaction has been estimated at 0.9 cases per 100,000 exposures (Krause 2010). The term anaphylactoid reaction refers to a syndrome that albeit clinically similar to anaphylaxis differs from true hypersensitivity reactions by mast cell or basophil degranulation which is independent from immunoglobulin-E mediation, not requiring previous sensitisation, and not consistently recurring in an experienced patients (Hong et al 2002). Mild symptoms include urticaria, pruritus, dizziness, mild dyspnea, nausea and vomiting and these are usually self-limiting and resolving with minimal medical therapy. In severe cases, symptoms such as hypotension, bronchospasm, laryngeal edema, abdominal cramps, pulmonary edema, syncope, and serious arrhythmias can occur and lead to death and therefore require intensive treatment. In patients who are at high risk of an anaphylactoid reaction to contrast media, H1 antihistamines and corticosteroids prior to the administration of ionic contrast may be useful in preventing anaphylactoid reactions to contrast agents (Delaney et al 2006). The treatment of anaphylactoid reactions depends on the severity of symptoms and clinical findings. Monitoring of the respiratory status and oxygen concentration is very important. If mild bronchospasm occurs, patient can be treated with oxygen supplementation and/or bronchodilator inhalation. In moderate cases, 0.1-0.3 mL of 1:1000 epinephrine should be subcutaneously administered carefully, especially in patients with cardiac disease. In more severe cases, 1 mL of 1:10,000 epinephrine can be administered intravenously for 5 minutes, which can be repeated every 10 minutes. Additionally, antihistamines may be administered. Hypotension is another serious side effect of contrast agents. Immediate oxygen supplementation and isotonic fluid supplement is necessary, and if ineffective, dopamine at an infusion rate of 2-20 μgm/kg/min can be administered.

2.1.2 Non-anaphylactoid reactions

Early (<24 hours) and late (24 hours ~ 7 days) reactions may occur after injection of contrast agents. The mechanisms of the late reactions are unknown and their manifestations are very diverse and non-specific, including flulike symptoms such as general weakness, headache, fever, chill, vomiting, abdominal pain, constipation or diarrhea, pruritus and rash. Most symptoms are self-limiting and respond well to symptomatic treatment and fluid administration.

Hypotension and bradycardia as consequence of vasovagal stimulation associated with high-osmolar contrast infusion are common. Isotonic fluid and atropine administration (0.5~1 mg, intravenously, repeated every 3-5 minutes) are effective in most cases. Life threatening cardiac arrhythmias such as ventricular tachycardia and ventricular fibrillation can occur after rapid injection of contrast media, especially in patients with acute myocardial infarction. Careful ECG monitoring after first contrast injection and immediate cardioversion or defibrillation should be performed.

Contrast-induced nephropathy (CIN), an important complication in the use of contrast media, is associated with increased frequency of late cardiovascular events after coronary intervention as well as increased risk of death. The commonly used definition of CIN is a rise in serum creatinine level of 0.5 mg/dL or a 25% increase from baseline value, assessed at 48 hours after angiography (Solomon et al 2010). The incidence of CIN in patients undergoing coronary intervention varies depending on the definition, preventive management, baseline renal function and procedures, and it ranges between 2~37% (Solomon et al. 2010, Gruberg et al 2000). There are several known risk factors for CIN (Table 2). The type of contrast media used is one of the important factors for the development or aggravation of renal failure. A meta-analysis showed that low-osmolarity contrast media was associated with significantly lower rates of CIN than high-osmolarity contrast media, especially in patients with pre-existing renal failure (Barrett et al 1993). Also, iso-osmolar contrast media have been shown to be associated with a lower risk of CIN than low-osmolar contrast media in patients with high risk for the development of CIN.

Patient comorbidities	Diabetes mellitus Congestive heart failure Acute hypotension Anemia Myocardial infarction Nephrotoxic drugs Volume depletion Reduced renal function (eGFR <60 mL/min/1.73 ^{m})
Procedural factors	Contrast volume Type of contrast Periprocedural hypotension

Table 2. Risk factors for contrast-induced nephropathy(Solomon et al. 2010, McCullough 2008)

The pathophysiology of CIN remains unknown; however, it is believed to result from release of acute vasoconstrictors induced by adenosine, endothelin, prostaglandin leading to ischemic injury and death of renal tubular cells (McCullough 2008). Although more clinical studies are needed, some effective preventive measures have been suggested based on postulated mechanisms and clinical trial results (Table 3). Volume expansion is the easiest and most effective method although there are limited data on optimal solution and volume. Although many pharmacological agents including antioxidants, ascorbic acid, statins, prostaglandins, aminophylline/theophyllines and N-acetylcysteine (NAC) have been suggested for the prevention of CIN, none has been proven effective. Also, there are inconsistent data regarding the renal protective effect of hydration, N-acetylcysteine, and theophylline. Among them, NAC is considered as a cost effective and safe agent, and the combination of volume expansion and NAC is more effective than NAC alone (Briguori et al 2007). A meta-analysis showed N-acetylcysteine as more renoprotective than hydration alone; theophylline also might reduce risk for contrast-induced nephropathy however the detected association did not achieve statistical significance (Kelly et al 2008).

Pre- and post-procedure	Hold nephrotoxic agents - Anti-inflammatory drugs - High dose diuretics - Aminoglycosides Volume expansion (Isotonic saline with/without bicarbonate solution) - 1.0 mL /kg/hr, 12 hours before and 12 hours after procedure - Urine flow : >150 mL/hr N-acetylcysteine - 1200 mg oral bid pre-and post-procedure
During procedure	Use iso- or low-osmolar contrast Lowest dose of contrast
Post-procedure	Dialysis and hemofiltration

Table 3. Suggestive preventive measures for contrast-induced nephropathy in patients at risk

2.2 Cholesterol embolization syndrome

Cholesterol embolization syndrome (CES), known as blue toe syndrome, is caused by systemic embolization of cholesterol crystals from aortic atherosclerotic plaques. CES is suggested by the gradual onset of peripheral cutaneous manifestations, livedo reticularis, accompanied by progressive increases in blood urea nitrogen and creatinine levels following an arterial catheterization procedure. The aortic plaques easily come off the aortic wall and embolize to the brain, eyes, kidneys and extremities. Eosinophilia which is present in up to 80% of cases might be an important clue to early detection of cholesterol embolization syndrome (Wilson et al 1991). The clinical incidence is 0.09~1.4%, varying according to the aggressiveness of procedures such as diagnostic angiography, coronary intervention and peripheral vascular intervention (Fukumoto et al 2003, Scolari et al 1996). Elevation of baseline plasma C-reactive protein (CRP) level is a risk factor independently associated with CES indicating an important association between systemic inflammation and CES (Fukumoto et al. 2003). The clinical presentation varies from asymptomatic to multi-organ failure. In-hospital mortality is 16% which is increased to 70~90% in patients with diffuse embolism and multi-organ failure (Fine et al 1987). When CES is suspected, it is recommended to discontinue anticoagulation because several case reports have suggested that patients are more likely to develop CES when they are anticoagulated (Bruns et al 1978). Most of the treatments are supportive with symptomatic measures.

2.3 Stroke

The cerebral embolism rate associated with coronary angiography is dependent on the clinical characteristics of the patients, catheterization methods, imaging modalities for the diagnosis, and clinical severity. In one series, silent ischemic cerebral lesions detected by diffusion-weighted MRI were found in 5-22% patients after cardiac catheterization (Hamon et al 2006, Busing et al 2005). After diagnostic coronary angiography via femoral approach, stroke occurred in 0.11%, with a persistent neurological defect in only 0.04% (Ammann et al 2003). Although radial access for coronary angiography is more prone than femoral access to generating more particulate cerebral microemboli which can pass the right middle cerebral artery, femoral and radial access are associated with similar rates of stroke.

3. Local complications

Local vascular puncture and closure necessary in all catheterization procedures can cause a variety of local complications, ranging from minor problems resolving with time to major complications with long-term sequelae. For the individual patient, the risk is dependent upon cardiovascular anatomy, the experience of the operator, and the type of procedure being performed. Immediate detection and proper treatment is vital for the prevention of catastrophic events.

3.1 Local hematoma and bleeding

Local bleeding and hematoma at the arterial puncture site are the most common complications of angiography. Small hematomas at the femoral puncture site are relatively common and usually insignificant; however, severe bleeding and hematoma requiring transfusion occur in 1.5~5.8% of the cases. Most hematomas occur within 12 hours after sheath removal. Immediate bleeding occurring after sheath insertion is induced by arterial laceration at the site of the atherosclerotic vessel wall. Otherwise, delayed bleeding after sheath removal is due to inappropriate compression or coagulation disorders. Clinically, risk factors are old age, female gender, high blood pressure, use of large sized sheaths, long procedural times and use of anticoagulants and glycoprotein IIb/IIIa receptor antagonists before or after procedures. Many arterial closure devices are available as an alternative to traditional mechanical compression. Although these devices have the potential to reduce the time to hemostasis, facilitate patient mobilization and decrease hospital length of stay, the incidence of access-site-related complications is similar or somewhat higher compared with mechanical compression (Nikolsky et al 2004, Biancari et al 2010). Local bleeding is transformed to hematoma, which spontaneously resolves in 1~2 weeks in small hematomas, or in several weeks or months in large hematomas. Table 4 describes the general recommendations for postprocedural hemostasis after femoral artery access listed in the American College of Cardiology/Society for Cardiac Angiography and Interventions Clinical Expert Consensus Document on Cardiac Catheterization Laboratory Standards (Bashore et al 2001).

Situation	Recommendation
Following hemostatic closure device	1–2 h recumbent in position of comfort, then ambulate 3 30 min before discharge
Following removal of venous sheath	1 h with leg straight, then ambulate 3 30 min before discharge
Following removal of femoral arterial sheath (ACT ,175 s)	
Manual compression	10–20 min (until hemostasis achieved)
Clamp	15 min to 1 h to achieve hemostasis
Bedrest	Leg straight, slight head elevation X 2–6 h
Ambulation	30 min to 1 h before discharge

Table 4. General recommendations regarding postprocedural hemostasis after prior femoral artery access(Bashore et al. 2001)

3.2 Pseudoaneurysm

After removal of the sheath and compression, the puncture site is surrounded and blocked by local hematoma. Inappropriate compression favours come-and-go blood flow between artery lumen and aneurysm surrounded by hematoma. Femoral peudoaneurysm is the second most common complication occurring in 0.1% to 0.2% of diagnostic angiograms and 3.5% to 5.5% of interventional procedures (Demirbas et al 2005, Kronzon 1997). If hemostasis is achieved using manual compression, the pseudoaneurysm rate is higher in superficial femoral artery than common femoral artery access, however rates are similar when using closure devices (Gutzeit et al 2011). In patients with acute coronary syndrome who are undergoing emergency angiography and possible intervention, pseudoaneurysm rate needing closure is lower in radial compared with femoral angiography (HR 0·30, 95% CI 0·13–0·71; p=0·006) (Jolly et al 2011). Small femoral pseudoaneurysm is usually filled with clots and does not require treatment, however, larger femoral pseudoaneurysms may lead to secondary complications including rupture, local pain and compression of the adjacent femoral vein or nerve (Kronzon 1997). Color Doppler ultrasonography is the best diagnostic tool with a positive diagnostic rate of 95%, however other imaging modalities such as 3-dimentional CT angiography and angiography are useful. Using color-Doppler ultrasonography, flow inside the aneurysm sac and the "to-and-fro flow" at the neck of the lesion is definitely diagnostic. Application of good external compression after sheath removal, selecting a small-bore introducer and sheath removal at a low activated clotting time (<200 sec) are important factors preventing pseudoaneurysm. Ultrasonography guided compression of the communicating canal of the pseudoaneurysm stops the blood flow and leads to clotting and obliteration with a success rate of 84-93% in patients without anticoagulation (Lange et al 2001, Gabriel et al 2007, Schaub et al 1994). Ultrasound-guided thrombin injection is another effective means with a success rate of 97-100% (Schneider et al 2009, Weinmann et al 2002). Other endovascular approaches, such as stent graft repair and coil embolization, are also available. Open surgical repair should be considered after non-surgical procedure failure.

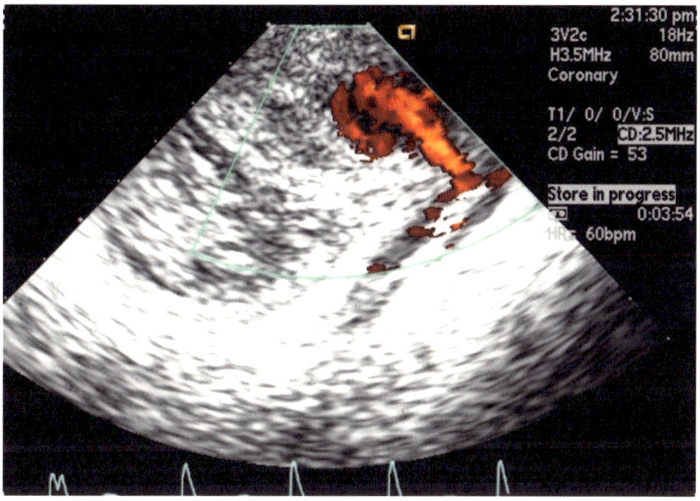

Fig. 1. Doppler ultrasonography image showing a flow jet from superficial femoral artery to pseudoaneurysm surrounded by huge hematoma

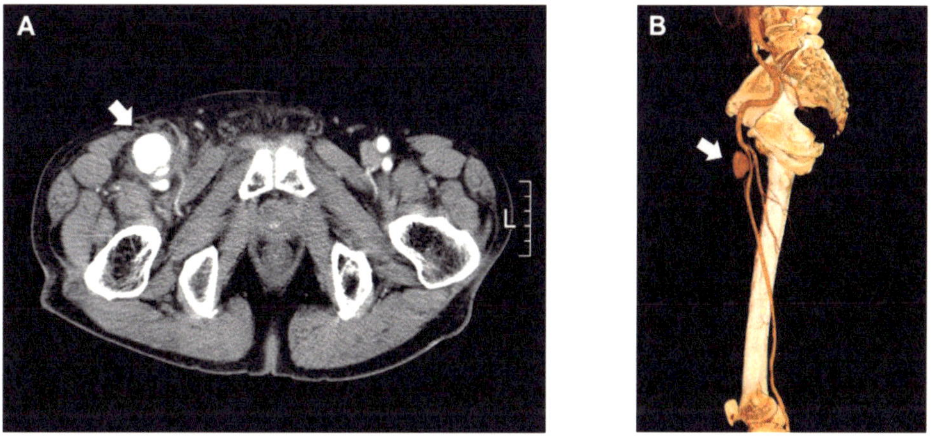

Fig. 2. Computerized tomographic (CT) findings of pseudoaneurysm in a patient who underwent coronary angiography. A: Contrast enhanced pseudoaneurysm (arrow) is seen at anterior aspect of the superficial femoral artery. B: Three-dimensional reconstruction of the same patient showing saccular pseudoaneurysm (arrow), superficial femoral artery and anteria profunda femoris.

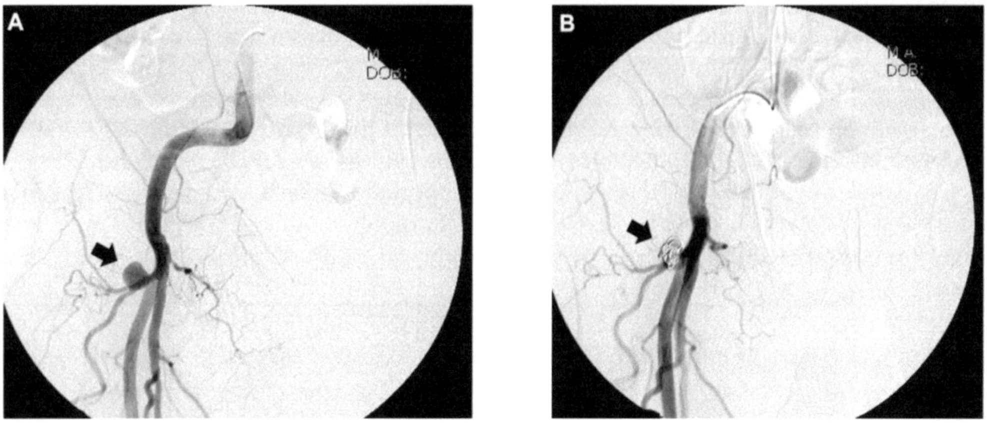

Fig. 3. Angiographic findings of pseudoaneurysm before (A) and after (B) coil embolization.

3.3 Arteriovenous fistula

Although iatrogenic femoral arteriovenous fistula is very rare with an incidence of 0.22%, it is a significant complication after femoral puncture technique (Sidawy et al 1993). The fistulas originating at the superficial femoral artery or at the profunda femoris artery drain to the superficial femoral, profunda femoris vein or its lateral circumflex branch. Below the femoral artery bifurcation, profunda femoralis vein crosses laterally behind the proximal superficial femoral artery and then lies in a posterior location to the profunda femoris artery. Therefore, it is important to avoid a low groin puncture by identifying the level of the inguinal ligament or localizing the distal half of the femoral head by fluoroscopy (Sidawy et al. 1993, Lamar R 1990). Early angiography and surgical correction are recommended for optimal results.

3.4 Retroperitoneal hematoma

Retroperitoneal hematoma occurs in less than 1% of cases of percutaneous coronary intervention. Clinical signs and symptoms include decreased haematocrit, back or inguinal pain, abdominal pain, diaphoresis, bradycardia and hypotension. Early recognition of retroperitoneal hematoma is very important because the diagnosis is often delayed as symptoms are nonspecific and difficult to recognize because blood silently tracks in the loose retroperitoneal fatty tissue. Factors predisposing to retroperitoneal hematoma are female gender, low body surface area, and higher femoral artery puncture (Farouque et al 2005). It can be easily detected on computerized tomography as an abnormal, high-density soft-tissue mass originating at the puncture site and contiguous with the retroperitoneum with resultant compression or distortion of the normal retroperitoneal structures. There is lack of clinical evidence for the best management of retroperitoneal haematoma. Inguinal compression is not effective in most cases. Retroperitoneal hematoma after femoral artery puncture can usually be treated by volume replacement, correction of coagulopathy and blood transfusion. A small subset of patients who are unresponsive to volume resuscitation require open repair of bleeding vessel (Kent et al 1994).

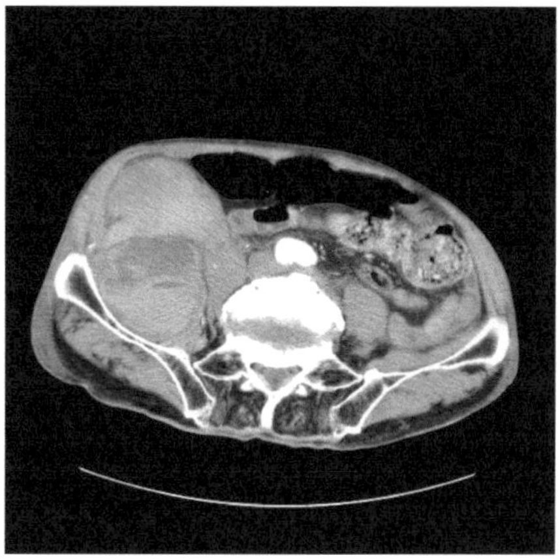

Fig. 4. Contrast-enhanced CT scan showing retropelvic hematoma one day after coronary angiography via right femoral artery

3.5 Spasm

Arterial spasm near the puncture site occurs when arterial size is too small for the sheath. The transradial approach for coronary angiography or angioplasty is increasingly being used as an alternative to femoral access due to its low rate of local complications. Arterial spasm is the most common complication of this technique especially in female patients. Use of hydrophilic coated sheath, but not long sheath, reduces the incidence of radial artery spasm during transradial coronary procedures (Rathore et al 2010). Intra-arterial or subcutaneous infusion of nitroglycerin reduces arterial spasm and facilitates introduction of catheters (Candemir et al 2009).

4. Conclusion

It is critical to make every attempt at minimizing occurrence of complications during and after coronary angiography and interventional procedures; beyond operator's experience and the patient factors noted, this involves care and attentiveness. The impact of improved understanding and techniques in intervention should be added to management considerations. Coronary angiography and intervention is continuously evolving and knowledge acquired through clinical experience and availability of new devices should therefore allow safer procedures in the future.

5. References

Ammann P, Brunner-La Rocca HP, Angehrn W, Roelli H, Sagmeister M and Rickli H (2003). Procedural complications following diagnostic coronary angiography are related to the operator's experience and the catheter size. *Catheter Cardiovasc Interv* 59. 13-8.

Barrett BJ and Carlisle EJ (1993). Metaanalysis of the relative nephrotoxicity of high- and low-osmolality iodinated contrast media. *Radiology* 188. 171-8.

Bashore TM, Bates ER, Berger PB, Clark DA, Cusma JT, Dehmer GJ, Kern MJ, Laskey WK, O'Laughlin MP, Oesterle S, Popma JJ, O'Rourke RA, Abrams J, Bates ER, Brodie BR, Douglas PS, Gregoratos G, Hlatky MA, Hochman JS, Kaul S, Tracy CM, Waters DD and Winters WL, Jr. (2001). American College of Cardiology/Society for Cardiac Angiography and Interventions Clinical Expert Consensus Document on cardiac catheterization laboratory standards. A report of the American College of Cardiology Task Force on Clinical Expert Consensus Documents. *J Am Coll Cardiol* 37. 2170-214.

Biancari F, D'Andrea V, Di Marco C, Savino G, Tiozzo V and Catania A (2010). Meta-analysis of randomized trials on the efficacy of vascular closure devices after diagnostic angiography and angioplasty. *Am Heart J* 159. 518-31.

Briguori C, Airoldi F, D'Andrea D, Bonizzoni E, Morici N, Focaccio A, Michev I, Montorfano M, Carlino M, Cosgrave J, Ricciardelli B and Colombo A (2007). Renal Insufficiency Following Contrast Media Administration Trial (REMEDIAL): a randomized comparison of 3 preventive strategies. *Circulation* 115. 1211-7.

Bruns FJ, Segel DP and Adler S (1978). Control of cholesterol embolization by discontinuation of anticoagulant therapy. *Am J Med Sci* 275. 105-8.

Busing KA, Schulte-Sasse C, Fluchter S, Suselbeck T, Haase KK, Neff W, Hirsch JG, Borggrefe M and Duber C (2005). Cerebral infarction: incidence and risk factors after diagnostic and interventional cardiac catheterization--prospective evaluation at diffusion-weighted MR imaging. *Radiology* 235. 177-83.

Candemir B, Kumbasar D, Turhan S, Kilickap M, Ozdol C, Akyurek O, Atmaca Y and Altin T (2009). Facilitation of radial artery cannulation by periradial subcutaneous administration of nitroglycerin. *J Vasc Interv Radiol* 20. 1151-6.

Delaney A, Carter A and Fisher M (2006). The prevention of anaphylactoid reactions to iodinated radiological contrast media: a systematic review. *BMC Med Imaging* 6. 2.

Demirbas O, Batyraliev T, Eksi Z and Pershukov I (2005). Femoral pseudoaneurysm due to diagnostic or interventional angiographic procedures. *Angiology* 56. 553-6.

Farouque HM, Tremmel JA, Raissi Shabari F, Aggarwal M, Fearon WF, Ng MK, Rezaee M, Yeung AC and Lee DP (2005). Risk factors for the development of retroperitoneal hematoma after percutaneous coronary intervention in the era of glycoprotein IIb/IIIa inhibitors and vascular closure devices. *J Am Coll Cardiol* 45. 363-8.

Fine MJ, Kapoor W and Falanga V (1987). Cholesterol crystal embolization: a review of 221 cases in the English literature. *Angiology* 38. 769-84.

Fukumoto Y, Tsutsui H, Tsuchihashi M, Masumoto A and Takeshita A (2003). The incidence and risk factors of cholesterol embolization syndrome, a complication of cardiac catheterization: a prospective study. *J Am Coll Cardiol* 42. 211-6.

Gabriel M, Pawlaczyk K, Waliszewski K, Krasinski Z and Majewski W (2007). Location of femoral artery puncture site and the risk of postcatheterization pseudoaneurysm formation. *Int J Cardiol* 120. 167-71.

Gruberg L, Mintz GS, Mehran R, Gangas G, Lansky AJ, Kent KM, Pichard AD, Satler LF and Leon MB (2000). The prognostic implications of further renal function deterioration within 48 h of interventional coronary procedures in patients with pre-existent chronic renal insufficiency. *J Am Coll Cardiol* 36. 1542-8.

Gutzeit A, Graf N, Schoch E, Sautter T, Jenelten R and Binkert CA (2011). Ultrasound-guided antegrade femoral access: comparison between the common femoral artery and the superficial femoral artery. *Eur Radiol* 21(6). 1323-8

Hamon M, Gomes S, Oppenheim C, Morello R, Sabatier R, Lognone T, Grollier G, Courtheoux P and Hamon M (2006). Cerebral microembolism during cardiac catheterization and risk of acute brain injury: a prospective diffusion-weighted magnetic resonance imaging study. *Stroke* 37. 2035-8.

Hong SJ, Wong JT and Bloch KJ (2002). Reactions to radiocontrast media. *Allergy Asthma Proc* 23. 347-51.

Jolly SS, Yusuf S, Cairns J, Niemela K, Xavier D, Widimsky P, Budaj A, Niemela M, Valentin V, Lewis BS, Avezum A, Steg PG, Rao SV, Gao P, Afzal R, Joyner CD, Chrolavicius S and Mehta SR (2011). Radial versus femoral access for coronary angiography and intervention in patients with acute coronary syndromes (RIVAL): a randomised, parallel group, multicentre trial. *Lancet* 377(9775). 1409-20

Kelly AM, Dwamena B, Cronin P, Bernstein SJ and Carlos RC (2008). Meta-analysis: effectiveness of drugs for preventing contrast-induced nephropathy. *Ann Intern Med* 148. 284-94.

Kent KC, Moscucci M, Mansour KA, DiMattia S, Gallagher S, Kuntz R and Skillman JJ (1994). Retroperitoneal hematoma after cardiac catheterization: prevalence, risk factors, and optimal management. *J Vasc Surg* 20. 905-10; discussion 910-3.

Krause RS (2010). Anaphylaxis: *e*-Medicine from WebMD

Kronzon I (1997). Diagnosis and treatment of iatrogenic femoral artery pseudoaneurysm: a review. *J Am Soc Echocardiogr* 10. 236-45.

Lamar R BR, Rama K. (1990). Femoral arteriovenous fistula as a complication of percutaneous transluminal coronary angioplasty. A report of five cases. *Am Surg* 56. 702-6.

Lange P, Houe T and Helgstrand UJ (2001). The efficacy of ultrasound-guided compression of iatrogenic femoral pseudo-aneurysms. *Eur J Vasc Endovasc Surg* 21. 248-50.

McCullough PA (2008). Contrat-induced acute kidney injury. *J Am Coll Cardiol* 51. 1419-28.

Nikolsky E, Mehran R, Halkin A, Aymong ED, Mintz GS, Lasic Z, Negoita M, Fahy M, Krieger S, Moussa I, Moses JW, Stone GW, Leon MB, Pocock SJ and Dangas G (2004). Vascular complications associated with arteriotomy closure devices in patients undergoing percutaneous coronary procedures: a meta-analysis. *J Am Coll Cardiol* 44. 1200-9.

Rathore S, Stables RH, Pauriah M, Hakeem A, Mills JD, Palmer ND, Perry RA and Morris JL (2010). Impact of length and hydrophilic coating of the introducer sheath on radial artery spasm during transradial coronary intervention: a randomized study. *JACC Cardiovasc Interv* 3. 475-83.

Schaub F, Theiss W, Heinz M, Zagel M and Schomig A (1994). New aspects in ultrasound-guided compression repair of postcatheterization femoral artery injuries. *Circulation* 90. 1861-5.

Schneider C, Malisius R, Kuchler R, Lampe F, Krause K, Bahlmann E and Kuck KH (2009). A prospective study on ultrasound-guided percutaneous thrombin injection for treatment of iatrogenic post-catheterisation femoral pseudoaneurysms. *Int J Cardiol* 131. 356-61.

Scolari F, Bracchi M, Valzorio B, Movilli E, Costantino E, Savoldi S, Zorat S, Bonardelli S, Tardanico R and Maiorca R (1996). Cholesterol atheromatous embolism: an increasingly recognized cause of acute renal failure. *Nephrol Dial Transplant* 11. 1607-12.

Sidawy AN, Neville RF, Adib H and Curry KM (1993). Femoral arteriovenous fistula following cardiac catheterization: an anatomic explanation. *Cardiovasc Surg* 1. 134-7.

Solomon R and Dauerman HL (2010). Contrast-induced acute kidney injury. *Circulation* 122. 2451-5.

Sutton AG FP, Grech ED, Hall JA, Stewart MJ, Davies A, de Belder MA (2001). Early and late reactions after the use of iopamidol 340, ioxaglate 320, and iodixanol 320 in cardiac catheterization. *Am Heart J* 141. 677-83.

Weinmann EE, Chayen D, Kobzantzev ZV, Zaretsky M and Bass A (2002). Treatment of postcatheterisation false aneurysms: ultrasound-guided compression vs ultrasound-guided thrombin injection. *Eur J Vasc Endovasc Surg* 23. 68-72.

Wilson DM, Salazer TL and Farkouh ME (1991). Eosinophiluria in atheroembolic renal disease. *Am J Med* 91. 186-9.

10

Coronary Angiography and Contrast-Induced Nephropathy

Omer Toprak
Balikesir State Hospital, Department of Nephrology, Balikesir Turkey

1. Introduction

Radiologic procedures such as coronary angiography utilizing intravascular contrast media (CM) injections are being widely applied for diagnostic and therapeutic purposes. These led to a parallel increase in the incidence of contrast-induced nephropathy (CIN). Renal failure requiring dialysis after contrast media administration is associated with a 40% in-hospital mortality rate and has a 2-year mortality rate of 80%. Approximately $180 million are spent annually to manage CIN in the US. The large number of patients who are severely affected by CIN underscores the importance of addressing known risk factors and preventions for CIN. Patients at risk for CIN can often be identified with a routine medical history, physical examination and laboratory analysis before the procedure. Two of the major risk factors of CIN are pre-existing renal failure and diabetes mellitus. After the high-risk patient population has been identified and risk factors addressed, the next step in preventing CIN is the use of different prophylactic therapies. The following chapter provides an overview of current risk factors and preventive methods of CIN.

2. Definition, differential diagnosis and incidence of CIN

The most commonly used definition for CIN in clinical trial is the elevation of serum creatinine by ≥0.5mg/dl or ≥25% occurring within 48 hours after administration of CM, and the absence of an alternative etiology. Serum creatinine is the standard marker to detect CIN. However, serum creatinine demonstrates major limitations. Using the Cockcroft-Gault and the Modification of Diet in Renal Disease equations are useful in estimation of the GFR. Serum cystatin C has been proposed as an alternative endogenous marker of GFR showing higher correlation to standard clearance methods such as inulin or iohexol clearance. Serum cystatin C may detect CIN one to two days earlier than creatinine. Also, recent studies documented that serum and urine neutrophil gelatinase-associated lipocalin is an early predictive biomarker of CIN in patients underwent coronary angiography (Shaker et al., 2010). Cholesterol atheroemboli, volume depletion, and interstitial nephritis should consider in differential diagnosis of CIN. Before coronary angiography, the volume status of high-risk patients can be assessed through the inferior vena cava index or bioimpedance spectroscopy. The incidence of CIN is reported to be 0.6-2.3% in general population who do not have any risk factor for CIN, but the incidence can be increased to 90% in patients at high risk for CIN (Toprak, 2007).

2.1 Pathophysiology of CIN

The pathogenesis of CIN is unclear. The proposed mechanisms are medullary hypoxia due to decreased renal blood flow secondary to renal artery vasoconstriction, tubular obstruction and direct tubular toxicity of the CM due to apoptosis and oxidative damage. Endothelial dysfunction and renal microcirculatory alterations also may play a role. The development of CIN is affected by changes in renal hemodynamics, such as increased activity of renal vasoconstrictors and decreased activity of renal vasodilators. Other factors that may decrease renal blood flow include increased viscosity of CM and increased erythrocyte aggregation induced by CM, which results in diminished oxygen delivery. Contrast agents have been found to reduce antioxidant enzyme activity, and direct cytotoxic effects mediated by oxygen free radicals. Apoptosis is also involved as a result of cellular injury. Hyperosmolar contrast agents induce renal hemodynamic changes caused by osmolar-driven solute diuresis with activation of tubuloglomerular feedback or an increase in tubular hydrostatic pressures, which may cause compression of the intrarenal microcirculation and a decreased GFR. Also hyperosmolar contrast agents have direct toxic effects on renal epithelial cells. In addition, DNA fragmentation was increased in cells exposed to hyperosmolar CM.

2.2 Clinical course and outcomes

CIN may range in severity from asymptomatic, nonoliguric transient renal dysfunction to oliguric severe renal failure that necessitates permanent dialysis. CIN is reported to be the third leading cause of in-hospital acute renal failure after hypotension and surgery. Approximately $180 million is spent annually to manage CIN in the US. Dangas et al. showed that in-hospital outcomes such as death (6.3% vs 0.8%), cardiac death (4.0% vs 0.5%), coronary artery bypass grafting (5.8% vs 0.5%), major adverse cardiac event (9.3% vs 1.1%), packed red cell transfusion (28% vs 6%), vascular surgery of access site (5.6% vs 2.6%), post-procedure length of stay (6.8±7.1 vs 2.3±2.5) were significantly higher in CIN developed patients compare with control ($p<0.0001$). In cumulative one-year outcome death, out-of-hospital death and major adverse cardiac events were significantly higher in CIN developed patients ($p<0.0001$) (Dangas et al., 2005). In a study of acute myocardial infarction patients undergoing primary angioplasty, it was found that CIN developed patients have significantly higher incidence of high-rate atrial fibrillation ($p=0.01$), high-degree conduction disturbances requiring permanent pacemaker ($p=0.04$), acute pulmonary edema ($p=0.008$), respiratory failure requiring mechanical ventilation ($p<0.0001$), cardiogenic shock requiring intra-aortic balloon ($p<0.0001$), and acute renal failure requiring renal replacement therapy ($p<0.0001$) (Marenzi et al., 2004).

2.3 Risk factors for CIN

Specific factors that increase the risks for development of CIN are related to the patient, the contrast media, and the procedure (Table 1).

2.3.1 Patient-related risk factors

Older age

The possible reasons of the high incidence of CIN in elderly were age-related changes in renal function, more difficult vascular access following tortuosity, calcification of the vessels

Risk Factors	Odds Ratio (95%CI)	p Value
Kidney Related Risk Factors		
Pre-existing renal failure		
Preprocedural creatinine 2.0-2.9 mg/dl	7.37 (4.78-11.39)	<0.0001
Preprocedural creatinine ≥ 3mg/d	12.82 (8.01-20.54)	<0.0001
Diabetes mellitus-Diabetic nephropathy		
Preprocedural creatinine≤ 1.1mg/dl	1.86 (1.20-2.89)	0.005
Preprocedural creatinine 1.2-1.9 mg/dl	2.42 (1.54-3.79)	<0.001
Use of nephrotoxic drugs		
Low effective circulatory volume	1.19 (0.72-1.95)	0.05
Cardiovascular System Related Risk Factors		
Class III-IV congestive heart failure	2.20 (1.60-2.90)	<0.0001
Left ventricle ejection fraction<40%	1.57 (1.14-2.16)	0.005
Acute myocardial infarction ≤ 24 h	1.85 (1.31-2.63)	0.0006
Hypertension	2.00 (1.40-2.80)	0.0001
Periprocedural hypotension	2.50 (1.70-3.69)	<0.00001
Multi-vessel coronary involvement	3.24 (1.07-9.82)	0.038
Peripheral vascular disease	1.90 (1.40-2.70)	<0.0001
Preprocedure shock	1.19 (0.72-1.96)	0.05
Using intra-aortic balloon pump	15.51 (4.65-51.64)	<0.0001
Bypass graft intervention	4.94 (1.16-20.9)	0.03
Time-to-reperfusion ≥6 h	2.51 (1.01-6.16)	0.04
Pulmonary edema	2.56 (1.42-4.52)	0.001
Demographic Risk Factors		
Age >75 years	5.28 (1.98-14.05)	0.0009
Female gender	1.4 (1.25-1.60)	0.0001
Contrast Media Related Risk Factors		
High total dose of contrast agent (>300 ml)	2.8 (1.17-6.68)	0.02
Osmolality (Low- vs. high-osmolality)	0.50 (0.36-0.68)	
Short duration of two contrast administration	4.4 (2.9-6.5)	<0.0001
Other Possible Risk Factors		
Procedural success	0.27 (0.19-0.38)	<0.0001
Baseline hematocrit	0.95 (0.92-0.97)	<0.00001
Hyperuricemia	4.71 (1.29-17.21)	0.019
ACE inhibitors	3.37 (1.14-9.94)	0.028
Angiotensin Receptor Blockers	2.70 (1.25-5.81)	0.011
Metabolic Syndrome	426 (1.19-15.25)	0.026
Hypoalbuminemia	5.79 (1.71-19.64)	0.005
Hypercholesterolemia		
Renal transplant		
Multiple myeloma		
Diuretics		
Intra-arterial contrast administration		
Sepsis, cirrhosis		

Table 1. Risk factors for the development of contrast-induced nephropathy

requiring greater amount of CM, defective prostaglandin synthesis, and the presence of renovascular disease. Furthermore, hypovolemia is very common in elderly patients. In a prospective study in which elderly patients (≥70 years) were subjected to cardiac catheterization, 11% developed CIN (Rich & Crecelius, 1990). In another study, CIN incidence was 17% in elderly patients (>60 years) as compared with 4% in younger patients (Kohli et al., 2000). In 208 patients with acute myocardial infarction who underwent coronary intervention, it was found that an age of ≥75 years was an independent risk for CIN (OR=5.28, p=0.0009) (Marenzi et al., 2004).

Gender

In a retrospective study of 8628 patients who underwent PCI, female sex was an independent predictor of CIN (OR=1.4, p<0.0001). One-year outcome analyses by gender showed a higher mortality among females than among males in a cohort of CIN patients (14% vs 10%, p=0.05) (Iakovou et al., 2003). The findings of this study contradict those of a previous randomized controlled trial of ionic vs nonionic CM, in which a multivariate analysis identified male gender as an independent risk factor for CIN (Rudnick et al., 1995). Whether female gender is truly an independent predictor of CIN will require further confirmatory studies.

Pre-existing renal disease

The major risk factor for CIN is a GFR<60 ml/min/1.73 m^2. Chronic kidney disease is associated with decreased vasodilatory response, which is important in developing CIN, and in patients with renal insufficiency, the clearance of CM is slower than in normal subjects. In a study of 7586 patients who underwent coronary intervention, CIN developed in 22.4% of the patients who had serum creatinine levels of 2.0 to 2.9 mg/dl and in 30.6% of those with serum creatinine levels of 3.0 mg/dl or higher, compared with 2.4% of patients with serum creatinine levels <1.1 mg/dl (Rihal et al., 2002). Two other studies (Moore et al., 1992; Barrett et al., 1992) reported that the incidence of CIN increased from 4% to 20% as the baseline serum creatinine increased from 1.2 to 2.9 mg/dl. In another study, the incidence of CIN increased from 8% to 92% as the serum creatinine increased from 1.5 to 6.8 mg/dl. Furthermore, the probability of CIN requiring dialysis increases from 0.04% to 48% as the baseline GFR decreases from 50 to 10 ml/min (McCullough et al., 1997).

Diabetes mellitus

Patients with diabetes constitute an important group at high risk of developing CIN. Patients with diabetic nephropathy and a mean serum creatinine of 6.8 mg/dl had a 92% incidence of CIN after coronary angiography (Weinrauch et al., 1977). Patients with diabetes who have advanced chronic renal failure because of causes other than diabetic nephropathy are at significantly higher risk of developing CIN like diabetic nephropathy. On the other hand, studies have shown that when pre-existing renal disease is present, patients with and without diabetes are similarly at risk of CIN, which correlates with the degree of renal disease. Some authors have suggested that DM in the absence of nephropathy, particularly in insulin-dependent patients with diabetes, is associated with an increased risk of CIN (McCullough et al., 1997; Toprak 2007). In a study, it was found that the incidence of CIN was rather low (2%) in patients with neither diabetes nor azotemia, significantly higher (16%) in individuals with diabetes but preserved renal function, and much higher (38%) in patients who had both diabetes and azotemia (Lautin et al., 1991). In another study, the incidence of CIN was found to be 2% in patients without diabetes and 3.7% in patients with diabetes with a baseline creatinine of 1.1 mg/dl or less (OR=1.86, p=0.005). When renal function is mildly impaired (serum creatinine level 1.2 to 1.9 mg/dl), the risk of CIN in patients with diabetes mellitus increases to 4.5% (OR=2.42, p<0.001) (Rihal et al., 2002). Other studies have failed to corroborate this connection (Parfrey et al., 1989). However, given that, those with diabetes alone were found to be at slightly higher risk of CIN than the general population.

Pre-diabetes

In a study of 421 patients who underwent coronary angiography with renal insufficiency, we presented that pre-DM increase the incidence of CIN 2.1-fold in comparison to patients with normal fasting glucose (NFG) but pre-DM is not as strong as DM as a risk of developing CIN. CIN occurred in 20% of the DM (RR=3.6, p=0.001), 11.4% of the pre-DM (RR 2.1, p=0.314) and 5.5% of the NFG group. The decrease of GFR was higher in DM and pre-DM (p=0.001 and p=0.002, respectively). Length of hospital stay was 2.45 ± 1.45 day in DM, 2.27 ± 0.68 day in pre-DM, and 1.97 ± 0.45 day in NFG (p<0.001, DM vs. NFG and p=0.032, pre-DM vs. NFG). The rate of major adverse cardiac events was 8.7% in DM, 5% in pre-DM, and 2.1% in NFG (*P*=0.042, DM vs. NFG). Hemodialysis was required in 3.6% of DM, and 0.7% in pre-DM (*P*=0.036, DM vs. NFG), and the total number of hemodialysis sessions during 3 months was higher in DM and pre-DM (*P*<0.001). Serum glucose ≥124 mg/dl was the best cut-off point for prediction of CIN (Toprak et al., 2007).

Congestive heart failure and reduced left ventricular ejection fraction

Studies have shown that reduced left ventricular ejection fraction (LVEF) (≤49%) and advanced congestive heart failure are independent risk factors for CIN. In a study, Dangas et al. showed that LVEF below 40% is an independent predictor of CIN (Dangas et al., 2005). We have previously reported that if the LVEF is greater than 30%, this condition does not show any significant effect on the development of CIN (Toprak et al., 2003). In a study it was shown that congestive heart failure was an independent risk for CIN (OR=1.53, p=0.007) (Rihal et al., 2002). In a cohort study it was found that congestive heart failure is a risk for CIN in patients who underwent PCI (OR=2.2, p<0.0001) (Bartholomew et al., 2004).

Hypertension

Hypertension has been categorized as a risk factor for CIN in some research. In a study of 8628 patients who underwent percutaneous interventions, hypertension was found to be an independent predictor of CIN (OR=1.2, p=0.0035) (Iakovou et al., 2003). In another cohort study, hypertension was a risk for CIN in patients who underwent PCI (OR=2.0, p=0.0001) (Bartholomew et al., 2004).

ACE Inhibitors and angiotensin receptor blockers

ACE inhibitors have been identified as a risk factor for CIN because of their potential to reduce renal function. On the other hand, some small studies have shown that the nephrotoxicity of CM may be reduced because of decreased renal vasoconstriction by inhibition of angiotensin II. In a randomized controlled study with 71 patients with diabetes who underwent coronary angiography randomized to captopril or control, 25-mg captopril was given three times daily. There was a significant decrease in CIN in the patients who received captopril compared with the control group (6% vs 29%, respectively, p<0.02) (Gupta et al., 1999). We have performed a randomized controlled study in 80 patients with serum creatinine below 2 mg/dl who underwent coronary angiography. Captopril was administered in 48 patients before coronary angiography. Five patients (10.4%) in the captopril group developed CIN, compared with only one patient (3.1%) in the control group (p=0.02) (Toprak et al., 2003). In a study of 230 patients with renal insufficiency and age ≥65 years we found that chronic ACE inhibitor administration was a risk for developing CIN. CIN occurred in 17 patients (15.6%) in the ACE inhibitor group and 7 patients (5.8%) in the control group (p=0.015). Chronic ACE inhibitor administration was a risk indicator of CIN (OR=3.37, p=0.028) (Cirit et al., 2006). In another study, 421 patients with renal insufficiency who underwent coronary angiography, use of ACE inhibitors or ARB was a risk for CIN in multivariate analysis (OR=2.7, p=0.011) (Toprak et al., 2007). In a recent study, the impact of renin-angiotensin and aldosterone system blockade on the frequency of CIN was assessed retrospectively. Patients treated with ACE inhibitors or ARB (n=269) and were not treated with them (n=143) underwent coronary angiography included to the study. CIN developed 11.9% in ACE-inhibitor using group and 4.2% in control group (p=0.006). Use of ARB or ACE inhibitors was found as a risk for CIN (OR=3.08, p=0.016) (Kiski et al., 2010). Checking the use of ACE inhibitors or ARB before coronary angiography seems to be a useful guide in tracking risk assessment for CIN.

Nephrotoxic drugs

Sulfonamides, aminoglycosides, and their combination with furosemide are particularly potent. Cyclosporin A may intensify medullary hypoxia, and cisplatin can attach to sulfhydryl groups. Mannitol can increase the metabolic workload in the kidney, and amphotericin B can cause the effect of a combination of mannitol and cyclosporine A. However, the individual roles of these medications as independent risk factors of CIN have not been determined in large trials. Nonetheless, it seems quite likely that nonselective NSAIDs and selective COX-2 inhibitors decrease the vasodilatory prostaglandins in the kidney and potentiate the vasoconstrictive effect of CM.

Multiple myeloma

The pathomechanism of this process has been explained by the precipitation of CM molecules together with Tamm–Horsfall proteins and other abnormal proteins, tubular epithelial cells damaged and desquamated as a result of ischemia, direct contrast toxicity, or disturbed function of integrins. In studies conducted on animals, intratubular light chains, particularly in the setting of intravascular volume depletion, have been found to augment the nephrotoxic potential of CM (Holland et al., 1985). Studies showed an incidence of CIN of only 0.6–1.25% in patients with myeloma if dehydration is avoided (McCarthy & Becker, 1992).

Metformin

The oral antidiabetic agent metformin is not itself nephrotoxic, but it is known that patients who are receiving metformin may develop lactic acidosis as a result of CIN. A decline in renal function after contrast exposure could adversely affect the clearance of metformin. The complication was almost always observed in diabetic patients with decreased renal function before injection of CM. It seems safer to instruct patients especially at high risk for CIN not to take this drug for 48 h or so after CM administration and resume taking the drug only if there are no signs of nephrotoxicity.

Hypercholesterolemia

In the literature, there are limited studies on the relationship between hypercholesterolemia and CIN. According to these studies, hypercholesterolemia aggravates CIN through the reduced production of nitric oxide (Yang et al., 2004). Altered nitric oxide-dependent renal vasodilatation, which is important in the pathogenesis of CIN, is prevalent in hypercholesterolemia.

Hyperuricemia

It has been suggested that tubular obstruction by uric acid plays a role in the pathogenesis of CIN. In a prospective cohort study we evaluated 266 patients who undergoing elective coronary angiography and we found that patients with hyperuricemia are at risk of developing CIN (OR=4.71, $p=0.019$). CIN occurred in 15.1% of the hyperuricemic group and 2.9% of the normouricemic group ($p<0.001$). Length of hospital stay ($p<0.001$) and CIN requiring renal replacement therapy ($p=0.017$) were significantly higher in hyperuricemic group. Serum uric acid ≥7 mg/dl in males and ≥5.9 mg/dl in females were found the best cut-off value for prediction of CIN (Toprak et al., 2006).

Multivessel coronary involvement, peripheral vascular disease, and renal artery stenosis

Factors related to accelerated or diffuse atherosclerosis are linked to the development of CIN. The treatment of multivessel disease, challenging chronic total occlusions and extensively diseased coronary segments, may require high doses of CM for providing an optimal image quality, thus enhancing the potential toxic effects on the renal function. If a patient has multivessel coronary involvement, the other vessels in the body, such as the renal artery, can be involved. In a study of 177 patients who underwent cardiac catheterization, subjects were also evaluated for renal artery stenosis. Coronary artery disease was detected in 110 patients (62%), and significant renal artery stenosis was detected in 19 patients (11%). Using multivariate analysis, it was found that the extent of coronary artery disease was an independent predictor of renal artery stenosis (Weber-Mzell et al., 2002). In a study a total of 5571 patients who underwent PCI were evaluated for CIN risk factors, and it was found that multivessel coronary involvement was only a univariate predictor of CIN ($p=0.003$) (Mehran et al., 2004). In two other cohort studies it was found that peripheral vascular disease is a risk for CIN in patients who underwent PCI (OR=1.9, $p<0.0001$ and OR=1.71, $p=0.001$, respectively) (Bartholomew et al., 2004; Rihal et al., 2002). In a study a total of 219 non-diabetic patients who underwent coronary angiography we have found that multivessel coronary involvement is a risk for CIN (OR=3.24, $p=0.038$) (Toprak et al., 2006).

Hypovolemia

Decreased effective circulating volume and reduced renal perfusion potentiate renal vasoconstriction after administration of intravascular CM. The toxic effects of CM on the renal tubular lumen may be exacerbated in hypovolemia. At present the most convincing preventive procedure of CIN is adequate hydration with isotonic saline or sodium bicarbonate, and intravenous hydration seems to have better results than does oral hydration. Before angiography, the volume status of patients can be assessed through the inferior vena cava index, mean atrial pressure, noninvasive pulmonary-capillary wedge pressure or bioimpedance spectroscopy (Toprak & Cirit, 2005).

Renal transplantation

Patients with renal transplantation may be at a higher risk of CIN due to concomitant use of cyclosporine and higher prevalence of diabetes and renal insufficiency. In a study, 33 patients with a functioning renal allograft who underwent different contrast studies, the incidence of CIN was 21.2% (Ahuja et al., 2000).

Acute myocardial infarction

A study by Rihal et al. showed that acute myocardial infarction within 24 h before administration of the CM is a risk factor for CIN (OR=1.85, p=0.0006). This study demonstrates that CIN is a frequent complication in acute myocardial infarction, even in patients with a normal baseline renal function. (Rihal et al., 2002). In a study of 208 acute myocardial infarction patients who underwent primary PCI, anterior acute myocardial infarction was significantly higher in patients who developed CIN (p=0.0015). However, in multivariate analysis, anterior acute myocardial infarction (OR=2.17, p=0.09) was not a risk for CIN (Marenzi et al., 2004). In 2082 percutaneous interventions for acute myocardial infarction, it was reported a more than seven-fold (3.2% vs 23.3%) increase in 1-year mortality in patients who developed CIN (Sadeghi et al., 2003).

Low hematocrit level

A baseline hematocrit value of less than 39% for men and less than 36% for women is a risk for CIN. The relationship between low hematocrit levels and CIN has been investigated in a prospective study of 6773 patients who underwent PCI (Nikolsky et al., 2005). A lower baseline hematocrit was an independent predictor of CIN; and each 3% decrease in baseline hematocrit resulted in a significant increase in the odds of CIN in patients with and without chronic kidney disease (11% and 23%, respectively). Dangas et al. showed that the baseline hematocrit level is an independent predictor of CIN in patients with chronic kidney disease (OR=0.95, p<0.00001) (Dangas et al., 2005).

Low serum albumin

Hypoalbuminemia impairs endothelial function, enhances renal vasoconstriction, impairs the synthesis and release of nitric oxide, and decreases antioxidant enzyme activity. In a study, low serum albumin (<3.5 g/dl) was identified as a risk factor for CIN in patients 70 years of age or older who underwent cardiac catheterization (Rich, et al., 1990). Also we have found that in 230 patients who underwent coronary angiography with renal insufficiency, serum albumin level ≤3.5 g/dl was a risk factor for CIN (OR=5.79, p=0.005) (Cirit et al., 2006).

Hypotension, sepsis, cirrhosis, and pulmonary edema

A systolic blood pressure of less than 80 mm Hg for at least 1 h that requires inotropic support with medications is a risk factor for CIN. A study by Dangas et al showed that periprocedural hypotension and pulmonary edema are independent predictors of CIN in patients with chronic kidney disease (OR=2.50, p<0.00001 and OR=2.56, p=0.001, respectively) (Dangas et al., 2005) Sepsis, through direct damage by bacterial toxins to renal tubules and impairment of circulation, has also been reported as a risk factor. Reduction of effective intravascular volume caused by liver cirrhosis has been reported as contributing to pre-renal reduction in renal perfusion, thus enhancing the ischemic insult of CM (Toprak, 2007).

Metabolic syndrome, impaired fasting glucose and hypertriglyceridemia

In a prospective cohort study of 219 non-diabetic elderly patients with reduced kidney function who underwent elective coronary angiography, we reported that metabolic syndrome was a risk indicator of CIN (OR=4.26, p=0.026). CIN occurred in 14% of the metabolic syndrome group and 3.6% of the non-metabolic syndrome group (relative risk 3.93, p=0.007). Impaired fasting glucose (OR=4.72, p=0.007), high triglyceride (OR=4.06, p=0.022); and multi-vessel involvement (OR=3.14, p=0.038) in the metabolic syndrome group were predictors of CIN (Toprak et al., 2006).

2.3.2 Procedure-related risk factors

Short duration of the two contrast administration and urgent/emergency procedure

In those who have no risk factors for CIN, angiography should be delayed more than 48 hours after a previous exposure to intravascular contrast media. In patients with diabetes or preexisting renal disease, this time interval should be increased to more than 72 hours. In a cohort study, urgent/emergency procedure was found as a predictor of CIN (OR=4, p<0.0001) (Bartholomew et al., 2004). The higher risk of developing CIN in patients with urgent status was irrespective of baseline renal function.

Use of intra-aortic balloon pump

In 208 consecutive acute myocardial infarction patients undergoing percutaneous coronary intervention, use of intra-aortic balloon pump was a risk predictor of CIN (OR=15.51, p<0.0001) (Marenzi et al., 2004). In a study, it has demonstrated that, intra-aortic balloon pump use is an independent predictor of CIN in patients with chronic kidney disease (OR=2.27, p=0.004) (Dangas et al., 2005). In another study, it was found that the use of intra-aortic balloon pump was a risk factor for CIN requiring dialysis after PCI (OR=1.94) (Gruberg et al., 2001). In another derivation and validation cohort study, intra-aortic balloon pump use was a risk for CIN in patients undergoing coronary intervention (OR=5.1, p<0.0001) (Bartholomew et al., 2004).

Bypass graft intervention and delayed reperfusion

Procedures with bypass angiography and intervention may be associated with higher complexity, longer duration, and limited success, thus indicating an unstable post-procedural period with impaired cardiac output. Gruberg et al. showed that the risk of CIN requiring dialysis after PCI was increased with bypass graft intervention (OR=4.94) (Gruberg et al., 2001). In a study of 208 acute myocardial infarction patients undergoing primary PCI, the risk of CIN was increased if the time-to-reperfusion is ≥6 h (OR=2.51, p=0.04) (Marenzi et al., 2004)

2.3.3 Contrast medium-related risk factors

Increased dose of contrast medium

According to different sources, the relatively safe cutoff point of contrast amount varies from 70 ml up to 220ml. However, doses as low as 20 to 30 ml are capable of inducing CIN. In a study that patients undergoing coronary angiography, each 100 ml of contrast medium administered was associated with a significant increase of 12% in the risk of CIN (OR=1.12, p=0.02) (Rihal et al., 2002). Marenzi et al. showed that contrast volume >300 ml is an independent risk for CIN (OR=2.80, p=0.02) (Marenzi et al., 2004). In another study patients with preexisting renal failure revealed a 10-fold risk of CIN when more than 125 ml of contrast media was administered (Taliercio et al., 1986).

High-osmolar and ionic CM

In a large study which comparing the non-ionic low-osmolality agent iohexol to the ionic high-osmolality agent meglumine/sodium diatrizoate in patients with pre-existing renal dysfunction undergoing angiography, patients with renal insufficiency receiving diatrizoate were 3.3 times as likely to develop CIN compared to those receiving iohexol (Rudnick et al., 1995). NEPHRIC trial is a randomized, prospective study comparing the nonionic iso-osmolar CM iodixanol with the nonionic low-osmolar CM iohexol in 129 renal impairment patients with diabetes undergoing coronary or aorto-femoral angiography. The incidence of CIN was 3% in the iodixanol group and 26% in the iohexol group ($p=0.002$) (Aspelin et al., 2003). In another randomized study, the renal tolerance of iodixanol and iohexol was compared in 124 patients with creatinine >1.7 mg/dl. The incidence of CIN was 3.7% in iodixanol group and 10% in iohexol group ($p>0.05$) (Chalmers et al., 1999). The available data do not provide clear evidence that the whole iso-osmolar CM class offers an improvement over the low-osmolar CM class. Other studies with iodixanol in renal failure patients have shown a higher incidence of CIN than that observed in the NEPHRIC study (21% in the RAPPID trial, 30% in the CONTRAST trial) (Baker et al., 2003: Stone et al., 2003). In addition to their osmolarity, contrast medias are characterized as ionic versus non-ionic. Small clinical trials of low-risk patients undergoing coronary angiography have shown little difference in the risk of CIN between the 2 types of CM. However, a randomized trial of 1196 patients undergoing coronary angiography showed that non-ionic CM reduced the incidence of CIN in patients with preexisting renal disease with or without diabetes (Rudnick et al., 1995). In addition, symptomatic or hemodynamic adverse drug events have been shown to occur less often with non-ionic, low-osmolality CM compared with ionic, high-osmolality CM. In high-risk patients, it is reasonable to don't use the high-osmolar and ionic CM to minimize the risk of CIN.

Intra-arterial administration of the contrast media

Intra-arterial contrast administration is a risk for CIN. This effect is thought to be due to the fact that the acute intra renal concentration of CM is much higher after intra arterial rather than intravenous injection.

2.3.4 Scoring method to predict high risk patients for CIN

Mehran et al. developed a simple scoring method that integrates eight baseline clinical variables to assess the risk of CIN after percutaneous coronary intervention (PCI). These are hypotension (score 5), use of intra-aortic balloon pump (score 5), congestive heart failure (score 5), serum creatinine>1.5 mg/dl (score 4), age>75 years (score 4), anemia (score 3), diabetes mellitus (score 3), and volume of CM (score 1 per 100 ml). If the total score is 5 or less, the risk category is low; if the total score is 16 or higher, the risk category is very high (Mehran et al., 2004)

2.4 Prevention strategies for CIN

Extracellular volume expansion with intravenous saline or sodium bicarbonate, minimizing the dose of CM, using low-osmolar non-ionic CM instead of high osmolar ionic CM, stopping the intake of nephrotoxic drugs and avoiding short intervals between procedures requiring CM have all been shown to be effective in reducing CIN. Alternatives to ordinary CM, such as carbon dioxide or gadolinium chelates, can be used in patients at high risk of CIN (Table 2).

Volume expansion

Volume expansion is the single most important measure that has been documented to be beneficial in preventing CIN. A standardized saline hydration protocol has been proven

Clinical evidence advocating their use	**Don't use**	**With conflicting or limited evidence**
Extracellular volume expansion	Nonsteroidal anti-inflammatory drugs, COX-2 inhibitors, aminoglycoside, cisplatin	Acetylcystein
Saline or sodium bicarbonate	Loop diuretics	Theophylline
Low or iso-osmolar contrast	Mannitol	Calcium channel blockers
Minimizing the dose of contrast	Multiple use of contrast within 72 h	Fenoldopam
Alternative imaging techniques	Large doses of contrast	Captopril
Monitoring serum creatinine	High-osmolar contrast	Ascorbic acid
Delaying contrast procedures until hemodynamic status is corrected	Metformin usage especially in patients with renal failure	Atrial natriuretic peptide
≥48 h between contrast procedures		Endothelin antagonist
		PGE1
		Hemofiltration
		Nebivolol
		Statins
		B-type natriuretic peptide
		Pentoxifylline

Table 2. Prevention strategies for contrast-induced nephropathy in high-risk patients

effective in reducing the risk of CIN and should be used routinely. The most widely accepted protocol is administering isotonic saline at 1 to 1.5 ml/kg/h beginning 6 to 12 hours prior to the procedure and continuing for up to 12 hours following contrastadministration. In a randomized trial, two different hydration regimens were compared in 1620 patients undergoing coronary interventions. They showed that the incidence of CIN was significantly lower among patients given an isotonic saline solution than among those given a hypotonic saline solution (0.7% vs. 2.0% respectively, $p=0.04$) (Mueller et al., 2002). In another trial, a total of 119 patients with serum creatinine exceeding 1.1 mg/dl were randomized to receive isotonic solution of sodium bicarbonate (n=59) or isotonic saline (n=60) at a rate of 3 ml/kg/h for 1 hour before and 1 ml/kg/h for 6 hours after contrast administration. CIN developed in only 1 patient (1.7%) compared with 8 patients (13.6%) in the saline group ($p=0.02$) (Merten et al., 2004). The authors postulated that a reduction in oxidative injury may have conferred protection against CIN. However, further studies are required to clarify the role of hydration with sodium bicarbonate in preventing CIN. In a prospective study, the effect of combination intravenous and oral volume supplementation on the development of CIN was studied in 425 patients undergoing percutaneous coronary intervention. Patients were randomly assigned to receive hydration with either isotonic or half-isotonic. In addition patients were encouraged to drink plenty of fluids (at least 1500 ml). They found that applying the combination of intravenous and oral volume supplementation results in a very low incidence of CIN (1.4%)

(Mueller et al., 2005). Most studies have found that hydration alone is better than hydration combined with a diuretic. In a study, 78 patients with serum creatinine >1.6 mg/dl were randomized to three groups: hydration alone, hydration with mannitol and hydration with furosemide. Half-isotonic saline was used for hydration. CIN occurred in 11%, 28% and 40% of patients in the three groups, respectively (p=0.02), thus showing that forced diuresis is of no benefit in preventing CIN. In a meta-analysis it was found that the administration of sodium bicarbonate is superior to the administration of saline alone in the prevention of CIN (Solomon et al., 1994). However, further controlled clinical trials are needed due to significant study heterogeneity and publication bias. The effectiveness of sodium bicarbonate treatment to prevent CIN in high-risk patients remains uncertain.

N-acetylcysteine

It had been postulated that antioxidant N-acetylcysteine (NAC) might scavenge oxygen free radicals, thus attenuate the cytotoxic effects of CM. NAC may also have direct vasodilating effects on the kidneys through an increase in the biologic effects of nitric oxide. Tepel et al. were evaluated the effects of NAC (600 mg orally twice daily), at first time, in 83 patients undergoing computed tomography. Two percent of the patients in the NAC group had CIN versus 21% in the placebo group (p=0.01) (Tepel et al., 2000). Since then, a number of trials have been published. Results from these trials have been inconsistent. In a randomized, placebo-controlled study it was found that NAC is protective against CIN Fifty-four patients were randomized to receive either 600 mg of NAC twice daily for 4 doses or placebo. The incidence of CIN was 8% in the NAC group versus 45% in the placebo group (p=0.005) (Diaz-Sandoval et al., 2002). In addition to oral administration, intravenous administration of NAC to protect against CIN has also been evaluated. In a study, Baker et al. randomly assigned 80 patients to receive either NAC infusion (n=41) versus saline infusion (n=39). CIN developed in only 2 (5%) of patients in the NAC group compared with 8 (21%) in the saline group (p=0.04) (Baker et al., 2003). The authors concluded that NAC infusion protects against CIN. In a meta-analysis, evaluating more than 800 patients at high risk of developing CIN also documented a positive impact of NAC prophylaxis on CIN (Birck et al., 2003). In another meta-analysis, nine randomized controlled trials were included and the difference in mean change in creatinine between the NAC treated group and controls was -0.27 mg/dl. The relative risk of developing CIN was 0.43 in subjects randomized to NAC. They suggest that NAC helps prevent declining renal function and CIN (Liu et al., 2005). In contrast to these reports, some studies failed to find a significant effect of NAC on the occurrence of CINA total of 183 patients with preexisting renal insufficiency undergoing contrast study were randomly assigned to receive NAC at a dose of 600 mg twice daily on the day before and the day of the contrast study plus saline infusion or saline alone. The incidence of CIN was 6.5% in the NAC group versus 11% in the control group (p=0.22) (Briguori et al., 2002). In a multi centric double blind clinical trial 156 patients undergoing coronary angiography or percutaneous coronary intervention with creatinine clearance <50 ml/min were randomly assigned to receive N-acetylcysteine 600 mg orally twice daily for two days or placebo. Sixteen patients developed CIN. Eight of 77 patients (10.4%) in the NAC group and eight of 79 patients (10.1%) in the placebo group (p=1.00). No difference was observed in the change in endogenous creatinine clearance, p=0.28). They concluded that oral NAC did not prevent CIN in patients at low to moderate risk undergoing cardiac catheterisation with ionic low osmolality CM (Gomes et al., 2005). In another study, 50 patients undergoing elective diagnostic coronary angiography with serum creatinine values above 1.3 mg/dl were included and CIN was detected in 3 of 25 patients (12%) in the NAC group and 2 of 25 patients (8%) in the control group ($p>0.05$). It was detected that in patients planned to undergo elective diagnostic coronary angiography with renal dysfunction, oral NAC and hydration before the procedure was not more effective than hydration alone in the prevention of CIN (Gulel et al., 2005). A direct renoprotective effect of NAC remains questionable. To date, only a few trials described the effects of NAC not only on serum creatinine but also on clinical end points. The serum creatinine can be decrease in administration of NAC without renoprotective effect. In a prospective study, NAC was given at a dose of 600 mg every 12 h for a total of four doses to the volunteers with a normal renal function who did not receive contrast agent. There was a significant decrease of the mean serum creatinine ($p<0.05$) and a significant increase of the GFR ($p<0.02$), whereas the cystatin C concentration did not change significantly (Hoffmann et al., 2004). In patients undergoing emergency diagnostic procedures, in whom a full hydration protocol is not possible, an abbreviated hydration regimen plus oral or intravenous administration of NAC can be recommended. NAC may be of benefit mostly in high-risk patients. If NAC is to be used as a preventative measure, it should be given at a dose of 600 mg orally twice daily on the day before and day of the procedure.

Ascorbic acid

Prophylactic oral administration of ascorbic acid may protect against CIN. In a randomized, placebo-controlled trial in 231 patients with serum creatinine concentration ≥1.2 mg/dl who undergoing coronary angiography showed that the use of ascorbic acid was associated with a significant reduction in the rate of CIN. CIN occurred in 11 of the 118 patients (9%) in the ascorbic acid group and in 23 of the 113 patients (20%) in the placebo group (OR=0.38; $p=0.02$) (Spargias et al., 2004). Further prospective studies are needed to validate these preliminary results.

Fenoldopam

Fenoldopam mesylate is a selective dopamine-1 receptor agonist that produces systemic, peripheral and renal arterial vasodilatation. Several investigators have reported a positive impact of fenoldopam against CIN in small studies. In a placebo-controlled, double-blind, multicenter trial, 315 patients with creatinine clearance of less than 60 ml/min were randomized to receive fenoldopam infusion [0.05 μg/kg/min titrated to 0.1 μg/kg/min (n=157)] or matching placebo (n=158). CIN occurred in 33.6% of patients in the fenoldopam group compared with 30.1% of patients in the placebo group ($p=0.61$) (Stone et al., 2003). The authors concluded that fenoldopam did not protect against CIN. In 2 other large studies comparing fenoldopam with NAC treatment with fenoldopam either had a similar, non significant effect as that of NAC or was inferior to it (Allaqaband et al., 2002; Briguori et al., 2004). Therefore, the routine use of fenoldopam cannot be recommended at the present time.

Adenosine antagonists

CM stimulate the intrarenal secretion of adenosine, which binds to the renal adenosine receptor and acts as a potent vasoconstrictor, reducing renal blood flow and increasing the generation of oxygen free radicals as it is metabolized to xanthine and hypoxanthine. Theophylline and aminophylline, adenosine antagonists, have also been studied in the prevention of CIN in a number of trials. Studies with these agents have used varying doses and dosage forms and yielded conflicting results (Erley et al., 1999; Kapoor et al., 2001).

Based on the conflicting information found in clinical studies, adenosine antagonists should not be routinely used in patients as a preventative measure at this time.

Calcium channel blockers

The calcium channel antagonists verapamil and diltiazem have been found to attenuate the renal vasoconstrictor response after exposure to CM. However, when the efficacy of the felodipine, nitrendipine and nifedipine was evaluated, results were inconsistent. Two small studies performed the use of sublingual nifedipine given prior to contrast administration. Patients (n=20) who received sublingual nifedipine did not have a significant increase in serum creatinine, while those in the placebo group did (Rodicio et al., 1990). In another study, patients (n=30) who received nifedipine had an increase in renal plasma flow following administration of contrast, while patients in the placebo group had a decrease in renal flow (Russo et al., 1990). One other study showed that nitrendipine use cause a significant reduction in the GFR in the placebo group compared to little or no change in GFR in the nitrendipine group (Neumayer et al., 1989). In another study, 27 patients with normal to moderately reduced renal function underwent femoral angiography randomized to receive either oral felodipine or placebo. Patients in the felodipine group had a significant increase in serum creatinine from baseline, while patients in the placebo group did not demonstrate a similar increase (Spangberg-Viklund et al., 1996). More large-scale trials are needed before calcium channel blockers can be routinely recommended in patients prior to contrast administration.

Prostaglandin E_1

PGE_1 has vasodilatory effects that may be beneficial in preventing CIN. In one study, 130 patients were randomly assigned to receive either placebo or one of three doses of PGE_1. The increase in serum creatinine level was smaller in all of the three PGE_1 groups than in the placebo group, but the difference was significant only in the medium-dose (20 ng/kg/min) of PGE_1 group (Koch et al., 2000). More studies need to be done to better understand the role of prostaglandin E1, but results from this pilot study appear promising.

Atrial natriuretic peptide (ANP)

ANP may prevent CIN by increasing renal blood flow. In a study, ANP was included in one of the four arms. In which dopamine, mannitol, and ANP caused an increase in CIN in diabetic patients as compared to saline alone (Weisberg et al., 1994). In another trial patients were randomized to one of four treatment arms: fluid alone or one of three doses of ANP. Results showed no statistically significant differences in the incidence of CIN between any of the four treatment arms (Kurnik et al., 1998) Based on these results and the limited clinical data, ANP cannot be advocated in the prevention of CIN.

Endothelin antagonists

Endothelin-1 is a potent endogenous vasoconstrictor, is thought to play a role in the development of CIN. Endothelin-1 has two primary receptors. In animal studies, endothelin-A antagonists were shown to reduce the incidence of CIN (Liss et al., 2003). However, in a randomized study of 158 patients, the use of a mixed endothelin-A and B antagonist was associated with a significantly higher incidence of CIN than was placebo (56% vs. 29%, $p=0.002$) (Wang et al., 2000). Endothelin antagonists currently have no role in prevention of CIN.

Low-dose of dopamine

At low doses (1-3 mcg/kg/min), dopamine activates two types of dopamine (DA) receptors, DA-1 and DA-2. Activation of the DA-1 receptor results in an increase in natriuresis and renal blood flow. Since dopamine, at low doses, is believed to be more selective for the DA-1 receptors, it has been investigated in the prevention of CIN. Kapoor et al. randomized 40 patients with diabetes scheduled to undergo a coronary angiography to either dopamine or placebo control. None of the patients in the dopamine group developed CIN compared to 50% of patients receiving placebo (Kapoor et al., 2002). In another prospective, randomized trial, Hans et al. evaluated 55 patients (40% had diabetes) with chronic renal insufficiency. Patients were randomized to receive dopamine or an equal volume of saline. The group receiving dopamine had a significantly lower incidence of CIN as compared to the control group (Hans et al., 1998). In contrast to the trials showing a potential benefit of dopamine, other studies have failed to demonstrate this benefit. Abizaid et al. performed a randomized, prospective study involving patients with renal insufficiency who underwent coronary angioplasty. Patients were randomized to continue with the saline, receive aminophylline in addition to the saline, or receive dopamine plus saline. In the dopamine plus saline group, 50% of patients developed CIN, while only 30% of the patients in the saline-alone group developed CIN. This difference did not reach statistical significance, but it appeared that use of dopamine might worsen outcomes (Abizaid et al., 1999). Low-dose dopamine use cannot be supported at this time.

Statins

Whether additional benefits can be achieved with the use of statin in decreasing the risk of CIN remains undetermined. In a recent meta analysis of randomised controlled trials comparing statin pretreatment with non-statin pretreatment for the prevention of CIN, it was found that, the incidence of CIN was not significantly lower in statin pretreatment group as compared with control group (RR=0.76, p=0.30) (Zhang et al., 2011). The current cumulative evidence suggests that statin pretreatment may neither prevent CIN nor reduce the need for renal replacement therapy.

Hemofiltration and hemodialysis

Currently available data do not support use of prophylactic hemodialysis for prevention of CIN. In a trial of 113 patients, reported that CIN occurred in 24% of the hemodialysis group as compared with 16% of non-hemodialysis group (Vogt et al., 2001). Clinically relevant events also were not different in two groups. Only continuous venovenous hemofiltration has been shown to protect against CIN. In a study, 114 patients with chronic renal failure undergoing percutaneous coronary intervention were divided in two groups: 56 patients received normal saline and 58 patients underwent hemofiltration at a rate of 1000 ml/h (Marenzi et al., 2003). Hemofiltration seems to have a protective effect, including significant reduction in in-hospital and 1-year mortality compared with routine hydration. The mechanisms of this benefit are not clear. Further studies are needed to confirm the results of this trial.

New types of contrast medias

Gadolinium-enhanced magnetic resonance coronary angiography is a non-invasive method for evaluation of coronary arteries. It has been suggested that gadolinum-based CM could be used in stead of iodinated CM for radiological examinations in patients with significant renal impairment. However, its use has been questioned on the basis of reports of nephrotoxicity and its association with nephrogenic systemic fibrosis, a rare and serious syndrome that involves fibrosis of skin, joints, eyes, and internal organs. In a study by Hoffmann et al. the effect of gadopentetate dimeglumine (iodine-based CM) was studied in 181 patients with normal renal function and the effect of gadolinium was studied in 198 patients with pre-excisting renal failure. There was no statistically significant change in serum creatinine concentration after gadopentetate dimeglumine. In contrary, serum creatinine levels decreased significantly after the administration of gadolinium ($p<0.01$) (Hoffmann et al., 2005). In a retrospective study, the safety of gadolinium was evaluated in 91 patients with stage 3 and 4 renal failure who underwent angiographic MRI procedures. Eleven of 91 patients developed CIN (12.1%) (Ergun et al., 2006). In another randomized study gadobutrol, a gadolinium-based CM, was compared with standard iohexol, an iodinated CM, in 21 patients with renal dysfunction. The incidence of CIN was 50% in gadobutrol group and 45% in iohexol group ($p=0.70$). In this study, gadolinium showed no benefit over iohexol in patients with severely impaired renal function (Erley et al., 2004). More studies need to be done to better understand the role of gadolinum on CIN. Ultrasound contrast agents are micro-bubbles which produce acoustic enhancement. They are pharmacologically almost inert and safe.

3. Conclusion

The development of CIN is associated with adverse outcomes including prolonged hospitalization, the potential need for renal replacement therapy, and most important, increased mortality. The treatment of established CIN is limited to supportive measures and dialysis. For this reason, screening for high-risk patients before CM including cardiac procedures and taking the appropriate prophylactic regimens is important in reducing CIN. Pre-existing renal dysfunction, especially when secondary to diabetic nephropathy, is the most important risk factor. Extra cellular volume expansion and use of low osmolar CM are the two most effective measures to prevent CIN. Acetylcysteine may use in high-risk patients, but this finding has not been uniform or always demonstrated by currently available trials.

4. References

Abizaid, AS., Clark, CE., Mintz, GS., Dosa, S., Popma, JJ., Pichard, AD., Satler, LF., Harvey, M., Kent, KM., & Leon, MB. (1999). Effects of Dopamine and Aminophylline on Contrast-Induced Acute Renal Failure after Coronary Angioplasty in Patients with Preexisting Renal Insufficiency. *The American Journal of Cardiology*, Vol.83, No.2, (January 1999), pp.260-263, ISSN 0002-9149

Ahuja, TS., Niaz, N., & Agraharkar, M. (2000). Contrast-Induced Nephrotoxicity in Renal Allograft Recipients. *Clinical Nephrology*, Vol.54, No.1, (July 2000), pp.11-14, ISSN 0301-0430

Allaqaband, S., Tumuluri, R., Malik, AM., Gupta, A., Volkert, P., Shalev, Y., & Bajwa, TK. (2002). Prospective Randomized Study of N-Acetylcysteine, Fenoldopam, and Saline for Prevention of Radiocontrast-Induced Nephropathy. *Catheterization and Cardiovascular Interventions*, Vol.57, No.3, (November 2002), pp.279-283, ISSN 1522-1946

Aspelin, P., Aubry, P., Fransson, SG., Strasser, R., Willenbrock, R., & Berg, KJ. (2003). Nephrotoxic Effects in High-Risk Patients Undergoing Angiography. *The New England Journal of Medicine*, Vol.348, No.6, (February 2003), pp.491-499, ISSN 0028-4793

Baker, CS., Wragg, A., Kumar, S., De Palma, R., Baker, LR., & Knight, CJ. (2003). A Rapid Protocol for the Prevention of Contrast-Inducted Renal Dysfunction: The RAPPID Study. *Journal of the American College of the Cardiology*, Vol. 41, No. 12, (June 2003), pp.2114-2118, ISSN 0735-1097

Bartholomew, BA., Harjai, KJ., Dukkipati, S., Boura, JA., Yerkey, MW., Glazier, S., Grines, CL., & O'Neill, WW. (2004). Impact of Nephropathy after Percutaneous Coronary Intervention and a Method for Risk Stratification, *The American Journal of Cardiology*, Vol.93, No.12, (June 2004), pp.1515-1519, ISSN 0002-9149

Barrett, BJ., Parfrey, PS., Vavasour HM., McDonald, J., Kent, G., Hefferton, D., O'Dea, F., Stone, E., Reddy, R., & McManamon, PJ. (1992). Contrast Nephropathy in Patients with Impaired Renal Function: High Versus Low Osmolar Media. *Kidney International*, Vol.41, No.5, (May 1992), pp. 1274–1279, ISSN 0085-2538

Birck, R., Krzossok, S., Markowetz, F., Schnulle, P., van der Woude, FJ., & Braun, C. (2003). Acetylcysteine for Prevention of Contrast Nephropathy: Meta-Analysis. *Lancet*, Vol.362, No.9384, (August 2003), pp.598-603, ISSN 0140-6736

Briguori, C., Manganelli, F., Scarpato, P., Elia, PP., Golia, B., Riviezzo, G., Lepore, S., Librera, M., Villari, B., Colombo, A., & Ricciardelli, B. (2002). Acetylcysteine and Contrast Agent-Associated Nephrotoxicity. *Journal of the American College of the Cardiology*, Vol.40, No.2, (July 2002), pp. 298-303, ISSN 0735-1097

Briguori, C., Colombo, A., Airoldi, F., Violante, A., Castelli, A., Balestrieri, P., Paolo Elia, P., Golia, B., Lepore, S., Riviezzo, G., Scarpato, P., Librera, M., Focaccio, A., & Ricciardelli, B. (2004). N-Acetylcysteine Versus Fenoldopam Mesylate to Prevent Contrast Agent-Associated Nephrotoxicity. *Journal of the American College of the Cardiology*, Vol.44, No.4, (August 2004), pp.762-765, ISSN 0735-1097

Chalmers, N., & Jackson, RW. (1999). Comparison of Iodixanol and Iohexol in Renal Impairment. *The British Journal of Radiology*, Vol.72, No.859, (July 1999), pp.701-703, ISSN 0007-1285

Cirit, M., Toprak, O., Yesil, M., Bayata, S., Postaci, N., Pupim, L., & Esi, E. (2006). Angiotensin-Converting Enzyme Inhibitors as a Risk Factor for Contrast-Induced Nephropathy. *Nephron Clinical Practice*, Vol.104, No.1, (August 2006), pp. c20-c27, ISSN 1660-2110

Dangas, G., Iakovou, I., Nikolsky, E., Aymong, ED., Mintz, GS., Kipshidze, NN., Lansky, AJ., Moussa, I., Stone, GW., Moses, JW., Leon, MB., & Mehran, R. (2005). Contrast-Induced Nephropathy After Percutaneous Coronary Interventions in Relation to Chronic Kidney Disease and Hemodynamic Variables. *The American Journal of Cardiology*, Vol.95, No.1, (January 2005), pp. 13-19, ISSN 0002-9149

Diaz-Sandoval, LJ., Kosowsky, BD., & Losordo, DW. (2002). Acetylcysteine to Prevent Angiography-Related Renal Tissue Injury (The APART Trial). *American Journal of Cardiology*, Vol.89, No.3, (February 2002), pp.356-358, ISSN 0002-9149

Ergun, I., Keven, K., Uruc, I., Ekmekci, Y., Canbakan, B., Erden, I., & Karatan, O. (2006). The Safety of Gadolinium in Patients with Stage 3 and 4 Renal Failure. *Nephrology Dialysis Transplantation*, Vol.21, No.3, (March 2006), pp. 697-700, ISSN 0931-0509

Erley, CM., Bader, BD., Berger, ED., Tuncel, N., Winkler, S., Tepe, G., Risler, T., & Duda, S. Gadolinium-Based Contrast Media Compared with Iodinated Media for Digital Subtraction Angiography in Azotaemic Patients. *Nephrology Dialysis Transplantation*, Vol.19, No.10, (October 2004), pp.2526-2531, ISSN 0931-0509

Erley, CM., Duda, SH., Rehfuss, D., Scholtes, B., Bock, J., Muller, C., Osswald, H., & Risler, T. (1999). Prevention of Radiocontrast Media-Induced Nephropathy in Patients with Pre-Existing Renal Insufficiency by Hydration in Combination with the Adenosine Antagonist Theophylline. *Nephrology Dialysis Transplantation*, Vol.14, No.5, (May 1999), pp.1146–1149, ISSN 0931-0509

Gomes, VO., Poli de Figueredo, CE., Caramori, P., Lasevitch, R., Bodanese, LC., Araujo, A., Roedel, AP., Caramori, AP., Brito, FS Jr., Bezerra, HG., Nery, P., & Brizolara, A. (2005). N-Acetylcysteine Does Not Prevent Contrast Induced Nephropathy after Cardiac Catheterisation with an Ionic Low Osmolality Contrast Medium: A Multicentre Clinical Trial. *Heart*, Vol.91, No.6, (June 2005), pp.774-778, ISSN 1355-6037

Gruberg, L., Mehran, R., Dangas, G., Mintz, GS., Waksman, R., Kent, KM., Pichard, AD., Satler, LF., Wu, H., & Leon, MB. (2001). Acute Renal Failure Requiring Dialysis after Percutaneous Coronary Interventions. *Catheterization and Cardiovascular Interventions*, Vol.52, No.4, (April 2001), pp.409-416, ISSN 1522-1946

Gulel, O., Keles, T., Eraslan, H., Aydogdu, S., Diker, E., & Ulusoy, V. (2005). Prophylactic Acetylcysteine Usage for Prevention of Contrast Nephropathy after Coronary Angiography. *Journal of Cardiovascular Pharmacology*, Vol.46, No.4, (October 2005), pp.464-467, ISSN 0160-2446

Gupta, RK., Kapoor, A., Tewari, S., Sinha, N., & Sharma, RK. (1999). Captopril for Preventing of Contrast-Induced Nephropathy in Diabetic Patients: A Randomized Study. *Indian Heart Jouurnal*, Vol.51, No.5, (September 1999), pp.521–526, ISSN 0019-4832

Hans, SS., Hans, BA., Dhillon, R., Dmuchowski, C., & Glover, J. (1998). Effect of Dopamine on Renal Function after Arteriography in Patients With Preexisting Renal Insufficiency. *The American Surgeon*, Vol.34, No.5, (May 1998), pp.1682-1688, ISSN 0003-1348

Hoffmann, U., Fischereder, M., Reil, A., Fischer, M., Link, J., & Kramer, BK. (2005). Renal Effects of Gadopentetate Dimeglumine in Patients with Normal and Impaired Renal Function. *European Journal of Medical Research*, Vol. 10, No.4, (April 2005), pp.149-154, ISSN 0949-2321

Hoffmann, U., Fischereder, M., Kruger, B., Drobnik, W.; & Kramer, BK. (2004). The Value of N-Acetylcysteine in the Prevention of Radiocontrast Agent-Induced Nephropathy Seems Questionable. *Journal of the American Society of Nephrology*, Vol.15, No.2, (February 2004), pp.407–410, ISSN 1046-6673

Holland, MD., Galla, JH., Sanders, PW., & Luke, RG. (1985). Effect of Urinary pH and Diatrizoate on Bence Jones Protein Nephrotoxicity in the Rat. *Kidney International*, Vol.27, No.1, (January 1985), pp. 46-50, ISSN 0085-2538

Iakovou, I., Dangas, G., Mehran, R., Lansky, AJ., Ashby, DT., Fahy, M., Mintz, GS., Kent, KM., Pichard, AD., Satler, LF., Stone, GW., & Leon, MB. (2003). Impact of Gender on the Incidence and Outcome of Contrast-Induced Nephropathy after Percutaneous Coronary Intervention. *The Journal of Invasive Cardiology*, Vol.15, No.1, (January 2003), pp. 18–22, ISSN 1042-3931

Kapoor, A., Kumar, S., Gulati, S., Gambhir, S., Sethi, RS., & Sinha, N. The Role of Theophylline in Contrast-Induced Nephropathy: A Case-Control Study. *Nephrology Dialysis Transplantation*, Vol. 17, No.11, (November 2002), pp.1936–1941, ISSN 0931-0509

Kapoor, A., Sinha, N., Sharma, RK., Shrivastava, S., Radhakrishnan, S., Goel, PK., & Bajaj R. (1996). Use of Dopamine in Prevention of Contrast Induced Acute Renal Failure: A Randomized Study. *International Journal of Cardiology*,Vol.53, No.3, (March 1996), pp.233-236, ISSN 0167-5273

Kiski, D., Stepper, W., Brand, E., Breithardt, G., & Reinecke, H. (2010). Impact of Renin-Angiotensin-Aldosterone Blockade by Angiotensin-Converting Enzyme Inhibitors or AT-1 Blockers on Frequency of Contrast Medium-Induced Nephropathy: A Post-Hoc Analysis from the Dialysis-Versus-Diuresis (DVD) Trial. . *Nephrology Dialysis Transplantation*, Vol.25, No.3, (May 2010), pp.759-64, ISSN 0931-0509

Koch, JA., Plum, J., Grabensee, B., & Modder, U. (2000). Prostaglandin E1: A New Agent for the Prevention of Renal Dysfunction in High Risk Patients Caused by Radiocontrast Media? *Nephrology Dialysis Transplantation*, Vol. 15, No.1, (January 2000), pp.43-49, ISSN 0931-0509

Kohli, HS., Bhaskaran, MC., Muthukumar, T., Thennarasu, K., Sud, K., Jha, V., Gupta, KL., & Sakhuja, V. (2000). Treatment-Related Acute Renal Failure in the Elderly: A Hospital-Based Prospective Study. . *Nephrology Dialysis Transplantation,* Vol.15, No.2, (February 2000), pp. 212-217, ISSN 0931-0509

Kurnik, BR., Allgren, RL., Genter, FC., Solomon, RJ., Bates, ER., & Weisberg, LS. (1998). Prospective Study of Atrial Natriuretic Peptide for the Prevention of Radiocontrast-Induced Nephropathy. *American Journal of the Kidney Diseases,* Vol.31, No.4, (April 1998), pp.674-680, ISSN 0272-6386

Lautin, EM., Freeman, NJ., Schoenfeld, AH., Bakal, CW., Haramati, N., Friedman, AC., Lautin, JL., Braha, S., Kadish, EG., & Sprayregen, S. (1991). Radiocontrast-Associated Renal Dysfunction: Incidence and Risk Factors. *AJR American Journal of Roentgenology,* Vol.157, No.1, (July 1991), pp. 49–58, ISSN 0033-8419

Liss, P., Carlsson, PO., Nygren, A., Palm, F., & Hansell, P. (2003). ET-A Receptor Antagonist BQ123 Prevents Radiocontrast Media-Induced Renal Medullary Hypoxia. *Acta Radiologica,* Vol.44, No.1, (January 2003), pp.111-117, ISSN 0284-1851

Liu, R., Nair, D., Ix, J., Moore, DH., & Bent, S. (2005). N-Acetylcysteine for the Prevention of Contrast-Induced Nephropathy. A Systematic Review and Meta-Analysis. *Journal of General Internal Medicine,* Vol.20, No.2, (Febrary 2005), pp.193-200, ISSN 0884-8734

McCarthy, CS., & Becker, JA. (1992). Multiple Myeloma and Contrast Media. *Radiology,* Vol.183, No.2, (May 1992), pp.519–521, ISSN 0033-8419

McCullough, PA., Wolyn, R., Rocher, LL., Levin, RN., & O'Neill, WW. (1997). Acute Renal Failure after Coronary Intervention: Incidence, Risk Factors, and Relationships to Mortality. *The American Journal of Medicine,* Vol.103, No.5, (November 1997), pp. 368–375, ISSN 0002-9243

Marenzi, G., Lauri, G., Assanelli, E., Campodonico, J., De Metrio, M., Marana, I., Grazi, M., Veglia, F., & Bartorelli, AL. (2004). Contrast-Induced Nephropathy in Patients Undergoing Primary Angioplasty for Acute Myocardial Infarction. *Journal of the American College of the Cardiology,* Vol.44, No.9, (November 2004), pp. 1780-1785, ISSN 0735-1097

Marenzi, G., Marana, I., Lauri, G., Assanelli, E., Grazi, M., Campodonico, J., Trabattoni, D., Fabbiocchi, F., Montorsi, P., & Bartorelli, AL. (2003). The Prevention of Radiocontrast-Agent-Induced Nephropathy by Hemofiltration. *The New England Journal of Medicine,* Vol.349, No.14, (October 2003), pp.1333-1340, ISSN 0028-4793

Mehran, R., Aymong, ED., Nikolsky, E., Lasic, Z., Iakovou, I., Fahy, M., Mintz, GS., Lansky, AJ., Moses, JW., Stone, GW., Leon, MB., & Dangas, G. (2004). A Simple Risk Score for Prediction of Contrast-Induced Nephropathy after Percutaneous Coronary Intervention: Development and Initial Validation. *Journal of the American College of Cardiology*. Vol.44, No.7, (October 2004), pp.1393-1399, ISSN 0735-1097

Merten, GJ., Burgess, WP., Gray, LV., Holleman, JH., Roush, TS., Kowalchuk, GJ., Bersin, RM., Van Moore, A., Simonton, CA 3rd., Rittase, RA., Norton, HJ., & Kennedy, TP.

(2004). Prevention of contrast-induced nephropathy with sodium bicarbonate: a randomized controlled trial. *Journal of the American Medical Association*, Vol.291, No.19, (May 2004), pp.2328-2334, ISSN 0098-7484

Moore, RD., Steinberg, EP., Powe, NR., Brinker, JA., Fishman, EK., Graziano, S., & Gopalan, R. (1992). Nephrotoxicity of High-Osmolarity vs Low-Osmolarity Contrast Media: Randomized Clinical Trial. *Radiology,* Vol.182, No.3, *(March* 1992), pp. 649–655, ISSN 0033-8419

Mueller, C., Seidensticker, P., Buettner, HJ., Perruchoud, AP., Staub, D., Christ, A., & Buerkle, G. (2005). Incidence of Contrast Nephropathy in Patients Receiving Comprehensive Intravenous and Oral Hydration. Swiss Medical Weekly, Vol.135, No.19, (May 2005), pp.286-290, ISSN 1424-7860

Mueller, C., Buerkle, G., Buettner, HJ., Petersen, J., Perruchoud, AP., Eriksson, U., Marsch, S., & Roskamm, H. (2002). Prevention of Contrast Media-Associated Nephropathy: Randomized Comparison of 2 Hydration Regimens In 1620 Patients Undergoing Coronary Angioplasty. *Archives of Internal Medicine*, Vol.162, No.3, (February 2002), pp.329-336, ISSN 0003-9926

Neumayer, HH., Junge, W., Kufner, A., & Wening, A. (1989). Prevention of Radiocontrast-Media-Induced Nephrotoxicity by the Calcium Channel Blocker Nitrendipine: A Prospective Randomized Clinical Trial. *Nephrology Dialysis Transplantation*, Vol.4, No.12, (April 1989), pp.1030-1036, ISSN 0931-0509

Nikolsky, E., Mehran, R., Lasic, Z., Mintz, GS., Lansky, AJ., Na, Y., Pocock, S., Negoita, M., Moussa, I., Stone, GW., Moses, JW., Leon, MB., & Dangas, G. Low Hematocrit Predicts Contrast-Induced Nephropathy After Percutaneous Coronary Interventions. *Kidney International*, Vol.67, No.2, (February 2005), pp.706-713, ISSN 0085-2538

Parfrey, PS., Griffiths, SM., Barrett, BJ., Paul, MD., Genge, M., Withers, J. Farid, N., & McManamon, PJ. (1989). Contrast Material-Induced Renal Failure in Patients with Diabetes Mellitus, Renal Insufficiency, or Both. A Prospective Controlled Study. *The New England Journal of Medicine,* Vol.320, No.3, (January 1989), pp.143-149, ISSN 0028-4793

Rich, MW., & Crecelius, CA. (1990). Incidence, Risk Factors, and Clinical Course of Acute Renal Insufficiency after Cardiac Catheterization in Patients 70 Years of Age or Older. A Prospective Study. *Archives of Internal Medicine*, Vol.150, No.6, (June1990), pp. 1237-1242), ISSN 0003-9926

Rihal, CS., Textor, SC., Grill, DE., Berger, PB., Ting, HH., Best, PJ., Singh, M., Bell, MR., Barsness, GW., Mathew, V., Garratt, KN., & Holmes, DR Jr. (2002). Incidence and Prognostic Importance of Acute Renal Failure after Percutaneous Coronary Intervention. *Circulation,* Vol.105, No.105, (May 2002), pp. 2259-2264, ISSN 0009-7322

Rodicio, JL., Morales, JM., & Ruilope, LM. (1990). Calcium Antagonists and the Kidney. *Nephrology Dialysis Transplantation*, Vol.5, No.2, (1990), pp.81-86, ISSN 0931-0509

Rudnick, MR., Goldfarb, S., Wexler, L., Ludbrook, PA., Murphy, MJ., Halpern, EF., Hill, JA., Winniford, M., Cohen, MB., & Van Fossen, DB. (1995). Nephrotoxicity of Ionic and Nonionic Contrast Media in 1196 Patients: A Randomized Trial. The Iohexol Cooperative Study. *Kidney International,* Vol.47, No.1, (January 1995), pp. 254-261, ISSN 0085-2538

Russo, D., Testa, A., Della Volpe, L., & Sansone, G. (1990). Randomised Prospective Study on Renal Effects of Two Different Contrast Media in Humans: Protective Role of a Calcium Channel Blocker. *Nephron,* Vo.55, No.3, (1990), pp.254-257, ISSN 0028-2766

Sadeghi, HM., Stone, GW., Grines, CL., Mehran, R., Dixon, SR., Lansky, AJ., Fahy, M., Cox, DA., Garcia, E., Tcheng, JE., Griffin, JJ., Stuckey, TD., Turco, M., & Carroll, JD. (2003). Impact of Renal Insufficiency in Patients Undergoing Primary Angioplasty for Acute Myocardial Infarction. *Circulation,* Vol.108, No.22, (December 2003), pp.2769-2775, ISSN 0009-7322

Shaker, OG., El-Shehaby, A., & El-Khatib, M. (2010). Early Diagnostic Markers for Contrast Nephropathy in Patients Undergoing Coronary Angiography. *Angiology,* Vol.61, No.8, (November 2010), pp. 731-736, ISSN 0003-3197

Solomon, R., Werner, C., Mann, D., D'Elia, J., & Silva, P. (1994). Effects of Saline, Mannitol and Furosemide to Prevent Acute Decreases in Renal Function Induced by Radiocontrast Agents. *The New England Journal of Medicine,* Vol. 331, No.21, (November 1994), pp.1416–1420, ISSN 0028-4793

Spangberg-Viklund, B., Berglund, J., Nikonoff, T., Nyberg, P., Skau, T., & Larsson, R. (1996). Does Prophylactic Treatment with Felodopine, a Calcium Antagonist, Prevent Low-Osmolar Contrast Induced Renal Dysfunction in Hydrated Diabetic and Nondiabetic Patients with Normal or Moderately Reduced Renal Function? *Scandinavian Journal of Urology and Nephrology,* Vol.30, No.1, (February 1996), pp.63-68, ISSN 0036-5599

Spargias, K., Alexopoulos, E., Kyrzopoulos, S., Iokovis, P., Greenwood, DC., Manginas, A., Voudris, V., Pavlides, G., Buller, CE., Kremastinos, D., & Cokkinos, DV. (2004). Ascorbic Acid Prevents Contrast-Mediated Nephropathy in Patients with Renal Dysfunction Undergoing Coronary Angiography or Intervention. *Circulation,* Vol.110, No.18, (November 2004), pp.2837-2842, ISSN 0009-7322

Stone, GW., McCullough, PA., Tumlin, JA., Lepor, NE., Madyoon, H., Murray, P., Wang, A., Chu, AA., Schaer, GL., Stevens, M., Wilensky, RL., & O'Neill, WW., CONTRAST Investigators. (2003). Fenoldopam Mesylate for the Prevention of Contrast-Induced Nephropathy: A Randomized Controlled Trial. *The Journal of the American Medical Association,* Vol.290, No.17, (November 2003), pp.2284-2291, ISSN 0098-7484

Taliercio, CP., Vlietstra, RE., Fisher, LD., & Burnett, JC. (1986). Risks for Renal Dysfunction with Cardiac Angiography. *Annals of Internal Medicine,* Vol.104, No.4, (April 1986), pp.501-504, ISSN 0003-4819

Tepel, M., van Der Giet, M., Schwarzfeld, C., Laufer, U., Liermann, D., & Zidek, W. (2000). Prevention of Radiographic-Contrast-Agent-Induced Reductions in Renal Function by Acetylcysteine. *The New England Journal of Medicine,* Vol.343, No.3, (July2000), pp.,180-184, ISSN 0028-4793

Toprak, O., Cirit, M., Tanrisev, M., Yazici, C., Canoz, O., Sipahioglu, M., Uzum, A., Ersoy, R., & Sozmen, EY. (2008). Preventive Effect of Nebivolol on Contrast-Induced Nephropathy in Rats. *Nephrology Dialysis Transplantation,* Vol.23, No.3, (March 2008), pp. 853-859, ISSN 0931-0509

Toprak, O. (2007). Conflicting and New Risk Factors for Contrast-Induced Nephropathy. *The Journal of Urology,* Vol. 178, No.6, (December 2007), pp. 2277-2283, ISSN 0022-5347

Toprak, O., Cirit, M., Yesil, M., Bayata, S., Tanrisev, M., Varol, U., Ersoy, R., & Esi, E. (2007). Impact of Diabetic and Pre-Diabetic State on Development of Contrast-Induced Nephropathy in Patients with Chronic Kidney Disease. *Nephrology Dialysis Transplantation,* Vol.22, No.3, (March 2007), pp. 819-826, ISSN 0931-0509

Toprak, O., Cirit, M., Yesil, M., Byrne DW, Postaci, N., Bayata, S., Majchrzak, KM., & Esi, E. (2006). Metabolic Syndrome as a Risk Factor for Contrast-Induced Nephropathy in Non-Diabetic Elderly Patients with Renal Impairment. *Kidney and Blood Pressure Research,* Vol.29, No.1, (June 2006), pp. 2-9, ISSN 1420-4096

Toprak, O., Cirit, M., Esi, E., Postaci, N., Yesil, M., & Bayata, S. (2007). Hyperuricemia as a Risk Factor for Contrast-Induced Nephropathy in Patients with Chronic Kidney Disease. *Catheterization and Cardiovascular Interventions,* Vol.67, No.2, (February 2006), pp. 227-235, ISSN 1522-1946

Toprak, O., & Cirit, M. (2006). Risk Factors and Therapy Strategies for Contrast-Induced Nephropathy. *Renal Failure,* Vol. 28, No. 5, (January 2006), pp. 365-381, ISSN 0886-022X

Toprak, O., & Cirit, M. (2005). Investigating the Volume Status Before Contrast Nephropathy Studies. *Nephrology Dialysis Transplantation,* Vol.20, No.2, (February 2005), pp. 464, ISSN 0931-0509

Toprak, O., Cirit, M., Bayata, S., Yesil, M., & Aslan, SL. (2003). The Effect of Pre-procedural Captopril on Contrast-Induced Nephropathy in Patients who Underwent Coronary Angiography. *Anadolu Kardiyoloji Dergisi,* Vol. 3, No.2, (June 2003), pp. 98-103, ISSN 1302-8723

Toprak, O., Cirit, M., Bayata, S., Aslan, SL., Sarioglu, F., & Cetinkaya, GS. (2003). Is There Any Relationship Between Left Ventricul Ejection Fraction and Contrast Induced Nephropathy? *Türkiye Klinikleri Journal of Medical Sciences,* Vol 23, No. 2, (March 2003), pp. 104-107 , ISSN 1300-0292

Vogt, B., Ferrari, P., Schonholzer, C., Marti, HP., Mohaupt, M., Wiederkehr, M., Cereghetti, C., Serra, A., Huynh-Do, U., Uehlinger, D., & Frey, FJ. (2001). Prophylactic Hemodialysis after Radiocontrast Media in Patients with Renal Insufficiency is Potentially Harmful. *The American Journal of Medicine,* Vol.111, No.9, (December 2001), pp.692-698, ISSN 0002-9243

Wang, A., Holcslaw, T., Bashore, TM., Freed, MI., Miller, D., Rudnick, MR., Szerlip, H., Thames, MD., Davidson, CJ., Shusterman, N., & Schwab, SJ. (2000). Exacerbation of Radiocontrast Nephrotoxicity by Endothelin Receptor Antagonism. *Kidney International,* Vol.57, No.4, (April 2000), pp.1675-1680, ISSN 0085-2538

Weber-Mzell, D., Kotanko, P., Schumacher, M., Klein, W., & Skrabal, F. (2002). Coronary Anatomy Predicts Presence or Absence of Renal Artery Stenosis. A Prospective Study in Patients Undergoing Cardiac Catheterization for Suspected Coronary Artery Disease. *European Heart Journal,* Vol.23, No.21, (November 2002), pp.1684–1691, ISSN 0195-668x

Weinrauch, LA., Healy, RW., Leland, OS Jr., Goldstein, HH., Kassissieh, SD., Libertino, JA., Takacs, FJ., & D'Elia, JA. (1977). Coronary Angiography and Acute Renal Failure in Diabetic Azotemic Nephropathy. *Annals of Internal Medicine,* Vol.86, No.1, (January 1977), pp.56-59, ISSN 0003-4819

Weisberg, LS., Kurnik, PB., & Kurnik, BR. (1994). Risk of Radiocontrast Nephropathy in Patients with and without Diabetes Mellitus. Kidney International, Vol.45, No.1, (January 1994), pp.259-265,ISSN 0085-2538

Yang, DW., Jia, RH., Yang, DP., Ding, GH., & Huang, CX. (2004). Dietary Hypercholesterolemia Aggravates Contrast Media-Induced Nephropathy. *Chinese Medical Journal,* Vol. 117, No.4 (April 2004), pp.542–546, ISSN 0366-6999.

Zhang, L., Zhang, L., Lu, Y., Wu, B., Zhang, S., Jiang, H., Ge, J., & Chen, H. (2011). Efficacy of Statin Pretreatment for the Prevention of Contrast-Induced Nephropathy: A Meta-Analysis of Randomised Controlled Trials. *International Journal of Clinical Practice,*Vol.65, No.5, (May 2011), pp.624-30, ISSN 1368-5031

11

Coronary Angiography in Patients with Chronic Kidney Disease

Luís Henrique Wolff Gowdak and
José Jayme Galvão de Lima
*Heart Institute (InCor), University of
São Paulo Medical School
Brazil*

1. Introduction

Cardiovascular disease, mostly coronary artery disease (CAD), remains an important cause of morbidity and mortality in patients with any degree of renal dysfunction. Presently, according to the United States Renal Data System, the size of the population with chronic kidney disease (CKD) stage V reached a new high in 2008, with almost 550,000 patients under treatment (U.S. Renal Data System, 2010). Sadly, it is expected that half of them will die from cardiovascular disease; moreover, it is noteworthy that even patients with less advanced stages of CKD are at greater risk of death from CAD than of reaching the final stages of renal failure that would eventually require renal replacement therapy (Sarnak et al., 2003). In these patients, about 50% to 60% of all cardiovascular deaths are due to acute myocardial infarction, sudden death, or ischemic heart disease (Herzog et al., 2008).

The interplay between CKD and CAD is a very complex one and can only be partly explained by the fact that patients with CKD share many of the so-called traditional risk factors also linked to CAD, such as long-standing diabetes, hypertension, low levels of HDL-cholesterol, and hypertriglyceridemia (McCullough, 2002a). Additionally, a pro-inflammatory state and high oxidative stress levels are usually seen in patients with advanced CKD, which may contribute to accelerated atherosclerosis, plaque instability, acute coronary syndromes, and myocardial fibrosis (Yerkey et al., 2004). The result of this clustering of traditional and nontraditional risk factors may explain the epidemiological observation that patients with CKD stage V have more than a 10-fold increased risk of death from CAD than a patient with 5 Framingham risk scores (McCullough, 2002b).

The prevalence of CAD in CKD patients undergoing dialysis varies with such factors as age, diabetic status, time of follow-up, and the diligence with which CAD is investigated. In a group of 4,024 new dialysis patients, including 44% with diabetes, 32% had a history of CAD (Foley, 2003), which is conceivably more than 3 times the figure corresponding to CAD in the general population (Levey & Eknoyan, 1999). The prevalence of angiographically confirmed CAD, on the other hand, defined as luminal reduction >50%, ranges from 24% in low-risk patients to 85% in older, diabetic patients (Goldsmith & Covic, 2001). Nevertheless, most of these data originated from studies in which coronary angiography was performed only in patients with clinical evidence and/or noninvasive studies suggestive of CAD, leaving out patients in whom asymptomatic, undiagnosed, significant CAD might be already present; therefore, the actual prevalence of CAD might even be higher.

Adding to the importance of CAD in patients with CKD, observational data also show that CAD remains a significant clinical problem even if a patient undergoes successful kidney transplantation (Aakhus et al., 2004). The annual risk of CVD death is 3.5% to 5% in renal transplant recipients, which is 50-fold higher than that in the general population (Ojo, 2006). Acute coronary syndrome is highly prevalent in the early posttransplant period, and on average, CVD mortality accounts for 30% and 75% of early and late posttransplant deaths, respectively.

Therefore, coronary angiography is a valuable tool, very often used in patients with CKD both in the acute as well as in the chronic setting of CAD, for the purpose of either the diagnosis of, or the treatment of CAD by means of percutaneous coronary intervention. The major challenges with coronary angiography relate to when is it appropriate to perform it as part of the cardiovascular assessment in patients with CKD and what are the risks associated with the procedure. The ultimate management of CAD, should it be found after the diagnostic procedure, is beyond the scope of this chapter.

2. Screening for coronary artery disease in patients with CKD

Based on the above considerations, screening for the presence and severity of CAD in patients with CKD, and especially in those being considered for renal transplantation, is a fundamental step during routine cardiovascular risk assessment; in the setting of kidney transplantation, for instance, numerous studies indicate that not only are the majority of serious cardiovascular events in renal transplant recipients related to CAD but also these events tend to occur during the first few months following transplant (Kahwaji et al., 2011). The last observation strongly suggests that relevant CAD could have been missed before patients were actually included on renal transplant waiting lists, although they had been screened for it during routine pretransplant workups according to current guidelines. According to the American Society of Transplantation recommendations (Kasiske et al., 2001), patients with diabetes, a prior history of ischemic heart disease or an abnormal ECG, or age ≥50 years should be considered at high risk for CAD and referred for a cardiac stress test, and only in those with a positive stress test, for coronary angiography.

This strategy, however, is under dispute for the now recognized reduced sensitivity and specificity of noninvasive testing in renal patients compared with that in the general population (Marwick et al., 1990; Schmidt et al., 2001; Welsh et al., 2011), a finding that prompted many investigators to recommend direct diagnostic coronary angiography in high-risk patients. In agreement with the last view, in a previous study, our group showed that significant CAD, as defined by coronary angiography, was the best predictor of cardiovascular events compared with radionuclide myocardial perfusion study or dobutamine-atropine stress echocardiography in renal transplant candidates (De Lima et al., 2003), even taking into account that coronary angiography is an expensive, invasive procedure, not free from complications. However, in the same investigation, we also found that the prevalence of significant CAD was less than 50%, suggesting a need for better screening mechanisms that could identify high-risk individuals in whom coronary angiography could be avoided without incurring an increased risk of future events.

2.1 The challenge of referring patients with CKD for coronary angiography

Tables 1 and 2 show the most recent guidelines for coronary angiography to establish the *diagnosis* in patients with suspected angina and for *risk stratification* in patients with chronic stable angina, respectively (Fraker Jr et al., 2007).

Invasive coronary angiography has received a Class I indication for patients with known or possible angina pectoris who have survived sudden cardiac death. For risk stratification in patients with chronic stable angina, coronary angiography should be performed in: a) patients with disabling (Canadian Cardiovascular Society classes III and IV) stable angina despite medical therapy; b) patients with high-risk criteria on noninvasive testing; c) patients with angina and symptoms and signs of heart failure; d) patients with clinical characteristics indicating a high likelihood of severe CAD.

Coronary angiography is indicated to establish the diagnosis of CAD in patients with suspected angina in those with...	Level of Evidence	Comment for Patients with CKD
Known or possible angina pectoris who have survived sudden cardiac death	B	Survival rates much lower than rates for the general population

Table 1. Class I indication of the AHA/ACC Guidelines for coronary angiography to establish a *diagnosis* in patients with suspected angina in the general population. Modified from Fraker Jr, et al. (2007).

Coronary angiography is indicated for risk stratification in patients with chronic CAD in those with...	Level of Evidence	Comment for Patients with CKD
Disabling chronic stable angina despite medical therapy	B	Uncommon clinical presentation for patients with CKD
High-risk criteria on noninvasive testing regardless of angina severity	B	Lower sensitivity than that in the general population
Angina who have survived sudden cardiac death or serious ventricular arrhythmia	B	Survival rates much lower than those in the general population
Angina and symptoms and signs of congestive heart failure	C	May be confused with hypertensive cardiomyopathy, fluid overload, subdialysis
Clinical characteristics that indicate a high likelihood of severe CAD	C	Lower specificity than that in the general population

Table 2. Class I indications of the AHA/ACC Guidelines for coronary angiography for *risk stratification* in patients with chronic stable angina. Modified from Fraker Jr, et al. (2007).

Although these guidelines have been extensively tested and validated in the general population, for patients with CKD the data supporting that approach is less robust. The main pitfalls of applying the same criteria recommended for patients with normal renal function to patients with CKD are briefly described below.

2.1.1 Clinical presentation

Although angina pectoris is usually a reliable indicator of the presence of CAD in the general population, it is not so among patients with CKD, particularly in the more advanced stages of renal failure. For instance, chest pain is commonly observed in the dialysis population; nevertheless, its characteristics make the discomfort often described as "atypical," and the pain does not correlate with the presence of significant CAD. In fact, fewer than 50% of dialysis patients with acute myocardial infarction present with chest pain, which likely explains why myocardial infarction is infrequently suspected on admission (Herzog et al., 2007). Reasons for the different presentations of ischemia are not well understood but may be related to associated diabetic or uremic neuropathy. Diagnosis of ischemia is further complicated by the fact that other symptoms of ischemia, such as dyspnea on exertion, fatigue, and hypotension, are common in dialysis patients and may be attributed to dialysis-related factors, such anemia, volume overload, acidosis, non-compliance with fluid intake or dialysis or to ultra-filtration during dialysis (Sosnov et al., 2006). Furthermore, silent ischemia occurs frequently in patients with CKD.

We previously found that, in a group of high-risk renal transplant candidates who underwent coronary angiography *per* protocol, regardless of symptoms, the prevalence of significant CAD was 40% in patients with, and 58% in patients without, angina (De Lima et al., 2003). Disabling symptoms, even in the presence of significant and extensive CAD, are quite uncommon in patients with CKD.

2.1.2 Noninvasive testing

2.1.2.1 Resting and exercise electrocardiogram

The interpretation of resting and exercise electrocardiograms for the diagnosis of CAD in patients on dialysis is often hampered by the presence of concurrent left ventricular hypertrophy, anemia, and electrolyte disturbances that may cause electrocardiographic changes resembling those of ischemia (Sharma et al., 2007). Also, most patients with CKD have poor physical stamina, limiting the utility of exercise electrocardiography as a diagnostic tool. The overall specificity and sensitivity of both tests for the diagnosis of CAD are lower (<50%) in patients with CKD than in the general population.

2.1.2.2 Myocardial perfusion assessment

Dipyridamole radionuclide stress testing with single-photon emission tomography (SPECT) has been widely used as a screening test for CAD in patients with a variety of clinical conditions. The reported specificity and sensitivity of the test are close to 70% and 80%, respectively. Among patients with CKD, however, the results are highly variable with sensitivity often <60% compared to that of coronary angiography (Holley et al., 1991; Sharma et al., 2007). The reasons for the unexpected low sensitivity and great variability of cardiac scintigraphy in patients with CKD are unclear but may reflect the increased levels of circulating adenosine, reduced coronary flow reserve, or left ventricular hypertrophy. Combined dipyridamole-exercise thallium imaging reportedly increases the sensitivity and specificity of the test.

Dobutamine-atropine stress echocardiography has been associated with better and more consistent results for detecting significant (>70%) coronary stenosis in patients with CKD,

with a sensitivity and negative predictive value between 70% and 80% (Herzog et al., 1999; Ferreira et al., 2007). However, the utility of this test is limited, because dobutamine often increases blood pressure, causing interruption of the test in about 15% of patients.
Until a few years ago, magnetic resonance imaging (MRI) had been used for assessment of myocardial function and detection of myocardial ischemia and scar tissue in patients with CKD (Andrade et al., 2009). Myocardial stress perfusion studies performed with MRI adequately detected CAD, and there was a good correlation between these results and those from coronary angiography and radionuclide studies (Andrade et al., 2004). Unfortunately, further development of this imaging modality was halted, because of the description of a serious complication related to the use of gadolinium-based contrast media in patients with CKD, called nephrogenic systemic fibrosis (Grobner, 2006). Thus, starting in 2007, the United States Food and Drug Administration issued a boxed warning about this progressive, debilitating and, occasionally fatal condition recommending that the use of gadolinium-based contrast agents should be avoided in patients with acute or chronic renal insufficiency with a glomerular filtration rate < $30 mL/min/1.73m^2$.

2.1.2.3 Coronary angiotomography

Multidetector-row computed tomography (MDCT) has been recently applied to the detection of CAD in patients with ESRD (Rosário et al., 2010). This method allows not only the detection of coronary calcifications but also the detailed visualization of the arterial wall and lumen, and therefore, may become an alternative to coronary angiography. Experience with this method in patients with CKD is still very limited.

2.1.2.4 Clinical implications

Thus, referring patients with CKD for coronary angiography is not an easy task (De Lima et al., 2010; Lentine et al., 2010). One could be very "conservative," only referring patients with overt, unequivocal symptoms of angina or extensive myocardial ischemia on noninvasive testing to undergo coronary angiography.
This approach would most likely yield a prohibitively large number of "false negatives," meaning that many patients with significant CAD will be deemed free of disease. It is quite easy to see the clinical implications of such an approach, especially for renal transplant candidates. Alternatively, one could be very "aggressive" and refer all patients with CKD stages IV or V for coronary angiography. We would be able to diagnose every single patient with CAD in adopting this strategy. The downside is that coronary angiography is a somewhat risky, costly procedure and as many as 50% to 60% of all patients will have no significant CAD at all and, therefore, will not be further referred for coronary interventions (percutaneous or surgical). Finally, patients still not on renal replacement therapy might not only not benefit from this strategy but might also have worsening of their residual renal function because of the contrast-induced nephropathy.
As a matter of fact, it is still unclear whether the benefits outweigh the harms of routine screening and prophylactic revascularization to prevent coronary artery disease (CAD) in asymptomatic kidney transplant candidates. To help clarify that issue, an ongoing randomized clinical trial is being performed to study the effect of CAD screening on major adverse cardiac events (Kasiske et al., 2011).

3. In whom should coronary angiography be performed?

The same indications presented in Tables 1 and 2 should be applied to patients with CKD. The greatest challenge facing the clinical cardiologist called upon to assess a patient with

CKD regarding the presence and severity of CAD is, based on the previous considerations, which additional patients should be referred for coronary angiography, especially those asymptomatic patients being assessed before renal transplantation.

In a previous study, we sought to determine the clinical predictors more closely related to CAD in 301 renal transplant candidates treated by hemodialysis (Gowdak et al, 2007). CAD (> 70% stenosis) was found in 45% of patients, and the clinical variables significantly associated with CAD were diabetes, peripheral vascular disease, and previous myocardial infarction. More important, the prevalence of CAD increased with the number of clinical predictors from 26% (none) to 100% (all present), while the incidence of events increased 2-, 4-, and 6-fold in those with diabetes, peripheral vascular disease, or previous myocardial infarction, respectively ($p < .0001$). This approach would allow reducing the prevalence of unnecessary angiography from 55% (when all patients undergo angiography) to 26%. However, we believe that missing the diagnosis of CAD in one-fourth of patients is still not totally satisfactory.

Another approach should be to restrict the use of coronary angiography as a predictive tool of cardiovascular events in patients with CKD in which this strategy is powerful enough to discern between patients at high- and low-risk, comparatively to either clinical stratification alone or to noninvasive testing. We compared the efficacy of clinical stratification, noninvasive testing, and coronary angiography in predicting cardiovascular events in patients with CKD being considered as potential renal transplant candidates (De Lima et al., 2006; Gowdak et al., 2008). We were able to show that, for patients considered at low-risk for CAD (age < 50 years, with no diabetes, and no history of cardiovascular disease), additional noninvasive or invasive testing, added no capability in predicting cardiovascular events beyond that given by clinical stratification. On the other hand, for patients at high-risk for CAD, defined by the presence of any 2 risk factors combined (age ≥ 50 years *or* diabetes *or* cardiovascular disease), noninvasive testing failed to identify patients at higher risk for cardiovascular events; indeed, the finding of significant CAD by angiography (luminal stenosis ≥ 70%) was the strongest predictor of events. For patients at intermediate-risk for CAD, defined by the presence of any single risk factor alone, noninvasive testing was a good tool in identifying patients at higher risk of events, should an abnormal myocardial perfusion scan be found. Figure 1 shows the proposed algorithm for risk stratification of CAD in renal transplant candidates.

4. Contrast-induced Acute Kidney Injury

Very often, the highlighted importance of coronary angiography for the diagnosis and/or management of CAD in patients with CKD is offset by the possibility of contrast-induced acute kidney injury (AKI) that may follow the use of any iodinated contrast media. Contrast-induced AKI is a common and potentially serious complication after the administration of contrast media in patients at risk for acute renal injury (McCullough, 2008). Unfortunately, the most important risk factor for contrast-induced AKI is an already compromised baseline renal function. The knowledge that not only contrast-induced AKI adversely affects the short- and long-term prognosis but also implies greater health costs prompted cardiologists to be particularly careful whenever coronary angiography is recommended to patients with any degree of CKD.

Many definitions currently exist in practice regarding contrast-induced AKI; it can be simply defined as an increase in serum creatinine (SCr) occurring within the first 24h after contrast exposure and peaking up to 5 days afterwards. The rise in Scr can be expressed either in absolute terms (0.5 to 1.0mg/dL) or as a proportional rise in SCr of 25% to 50% above the baseline value (Gleeson & Bulugahapitiya, 2004).

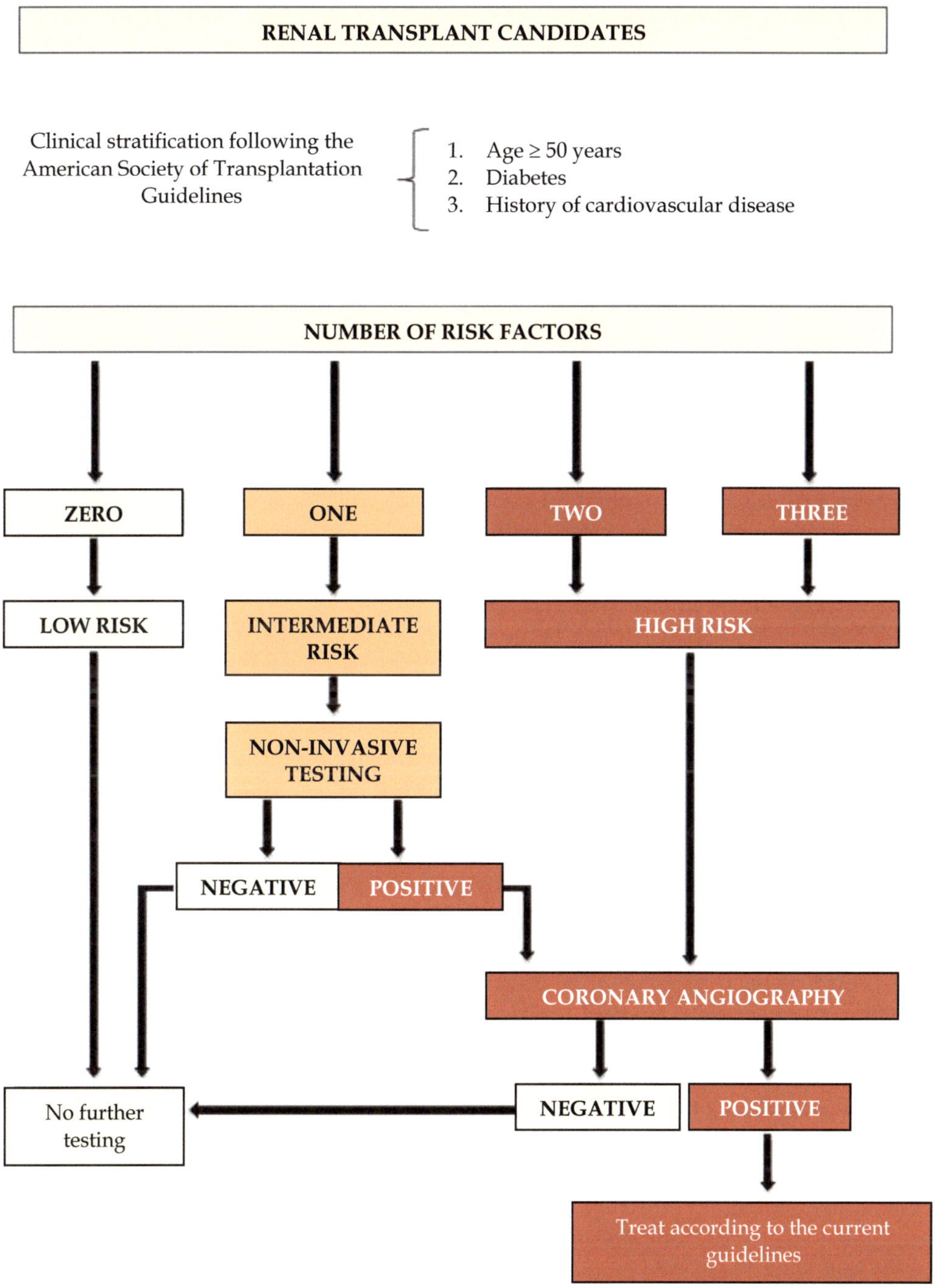

Fig. 1. Proposed algorithm for coronary angiography in patients with CKD awaiting renal transplantation.

The increase in SCr seen in patients with contrast-induced AKI is associated with a significant increase in the risk of death. In a large retrospective study comprising over 16,000 patients undergoing procedures, those who developed contrast-induced AKI had a 5.5-fold increased risk of death during hospitalization (Levy et al., 1996). Another study with more than 7,000 patients confirmed the short-term worse prognosis in patients with AKI but extended the greater risk of death up to 5 years after the procedure: the mortality rates at 1 year after development of contrast-induced AKI (12.1%) and at 5 years (44.6%) were higher compared with rates of 3.7% and 14.5%, respectively, in patients who did not develop contrast-induced AKI, indicating that the increased risk of death persisted in the long term (Rihal et al., 2002).

Besides the increased mortality, contrast-induced AKI also poses a high morbidity risk. Its occurrence has been linked to late cardiovascular events after percutaneous coronary intervention (such as myocardial infarction), bleeding requiring transfusion, and vascular complications. As a consequence of more serious adverse events, the in-hospital stay is longer with an estimated US$10,000 to US$12,000 added to the final bill during the first year (Subramanian et al., 2007).

4.1 Pathophysiology of contrast-induced Acute Kidney Injury

Centrally to the pathophysiology of contrast-induced AKI is the presence of a reduced nephron mass, a hallmark of chronic kidney disease. It has already been demonstrated that in patients with CKD, defined by an estimated glomerular filtration rate < $60mL/min/1.73m^2$, there is a considerable loss of nephron units, making the residual renal function prone to further declines with renal insults (Figure 2). When serum creatinine or eGFR is unavailable, then a survey may be used to identify patients at higher risk than the general population for contrast-induced AKI. Iodinated contrast, after causing a brief (minutes) period of vasodilation, causes sustained (hours to days) intrarenal vasoconstriction and ischemic injury. The ischemic injury sets off a cascade of events largely driven by oxidative injury causing death of renal tubular cells. If a sufficient mass of nephron units is affected, then a recognizable rise in serum creatinine will occur. Any superimposed insult, such as sustained hypotension in the catheterization laboratory, micro-showers of atheroembolic material from catheter exchanges or the use of intraaortic balloon counterpulsation, or a bleeding complication can amplify the injury processes occurring in the kidney (McCullough et al., 2006a).

Renal function must be assessed before administration of contrast medium so appropriate caution may be exercised to avoid additional risks. The National Kidney Foundation Kidney Disease Outcome Quality Initiative recommends that clinicians use an eGFR calculated from the SCr as an index of renal function rather than using SCr in stable patients. In such a situation when an eGFR cannot be obtained prior to the procedure, clinicians should inquire about risk markers for AKI after iodinated contrast (Table 3).

The presence of multiple contrast-induced AKI risk factors in the same patient or high-risk clinical scenarios can create a very high risk (~50%) for contrast-induced AKI and (~15%) acute renal failure requiring dialysis after contrast exposure.

In the setting of emergency procedures, where the benefit of very early imaging outweighs the risk of waiting, the procedure can be performed without knowledge of serum creatinine or eGFR.

Risk markers for contrast-induced acute kidney injury	
previous renal disease	diabetes mellitus
prior renal surgery	hypertension
proteinuria	gout
use of nephrotoxic drugs, such as nonsteroidal anti-inflammatory agents	

Table 3. A brief 7-item survey to identify patients at higher risk for AKI.

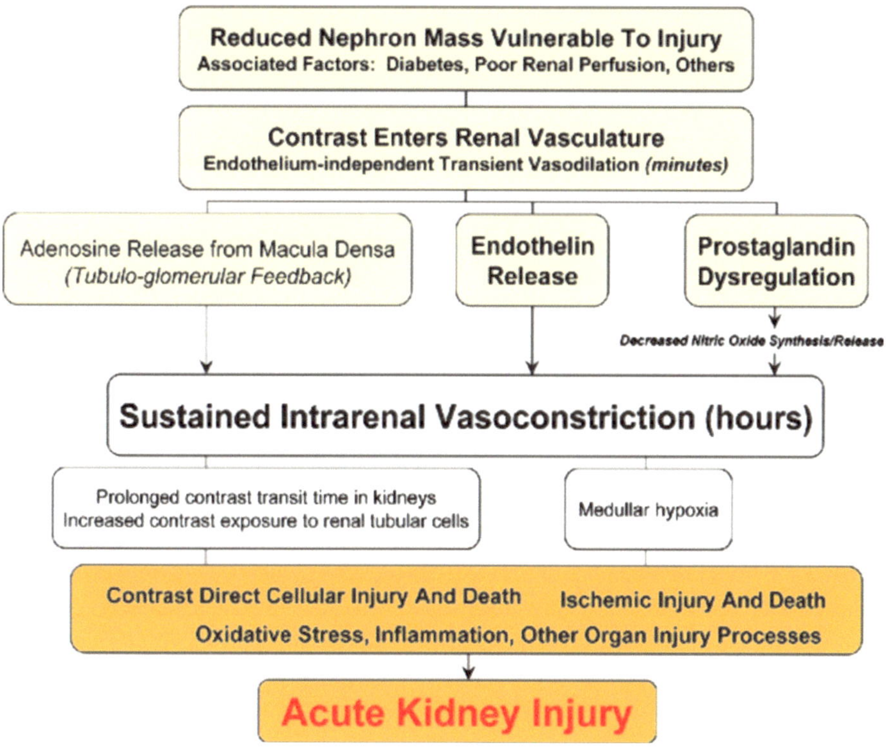

Fig. 2. Postulated pathophysiology of contrast-induced AKI (McCullough, 2008).

4.2 Contrast medium use

In patients at increased risk for contrast-induced AKI undergoing intraarterial administration of contrast, ionic high-osmolality agents pose a greater risk for contrast-induced AKI than low-osmolality agents (Barrett & Carlisle, 1993). Red blood cell deformation, systemic vasodilation, intrarenal vasoconstriction, as well as direct renal tubular toxicity are all more common in contrast agents with osmolality greater than that of blood.

Current evidence suggests that for intraarterial administration in high-risk patients with CKD, particularly those with diabetes mellitus, nonionic, iso-osmolar contrast is associated with the lowest risk of contrast-induced AKI. Iodixanol (an iso-osmolar contrast media) has been shown to have the lowest risk for contrast-induced AKI in patients with CKD and diabetes mellitus compared with low-osmolar contrast media (McCullough et al. 2006b). The *American College of Cardiology/American Heart Association* guidelines for the management of acute coronary syndromes in patients with CKD listed the use of iso-osmolar contrast media as a class I, Level of Evidence: A recommendation. The *National Kidney Foundation Kidney Disease Outcome Quality Initiative* guidelines have also recommended use of iso-osmolar contrast media in renal dialysis patients to minimize the chances of volume overload and complications before the next dialysis session.

Higher contrast volumes (~100 mL) are associated with higher rates of contrast-induced AKI in patients at risk. However, even small (~30 mL) volumes of iodinated contrast in very high-risk patients can cause contrast-induced AKI and acute renal failure requiring dialysis, suggesting the absence of a threshold effect (Manske et al., 1990). As a general rule, the volume of contrast received should not exceed twice the baseline level of eGFR in mL.

Finally, intraarterial administration of iodinated contrast appears to pose a greater risk of contrast-induced AKI above that with intravenous administration.

4.3 Strategies to further reduce the risk of contrast-induced Acute Kidney Injury

4.3.1 Volume expansion

Adequate intravenous volume expansion with isotonic crystalloid (1.0–1.5 mL/kg/h) for 3–12 h before the procedure and continued for 6–24 h afterwards can lessen the probability of contrast-induced AKI in patients at risk (Mueller et al., 2002). Achieving a good urine output (~150 mL/h) in the 6h after the procedure has been associated with reduced rates of AKI in one study. The data on oral as opposed to intravenous volume expansion as a contrast-induced AKI prevention measure are insufficient.

4.3.2 Pharmacologic agents

No adjunctive medical or mechanical treatment has been proven to be efficacious reducing the risk of AKI after exposure to iodinated contrast. With iodinated contrast, the pharmacologic agents tested in small trials that deserve further evaluation include the antioxidants ascorbic acid and N-acetylcysteine (NAC), aminophylline/theophylline, statins, and prostaglandin E1.

4.3.2.1 Ascorbic acid

Only ascorbic acid has been tested in a multicenter, blinded, placebo-controlled trial (n=231) and been shown to reduce rates of contrast-induced AKI. The dose of ascorbic acid (vitamin C over the counter) used in this trial was 3g orally the night before and 2g orally twice a day after the procedure (Spargias et al., 2004).

4.3.2.2 N-acetylcysteine

Although popular, NAC has not been consistently shown to be effective. Nine meta-analyses have been published, all documenting the significant heterogeneity between studies and pooled odds ratios for NAC approaching unity (Stacul et al., 2006). Importantly, only in those trials where NAC reduced SCr below baseline values because of decreased skeletal muscle production did renal injury rates appear to be reduced.

However, NAC as an antioxidant has been shown to lower rates of AKI and mortality after primary PCI in 1 trial. The recently published REMEDIAL (Renal Insufficiency Following Contrast Media Administration) trial suggested that the use of volume supplementation with sodium bicarbonate together with NAC was more effective than NAC alone in reducing the risk of AKI (Briguori et al., 2007; Brown et al., 2009). Dosing of NAC has varied in the trials; however, the most successful approach has been with 1,200 mg orally twice a day on the day before and after the procedure.

4.3.2.3 Other agents

Fenoldopam, dopamine, calcium-channel blockers, atrial natriuretic peptide, and L-arginine have not been shown to be effective in the prevention of contrast-induced AKI. Furosemide, mannitol, and an endothelin receptor antagonist are potentially detrimental (Stacul et al., 2006).

In general, cardiovascular patients undergoing procedures with iodinated contrast have either high risk for atherosclerosis or have the anatomic presence of disease. Therefore, the vast majority of patients should be on statin therapy with a common low-density lipoprotein cholesterol target of <70 mg/dL. Several studies have demonstrated that patients continuing on statins during cardiovascular procedures including PCI and coronary artery bypass grafting have lower rates of AKI (Khanal et al., 2005). All small, randomized trials published to date support this concept as well. Preservation of endothelial function at the level of the glomerulus and reductions in systemic inflammatory factors are postulated mechanisms by which statins may have renoprotective effects.

4.3.2.4 Dialysis and hemofiltration

Prophylactic hemodialysis or hemofiltration has not been validated as an effective strategy, even when carried out within 1 h or simultaneously with contrast administration.

Hemofiltration, however, performed 6 h before and 12 to 18 h after contrast deserves consideration, given reports of reduced mortality and need for hemodialysis in the postprocedure period in very high-risk patients (Marenzi et al., 2003).

4.3.2.5 Withdrawal of additional nephrotoxic drugs

Despite the lack of more robust data in this area, it is a reasonable practice to withhold nonsteroidal anti-inflammatory drugs, calcineurin inhibitors, high-dose loop diuretics, aminoglycosides, and other nephrotoxic agents if possible for several days before contrast exposure (McCullough, 2008). It is routine practice to withhold metformin before all contrast procedures, not because metformin itself is nephrotoxic but because in the setting of AKI if metformin is continued, lactic acidosis can develop leading to systemic complications and death. As a general rule, metformin should not be restarted until the clinician is confident that the patient has not developed AKI.

4.4 Management of patients receiving iodinated contrast media

An integrated proposed algorithm for the management of patients receiving iodinated contrast media is presented in Figure 3. Since there are no approved pharmaceutical agents for the prevention of this complication, the practitioner should be cautious with the use of any of the drugs suggested. We also recommend that all patients at risk for contrast-induced AKI should have follow-up serum creatinine and electrolyte monitoring daily while in the hospital, and then at 48 to 96h after discharge.

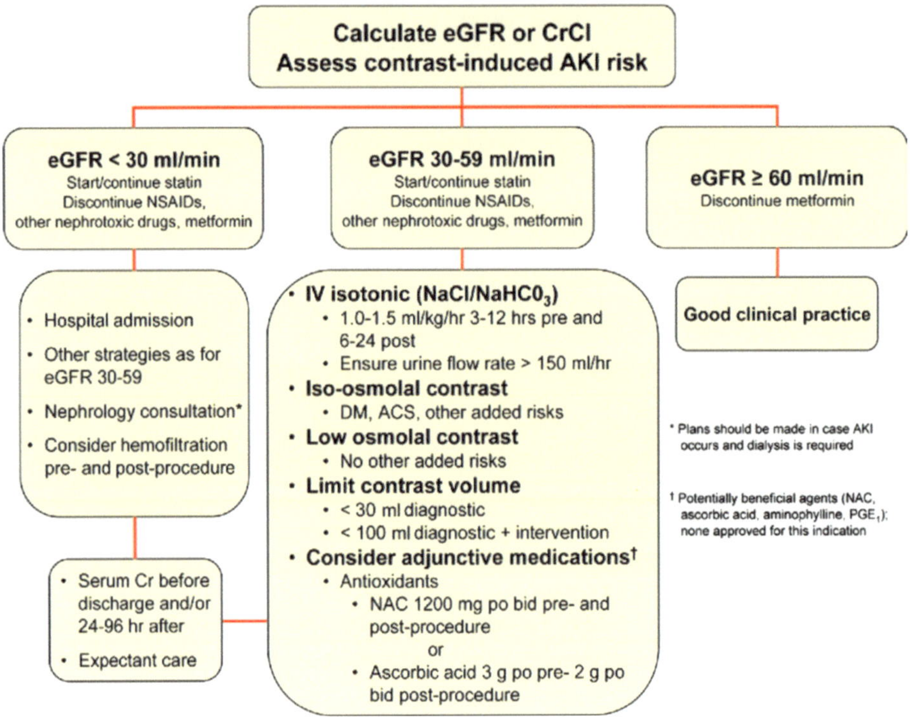

Fig. 3. Proposed algorithm for management of contrast-induced AKI (McCullough, 2008).

5. Conclusion

Patients with chronic kidney disease are at high-risk for CAD and, therefore, coronary angiography is very often needed to establish the diagnosis and severity of CAD. The major challenges in this regard are how to select those patients more likely to have significant CAD, in the absence of typical symptoms suggestive of CAD or myocardial perfusion defects disclosed by noninvasive testing. Moreover, the possibility of contrast-induced acute kidney injury should signal the need for a careful and more judicious decision-making approach by the cardiologist, working in tandem with the nephrologist, when trying to establish the risk-benefit ratio for each patient being considered for invasive assessment. Having decided that an invasive procedure is clearly needed, all preventive and therapeutic measurements should be applied to minimize the risk of worsening residual renal function.

6. References

Aakhus S, Dahl K & Widerøe TE (2004). Cardiovascular disease in stable renal transplant patients in Norway: morbidity and mortality during a 5-yr follow-up. *Clinical Transplantation*, Vol.18, No.5, pp.596-604.

Andrade JM, Rochitte CE, Gowdak LH, Paula FJ, Giorgi MCP, Parga JR, Avila LF, Ramires JAF & Lima JJG (2004). Evaluation of myocardial ischemia by magnetic resonance myocardial stress perfusion in renal transplant candidates: Comparison with SPECT and coronary angiography. *Journal of the American College of Cardiology*, Vol.43, No.5 (Supplement A), pp.353A-353A.

Andrade JM, Gowdak LH, Giorgi MC, de Paula FJ, Kalil-Filho R, de Lima JJ & Rochitte CE (2009). Cardiac MRI for detection of unrecognized myocardial infarction in patients with end-stage renal disease: comparison with ECG and scintigraphy. *American Journal of Roentgenolology*, Vol.193, No.1, pp.W25-32.

Barrett BJ & Carlisle EJ (1993). Metaanalysis of the relative nephrotoxicity of high- and low-osmolality iodinated contrast media. *Radiology*, Vol.188, No.1, pp.171-178.

Briguori C, Airoldi F, D'Andrea D, Bonizzoni E, Morici N, Focaccio A, Michev I, Montorfano M, Carlino M, Cosgrave J, Ricciardelli B & Colombo A (2007). Renal insufficiency following contrast media administration trial (REMEDIAL): a randomized comparison of 3 preventive strategies. *Circulation*, Vol.115, No.10, pp.1211–1217.

Brown JR, Block CA, Malenka DJ, O'Connor GT, Schoolwerth AC & Thompson CA (2009). Sodium bicarbonate plus N-acetylcysteine prophylaxis: a meta-analysis. *Journal of the American College of Cardiology Cardiovascular Interventions*, Vol.2, No.11, pp.1116-1124.

De Lima JJ, Sabbaga E, Vieira ML, de Paula FJ, Ianhez LE, Krieger EM & Ramires JA (2003). Coronary angiography is the best predictor of events in renal transplant candidates compared with noninvasive testing. *Hypertension*, Vol. 42, No.3, pp.263-268.

De Lima JJG, Paula FJ, Martinez Filho E, Meneghetti C, Cesar LAM, Ramires JAF, Krieger EM & Gowdak LHW (2006). Predicting cardiovascular events in patients with end-stage renal disease on the waiting list for renal transplantation - to invade or not to invade? *European Heart Journal*, Vol.27, Supplement 1, pp.10-10.

De Lima JJ, Wolff Gowdak LH, de Paula FJ, Ianhez LE, Franchini Ramires JA & Krieger EM (2010). Validation of a strategy to diagnose coronary artery disease and predict cardiac events in high-risk renal transplant candidates. *Coronary Artery Disease*, Vol.21, No.3, pp.164-167.

Ferreira PA, de Lima VC, Campos Filho O, Gil MA, Cordovil A, Machado CV, Pestana JO & Carvalho AC (2007). Feasibility, safety and accuracy of dobutamine/atropine stress echocardiography for the detection of coronary artery disease in renal transplant candidates. *Arquivos Brasileiros de Cardiologia*, Vol.88, No.1, pp.45-51.

Foley RN (2003). Clinical epidemiology of cardiac disease in dialysis patients: left ventricular hypertrophy, ischemic heart disease, and cardiac failure. *Seminars in Dialysis*, Vol.16, No.2, pp.111-117.

Fraker Jr TD, Fihn SD & Writing on behalf of the 2002 Chronic Stable Angina Writing Committee (2007). 2007 chronic angina focused update of the ACC/AHA 2002 guidelines for the management of patients with chronic stable angina: a report of the American College of Cardiology/American Heart Association Task Force on Practice Guidelines Writing Group to develop the focused update of the 2002 guidelines for the management of patients with chronic stable angina. *Journal of the American College of Cardiology*, Vol.50, No.23, pp.2264-2274.

Gleeson TG & Bulugahapitiya S (2004). Contrast-induced nephropathy. *American Journal of Roentgenology*, Vol.183, No.6, pp.1673-1789.

Goldsmith DJ & Covic A (2001). Coronary artery disease in uremia: Etiology, diagnosis, and therapy. *Kidney International*, Vol.60, No. 6, pp.2059-2078.

Gowdak LH, de Paula FJ, César LA, Martinez Filho EE, Ianhez LE, Krieger EM, Ramires JA & de Lima JJ (2007). Screening for significant coronary artery disease in high-risk renal transplant candidates. *Coronary Artery Disease*, Vol.18, No.7, pp.553-558.

Gowdak LHW, Arantes RL, De Paula FJ, Cesar LAM, Ianhez LE, Krieger EM & De Lima JJG (2008). Reviewing the American Society of Transplantation guidelines for cardiovascular risk stratification in renal transplant candidates. *Circulation*, Vol.118, No.12, pp.E462-E462.

Grobner T (2006). Gadolinium - a specific trigger for the development of nephrogenic fibrosing dermopathy and nephrogenic systemic fibrosis? *Nephrolology Dialysis Transplantation*, Vol.21, No.4, pp.1104-1108.

Herzog CA, Marwick TH, Pheley AM, White CW, Rao VK & Dick CD (1999). Dobutamine stress echocardiography for the detection of significant coronary artery disease in renal transplant candidates. *American Journal of Kidney Disease*, Vol.33, No.6, pp.1080-1090.

Herzog CA, Littrell K, Arko C, Frederick PD & Blaney M (2007). Clinical characteristics of dialysis patients with acute myocardial infarction in the United States: a collaborative project of the United States Renal Data System and the National Registry of Myocardial Infarction. *Circulation*, Vol.116, No.13, pp.1465-1472.

Herzog CA, Mangrum JM & Passman R (2008). Sudden cardiac death and dialysis patients. *Seminars in Dialysis*, Vol. 21, No.4, pp.300-307.

Holley JL, Fenton RA & Arthur RS (1991). Thallium stress testing does not predict cardiovascular risk in diabetic patients with end-stage renal disease undergoing cadaveric renal transplantation. *American Journal of Medicine*, Vol.90, No.5, pp.563-570.

Kahwaji J, Bunnapradist S, Hsu JW, Idroos ML & Dudek R (2011). Cause of death with graft function among renal transplant recipients in an integrated healthcare system. *Transplantation*, Vol. 91, No.2, pp.225-230.

Kasiske BL, Cangro CB, Hariharan S, Hricik DE, Kerman RH, Roth D, Rush DN, Vazquez MA, Weir MR & American Society of Transplantation (2001). The evaluation of renal transplantation candidates: clinical practice guidelines. *American Journal of Transplantation*, Vol. 1, Supplement 2, pp.3-95.

Kasiske BL, Israni AK, Snyder JJ, Camarena A & COST Investigators (2011). Design considerations and feasibility for a clinical trial to examine coronary screening before kidney transplantation (COST). *American Journal of Kidney Disease*, Mar 14, Epub ahead of print.

Khanal S, Attallah N, Smith DE, Kline-Rogers E, Share D, O'Donnell MJ & Moscucci M (2005). Statin therapy reduces contrast-induced nephropathy: an analysis of contemporary percutaneous interventions. *American Journal of Medicine*, Vol.118, No.8, pp.843-849.

Lentine KL, Hurst FP, Jindal RM, Villines TC, Kunz JS, Yuan CM, Hauptman PJ & Abbott KC (2010). Cardiovascular risk assessment among potential kidney transplant candidates: approaches and controversies. *American Journal of Kidney Disease*, Vol.55, No.1, pp.152-167.

Levey AS & Eknoyan G (1999). Cardiovascular disease in chronic renal disease. *Nephrology Dialysis Transplantation*,. Vol. 14, No.4, pp.828-833.

Levy EM, Viscoli CM & Horwitz RI (1996). The effect of acute renal failure on mortality. A cohort analysis. *Journal of the American Medical Association*, Vol.275, No.19, pp.1489-1494.

Manske CL, Sprafka JM, Strony JT & Wang Y (1990). Contrast nephropathy in azotemic diabetic patients undergoing coronary angiography. *American Journal of Medicine*, Vol.89, No.5, pp.615-620.

Marenzi G, Marana I, Lauri G, Assanelli E, Grazi M, Campodonico J, Trabattoni D, Fabbiocchi F, Montorsi P & Bartorelli AL (2003). The prevention of radiocontrast agent-induced nephropathy by hemofiltration. *The New England Journal of Medicine*, Vol.349, No.14, pp.1333-1340.

Marwick TH, Steinmuller DR, Underwood DA, Hobbs RE, Go RT, Swift C & Braun WE (1990). Ineffectiveness of dipyridamole SPECT thallium imaging as a screening technique for coronary artery disease in patients with end-stage renal failure. *Transplantation*, Vol.49, No.1, pp.100-103.

McCullough PA (2002a). Scope of cardiovascular complications in patients with kidney disease. *Ethnicity and Disease*, Vol.12, No.4, pp.S3-44-48.

McCullough PA (2002b). Cardiorenal risk: An important clinical intersection. *Reviews in Cardiovascular Medicine*, Vol.3, No.2, pp.71-76.

McCullough PA, Adam A, Becker CR, Davidson C, Lameire N, Stacul F, Tumlin J & CIN Consensus Working Panel (2006a). Risk prediction of contrast-induced nephropathy. *American Journal of Cardiology*, Vol.98, No.6A, pp.27K-36K.

McCullough PA, Bertrand ME, Brinker JA & Stacul F (2006b). A meta-analysis of the renal safety of isosmolar iodixanol compared with low-osmolar contrast media. *Journal of the American College of Cardiology*, Vol.48, No.4, pp.692–699.

McCullough PA (2008). Contrast-induced acute kidney injury. *Journal of the American College of Cardiology*, Vol.51, No.15, pp.1419-1428.

Mueller C, Buerkle G, Buettner HJ, Petersen J, Perruchoud AP, Eriksson U, Marsch S & Roskamm H (2002). Prevention of contrast media-associated nephropathy: randomized comparison of 2 hydration regimens in 1620 patients undergoing coronary angioplasty. *Archives of Internal Medicine*, Vol.162, No.3, pp.329-336.

Ojo AO (2006). Cardiovascular complications after renal transplantation and their prevention. *Transplantation*, Vol.82, No.5, pp. 603-611.

Rihal CS, Textor SC, Grill DE, Berger PB, Ting HH, Best PJ, Singh M, Bell MR, Barsness GW, Mathew V, Garratt KN & Holmes Jr DR (2002). Incidence and prognostic importance of acute renal failure after percutaneous coronary intervention. *Circulation*, Vol.105, No.19, pp.2259-2264.

Rosário MA, Lima JJ, Parga JR, Avila LF, Gowdak LH, Lemos PA & Rochitte CE (2010). Coronary calcium score as predictor of stenosis and events in pretransplant renal chronic failure. *Arquivos Brasileiros de Cardiologia*, Vol.94, No.2, pp.252-260.

Sarnak MJ, Levey AS, Schoolwerth AC, Coresh J, Culleton B, Hamm LL, McCullough PA, Kasiske BL, Kelepouris E, Klag MJ, Parfrey P, Pfeffer M, Raij L, Spinosa DJ & Wilson PW; American Heart Association Councils on Kidney in Cardiovascular Disease, High Blood Pressure Research, Clinical Cardiology, and Epidemiology and Prevention (2003). Kidney disease as a risk factor for development of cardiovascular disease: a statement from the American Heart Association Councils on Kidney in Cardiovascular Disease, High Blood Pressure Research, Clinical Cardiology, and Epidemiology and Prevention. *Circulation*, Vol.108, No.17, pp.2154-2169.

Sharma R, Pellerin D & Brecker SJ (2007). The detection of myocardial ischemia in end-stage renal disease. *Current Opinion in Investigational Drugs*, Vol.8, No.3, pp.232-236.

Schmidt A, Stefenelli T, Schuster E & Mayer G (2001). Informational contribution of noninvasive screening tests for coronary artery disease in patients on chronic renal replacement therapy. *American Journal of Kidney Disease*, Vol.37, No.1, pp.56-63.

Sosnov J, Lessard D, Goldberg RJ, Yarzebski J & Gore JM (2006). Differential symptoms of acute myocardial infarction in patients with kidney disease: a community-wide perspective. *American Journal of Kidney Disease*, Vol.47, No.3, pp.378-384.

Spargias K, Alexopoulos E, Kyrzopoulos S, Iokovis P, Greenwood DC, Manginas A, Voudris V, Pavlides G, Buller CE, Kremastinos D & Cokkinos DV (2004). Ascorbic acid prevents contrast-mediated nephropathy in patients with renal dysfunction undergoing coronary angiography or intervention. *Circulation*, Vol.110, No.18, pp.2837-2842.

Stacul F, Adam A, Becker CR, Davidson C, Lameire N, McCullough PA, Tumlin J & CIN Consensus Working Panel (2006). Strategies to reduce the risk of contrast-induced nephropathy. *American Journal of Cardiology*, Vol.98, No.6A, pp.59K–77K.

Subramanian S, Tumlin J, Bapat B & Zyczynski T (2007). Economic burden of contrast-induced nephropathy: implications for prevention strategies. *Journal of Medical Economics*, Vol.10, No.2, pp.119-134.

U.S. Renal Data System (2010). USRDS 2010 Annual Data Report: Atlas of Chronic Kidney Disease and End-Stage Renal Disease in the United States, National Institutes of Health, National Institute of Diabetes and Digestive and Kidney Diseases, Bethesda, MD. Accessed: Apr 26, 2011, Available from: <http://www.usrds.org>

Welsh RC, Cockfield SM, Campbell P, Hervas-Malo M, Gyenes G & Dzavik V (2011). Cardiovascular assessment of diabetic end-stage renal disease patients before renal transplantation. *Transplantation*, Vol.91, No.2, pp.213-218.

Yerkey MW, Kernis SJ, Franklin BA, Sandberg KR & McCullough PA (2004). Renal dysfunction and acceleration of coronary disease. *Heart*, Vol. 90, No. 8, pp.961-966.

12

Cardiac Catheterization and Coronary Angiography in Patients with Cardiomyopathy

Ali Ghaemian
Mazandaran University of Medical Sciences
Iran

1. Introduction

Cardiomyopathies are a group of heart diseases that influence muscles directly and are not related to congenital, valvular, and pericardial diseases (Salehifar et al., 2008). Cardiomyopathies are usually classified on the basis of structural or functional causes. Thus, dilated cardiomyopathy is characterized by an enlarged ventricular chamber size and reduced cardiac contractility, hypertrophic cardiomyopathy is characterized by hypertrophy of the ventricular walls and increased cardiac performance and finally the restrictive form is characterized by stiff ventricular walls which restrict diastolic filling of the ventricle while systolic performance is not impaired (Ammash et al., 2000; Dec & Fuster ,1994). The classification by the American Heart Association Scientific Statement panel divides cardiomyopathy into primary and secondary causes (Maron et al., 2006).In this classification primary cardiomyopathies are subdivided into genetic, mixed and acquired groups.

2. Dilated cardiomyopathy

Dilated cardiomyopathy (DCM) is characterized by enlargement of one or both ventricles accompanied by impaired myocardial systolic function.DCM is the most common cardiomyopathy. Patients with DCM usually have symptoms and signs of congestive heart failure and there are many cardiac and systemic causes leading to DCM. However, in about 50 percent or more of the patients with DCM, the etiology can not be identified. Thus, the patient is called as having an idiopathic DCM (Felker et al., 2000).

2.1 Natural history and prognosis

Because of different etiologies patients have variable presentations. Asymptomatic patients with left ventricular dysfunction to advanced stages of heart failure are two sides of the spectrum of presentations of the patients. The annual mortality ranges between 10 and 50 percents (Levy et al., 2006).While survival of some patients is good, some cardiomyopathy patients have poor prognosis. For example, cardiomyopathy patients with human immunodeficiency virus and amyloidosis do not have long-term survival (Levy et al., 2006). Patients with idiopathic DCM have variable natural history. Some patients may be stable over years or even decades. This stability may be in response to pharmacological or device therapy or it can be due to spontaneous reverse remodeling. On the other hand, the clinical stability of some patients deteriorates suddenly and the hemodynamic situation requires inotropic or mechanical support (Teuteberg et al.,2006).

2.2 Etiology

DCM is the major cause of congestive heart failure (CHF).Other most frequent specific Cardiomyopathies causing CHF include ischemic or hypertensive cardiomyopathies and nonsystolic heart failure (Owan et al.,2006).In DCM after excluding the specific disease about 50 percent is called idiopathic DCM(Felker et al., 2000).However, some of these idiopathic DCM cases are caused by genetic abnormalities or some environmental etiologies that are not diagnosed at the time of primary presentation and with more imaging or molecular evaluation, many of these idiopathic cases will have a specific etiology.

2.3 Specific forms of dilated cardiomyopathy

There are many important causes of secondary CMP including alcohol, HIV infection, metabolic impairments and cardiotoxic drugs such as doxorubicin. There are four specific causes of dilated CMP with more probability of recovery.

2.3.1 Tachycardia-induced cardiomyopathy

Patients with recurrent or permanent tachycardia such as atrial fibrillation or supraventricular tachycardia may develop CHF or DCM. Atrial fibrillation is a frequent disease among patients affected by CHF (Ghaemian et al., 2011).There is a high probability of recovery by controlling the arrhythmia (Redfield et al., 2000).Thus , patients should be treated to restore normal sinus rhythm.

2.3.2 Peripartum cardiomyopathy

This form of cardiomyopathy presents between 6 months to the last month of pregnancy (Elkayam et al., 2001).Usually the prognosis is good. However, women who recover the first attack are at increased risk of recurrence during the next pregnancies.

2.3.3 Broken heart or tako-tsubo syndrome

This CMP is usually caused by a stressful condition. This CMP is more common in women and the patients usually recover with treatment. Electrocardiogram may show findings of myocardial infarction, but in coronary angiography epicardial coronary arteries do not show stenosis.

2.3.4 Alcoholic cardiomyopathy

This form of CMP usually is related to the amount of consumption of alcohol with recovery by cessation of alcohol. The mechanism usually is direct toxicity of the alcohol (Fernandez-sola et al.,2006).This CMP is more common in men, patients usually have a history of excessive consumption of alcohol for more than 10 years. Patients may have a fulminant course with biventricular failure. Alcohol may precipitate some arrhythmias including atrial fibrillation or supraventricular tachycardia. Many electrocardiographic abnormalities including QT interval prolongation are common. Hemodynamic and echocardiographic findings are similar to those of DCM patients. Cessation of consumption of the alcohol is the main component of treatment.

2.4 Clinical presentation of the dilated cardiomyopathy

DCM is more frequent in middle age man, but it affects all ages. The incidence if ischemic CMP is higher than DCM. The clinical presentation of patients with DCM is variable. While some patients gradually become symptomatic, others may develop symptoms over only weeks and yet some of them have fulminant course of congestive heart failure (McCarthy et al., 2000).The most frequent symptoms of patients are dyspnea and fatigue.

2.5 Laboratory evaluation

Screening the biochemical testing including serum electrolytes, calcium, phosphorus and serum creatinine is necessary. Rheumatological tests such as antinuclear antibody (ANA) and erythrocyte sedimentation rate should also be obtained. Endocrine tests including thyroid function test and urinary examination of catecholamine levels may be helpful. Serum troponin levels to assess myocardial necrosis and brain natriuretic peptide levels are usually obtained.

2.5.1 Electrocardiography

Nonspecific electrocardiographic changes include sinus tachycardia, interventricular conduction delay and poor R progression and left bundle branch block. Other electrocardiographic abnormalities such as ST segment and T wave abnormalities may also be seen. Patients may show a wide spectrum of supraventricular and ventricular arrhythmia.

2.5.2 Echocardiography

By two-dimensional echocardiography ventricular size and function are usually evaluated. Doppler echocardiography is helpful to evaluate valvular stenosis or regurgitation and restrictive filling patterns. Dobutamine stress echocardiography is helpful to differentiate ischemic from idiopathic DCM and also to assess contractile reserve of myocardium.

2.5.3 Radionuclide imaging

This imaging technique is useful to identify ischemic CMP and also can assess cardiac function and ejection fraction of both ventricles.

2.5.4 Magnetic Resonance Imaging (MRI)

Cardiac MRI is useful to diagnose some specific CMPs such as myocarditis, amyloidosis, sarcoidosis and infiltrative and inflammatory cardiomyopathies and arrhythmogenic right ventricular dysplasia (Maceira et al., 2005; Mahrholdt et al.,2004; Tandri et al., 2005).

3. Ischemic cardiomyopathy

When myocardial dysfunction is secondary to occlusion of the coronary arteries, the term ischemic CMP is used and is the most common cause of heart failure. Based on the pathophysiological processes ischemic CMP may be classified into three groups. The first one is called myocardial hibernation. In this form of ischemic CMP a reduced coronary flow will result in persistent contractile dysfunction and revascularization procedures will usually restore myocardial function, at least partially. Myocardial stunning is the second form of ischemic CMP. In this form the contractile dysfunction of the viable myocardium is transient and is usually caused by reduced sensitivity of contractile proteins to calcium.

Finally in the third type, the contractile dysfunction is secondary to irreversible cell death of the myocardium.

3.1 Revascularization in ischemic CMP

In patients with ischemic CMP revascularization is beneficial only when the myocardium is viable and revascularization procedures cause an improvement in left ventricular function. In patients with severe left ventricular dysfunction, but with viable myocardium, coronary artery revascularization results in an average 8 to 10 percent of improvement in left ventricular ejection fraction (Kumpati et al.,2001).This will be associated with improvement in clinical situation and survival of the patients. However, if the viable myocardium is not considerable improvement of left ventricular function will not occur. It has been reported that 20 to 25 percent or more of the myocardium is the threshold of myocardial viability for which surgery is indicated (De Bonis & Alfieri 2006).Patients with ischemic CMP should be examined for detection of myocardial viability.Thallium-201 single-photon emission computed tomography (SPECT) and dobutamine stress echocardiography are usually used for this purpose. When both of these two methods predicated viability, the global left ventricular ejection fraction rose from 35 to 40 percent after operation (Starling et al., 2003).In other reports positron emission tomography (PET) was better than SPECT to predict improvement of left ventricular ejection fraction after revascularization (Pagano et al., 1999;Starling et al., 2003). In a meta-analysis of 24 studies in patients with ischemic CMP revascularization decreased the risk of death by 79.6 percent in patients with viable myocardium detected by SPECT, dobutamine echocardiography or positron emission tomography (Bishay et al., 2000). Thus, in patients with heart failure secondary to coronary artery disease coronary angiography and viability study should be performed.

4. Right and left heart catheterization

Catheterization of the right and left side of the heart are usually performed to examine the hemodynamics of the heart i.e. to measure intracardiac pressure, cardiac outputs, and vascular resistances. In patients with heart failure, respiratory failure, valvular heart disease, pericardial disease, restrictive or hypertrophic cardiomyopathies hemodynamic assessment is of great value for the diagnosis and management of the patients. If necessary angiographic procedures such as left or right ventriculography, pulmonary angiography, and aortography may be performed during cardiac catheterization. Besides, selective angiographic procedures include native coronary, coronary bypass graft and carotid angiography.

4.1 Hemodynamic evaluation

Catheterization laboratories use disposable, fluid – filled transducers to measure pressure. For hemodynamic evaluation, the right heart catheter is placed in the pulmonary artery and a pigtail catheter in the aorta. Cardiac out is usually measured by the thermodilution method. Oxymetric analysis is performed on the blood collected from the aorta and the pulmonary artery, cardiac output is calculated by the Fick method , the presence of a left- to - right shunt is also screened. Catheter of the aorta is advanced into the left ventricle and the right- sided catheter into pulmonary capillary wedge position and the pressures are measured simultaneously. Then the right sided catheter is withdrawn and all the pressures are recorded. With the simultaneous measurement of the pressure of right and left ventricles it is possible to screen for restrictive or constrictive physiology. Then by pulling back the left- sided catheter the pressure gradient across the aortic valve is determined.

4.2 Complications

Cardiac catheterization also is a safe procedure, potentially has some complications. In patients with left ventricular thrombus or aortic valve endocarditis it is better to avoid inserting catheters into the left heart. Catheter induced arrhythmia is another potential complication of right or left heart. Right or left bundle branch blocks may occur if the catheter is placed in the right ventricular outflow tract or crossed the aortic valve, respectively. Thus, patients with right or left bundle branch block are at potential risk of developing complete heart block during cardiac catheterization. Renal failure, contrast reactions, vascular complications are the more common complications of cardiac catheterization. The incidence of cerebrovascular accident, myocardial infarction, and death is less than 1 percent. Other rare complications include infection, chamber or vessel perforation, cholesterol embolism, air embolism, and radiation -induced skin injury.

4.3 Right heart catheterization

Right heart catheterization is performed from the right internal Jugular, femoral or subclavian veins using a balloon flotation catheter. For right heart catheterization fluoroscopy is not necessary and by attaching the catheter to a pressure transducer the operator can advance the catheter. Pressure is recorded in the right sided chambers and the pulmonary artery. With the catheter in the pulmonary artery, it is possible to measure thermodilution cardiac output and perform oximetry to detect a shunt and determine cardiac output by the Fick method. The catheter also can be advanced to a pulmonary capillary wedge position to obtain the wedge pressure. If by the pressure-guided technique catheter does not advance successfully and also when the right heart catheterization is performed from the femoral veins fluoroscopy is used. The normal pressure of the right atrium is 2 to 6 mmHg with positive "a" and "v" waves and negative "x" and "y" descents (Fig.1).

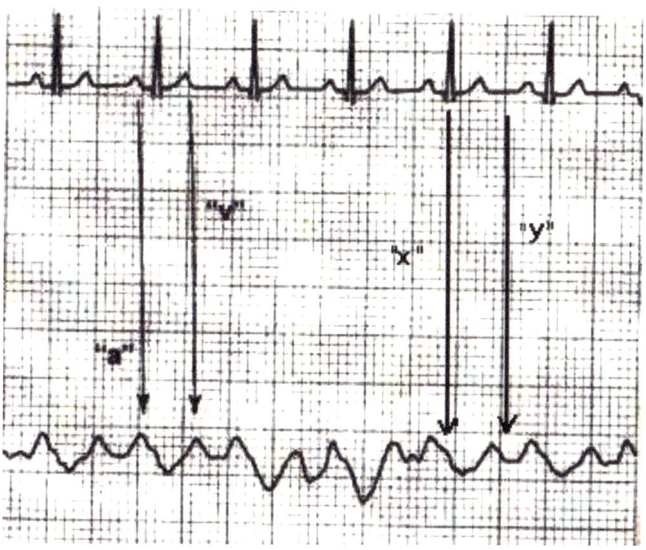

Fig. 1. Normal right atrial waveform

The atrial contraction increases the right atrial pressure producing the "a" wave. At the initial part of ventricular systole the downward motion of the tricuspid valve and the atrial relaxation produce the "x" descent. An inconsistent "c" waves after the "a" represents the motion of the tricuspid annulus toward the right atrium at the onset of the ventricular systole. The distance of the "c" from the "a" is the same as the PR interval in the electrocardiogram and first degree atrioventricular block produces a more visible "c" wave. The "x" descent represents the decrease of the right atrial pressure in ventricular systole which is followed by the "v" wave in atrial diastole when the right atrium is filled by venous return. The peak of the "v" wave occurs at the end of ventricular systole when the right atrium is maximally filled and is at the same time of T wave on the electrocardiogram. The final "y" descent represents the rapid emptying of the right atrium at the initial part of ventricular diastole when the tricuspid valve opens. As shown in Figure 2 the normal right ventricular systolic pressure is 20 to 30mmHg, and normal right ventricular end-diastolic pressure is 0 to 8 mmHg. The right ventricular pressure normally consists of a rapid rise of pressure followed by a decline during ventricular contraction and then rapid downward motion with ventricular relaxation. At the beginning of diastole the pressure is low and with ventricular filling increases gradually.

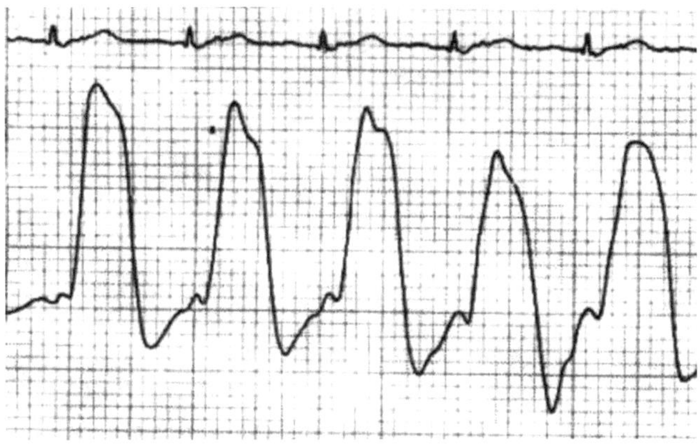

Fig. 2. Normal right ventricular waveform

The normal range of pulmonary artery systolic pressure is about 20 to 30 mmHg while the diastolic pressure is 4 -12 mmHg . As is shown in Figure 3 the pressure waveform of the pulmonary artery increase rapidly during systole and reaches a peak. However, during diastolic descent of the pressure there is a dicrotic notch.

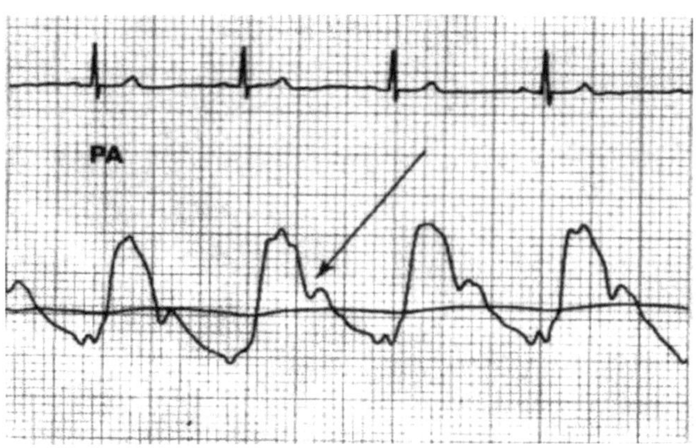

Fig. 3. Normal pulmonary artery waveform

During right heart catheterization the pulmonary capillary wedge pressure (PCWP) waveform is usually evaluated. The pressure waveform is better to obtain with an end-hole catheter. The end-hole catheter obstructs the antegrade flow into the pulmonary artery, so it reflects the left atrial pressure, or the PCWP. This pressure can be obtained by a Swan-Ganz catheter in the pulmonary artery. By inflating the balloon of this catheter and obstructing the flow, the PCWP is obtained. The normal mean pressure of the PCWP is about 2 to 14mmHg and consists of positive "a" and "v" and negative "x" and "y" waves (Fig.4).

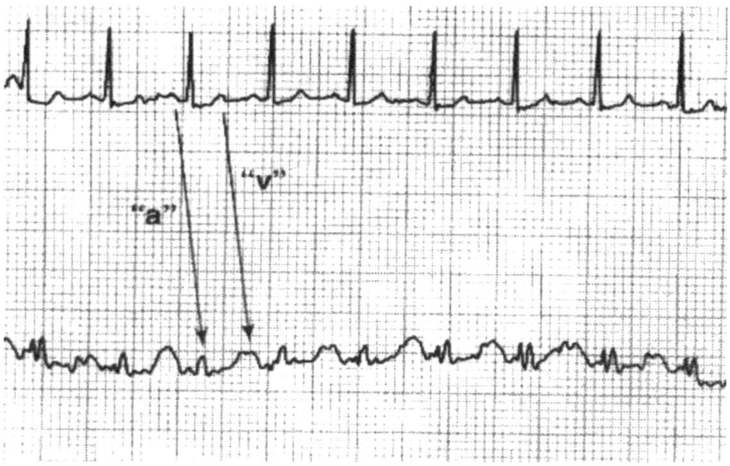

Fig. 4. Normal pulmonary capillary wedge pressure waveform

However, "c" wave which is sometimes seen in an atrial pressure is usually not seen in PCWP and also because the PCWP is the pressure transmitted through the pulmonary capillary bed, a time delay occurs between an electrocardiographic event and the onset of the relevant wave. For example the "a" wave of the right atrial pressure follows the P wave of the electrocardiogram by about 80 milliseconds while it is about 240 milliseconds in PCWP. Also, the peak of the "v" wave in PCWP tracing occurs after the T wave. Finally it should be noted that the oxygen saturation obtained from the catheter in the PCWP position is greater than 90%.

4.4 Left heart catheterization

Left heart catheterization is usually performed using a pigtail catheter. The catheter is advanced to the ascending aorta and then is positioned in the left ventricle. For this purpose, it may be necessary to rotate the catheter clockwise or counterclockwise gently to cross the valve. Occasionally a J- tipped stiff guide wire should be used.

The left ventricular waveform has a rapid upstroke during ventricular contraction and then during relaxation the pressure decreases (Fig.5).

At the initial part of the diastole the ventricular pressure is low and increases slowly until the end diastolic portion and the normal diastolic pressure is 8 to 16 mmHg. Left ventricular end -diastolic pressure is the pressure just before the abrupt increase in systolic pressure. Central aortic pressure waveforms normally have a rapid upstroke, a systolic peak followed by a dicrotic notch due to closure of the aortic valve (Fig.6).

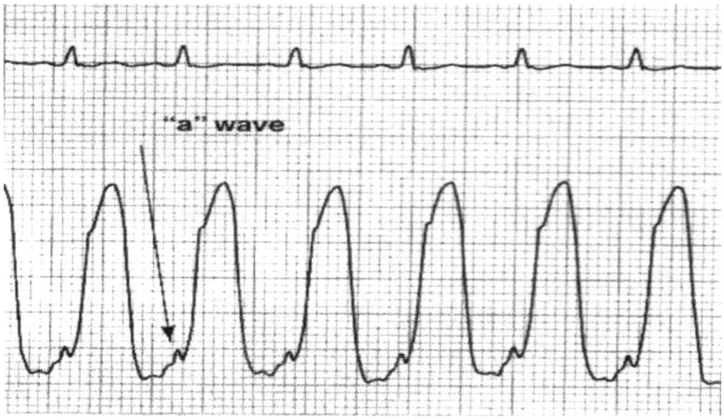

Fig. 5. Prominent "a" wave in left ventricular waveform

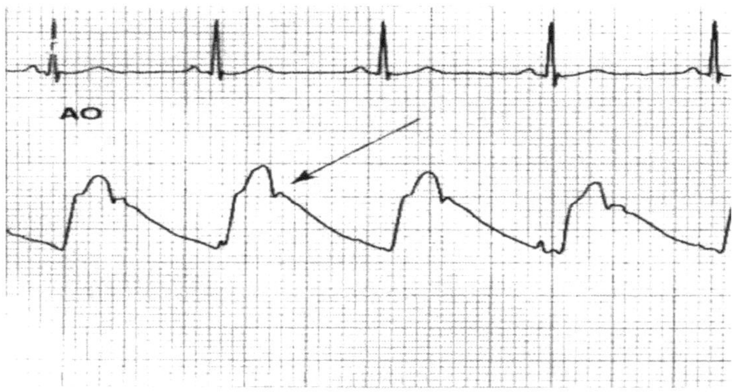

Fig. 6. Normal central aortic waveform

During hemodynamic evaluation for screening for the presence of a restrictive or constrictive physiology, simultaneous measurement of left and right ventricular pressures is performed. Normally peak systolic pressure changes during expiration and inspiration in the right and left ventricle parallel each other (Fig.7) and the diastolic pressures of the two ventricles differ by at least 5 mmHg during the respiratory cycle (Fig.8).

4.5 Hemodynamic calculations

During cardiac catheterization and hemodynamic evaluation, hemodynamic calculations are made. For example, calculation of the cardiac output by the Fick method, calculations of the pulmonary and peripheral vascular resistances, and calculations of the mitral and aortic valves areas can be obtained. However, most of the computerized hemodynamic data collection systems have the softwares to calculate these values automatically.

4.6 Trans - septal heart catheterization

In some situations it is not possible to enter the left ventricle via retrograde approach. For example, in the presence of a mechanical aortic valve at severe aortic stenosis it may be necessary to measure left ventricular pressure or perform left ventriculography and trans -

septal approach can be helpful. During some interventional procedures such as mitral balloon valvuloplasty, percutaneous mitral valve repairs with clips, some electrophysiologic procedures, and placement of a percutaneous left ventricular assist device may require trans -septal puncture.

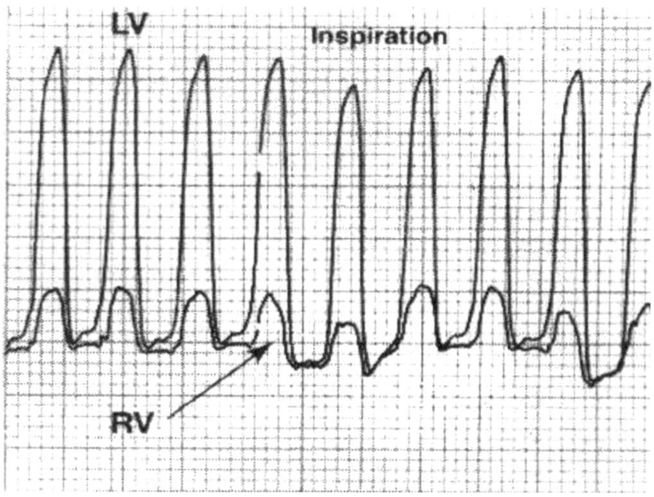

Fig. 7. Normal concomitant waveform of right ventricle and left ventricular in systole

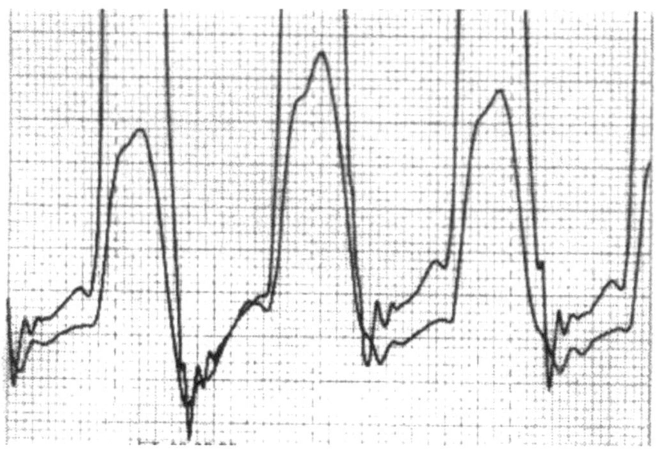

Fig. 8. Normal concomitant right and left ventricular waveform in diastole

During a trans-septal puncture the goal is usually to puncture the atrial septum at the fossa ovalis and the procedure is performed from the right femoral vein. At the same time a pigtail catheter is positioned on the aortic valve to identify the aorta by fluoroscopy. The puncture of the interatrial septum is performed using the Brockenbrough needle inserted into a dilator. After the puncture, a guidewire is advanced into the left atrium and the dilator is advanced over the wire in order to position the sheath within the left atrium and left atrial pressure is recorded. Then based on the procedure, the rest of the catheterization or intervention can be performed.

5. Abnormal hemodynamic waveforms in patients

In patients with left ventricular systolic dysfunction including dilated CMP the hemodynamic findings are nonspecific. Heart failure increases the pulmonary capillary wedge pressure and right-sided pressures. Chronic heart failure increases the pulmonary artery pressure because of reactive and fixed increases in pulmonary vascular resistance, leading to pulmonary hypertension and secondary tricuspid regurgitation and right heart failure. In patients with systolic dysfunction left ventricular end-diastolic pressure is increased and a prominent "a" wave may be seen (Fig 9).

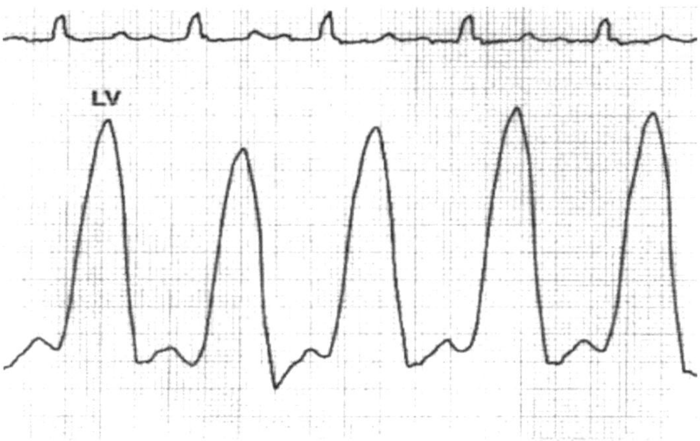

Fig. 9. Pressure waveform in a patient with left ventricular dysfunction showing a prominent "a" wave

In patients with advanced stages of left ventricular dysfunction, left ventricular pressure may have a delay to reach the systolic peak due to diminished contractility (Fig 10).

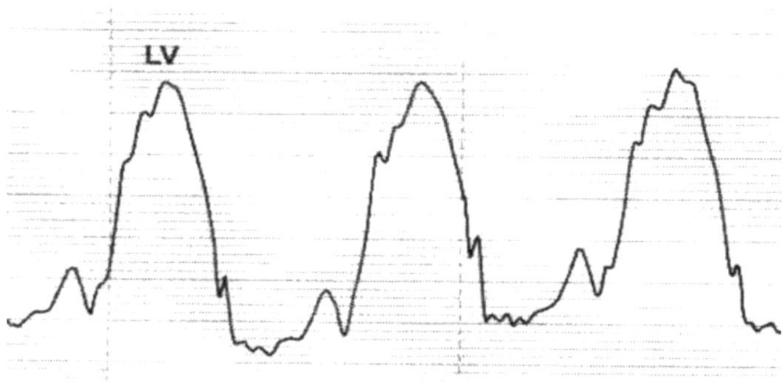

Fig. 10. Left ventricular pressure waveform in a patient with severe left ventricular dysfunction which have a triangular appearance

Another presentation of severely reduced left ventricular contractility is the appearance of pulsus alternans on the aortic or left ventricular pressure waveform (Fig 11).
Ambulatory patients with dilated CMP may have a relatively low normal resting cardiac output and a modest elevation in both right-and left-sided filling pressures. However, in advanced stages of heart failure, the systemic vascular resistance rises significantly in response to the reduced cardiac output. Also, in advanced heart failure in dilated CMP patients

biventricular failure is usually characteristic. The right atrial pressure waveform will demonstrate steep "x" and "y" descents indicative of severe volume overload and right ventricular systolic and diastolic dysfunction. Kussmaul sign, i.e., absence of the normal respiratory fall in the right atrial pressure is common and as a result of tricuspid regurgitation the "y" descent is steep. The PCWP waveform may demonstrate a prominent "v" wave. The left ventricular pressure waveform is characterized by an elevation in pressure throughout early diastole. The arterial tracing may show a narrow pulse pressure (pulsus parvus).

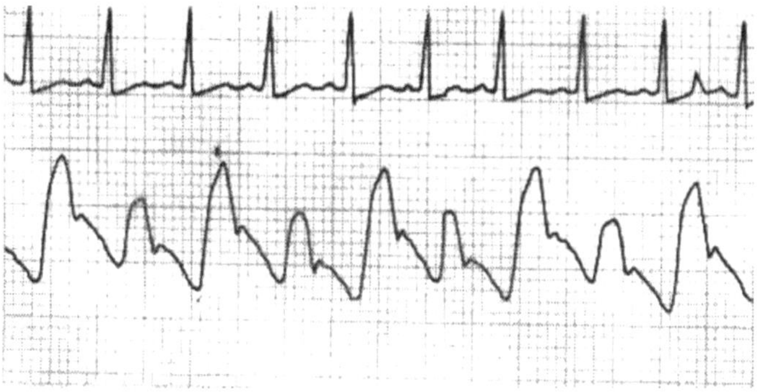

Fig. 11. Aortic pressure tracing in a patient with severe left ventricular dysfunction pulsus alternans

In patients with right-sided heart failure similar to left heart failure, pulsus alternans may be present in right-sided pressure waveforms (Fig 12).

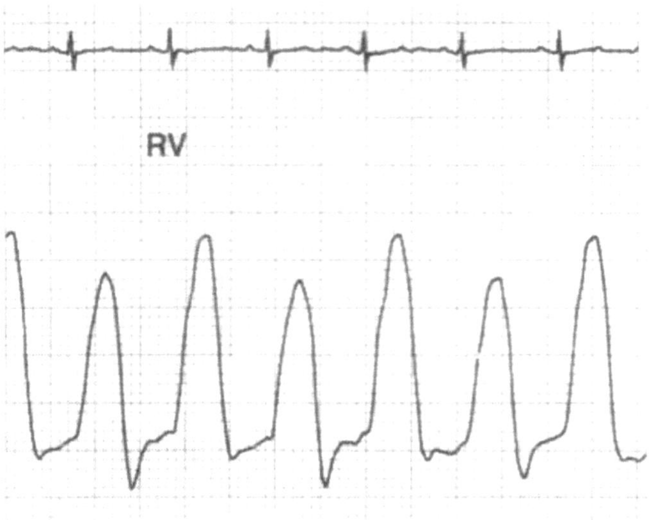

Fig. 12. Pulsus alternans in the right ventricular wave form in a patient with right-sided heart failure

In the case of tricuspid regurgitation secondary to pulmonary hypertension as in primary tricuspid regurgitation a prominent "v" wave on the right atrial waveform may appear (Fig 13) and in severe cases of tricuspid regurgitation ventricularization of the right atrial waveform may occur (Fig 14).

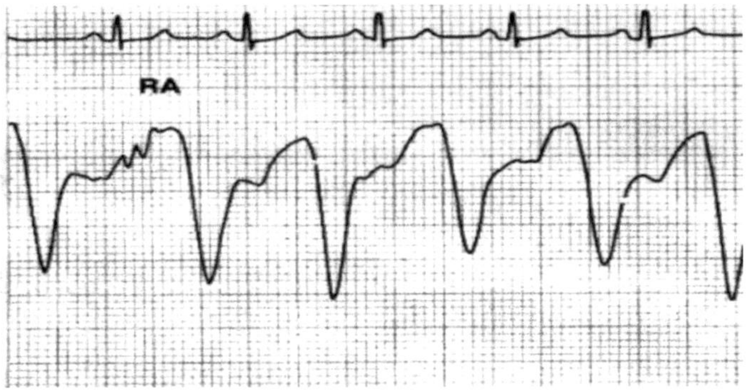

Fig. 13. Prominent "v" wave in the right atrial pressure in a patient with severe tricuspid regurgitation

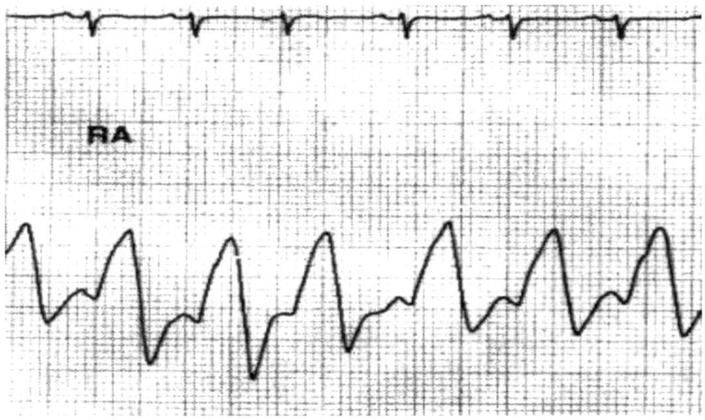

Fig. 14. Ventricularization of the right atrial waveform in a patient with severe tricuspid regurgitation

In patients with hypertrophic obstructive cardiomyopathy the systolic anterior motion of the mitral valve obstructs the left ventricular outflow tract causing a pressure gradient between the left ventricle and aorta (Fig 15). And the aorta pressure waveform may show the characteristic pattern of spike and dome configuration (Fig 16). In some cases the gradient may be absent at rest but can be provoked by decreasing the preload.

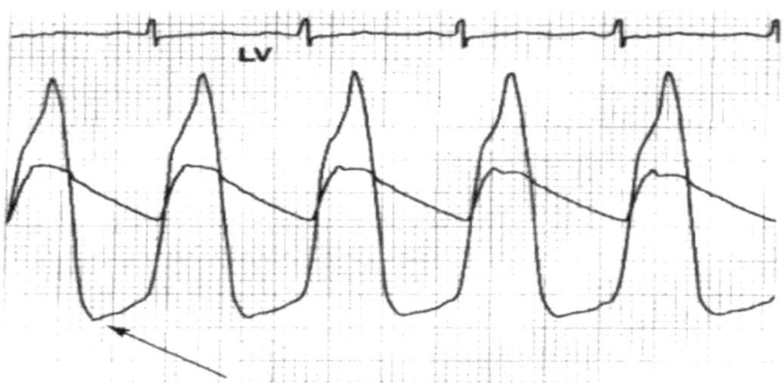

Fig. 15. Simultaneous left ventricular and aortic pressure waveform in a patient with hypertrophic obstructive cardiomyopathy which shows significant pressure gradients at rest

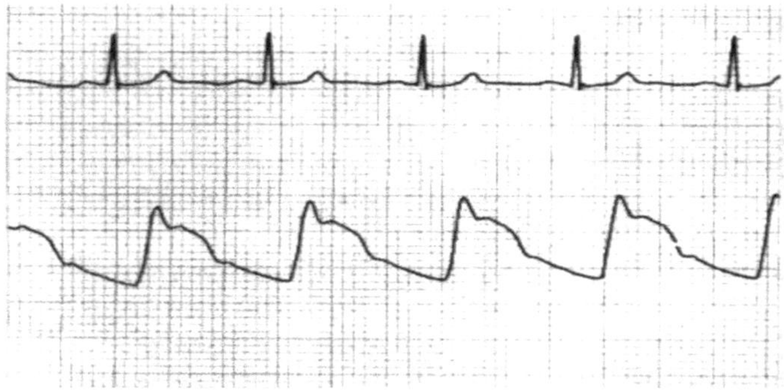

Fig. 16. Aortic pressure waveform showing "spike-and-dome" configuration

6. Left ventriculography

Left ventriculography is performed during a left heart catheterization to assess left ventricular function. Left ventriculography can also be helpful to identify the presence of mitral regurgitation, ventricular septal defect, and left ventricular hypertrophy. In patients with high pulmonary capillary wedge pressure or left ventricular end-diastolic pressure the injection of contrast may impose the patient to the risk of acute pulmonary edema. In addition, in patients with a mobile left ventricular thrombus seen on echocardiography it is better not to perform left ventriculography. Left ventriculography is commonly performed by a power injector and a pigtail catheter positioned in the mid ventricle.

For assessment of ventricular systolic function, ejection fraction is calculated via left ventriculography. Usually computer-based software is applied and the left ventricular end-diastolic and end-systolic contours are traced. Diastolic and systolic areas can be determined and based on the assumptions regarding the geometry of the heart, ventricular volumes are calculated and then the left ventricular ejection fraction can be calculated. Furthermore, in patients with coronary artery disease, regional left ventricular function can be assessed. Based on the distribution of the coronary arteries the left ventricle is divided into some segments. The contractions of the segments are evaluated. If the contraction of each segment is reduced it is classified as "hypokinetic" and if there is no contraction it is called "akinetic". Finally, if during systole the segment moves outward it is called "dyskinetic". In patients with hypertrophic cardiomyopathy, because of excessive hypertrophy, in left ventriculography cavity obliteration and a small ventricular end-systolic volume are commonly seen. In these patients if ventricular outflow tract obstruction also is present, systolic anterior motion of the mitral valve can be noted. Interestingly, in apical form of hypertrophic cardiomyopathy the ventriculogram appears with a "spade" - shaped contour. In patients with apical ballooning syndrome who have transient severe left ventricular dysfunction in the absence of coronary artery disease left ventriculography shows aneurysm of the left ventricle which predominantly affects the apex of the heart.

7. Right ventriculography

Right ventriculography is usually indicated in congenital heart disease. However, right ventriculography in adults may be helpful in the diagnosis of right ventricular dysplasia and determination of right ventricular systolic function. In patients with arrhythmogenic right ventricular dysplasia several findings associated with this disorder have been noted. However, there is no pathognomonic feature in right ventriculography in these patients.

8. Coronary angiography

Coronary angiography is considered the gold standard for diagnosing coronary artery disease and can be useful to differentiate ischemic from dilated forms of cardiomyopathies. During coronary angiography the dominant vessel and also the vascular territories for each artery can be identified. Obstructive coronary artery disease is usually defined by angiography when a greater than 50% diameter narrowing is seen. When the lesions narrow the lumen by more than 70%, they are generally believed to be hemodynamically significant. However, there are some limitations regarding the usefulness of coronary angiography in diagnosing coronary artery disease. Coronary angiography only assesses the arterial lumen, while atherosclerosis is a disease of the arterial wall. There may be a substantial amount of plaque in the arterial wall before it is evident by angiography. Thus, a normal coronary arteriogram does not exclude the presence of coronary artery disease. Second, there is a wide range of interobserver variability in interpreting the coronary arteriogram of a patient. Third, depending on the image quality, the operator technique, patient body habitus, the vessel tortuosity, and the presence of overlapping segments, the ability of the angiography to assess a lesion may be affected. Finally, for identification of a luminal narrowing a reference normal segment of the vessel is usually used for comparison. In patients with diffuse coronary lesions, a true normal segment is not present and the arterial lumen may appear uniform.

Ischemic cardiomyopathy results following severe coronary artery disorders and usually angiography must be performed for proper diagnosis (Shokrzadeh et al., 2008). Coronary atherosclerosis usually causes narrowing of the lumen of the coronary arteries in advanced stages. In the early stages of atherosclerosis, compensatory enlargement of the artery maintains the coronary artery lumen. Thus, coronary angiography which only assesses the arterial lumen can not detect the early stages of atherosclerosis. However, techniques such as intravascular ultrasound provide images of arterial wall and detect coronary atherosclerosis in earlier stages. Coronary atherosclerosis can be detected anywhere along the course of the artery.

There are many indications for performing coronary angiography. For example, in different clinical situations such as myocardial infarction, acute coronary syndromes stable angina, patients with valvular or congenital heart diseases coronary angiography may be useful to define coronary artery anatomy. However, coronary angiography should not be performed in patients who do not want to undergo revascularization, patients with severe left ventricular dysfunction in whom revascularization is not likely to improve ventricular function, patients with acute bleeding, unexplained fever, and in patients with severe coagulopathy.

9. Conclusion

Cardiac catheterization is performed in patients with heart failure to assess the etiology, to evaluate the hemodynamic status of the patient, and to define therapeutic responses. While the major part of the hemodynamic evaluation is assessed in the supine state, exercise conditions can also be evaluated. After hemodynamic evaluation of the patient angiography should be performed to define the coronary anatomy and if needed left ventriculography to assess ventricular contractility. Ventriculography is also helpful to define ventricular size and mitral regurgitation, although most patients will have had complete echocardiographic study prior to catheterization. In the absence of coronary artery disease to explain ventricular dysfunction, an endomyocardial biopsy should be considered for a specific diagnosis.

10. Acknowledgement

I wish to thank Dr Safoora Masoumi for her help in providing this chapter.

11. References

Ammash, NM., Seward, JB., Bailey, KR., Edwards, WD., & Tajik, AJ. (2000).Clinical profile and outcome of idiopathic restrictive cardiomyopathy. *Circulation,* Vol. 101, No.21, (may 2000), pp.2490-2496, ISSN 0009-7322

Bishay, ES., McCarthy, PM., Cosgrove, DM., Hoercher, KJ., Smedira, NG., Mukherjee, D., White, J., & Blackstone, EH.(2000). Mitral valve surgery in patients with severe left ventricular dysfunction. *Eur J Cardiothorac Surg,* Vol.17, No.3, (Mar 2000), pp.213-221, ISSN 1010-7940

De Bonis, M., & Alfieri, O.(2006). Surgery insight: Surgical methods to reverse left ventricular remodeling. *Nat Clin Pract Cardiovasc Med,* Vol.3, No.9, (Sep 2006), pp.507-513, ISSN 1759-5002

Dec, GW., & Fuster, V.(1994). Idiopathic dilated cardiomyopathy. *N Engl J Med,* Vol. 331, No.23, (Dec 1994), pp.1564-1575, ISSN 0028-4793

Elkayam, U., Tummala, PP., Rao, K., Akhter, MW., Karaalp, IS., Wani, OR., Hameed, A., Gviazda, I., & Shotan A.(2001) Maternal and fetal outcomes of subsequent pregnancies in women with peripartum cardiomyopathy. *N Engl J Med,* Vol.344, No.21(May 2001), pp.1567-1571, ISSN 0028-4793

Felker, GM., Thompson, RE., Hare, JM., Hruban, RH., Clemetson, DE., Howard, DL., Baughman, KL., & Kasper, EK. (2000) Underlying causes and long-term survival in patients with initially unexplained cardiomyopathy. *N Engl J Med,* Vol.342, No.15, (Apr 2000), pp.1077-1084, ISSN 0028-4793

Fernández-Solà, J., Fatjó, F., Sacanella, E., Estruch, R., Bosch, X., Urbano-Márquez, A., & Nicolás, JM.(2006) Evidence of apoptosis in alcoholic cardiomyopathy. *Hum Pathol,* Vol.37, No.8(Aug 2006), pp.1100-1110, ISSN 0046-8177

Ghaemian, A., Salehifar, E., Jalalian, R., Ghasemi, F., Azizi, S., Masoumi, S., Shiraj, H., Mohammadpour, RA., & Bagheri GA.(2011). Zinc and Copper Levels in Severe Heart Failure and the Effects of Atrial Fibrillation on the Zinc and Copper Status. *Biol Trace Elem Res,* [Epub ahead of print], (2011 Jan), DOI 10.1007/s12011-011-8956-6

Kumpati, GS., McCarthy, PM., & Hoercher, KJ.(2001). Surgical treatments for heart failure. *Cardiol Clin,* Vol.19, No .4, (Nov 2001), pp. 669-681, ISSN 0160-9289

Levy, WC., Mozaffarian, D., Linker, DT., Sutradhar, SC., Anker, SD., Cropp, AB., Anand, I., Maggioni, A., Burton, P., Sullivan, MD., Pitt, B., Poole-Wilson, PA., Mann, DL., & Packer, M.(2006) The Seattle heart failure model-Prediction of survival in heart failure.*Circulation,* Vol.113, No.11, (Mar 2006), pp.1424-1433, ISSN 0009-7322

Maceira, AM., Joshi, J., Prasad, SK., Moon, JC., Perugini, E., Harding, I., Sheppard, MN., Poole-Wilson, PA., Hawkins, PN., & Pennell DJ. (2005).Cardiovascular magnetic resonance in cardiac amyloidosis. *Circulation,* Vol .111, No.2, (Jan 2005), pp.186-193, ISSN 0009-7322

Mahrholdt, H., Goedecke, C., Wagner, A., Meinhardt, G., Athanasiadis, A., Vogelsberg, H., Fritz, P., Klingel, K., Kandolf, R., & Sechtem U.(2004) Cardiovascular magnetic resonance assessment of human myocarditis-A comparison to histology and molecular pathology. *Circulation*, Vol. 109, No.10, (Mar 2004), pp. 1250-1258, ISSN 0009-7322

Maron, BJ., Towbin, JA., Thiene, G., Antzelevitch, C., Corrado, D., Arnett, D., Moss, AJ., Seidman, CE., Young, JB., American Heart Association., Council on Clinical Cardiology., Heart Failure and Transplantation Committee., Quality of Care and Outcomes Research and Functional Genomics and Translational Biology Interdisciplinary Working Groups., & Council on Epidemiology and Prevention.(2006). Contemporary definitions and classification of the cardiomyopathies—An American Heart Association Scientific Statement from the Council on Clinical Cardiology, Heart Failure and Transplantation Committee; Quality of Care and Outcomes Research and Functional Genomics and Translational Biology Interdisciplinary Working Groups; and Council on Epidemiology and Prevention. *Circulation,* Vol.113, No.14, (Apr 2006), pp 1807-1816, ISSN 0009-7322

McCarthy, RE., Boehmer, JP., Hruban, RH., Hutchins, GM., Kasper, EK., Hare, JM., & Baughman KL.(2000). Long-term outcome of fulminant myocarditis as compared with acute (nonfulminant) myocarditis. *N Engl J Med,* Vol.342, No.10, (Mar 2000), pp. 690-695, ISSN 0028-4793

Owan, TE., Hodge, DO., Herges, RM., Jacobsen, SJ., Roger, VL., & Redfield MM.(2006) Trends in prevalence and outcome of heart failure with preserved ejection fraction. *N Engl J Med,* Vol.355, No.3, (Jul 2006), pp.251-259, ISSN 0028-4793

Pagano, D., Bonser, RS., & Camici, PG. (1999) .Myocardial revascularization for the treatment of post-ischemic heart failure. *Curr Opin Cardiol,* Vol.14, No.6, (Nov 1999), pp.506-509, ISSN 0268-4705

Redfield, MM., Kay, GN., Jenkins, LS., Mianulli, M., Jensen, DN., & Ellenbogen, KA.(2000) Tachycardia-related cardiomyopathy: A common cause of ventricular dysfunction in patients with atrial fibrillation referred for atrioventricular ablation. *Mayo Clinic Proc,* Vol.75, No.8(Aug 2000), pp.790-795, ISSN 0025-6196

Salehifar, E., Shokrzadeh, M., Ghaemian, A., Aliakbari, S., & Saeedi Saravi, SS.(2008). The study of Cu and Zn serum levels in idiopathic dilated cardiomyopathy (IDCMP) patients and its comparison with healthy volunteers. *Biol Trace Elem Res,* Vol.125, No.2, (Nov 2008), pp.97-108 ISSN 0163-498

Shokrzadeh, M., Ghaemian, A., Salehifar, E., Aliakbari, S., Saravi, SS., & Ebrahimi, P.(2009). Serum zinc and copper levels in ischemic cardiomyopathy. *Biol Trace Elem Res,* Vol.127, No.2, (Feb 2009), pp.116-123, ISSN 0163-498

Starling, RC., McCarthy, PM., & Yamini, MH.(2003). Surgical treatment of chronic congestive heart failure, In: *Heart Failure: A Companion to Braunwald's Heart Disease,* D.L. Mann, (Ed.), pp.717-736, WB Saunders, ISBN 0721694454 Philadelphia

Tandri, H., Saranathan, M., Rodriguez, ER., Martinez, C., Bomma, C., Nasir, K., Rosen, B., Lima, JA., Calkins, H., & Bluemke DA.(2005). Noninvasive detection of myocardial fibrosis in arrhythmogenic right ventricular cardiomyopathy using delayed-enhancement magnetic resonance imaging. *J Am Coll Cardiol,* Vol.45, No.1, (Jan 2005), pp.98-103, ISSN 0735-1097

Teuteberg, JJ., Lewis, EF., Nohria, A., Tsang, SW., Fang, JC., Givertz, MM., Jarcho, JA., Mudge, GH., Baughman, KL., & Stevenson LW.(2006) Characteristics of patients who die with heart failure and a low ejection fraction in the new millennium. *J Cardiac Fail,* Vol .12, No. 1, (Feb 2006), pp.47-53, ISSN 071-9164

13

Contrast-Induced Nephropathy in Patients with Type 2 Diabetes Mellitus and Coronary Artery Disease: Update and Practical Clinical Applications

Richard E. Katholi and Charles R. Katholi
Southern Illinois University School of Medicine and University of Alabama at Birmingham School of Medicine USA

1. Introduction

Contrast-induced nephropathy (CIN) is an injury to the kidney as a result of exposure to intravascular iodinated contrast medium. It represents an increasing health care burden and challenge as the frequency of diagnostic imaging and interventional studies increase, particularly among populations at risk of developing CIN. As the population ages, decreased renal function and increased atherosclerotic cardiovascular disease become more prevalent. An increasing incidence of obesity with resultant metabolic syndrome and/or type 2 diabetes mellitus also increases the population at risk for CIN (Toprak et al., 2006). Coronary artery disease is a major complication of type 2 diabetes mellitus. Thus, patients with type 2 diabetes mellitus often require coronary angiography and coronary intervention and are at risk of CIN.

2. Contrast-induced nephropathy in patients with type 2 diabetes mellitus and coronary artery disease

For clinical and research purposes, CIN is defined as an acute decline in renal function (rise in serum creatinine by 25% or greater than 0.5 mg/dL from baseline or fall in estimated glomerular filtration rate (eGFR) by greater than 25%) after systemic contrast medium administration in the absence of other causes. Typically, CIN onset occurs within 24-48 hours of exposure, serum creatinine levels peak in 3-5 days, and renal function returns to baseline in 7-21 days. If renal function does not return to baseline, other causes of acute renal injury, like atheroembolism or hypotension, should be suspected (Saleem et al., 1996). CIN is associated with both short-and long-term adverse outcomes, including the need for renal replacement therapy, increased length of hospital stay, major cardiac adverse events, and mortality. The incidence of CIN is less than 5% in patients with normal renal function and 15-50% in patients with baseline renal dysfunction (eGFR less than 60 mL/min/1.73m^2). The increased risk of CIN in diabetic patients with reduced renal function is well documented (Parfrey et al., 1989). Yet, diabetic patients without overt renal dysfunction are also at risk as compromised renal function may not manifest until an acute renal insult results from the administration of contrast medium. CIN carries short-term and long-term mortality. Acute renal failure after coronary intervention is associated with a 36% in-hospital mortality rate and a 19% 2-year survival rate. Thus, understanding why patients with type 2 diabetes are at increased risk of CIN and controlling factors to decrease the risk of CIN, has major short- and long-term benefits to patients with type 2 diabetes (Nikolsky et al., 2004). Most clinical studies on CIN have mainly been in patients with type 2 diabetes mellitus rather than type 1 diabetes mellitus and, thus, the remarks in this chapter will be confined to patients with type 2 diabetes kidney disease.

2.1 Mechanisms of contrast-induced nephropathy in patients with type 2 diabetes mellitus

The pathogenesis of CIN is complex with a cascade of contributing factors that are not fully understood. Factors contributing to CIN in patients with type 2 diabetes mellitus include decreased GFR, endothelial dysfunction and increased reactivity to intrarenal adenosine (Pfueger et al., 2000). After injection of contrast medium, renal blood flow increases transiently, followed by a more prolonged decrease, particularly at the corticomedullary junction of the kidney. The outer medulla is particularly susceptible to ischemic injury because of its high metabolic activity and low prevailing oxygen tension. Associated with the decrease in renal blood flow, there is a decrease in glomerular filtration rate due to afferent renal arteriolar vasoconstriction which is calcium-dependent with increased intrarenal adenosine and increased endothelin-1 activity as likely mediators of the vasoconstriction (Arakawa et al., 1996). The risk of CIN increases if there are inadequate compensatory vasodilatory responses, such as prostaglandins (E2 and I2) and nitric oxide.

Renal tubular cellular injury, in part, is mediated by generation of oxygen-free radicals. Intrarenal adenosine accumulates due to the depletion of adenosine triphosphate as a consequence of proximal tubular stress due to osmotic load and the large size of contrast media molecules. The renal toxicity from the direct effects of contrast media is reversible. It has been shown *in vitro* that renal tubular cells respond to contrast media exposure by increasing the concentrations of extracellular adenosine and by decreasing the activity of mitochondrial enzymes without altering viability. A late effect of intrarenal adenosine is oxygen-free radical production due to the catabolism of intrarenal adenosine to xanthine.

A role for intrarenal adenosine as a renal vasoconstrictor and substrate for oxygen-free radical formation is supported in human studies. Adenosine increases in urine following contrast medium; the magnitude of adenosine release and depression of creatinine clearance is proportional to the osmolality of the contrast agent, essentially a dose response relationship. Further, an inhibitor of adenosine uptake, dipyridamole, exacerbates the fall in GFR after contrast medium. In addition, blockade of the renal arterial adenosine receptors with theophylline attenuates the fall in GFR following contrast medium. Finally, following pretreatment with allopurinol (a xanthine oxidase inhibitor), urinary xanthine increases and the fall in GFR after contrast medium is lessened.

Endothelin is a potent renal afferent arteriolar vasoconstrictor, like intrarenal adenosine. Intravascular administration of contrast medium induces exacerbated release of urinary endothelin in patients with impaired renal function. Human studies show no significant increase in plasma endothelin levels until a volume of contrast media administered is greater than 150 mL (Clark et al., 1997). However, in diabetic patients or in patients with renal insufficiency, significant endothelin levels are detected when less than 100 mL of contrast medium are administered intraarterially.

In patients with normal GFR, the risk of CIN is likely less, not only because of more rapid clearance of contrast medium from the kidney (less time for generation of oxygen-free radicals), but, presumably, because of the presence of a variety of endogenous vasodilators that protect against renal ischemia, including prostaglandins (E2 and I2), atrial natriuretic peptide and nitric oxide. In patients with GFR of less than 60 mL/min/1.73 m2, the risk of CIN increases with prolonged clearance of contrast medium.

In summary, patients with type 2 diabetes mellitus appear to be at increased risk of CIN, not only because chronic renal disease is common in these patients, but also because there appears to be a greater vasoconstriction of the renal afferent arterioles to intrarenal adenosine and suppressed nitric oxide bioavailability in the kidney due to endothelial dysfunction (Komers & Anderson, 2003). Recent reports indicate that severe renal dysfunction need not be present to create a risk of CIN in diabetic patients with measured creatinine clearance of 100 mL/min and receiving proper hydration (Hardiek et al., 2008).

2.1.1 Prevention strategies to attenuate contrast-induced nephropathy in patients with type 2 diabetes mellitus and coronary artery disease

Since treatment of CIN after it has occurred is ineffective, efforts to prevent or attenuate the injury are the focus of ongoing investigations. Early diagnosis and careful long-term treatment of patients with type 2 diabetes mellitus and coronary artery disease includes 81 mg aspirin daily, angiotensin-converting enzyme inhibitor therapy or angiotensin II receptor blocker therapy and 3-hydroxyl-methylglutaryal coenzyme A reductase inhibitor therapy. Ideal goals for vascular risk factor modification include blood pressure of 130/80 mmHg or better, LDL cholesterol less than 70 mg/dL and hemoglobin A1C less than 7%. Successful accomplishment of these goals should decrease the progression of macro- and microvascular complications. In addition, if these goals are accomplished, endothelial function should be better. If the patient suddenly develops an acute coronary syndrome, the ability of the kidney to have a compensatory vasodilatory response in response to contrast medium should decrease the risk of CIN. Based on the assumption that acute renal adenosine and/or endothelia-medicated vasoconstriction and endothelial dysfunction are major interrelated pathogenic events in CIN, a type 2 diabetic patient meeting therapeutic goals should be at lower risk when coronary angiography and/or coronary intervention are required. When a patient with type 2 diabetes presents with an acute coronary syndrome, hyperglycemia is common, and increased risk of mortality in patients has been observed (Kosiborod & McGuire, 2010). Well-designed, large clinical outcome trials are required for better guidance as far as how hyperglycemia in the acute situation should be managed. Observational studies suggest that hypoglycemia should be avoided (Zoungas et al., 2010). Guidelines now recommend a therapeutic target of glucose control at 140 to 180 mg/dL in the critically ill patient which is a more liberal approach than prior recommendations (O'Keefe et al., 2011). Previously recommended more aggressive glucose lowering (including normalization of blood sugar) was not shown to have additional benefit and appeared to be harmful because of the increased incidence of hypoglycemia.

As mechanisms for CIN in patients with type 2 diabetes mellitus are better understood, there is a growing list of medications that may exacerbate the risk of CIN. Many of these medications are taken by patients with cardiovascular disease and should be addressed prior to proceeding with angiography. Medications that increase the risk of a patient developing CIN include nonsteroidal anti-inflammatory drugs which inhibit compensatory renal prostaglandin synthesis, diuretics that dehydrate the kidney and increase the risk of

medullary ischemia, and dipyridamole that blocks the normal cellular uptake of adenosine resulting in a greater renal adenosine – mediated vasconstrictive response.
In patients with type 2 diabetes mellitus requiring elective angiography, nonsteroidal anti-inflammatory medicines, diuretics and dipyridamole should be held prior to the procedure. While nonsteroidal anti-inflammatory medications are considered the cornerstone for managing the pain of osteoarthritis and other painful conditions, recent meta-analysis indicate significantly increased risk of myocardial infarction, stroke or death from cardiovascular disease compared to placebo with the chronic use of these medications. Contrary to some previous reports, the current meta-analysis found no suggestion that this increased cardiovascular risk is specific to cyclo-oxygenase-2 inhibitors. Data were available for naproxen, ibuprofen, diclofenac, celecoxib, etoricoxib, rofecoxib and lumiracoxib. Overall, naproxen appeared to be the least harmful nonsteroidal anti-inflammatory medication in terms of cardiovascular outcomes. Risks were greatest with ibuprofen, diclofenac, etoricoxib and lumiracoxib. Thus, chronic use of nonsteroidal anti-inflammatory medications in patients with type 2 diabetes who are at increased cardiovascular risk is discouraged. In regard to dipyridamole, recent data suggests superiority of clopidogrel over dipyridamole in patients who have suffered a cerebral vascular accident. Increasingly clopidogrel rather than dipyridamole is the recommended antiplatelet agent in addition to 81 mg aspirin in patients with type 2 diabetes after transient ischemic attacks or cerebral vascular accidents. Thus, if the patient with type 2 diabetes mellitus needs emergency angiography, the risk of dipyridamole contributing to CIN would no longer exist.
Patients with type 2 diabetes mellitus have a significantly greater risk of macrovascular disease, including coronary heart disease, stroke and peripheral vascular disease, in addition to the microvascular complications, such as retinopathy, neuropathy and nephropathy. Despite evidence of benefit for reduction of microvascular disease with glycemic control, to date, there is no such evidence for the role of glycemic control in macrovascular event reduction. In newly diagnosed patients with type 2 diabetes, besides initiation of diet, exercise and weight reduction, metformin is usually the recommended initial therapy unless contraindicated, such as renal disease (serum creatinine greater than 1.5 mg/dL in males and greater than 1.4 mg/dL in females). Although not relevant to CIN prevention, metformin should be temporarily discontinued at the time of or prior to use of contrast medium or major surgical procedures and withheld for 48 hours after the procedure. Metformin should be restarted after renal function has been reevaluated and found to be normal (Goergen et al., 2010). While the mortality rate for patients who develop lactic acidosis can be quite high, the actual number of people dying from metformin-induced lactic acidosis after contrast medium exposure is quite low using these guidelines.
Cigarette smoking is the most common cause of preventable morbidity and mortality in developed countries. In addition to it being a major risk factor for cardiovascular disease, lung disease and cancer, cigarette smoking is now recognized as an important independent risk factor of chronic kidney disease, including diabetic nephropathy, by increasing the rate of transition from microalbuminuria to proteinuria and promoting the progression to end-stage renal disease (Phisitkul et al., 2008). Furthermore, a recent cross-sectional analysis of participants in the National Health and Nutrition Examination Survey demonstrated a strong association between exposure to secondhand smoke and proteinuria, suggesting that passive smokers are also at increased risk of chronic kidney disease (Obert et al., 2011). Several clinical and experimental studies have demonstrated the role of transforming growth factor-beta in the pathogenesis of chronic kidney disease, including diabetic

nephropathy. This cytokine is largely profibrotic and plays a significant role in diabetic nephropathy by increasing the production of extracellular matrix proteins, including fibronectin and collagen, in the glomerulus. It is also known that one cigarette paralyzes the ability of the endothelium to make nitric oxide for up to 24 hours. Thus, patients with type 2 diabetes mellitus should be counseled to discontinue smoking. Emphasizing that recommendation prior to elective angiography may decrease the incidence of CIN.

Another class of medication that warrants discussion in the long-term treatment of patients with type 2 diabetes mellitus, not only for the long-term metabolic advantages, but also because of the risk of CIN is beta-blocker therapy. Both nonselective and selective traditional beta-blockers have been shown to increase insulin resistance, facilitate weight gain of approximately 1 kilogram per six months and worsen hypertriglyceridemia by approximately 13%. In contrast, carvedilol in hypertensive diabetic patients has been found to have a neutral effect on insulin resistance, weight and triglycerides (Bakris et al., 2004). This favorable metabolic profile also suggests that carvedilol is a better choice compared to traditional beta-blockers in these high risk patients. Recent trials emphasize the class heterogeneity that exists for beta-blockers and provide a strong basis for preferred use of carvedilol in patients with type 2 diabetes. Carvedilol is a unique molecule that combines the properties of a nonspecific beta-blocker and a specific alpha-1-blocker in a ratio of 2:3. Carvedilol also possesses antioxidant properties. In hypertensive diabetic patients, carvedilol compared to metoprolol tartrate has been shown to reduce existing microalbuminuria and to decrease the risk of progression to microalbuminuria. These results suggest improved endothelial function and may be related to improvement in insulin resistance or an effect on oxidant stress in the kidney. Thus, in patients with type 2 diabetes mellitus that require beta-blocker therapy, carvedilol has become the recommended beta-blocker. There are also data to suggest that carvedilol compared to traditional beta-blockers attenuates CIN. Proposed mechanisms include unopposed alpha-medicated renal vasoconctriction causing more ischemia when on traditional beta-blockers and/or improved endothelial function due to the antioxidant properties of carvedilol.

There are other medicines that may attenuate the risk of CIN. Calcium-channel blocking medications attenuate both the magnitude and duration of renal vasoconstriction after contrast medium administration (Russo et al., 1990). In patients with type 2 diabetes mellitus and hypertension and/or angina requiring calcium-channel blocking medications, these medications should be continued if contrast medium administration is planned.

The adenosine receptor antagonists, theophylline and aminophylline, attenuate the decrease in GFR seen after contrast medium. Since patients with type 2 diabetes mellitus have an increased reactivity to intrarenal adenosine, theophylline prior to contrast medium administration warrants special consideration. The kidney responds to contrast media-induced stress with a tubuloglomercular feedback response which is largely medicated by adenosine when less than 100 mL of contrast medium is administered. This mechanism has been confirmed by both animal and clinical studies. Pretreatment with long-acting theophylline 3 mg/kg orally at least 30 minutes before contrast medium administration and 12 hours later in addition to hydration has been shown to attenuate the depression of creatinine clearance. It is critical that theophylline be administered before contrast medium injection, but prolonged treatment after angiography is unnecessary. Theophylline prophylaxis is effective, safe, and inexpensive. This dose of theophylline is manyfold greater than the minimum dose required to block renal vascular adenosine receptors and is well below that shown to affect renal cyclic nucleotide phosphodiesterase activity (Vassallo &

Lipsky, 1998). This dose of theophylline causes transient plasma theophylline levels of 7 mcg/mL which is below therapeutic levels required for treatment of asthma and unlikely to cause serious gastrointestinal, neurological, or cardiovascular adverse effects (Cooling, 1993; Shannon, 1999).

Adenosine receptor antagonists, theophylline and aminophylline, prophylaxis to attenuate CIN has not been strongly adopted except in patients at high risk for CIN. Some controlled trials have shown a significant reduction in the risk for CIN while others have shown no reduction (Abizaid et al., 1999; Erley et al., 1999; Erley et al., 1994; Gandhi et al., 1992; Huber et al., 2001; Huber et al., 2002; Huber et al., 2003; Kolonko et al., 1998; Shammas et al., 2001). However, these studies have been limited by small sample size, variation in timing and dosage of drug administration, and variation in the definition of CIN. Three meta-analyses have dealt specifically with the clinical use of theophylline for the prevention of CIN. Each of these gave extensive information concerning the way that the papers which were included were chosen, exactly what factors were chosen for matching across studies and which factors did not match. In addition, statistics were presented which addressed the concerns about selection bias and efforts were made to adjust for non-matching factors to the extent possible. No attempt will be made to describe each of these studies completely, however, we will give some summary information concerning each of them. One meta-analysis identified 10 studies in which theophylline was used for the prevention of CIN (Ix et al., 2004). Of the ten, seven were found to fulfill all the inclusion criteria and these constituted the final sample for the analysis. The studies included were reported between 1994 and 2003 and included a number of different protocols for the administration of the theophylline. The final conclusion reached by these investigators was that the prophylactic administration of theophylline appears to protect against contrast-induced declines in kidney function. They also reported that "the protective benefits appeared robust regardless of the study design, form or volume of contrast medium delivered, and the presence or absence of intravenous volume expansion." The investigators did indicate that they were unable to determine (given the available data) if theophylline reduced the number of patients who experienced large increases in serum creatinine concentrations or required dialysis. Another meta-analysis identified nine studies which met the study criteria for their protocol (Bagshaw & Ghali, 2005). Their conclusion was that the data they considered indicated that there is promising evidence supporting the use of theophylline for the prevention of CIN but the evidence is still not conclusive. They suggested that what was required to answer this question was a larger, well designed clinical trial for confirmation and assessment of risks before theophylline could be recommended routinely for the prevention of CIN. They also noted from their analysis of these papers that such a trial should include a hydration protocol and the routine use of low or iso-osmolar nonionic contrast media since those are now the current standards of care. These two meta-analyses focused primarily on theophylline and a comparison of the choices of papers from the two studies shows that seven papers included in the initial meta-analysis were also included in the nine chosen by the second meta-analysis. The latter authors included two papers which were in the same search time frame as the initial meta-analysis but were not selected under that study protocol. A third meta-analysis covered a number of drugs aimed at reducing the incidence of CIN (Kelly et al., 2008). The primary drug considered was N-acetylcysteine with theophylline being more secondary to the study. Only six of the studies considered dealt primarily with theophylline. Of the six considered, five were part of the set of studies considered by the second meta-analysis while four of them coincided with those used in the initial meta-analysis. The sixth paper which was unique to this analysis appeared in 2006 which was out of the range of years covered by the other two papers. One of the six papers common to both was not included by the initial meta-analysis. The conclusion of this paper with respect to the efficacy of theophylline was that it produced a large risk reduction but did not achieve statistical significance. Of these three meta-analyses, the first two are most comparable. Both reach the same conclusion. Each of these papers used slightly different statistical methods. Both contained a thorough discussion of the selection criteria used to choose the papers included and measures to check for selection bias. The general conclusions were favorable with the hypothesis that theophylline is protective against CIN. Unfortunately, neither group of authors was willing to report a definitive answer. There are some areas where the studies under review by these authors differed. One was in the area of how the theophylline was administered: as a fixed dose regardless of body weight or as a dose adjusted per kilogram of body weight. The broad conclusion reached is that a large, carefully designed clinical trial needs to be conducted to reach a final conclusion. The trial should be stratified according to ancillary risk factors such as age and diabetes. In addition, the effect of the dosing protocol and hydration methods needs to be considered. Finally, since it is known that certain beverages like coffee and tea also block adenosine vascular receptors, a study testing the benefit of theophylline should exclude other xanthine exposure during the time before contrast medium administration and for the 48 hours after while the subject is being followed.

Studies suggest two mechanisms by which intrarenal adenosine contributes to CIN. Early depression of renal function after contrast medium exposure is caused by A_1 receptor-mediated renal afferent arteriolar vasoconstriction and A_2 receptor-mediated efferent arteriolar vasodilatation resulting in decreased glomerular perfusion pressure. Later depression of renal function after contrast medium exposure is caused by oxygen-free radical production, in part, due to intrarenal adenosine catabolism to xanthine. Pretreatment with theophylline may attenuate CIN by maintaining GFR such that contrast medium is cleared from the kidney more rapidly, thus, decreasing direct cytotoxic effects from contrast medium and decreasing the potential for intrarenal adenosine-mediated oxygen-free radical production. Pretreatment with allopurinol has also been shown to attenuate CIN. To be effective, it is crucial to administer allopurinol at least 24 hours prior to exposure to contrast medium. Pretreatment allows time for production of oxypurinol, the chief metabolite of allopurinol, which is a much more potent xanthine oxidase inhibitor. Allopurinol administered in this fashion was renally protective. Decreasing renal xanthine oxidase decreases the catabolism of intrarenal adenosine to xanthine resulting in decreased oxygen-free radical production and less renal tubular cell injury.

Patients with type 2 diabetes mellitus are usually on angiotensin-converting enzyme inhibitors, angiotensin II receptor blockers and/or direct renin inhibitor to decrease the progression of renal disease. Whether these agents need to be held or should be continued when contrast medium is administered requires clinical judgment. Intrarenal angiotensin II enhances adenosine-mediated vasoconstriction so theoretically blockade of the renin-angiotensin system should attenuate the risk of CIN. In support of this concept, preprocedure angiotensin-converting enzyme inhibitor use has been shown to lower the risk for CIN in patients with chronic renal disease (Dangas et al., 2005). Another clinical trial showed that periprocedural captopril, compared with an untreated control group, reduced the risk of CIN in patients with type 2 diabetes mellitus (Gupta et al, 1999). However, if an unstable patient has low cardiac output or hypotension, renin-angiotensin system blockade is known to worsen glomerular perfusion (i.e. intrarenal angiotensin II is needed). In such patients, angiotensin-converting inhibitor therapy has increased the risk of CIN (Cirit et al., 2006; Holscher et al., 2008; Louis et al., 1996; Rosenstock et al., 2008). Given the long-term benefit of angiotensin-converting enzyme inhibitor and angiotensin II receptor antagonists, most believe these medications should be continued in patients with diabetes mellitus and chronic kidney disease requiring contrast medium administration unless the patient is hemodynamically unstable. However, if angiotensin-converting enzyme inhibitors or angiotensin II receptor blockers are held before contrast medium administration, they should be restarted when renal function is considered stable.

Recent research suggests that 3-hydroxy-methylglutaryl coenzyme A reductase inhibitors, or statins, may reduce the risk of CIN because they have beneficial effects on endothelial function, maintain nitric oxide production and reduce oxidative stress (Adel et al., 2010). Recent retrospective reviews of patients with renal impairment undergoing angiography suggests that the risk of CIN was lower in patients in whom a statin was initiated before the procedure (Khanal et al., 2005). These findings reinforce the rationale for the introduction of statin therapy before undergoing diagnostic or interventional coronary angiography, particularly in patients with type 2 diabetes mellitus (Attallah et al., 2004).

Hypomagnesemia, serum magnesium level less than 2 mEq/L, may also be a correctable risk factor for CIN in patients with renal dysfunction. Patients with type 2 diabetes mellitus frequently become hypomagnesemic due to poor control with glycosuria, the development of an acquired renal tubular defect and from chronic diuretic therapy. All three conditions decrease the renal tubular reabsorption of magnesium. Detecting hypomagnesemia and correcting it prior to angiography or coronary intervention may be indicated. The renal protective effect of magnesium is likely multifactorial. Besides its role as an antioxidant and as a coenzyme for compensatory sodium-potassium adenosine triphosphatase, magnesium has calcium channel blocking properties.

The universally accepted prevention strategy for CIN is adequate intravenous volume expansion. Extracellular volume expansion plays a well established role in reducing the risk of CIN although few trials have directly addressed the ideal protocol. Intravenous volume expansion before and after the administration of contrast medium appears to be more effective than either bolus volume expansion during the procedure or removal of restrictions on oral fluid intake. Isotonic saline has been found to be better than 0.45% saline and is given intravenously before and after administration of contrast medium for a total of 24 hours. An additional strategy that is under study is for patients to receive prophylactic volume expansion with isotonic sodium bicarbonate solution (Merten et al., 2004). It is thought that an alkaline environment decreases oxygen-free radical formation in the renal tubule. The findings of several recent trials and a meta-analysis indicate that volume expansion with sodium bicarbonate is more effective than volume expansion with saline. However, recent reports argue against a clear benefit for sodium bicarbonate volume expansion but examination of the various trials suggests that the dose given to accomplish an alkaline environment in the renal tubule is important. Isotonic sodium bicarbonate solution, administered at 3 mL/kg/h for one hour prior to angiography and at 1 mL/kg/h for, at least, six hours afterward accomplishes that goal. A major robust, well-designed trial comparing volume expansion with sodium bicarbonate versus normal saline is ongoing. At this time, the CIN consensus working panel concludes that no adjunctive medical pretreatment has been validated as effective for preventing CIN. Use of furosemide, mannitol or an endothelin receptor antagonist is potentially detrimental. Felodipine, dopamine, atrial natriuretic peptide and L-arginine have not been shown to be effective. Potentially beneficial strategies for attenuating CIN include theophylline, allopurinol, ascorbic acid, oral and intravenous N-acetylcysteine, hemodialysis of contrast medium and venous capture of contrast medium.

In regard to pretreatment approaches to limit oxygen-free radical injury following contrast medium, four pharmacologic approaches warrant further study with adequately powered, appropriately designed, randomized trials of high-risk diabetic patients, perhaps combined with theophylline pretreatment. One of these is isotonic sodium bicarbonate solution with the length of post-procedure treatment determined by the volume of contrast medium administered. Maintaining an alkaline environment should decrease oxygen-free radical formation in the renal tubule. As discussed above, one source of oxygen-free radical production after contrast medium is the catabolism of intrarenal adenosine to xanthine. Allopurinol, a xanthine oxidase inhibitor, 4 mg/kg orally daily starting 24 hours before administration of contrast medium has shown benefit. This dose of allopurinol, if given 24 hours before elective procedures, is metabolized into oxypurinol which is a more effective xanthine oxidase inhibitor than allopurinol. This 24-hour pretreatment approach has been shown to attenuate the fall in GFR after contrast medium exposure. Besides limiting oxygen-free radical formation, allopurinol may also protect the kidney from contrast medium exposure by its ability to inhibit adenine nucleotide degradation (thus, preservation of adenine nucleotide is required for recovery from renal injury). Allopurinol has also been found to markedly decrease the vasodilatation response to intravenous adenosine in the renal vasculature. Less adenosine-mediated efferent renal arteriolar vasodilatation would preserve glomerular perfusion pressure. In view of the possible role of oxidase stress and oxygen-free radical generation in CIN, ascorbic acid as an antioxidant warrants further study (Spargias et al., 2004). N-acetylcysteine, as an antioxidant and renal vasodilator, has not been shown to be consistently effective when given orally (Solomon, 2009). Perhaps a larger oral dose is needed or intravenous administration may be required. Allopurinol, ascorbic acid and N-acetylcysteine, if proven beneficial, require pretreatment and would be less helpful in diabetic patients requiring emergency diagnostic and/or interventional contrast medium usage.

To decrease the risk of CIN requires careful patient screening and selection, adequate patient hydration, limiting the volume of contrast medium administered and choosing a safe, non-ionic, low osmolar contrast agent. Based on comparisons of contrast media in proximal renal tubular cell culture and in recent robust head-to-head prospective clinical trials in high risk patients, however, iso-osmolar iodixanol and low-osmolar iopamidol are comparable and appear to be the contrast agents of choice to reduce renal risk for CIN.

The direct cellular toxicities of commonly used contrast medium have been compared in renal proximal tubular cells in culture (Hardiek et al., 2001). All contrast media, whether high-osmolar or iso-osmolar, ionic or non-ionic, stress renal proximal tubular cells. When renal proximal tubular cells in culture are exposed to contrast media, they respond by increasing extracellular adenosine concentrations because of the depletion of adenosine triphosphate due to osmotic load and the large size of contrast medium molecules. The renal toxicity from the direct effects of contrast medium is reversible, as has been shown *in vitro* in studies in which renal tubular cells respond to contrast media exposure by decreasing the activity of mitochondrial enzymes without altering viability. While all contrast medium may reduce mitochondrial enzyme activity, differences among agents are seen with iopamidol and iodixanol being the least toxic and the two ionic contrast media, ioxaglate and diatrizoate, being the most toxic. The lesser the depression of mitochondrial function, the more rapidly renal proximal tubular cells can recover after contrast medium has been eliminated from the kidney suggesting that iopamidol and iodixanol are the least nephrotoxic molecules when studied in cell culture.

Earlier clinical trials comparing contrast medium risk in patients with type 2 diabetes for CIN had limitations that prevented valid conclusions: the studies were not blinded, the number of patients was small, the timing of outcome assessment was unclear, or the patients received contrast intra-arterially and/or intravenously. With proper hydration and identification of high-risk patients, the incidence of CIN after intra-arterial contrast medium administration is about 10%. More recent trials in high-risk diabetic patients given contrast medium intravenously suggest that the incidence of CIN is about 5%. More recent trials have been head-to-head, robust and prospective in high-risk patients with chronic renal failure (eGFR 59-20 mL/min) with intra-arterial contrast medium administration. Based on animal studies, concern about osmotoxicity in the pathogenesis of CIN emerged which led to the development of low-osmolar, and, later, iso-osmolar contrast medium. Of interest, in human prospective trials and meta-analysis, no specifically significant differences in nephrotoxicity between high-osmolar (1,400-2,000 mOsm/kg) and non-ionic low-osmolar (600-800 mOsm/kg) contrast have been found in patients with normal renal function (Solomon, 2005). Clinical trials published in the 1990s, however, showed that use of high-osmolar ionic monomer diatrizoate in patients with chronic renal disease who were undergoing coronary angiography had a higher incidence of CIN than that associated with non-ionic low-osmolar contrast medium. In general, lower osmolar contrast medium has now replaced diatrizoate for routine clinical use. It is less clear whether there are appreciable differences among various non-ionic low-osmolar contrast medium regarding the incidence of CIN. Because individual contrast medium has specific effects on renal tubular cells, head-to-head studies are required to compare the safer contrast medium in at risk patients undergoing angiography. With the development of the non-ionic iso-osmolar dimer, iodixanol, subsequent studies have evaluated whether a further reduction in osmolality would result in still more protection against CIN. In the first of these comparative studies ((Nephrotoxicity of High-Risk Patient Study of Iso-osmolar and Low-Osmolar Non-ionic Contrast Medium (NEPHRIC)) 129 patients with diabetes with chronic renal failure (baseline eGFR of 48 mL/min) and serum creatinine levels 1.5-3.5 mg/dL were randomized to the low-osmolar contrast medium iohexol or the iso-osmolar contrast medium, iodixanol (Aspelin et al., 2003). A higher rate of CIN defined as a serum creatinine rise of greater than 0.5 mg/dL after angiography was noted after iohexol (26.2%) than after iodixanol (3.1%).

Since the publication of NEPHRIC, subsequent prospective randomized trials involving high-risk patients with renal insufficiency and diabetes and the intra-arterial administration of contrast medium have not consistently found a lower incidence of CIN associated with iso-osmolar contrast medium. In general, a benefit favoring the non-ionic iso-osmolar dimer, iodixanol, is seen compared with the non-ionic low-osmolar monomer iohexol or the ionic low-osmolar dimer, ioxaglate. In contrast, when comparing non-ionic low-osmolar monomers, iopamidol or ioversol, in high-risk patients with iso-osmolar iodixanol, no additional protective effect is seen. There have been no head-to-head comparisons of iohexol with any other non-ionic, low-osmolar contrast agents in high-risk patients undergoing intra-arterial administration of contrast. Based on a recent systematic review of angiographic contrast medium in high-risk patients, however, the likely explanation of the

NEPHRIC findings is that low-osmolar, iohexol, appears to be more nephrotoxic than other low-osmolar contrast media, such as iopamidol and ioversol. Furthermore, a systematic review of angiographic contrast media in high-risk patients found no statistically significant difference in the risk of CIN between low-osmolar iopamidol and iso-osmolar iodixanol (Solomon, 2005). These comparisons in low-osmolar and iso-osmolar contrast medium administered intra-arterially in high-risk patients suggest that each molecule's safety must be based on robust clinical trials. These data also suggest that physical and/or chemical properties of each molecule, other than osmolarity, are implicated in the pathogenesis of CIN. Given this incidence of CIN, prospective randomized trials need larger patient populations to be properly powered to be certain of the conclusions. The recently published Cardiac Angiography in Renally-Impaired Patients (CARE) study fits these criteria by being a multicenter, double-blind, randomized study designed to prospectively compare the incidence of CIN after intra-arterial administration of low-osmolar iopamidol or iso-osmolar iodixanol in 414 patients with moderate to severe chronic kidney disease (eGFR of 20-59 mL/min/1.73 m^2) who underwent coronary angiography or percutaneous coronary intervention (Solomon et al., 2007). All patients received intravenous sodium bicarbonate prophylaxis. The primary endpoint was a post-dose serum creatinine increase of greater than 0.5 mL/dL over baseline. The renal effects of these two agents were comparable with no significant difference in occurrence of CIN and no significant difference in occurrence of CIN in the subgroup of chronic kidney disease patients with diabetes. More recently, a multicenter, randomized double-blind trial comparing the renal effects of non-ionic, iso-osmolar iodixanol versus non-ionic, low-osmolar iopamidol in 526 patients with impaired baseline renal function and diabetes undergoing diagnostic and/or therapeutic coronary angiography procedures was completed (Laskey et al., 2009). This trial showed overall rate of CIN in patients with chronic kidney disease and diabetes undergoing coronary angiographic procedures was 10.5%. There was no significant difference between iodixanol and iopamidol in either peak increase in serum creatinine or risk of CIN.

The renal effects of iodixanol and iopamidol are comparable in high-risk diabetic patients requiring contrast medium for diagnostic studies or intervention. The non-renal differences between these contrast agents should be considered when selecting an agent and when obtaining informed patient consent, however. Using a contrast medium with a higher iodine concentration per milliliter, such as iopamidol which has 370 mg/mL compared to iodixanol which has 320 mg/mL iodine content, may allow for a smaller volume to be used intravenously without sacrificing image quality. The higher iodine concentration of iopamidol may make complex plaques easier to appreciate during coronary angiography and intervention. Other considerations are that iodixanol is threefold more likely to cause contrast-induced delayed skin reactions compared to iopamidol. After percutaneous coronary intervention with bare-metal or drug-eluting stent placement, cardiac patients require antiplatelet therapy with clopidogrel, which may cause a rash within 5 to 7 days of treatment initiation, a timeline similar to that for delayed contrast-induced skin reactions. In clinical trials with clopidogrel, skin reactions are noted in 4.2% of patients. The choice of a contrast molecule, such as iopamidol, that is less likely to cause a delayed contrast-induced skin reaction makes decisions regarding the discontinuation of clopidogrel less frequent and more definitive. Finally, iopamidol is less expensive than iodixanol.

Gadolinium-based contrast agents were introduced, partly, because of the discovery that iodine-based contrast medium could cause CIN. However, recent reports suggest that gadolinium-based agents may also be nephrotoxic. Furthermore, after exposure to gadolinium-based contrast, some patients with renal insufficiency have developed nephrogenic systemic sclerosis with scleroderma-like changes in the skin, connective tissues and other organs, which has sometimes been fatal (Grobner & Prischl, 2007). In diabetic patients with chronic renal failure, the use of any contrast agent should be avoided, if possible, but, if required, small volumes of a contrast agent, such as iodixanol or iopamidol with proper hydration appears to be the safest clinical management to reduce renal and long-term patient risk.

Ongoing investigation is searching for even more sensitive markers that may predict the development of CIN after percutaneous coronary interventions in patients with normal serum creatinine values (Kato et al., 2008). Future studies should include cystatin C which is an alternative serum measurement of kidney function that approximates direct measures of GFR more precisely than creatinine because its serum concentrations are independent of muscle mass and do not appear to be affected by age or sex. Cystatin C may identify a preclinical risk of kidney dysfunction after contrast medium that is not detected by serum creatinine or eGFR (Perkins et al., 2005). More recently, the value of neutrophil gelatinase-associated lipocalin (NGAL) has been highlighted as a novel biomarker for the early detection of acute renal failure (Ling et al., 2008). NGAL, a member of the lipocalin family, was originally isolated from the supernatant of activated human neutrophils, but it is also expressed at a low level in human tissues, including the kidney. Because of its small molecular size and resistance to degradation, NGAL is readily excreted and detected in urine. Thus, NGAL is highly accumulated in human kidney cortical tubules, blood and urine after renal injuries. NGAL might represent an early, sensitive and noninvasive urinary marker for the detection of CIN. Initial studies of NGAL after percutaneous coronary intervention showed an earlier increase in serum than in urine probably because NGAL was released into the circulation secondary to inflammatory activation of neutrophils initiated by percutaneous coronary intervention. Moreover, since NGAL is increased in atherosclerotic plaques, it might also be released in the circulation during the PCI. It has been found that predictors of serum NGAL 2 hours after PCI were serum creatinine, cystatin C, length of the percutaneous coronary intervention and the presence of diabetes. These findings have important implications for the clinical management of diabetic patients undergoing PCI. Since patients after PCI are often discharged the next day and CIN often occurs subsequent to discharge, NGAL needs to be investigated as a potential early marker for nephrotoxicity. Further studies in type 2 diabetes mellitus patients with chronic renal failure undergoing contrast medium administration are warranted to assess the use of NGAL with respect to earlier detection of CIN so that patients can be advised properly and medicines, such as metformin and angiotensin-converting enzyme inhibitors or angiotensin II receptor blockers, can be restarted appropriately.

In patients undergoing cardiac catheterization, cystatin C may be useful in predicting before catheterization the risk of CIN. In contrast, urinary human liver-type fatty acid-binding protein (L-FABP) consistently appears to be the only marker for detecting transient renal tubular damage in patients with moderate renal disease. Thus, urinary L-FABP appears to be a useful marker of renal tubular damage caused by contrast medium. Other investigators have found that urinary intraleukin-18 (IL-18) is associated with the later cardiac outcomes in patients with CIN after coronary angiography. CIN, a form of acute kidney injury, has received increasing attention the past few years because of the recognition that CIN is associated with long-term adverse events. The increased incidence of adverse events after CIN is derived primarily from retrospective analysis of large data bases or observational studies of patients who have undergone coronary angiography and/or percutaneous coronary intervention. A cause-and-effect relationship cannot be determined from such data. Patients with an increased burden of cardiovascular risk factors before contrast medium exposure may be more likely to develop CIN and independent of the occurrence of CIN may have more long-term adverse events (Shlipak et al., 2005). Alternatively, the occurrence of CIN may in some as yet undefined manner alter the future likelihood of adverse events (i.e., CIN triggers a pathophysiologic pathway that leads to adverse events). The Cardiac Angiography in REnally-impaired patients (CARE) study has allowed the opportunity to explore the association of CIN with long-term adverse events (Solomon et al., 2009). Patients were followed for the year after the trial, and adverse events were collected. The rate of long-term adverse events was higher in individuals who developed CIN. After adjustment for baseline comorbidities and risk factors, the adjusted incident ratio for adverse events was twice as high in those with CIN compared to the patients who did not develop CIN. It is also noted that randomization to iopamidol reduced the incidence of CIN and adverse events compared to iodixanol. Parallel decrease of incidence of CIN and adverse events in the iopamidol arm of this randomized trial supports a causal role for CIN in late adverse events in diabetic patients undergoing coronary angiography and/or coronary intervention. Why a transient decrease in renal function results in long-term increased risk of cerebrovascular accident, myocardial infarction and death is an area of intense study. Some investigators report that traditional cardiovascular risk factors have greater associations with cardiovascular mortality than novel risk factors. Thus, in patients that develop CIN, continued treatment of hypertension, hyperlipidemia and diabetes is recommended. Since multiple studies have demonstrated the important role of nitric oxide in endothelial physiology and the pathogenesis of vascular disease, ongoing studies are examining endogenous nitric oxide synthase inhibitors, such as the amino acid asymmetric dimethylarginine, in the pathogenesis of late adverse events (Chirinos et al., 2008). Additional studies are required to assess the prognostic value of measuring for this endogenous nitric oxide synthase inhibitor and assessing whether interventions limiting its effect will benefit patients at risk for future cardiovascular events.

2.1.1.1 Risks and benefits of prevention strategies to attenuate contrast-induced nephropathy in patients with type 2 diabetes mellitus and coronary artery disease

The risks of a short course of theophylline, either orally or intravenously, is low. If a patient is on theophylline, one cannot give adenosine as a coronary vasodilator as part of a flow wire analysis to assess the functional significance of a coronary stenotic lesion (Casella et al., 2003; Yoon et al., 2009). However, intravascular ultrasound can be used as the guide for functional significance, and, thus, pretreatment with theophylline to attenuate CIN may be more important than losing this one technique of assessing functional coronary stenosis. Of the various potential strategies for attenuating CIN, theophylline can be administered orally or intravenously within 30 minutes of the procedure and be beneficial. Antioxidant strategies, such as allopurinol, ascorbic acid, or N-acetylcysteine require pretreatment and will be less helpful in patients requiring emergency diagnostic and/or interventional contrast medium usage.

Volume expansion with normal saline or sodium bicarbonate is the universally agreed upon strategy to attenuate CIN. Bicarbonate therapy was initially explored because the generation of oxygen-free radicals is pH dependent through the Haber-Weiss reaction (Merten et al., 2004). Alkalinization of the urinary space is achieved very quickly with intravenous infusion of sodium bicarbonate because normally there is little bicarbonate in the urine. Even a small increase in serum bicarbonate of 1 to 2 mEq/L will result in the 'dumping' of bicarbonate into the urine in most patients (Solomon, 2009). Such a change in serum is easily obtained with the infusion rate recommended. Sodium bicarbonate therapy is readily available, inexpensive, and safe. The question is whether it is efficacious for prevention of CIN. Of particular clinical interest from recent meta-analysis was the finding that sodium bicarbonate therapy is most effective in patients who experienced urgent or emergency contrast medium exposure (Meier et al., 2009). Presumably this selects a group of patients who are less likely to receive any other form of prophylaxis for CIN. This is of great potential importance for the emergency room and cardiac catheterization laboratory. Sodium bicarbonate therapy was also most effective in those receiving low osmolality contrast media compared with iso-osmolality contrast media. Low osmolality contrast is increasingly chosen because of its safety, lower costs, and higher iodine content. It has also been found that the addition of N-acetylcysteine to fluid expansion with sodium bicarbonate showed no additional reduction in the rate of CIN after the intra-arterial administration of iopamidol or iodixanol to high-risk patients with type 2 diabetes mellitus and chronic kidney disease (Staniloae et al., 2009).

CIN needs to be redefined using markers of kidney injury that are sensitive, specific, and predictive of adverse outcomes (Solomon, 2009). This will enable investigators to better address the question of how to attenuate this condition in the future. The most important question to be answered is whether prevention of kidney injury results in a change in short- and long-term adverse outcomes. Using iopamidol has been associated with a reduction in long-term adverse events (Solomon et al., 2007). The recent meta-analyses found that despite a reduction in the incidence of CIN, sodium bicarbonate therapy had no benefit on the need for dialysis or mortality (Meier et al., 2009). No matter how available, inexpensive, and safe a potential preventive therapy, to find an important role in clinical therapeutics, it must improve the 'downstream' adverse outcomes, an as yet elusive goal for the prevention and treatment of CIN (Solomon, 2009).

3. Conclusions

In summary, CIN remains an important clinical challenge in patients with type 2 diabetes mellitus with coronary artery disease. Reducing the incidence of CIN requires recognizing high risk patients, such as patients with type 2 diabetes mellitus. Long-term risk factor modification should improve endothelial function so a more normal renal compensatory response will occur should contrast medium administration be required. Lowest volume of iopamidol needed would appear to be the contrast agent of choice. In patients with type 2 diabetes mellitus, pretreatment with theophylline to block adenosine-mediated renal vasoconstriction combined with volume expansion with sodium bicarbonate to limit oxygen-free radical generation is a rational approach based on existing data. Appropriately designed robust randomized clinical trials combining pharmacologic approaches aimed at both the renal vasoconstriction and the oxygen-free radical generation are needed to confirm that this is the best preventive strategy in patients with type 2 diabetes mellitus.

4. Acknowledgement

Special thanks to Marcey R. Ervin and Sandy Sledge for preparation of the manuscript.

5. References

Abizaid, A. S., C. E. Clark, G. S. Mintz, S. Dosa, J. J. Popma, A. D. Pichard, L. F. Satler, M. Harvey, K. M. Kent, & M. B. Leon. (1999). Effects of dopamine and aminophylline on contrast-induced acute renal failure after coronary angioplasty in patients with preexisting renal insufficiency. *American Journal of Cardiology* 83 (2):pp. ISSN 260-263, A265, 0002-9149.

Adel, A., Z. Abdel-Salam, & W. Nammas. (2010). Low-dose statin therapy improves endothelial function in type 2 diabetic patients with normal serum total cholesterol: a randomized placebo-controlled study. *J Clin Hypertens (Greenwich)* 12 (10):pp. 820-825, ISSN 1751-7176.

Arakawa, K., H. Suzuki, M. Naitoh, A. Matsumoto, K. Hayashi, H. Matsuda, A. Ichihara, E. Kubota, & T. Saruta. (1996). Role of adenosine in the renal responses to contrast medium. *Kidney International* 49 (5):pp. 1199-1206, ISSN 0085-2538.

Aspelin, P., P. Aubry, S. G. Fransson, R. Strasser, R. Willenbrock, & K. J. Berg. (2003). Nephrotoxic effects in high-risk patients undergoing angiography. *New England Journal of Medicine* 348 (6):pp. 491-499, ISSN 1533-4406.

Attallah, N., L. Yassine, J. Musial, J. Yee, & K. Fisher. (2004). The potential role of statins in contrast nephropathy. *Clinical Nephrology* 62 (4):pp. 273-278, ISSN 0301-0430

Bagshaw, S. M., & W. A. Ghali. (2005). Theophylline for prevention of contrast-induced nephropathy: a systematic review and meta-analysis. *Archives of Internal Medicine* 165 (10):pp. 1087-1093, ISSN 0003-9926.

Bakris, G. L., V. Fonseca, R. E. Katholi, J. B. McGill, F. H. Messerli, R. A. Phillips, P. Raskin, J. T. Wright, Jr., R. Oakes, M. A. Lukas, K. M. Anderson, & D. S. Bell. (2004). Metabolic effects of carvedilol vs metoprolol in patients with type 2 diabetes mellitus and hypertension: a randomized controlled trial. *JAMA* 292 (18):pp. 2227-2236, ISSN 1538-3598.

Casella, G., J. Rieber, T. M. Schiele, H. U. Stempfle, U. Siebert, M. Leibig, K. Theisen, U. Buchmeier, & V. Klauss. (2003). A randomized comparison of 4 doses of intracoronary adenosine in the assessment of fractional flow reserve. *Zeitschrift fur Kardiologie* 92 (8):pp. 627-632, ISSN 0300-5860.

Chirinos, J. A., R. David, J. A. Bralley, H. Zea-Diaz, E. Munoz-Atahualpa, F. Corrales-Medina, C. Cuba-Bustinza, J. Chirinos-Pacheco, & J. Medina-Lezama. (2008). Endogenous nitric oxide synthase inhibitors, arterial hemodynamics, and subclinical vascular disease: the PREVENCION Study. *Hypertension* 52 (6):pp. 1051-1059, ISSN 1524-4563.

Cirit, M., O. Toprak, M. Yesil, S. Bayata, N. Postaci, L. Pupim, & E. Esi. (2006). Angiotensin-converting enzyme inhibitors as a risk factor for contrast-induced nephropathy. *Nephron Clin Pract* 104 (1):pp. c20-27, ISSN 1660-2110.

Clark, B. A., D. Kim, & F. H. Epstein. (1997). Endothelin and atrial natriuretic peptide levels following radiocontrast exposure in humans. *American Journal of Kidney Diseases* 30 (1):pp. 82-86, ISSN 0272-6386.

Cooling, D. S. (1993). Theophylline toxicity. *Journal of Emergency Medicine* 11 (4):pp. 415-425, ISSN 0736-4679.

Dangas, G., I. Iakovou, E. Nikolsky, E. D. Aymong, G. S. Mintz, N. N. Kipshidze, A. J. Lansky, I. Moussa, G. W. Stone, J. W. Moses, M. B. Leon, & R. Mehran. (2005). Contrast-induced nephropathy after percutaneous coronary interventions in relation to chronic kidney disease and hemodynamic variables. *American Journal of Cardiology* 95 (1):pp. 13-19, ISSN 0002-9149.

Erley, C. M., S. H. Duda, D. Rehfuss, B. Scholtes, J. Bock, C. Muller, H. Osswald, & T. Risler. (1999). Prevention of radiocontrast-media-induced nephropathy in patients with pre-existing renal insufficiency by hydration in combination with the adenosine antagonist theophylline. *Nephrology, Dialysis, Transplantation* 14 (5):pp. 1146-1149, ISSN 0931-0509.

Erley, C. M., S. H. Duda, S. Schlepckow, J. Koehler, P. E. Huppert, W. L. Strohmaier, A. Bohle, T. Risler, & H. Osswald. (1994). Adenosine antagonist theophylline prevents the reduction of glomerular filtration rate after contrast media application. *Kidney International* 45 (5):pp. 1425-1431, ISSN 0085-2538.

Gandhi, M. R., P. Brown, C. A. Romanowski, S. K. Morcos, S. Campbell, A. M. el Nahas, & T. A. Gray. (1992). The use of theophylline, an adenosine antagonist in the prevention of contrast media induced nephrotoxicity. *British Journal of Radiology* 65 (777):pp. 838, ISSN 0007-1285.

Goergen, S. K., G. Rumbold, G. Compton, & C. Harris. (2010). Systematic review of current guidelines, and their evidence base, on risk of lactic acidosis after administration of contrast medium for patients receiving metformin. *Radiology* 254 (1):pp. 261-269, ISSN 1527-1315.

Grobner, T., & F. C. Prischl. (2007). Gadolinium and nephrogenic systemic fibrosis. *Kidney International* 72 (3):pp. 260-264, ISSN 0085-2538.

Gupta, R. K., A. Kapoor, S. Tewari, N. Sinha, & R. K. Sharma. (1999). Captopril for prevention of contrast-induced nephropathy in diabetic patients: a randomised study. *Indian Heart Journal* 51 (5):pp. 521-526, ISSN 0019-4832.

Hardiek, K., R. E. Katholi, V. Ramkumar, & C. Deitrick. (2001). Proximal tubule cell response to radiographic contrast media. *Am J Physiol Renal Physiol* 280 (1):pp. F61-70, ISSN 0363-6127.

Hardiek, K. J., R. E. Katholi, R. S. Robbs, & C. E. Katholi. (2008). Renal effects of contrast media in diabetic patients undergoing diagnostic or interventional coronary angiography. *Journal of Diabetes and Its Complications* 22 (3):pp. 171-177, ISSN 1056-8727.

Holscher, B., C. Heitmeyer, M. Fobker, G. Breithardt, R. M. Schaefer, & H. Reinecke. (2008). Predictors for contrast media-induced nephropathy and long-term survival: prospectively assessed data from the randomized controlled Dialysis-Versus-Diuresis (DVD) trial. *Canadian Journal of Cardiology* 24 (11):pp. 845-850, ISSN 1916-7075.

Huber, W., B. Jeschke, M. Page, W. Weiss, H. Salmhofer, U. Schweigart, K. Ilgmann, J. Reichenberger, B. Neu, & M. Classen. (2001). Reduced incidence of radiocontrast-induced nephropathy in ICU patients under theophylline prophylaxis: a prospective comparison to series of patients at similar risk. *Intensive Care Medicine* 27 (7):pp. 1200-1209, ISSN 0342-4642.

Huber, W., C. Schipek, K. Ilgmann, M. Page, M. Hennig, A. Wacker, U. Schweigart, L. Lutilsky, C. Valina, M. Seyfarth, A. Schomig, & M. Classen. (2003). Effectiveness of theophylline prophylaxis of renal impairment after coronary angiography in patients with chronic renal insufficiency. *American Journal of Cardiology* 91 (10):pp. 1157-1162, ISSN 0002-9149.

Ix, J. H., C. E. McCulloch, & G. M. Chertow. (2004). Theophylline for the prevention of radiocontrast nephropathy: a meta-analysis. *Nephrology, Dialysis, Transplantation* 19 (11):pp. 2747-2753, ISSN 0931-0509.

Kapoor, A., S. Kumar, S. Gulati, S. Gambhir, R. S. Sethi, & N. Sinha. (2002). The role of theophylline in contrast-induced nephropathy: a case-control study. *Nephrology, Dialysis, Transplantation* 17 (11):pp. 1936-1941, ISSN 0931-0509.

Kato, K., N. Sato, T. Yamamoto, Y. K. Iwasaki, K. Tanaka, & K. Mizuno. (2008). Valuable markers for contrast-induced nephropathy in patients undergoing cardiac catheterization. *Circ J* 72 (9):pp. 1499-1505, ISSN 1346-9843.

Kelly, A. M., B. Dwamena, P. Cronin, S. J. Bernstein, & R. C. Carlos. (2008). Meta-analysis: effectiveness of drugs for preventing contrast-induced nephropathy. *Annals of Internal Medicine* 148 (4):pp. 284-294, ISSN 1539-3704.

Khanal, S., N. Attallah, D. E. Smith, E. Kline-Rogers, D. Share, M. J. O'Donnell, & M. Moscucci. (2005). Statin therapy reduces contrast-induced nephropathy: an analysis of contemporary percutaneous interventions. *American Journal of Medicine* 118 (8):pp. 843-849, ISSN 0002-9343.

Kolonko, A., A. Wiecek, & F. Kokot. (1998). The nonselective adenosine antagonist theophylline does prevent renal dysfunction induced by radiographic contrast agents. *J Nephrol* 11 (3):pp. 151-156, ISSN 1121-8428.

Komers, R., & S. Anderson. (2003). Paradoxes of nitric oxide in the diabetic kidney. *Am J Physiol Renal Physiol* 284 (6):pp. F1121-1137, ISSN 0363-6127.

Kosiborod, M., & D. K. McGuire. (2010). Glucose-lowering targets for patients with cardiovascular disease: focus on inpatient management of patients with acute coronary syndromes. *Circulation* 122 (25):pp. 2736-2744, ISSN 1524-4539.

Laskey, W., P. Aspelin, C. Davidson, M. Rudnick, P. Aubry, S. Kumar, F. Gietzen, & M. Wiemer. (2009). Nephrotoxicity of iodixanol versus iopamidol in patients with chronic kidney disease and diabetes mellitus undergoing coronary angiographic procedures. *American Heart Journal* 158 (5):pp. 822-828 e823, ISSN 1097-6744.

Ling, W., N. Zhaohui, H. Ben, G. Leyi, L. Jianping, D. Huili, & Q. Jiaqi. (2008). Urinary IL-18 and NGAL as early predictive biomarkers in contrast-induced nephropathy after coronary angiography. *Nephron Clin Pract* 108 (3):pp. c176-181, ISSN 1660-2110.

Louis, B. M., B. S. Hoch, C. Hernandez, N. Namboodiri, G. Neiderman, A. Nissenbaum, F. P. Foti, A. Magno, G. Banayat, F. Fata, N. L. Manohar, & H. I. Lipner. (1996). Protection from the nephrotoxicity of contrast dye. *Renal Failure* 18 (4):pp. 639-646, ISSN 0886-022X

Meier, P., D. T. Ko, A. Tamura, U. Tamhane, & H. S. Gurm. (2009). Sodium bicarbonate-based hydration prevents contrast-induced nephropathy: a meta-analysis. *BMC Med* 7:pp. 23, ISSN 1741-7015.

Merten, G. J., W. P. Burgess, L. V. Gray, J. H. Holleman, T. S. Roush, G. J. Kowalchuk, R. M. Bersin, A. Van Moore, C. A. Simonton, 3rd, R. A. Rittase, H. J. Norton, & T. P. Kennedy. (2004). Prevention of contrast-induced nephropathy with sodium bicarbonate: a randomized controlled trial. *JAMA* 291 (19):pp. 2328-2334, ISSN 1538-3598.

Nikolsky, E., R. Mehran, D. Turcot, E. D. Aymong, G. S. Mintz, Z. Lasic, A. J. Lansky, E. Tsounias, J. W. Moses, G. W. Stone, M. B. Leon, & G. D. Dangas. (2004). Impact of chronic kidney disease on prognosis of patients with diabetes mellitus treated with percutaneous coronary intervention. *American Journal of Cardiology* 94 (3):pp. 300-305, ISSN 0002-9149.

Obert, D. M., P. Hua, M. E. Pilkerton, W. Feng, & E. A. Jaimes. (2011). Environmental tobacco smoke furthers progression of diabetic nephropathy. *American Journal of the Medical Sciences* 341 (2):pp. 126-130, ISSN 1538-2990.

O'Keefe, J. H., M. Abuannadi, C. J. Lavie, & D. S. Bell. (2011). Strategies for optimizing glycemic control and cardiovascular prognosis in patients with type 2 diabetes mellitus. *Mayo Clinic Proceedings* 86 (2):pp. 128-138, ISSN 1942-5546.

Parfrey, P. S., S. M. Griffiths, B. J. Barrett, M. D. Paul, M. Genge, J. Withers, N. Farid, & P. J. McManamon. (1989). Contrast material-induced renal failure in patients with diabetes mellitus, renal insufficiency, or both. A prospective controlled study. *New England Journal of Medicine* 320 (3):pp. 143-149, ISSN 0028-4793.

Perkins, B. A., R. G. Nelson, B. E. Ostrander, K. L. Blouch, A. S. Krolewski, B. D. Myers, & J. H. Warram. (2005). Detection of renal function decline in patients with diabetes and normal or elevated GFR by serial measurements of serum cystatin C concentration: results of a 4-year follow-up study. *Journal of the American Society of Nephrology* 16 (5):pp. 1404-1412, ISSN 1046-6673.

Pflueger, A., T. S. Larson, K. A. Nath, B. F. King, J. M. Gross, & F. G. Knox. (2000). Role of adenosine in contrast media-induced acute renal failure in diabetes mellitus. *Mayo Clinic Proceedings* 75 (12):pp. 1275-1283, ISSN 0025-6196.

Phisitkul, K., K. Hegazy, T. Chuahirun, C. Hudson, J. Simoni, H. Rajab, & D. E. Wesson. (2008). Continued smoking exacerbates but cessation ameliorates progression of early type 2 diabetic nephropathy. *American Journal of the Medical Sciences* 335 (4):pp. 284-291, ISSN 0002-9629.

Rosenstock, J. L., R. Bruno, J. K. Kim, L. Lubarsky, R. Schaller, G. Panagopoulos, M. V. DeVita, & M. F. Michelis. (2008). The effect of withdrawal of ACE inhibitors or angiotensin receptor blockers prior to coronary angiography on the incidence of contrast-induced nephropathy. *International Urology and Nephrology* 40 (3):pp. 749-755, ISSN 0301-1623.

Russo, D., A. Testa, L. Della Volpe, & G. Sansone. (1990). Randomised prospective study on renal effects of two different contrast media in humans: protective role of a calcium channel blocker. *Nephron* 55 (3):pp. 254-257, ISSN 0028-2766.

Saleem, S., F. G. Lakkis, & M. Martinez-Maldonado. (1996). Atheroembolic renal disease. *Seminars in Nephrology* 16 (4):pp. 309-318, ISSN 0270-9295.

Shammas, N. W., M. J. Kapalis, M. Harris, D. McKinney, & E. P. Coyne. (2001). Aminophylline does not protect against radiocontrast nephropathy in patients undergoing percutaneous angiographic procedures. *Journal of Invasive Cardiology* 13 (11):pp. 738-740, ISSN 1042-3931.

Shannon, M. (1999). Life-threatening events after theophylline overdose: a 10-year prospective analysis. *Archives of Internal Medicine* 159 (9):pp. 989-994, ISSN 0003-9926.

Shlipak, M. G., L. F. Fried, M. Cushman, T. A. Manolio, D. Peterson, C. Stehman-Breen, A. Bleyer, A. Newman, D. Siscovick, & B. Psaty. (2005). Cardiovascular mortality risk in chronic kidney disease: comparison of traditional and novel risk factors. *JAMA* 293 (14):pp. 1737-1745, ISSN 1538-3598.

Solomon, R. (2005). The role of osmolality in the incidence of contrast-induced nephropathy: a systematic review of angiographic contrast media in high risk patients. *Kidney International* 68 (5):pp. 2256-2263, ISSN 0085-2538.

Solomon, R. (2009). Preventing contrast-induced nephropathy: problems, challenges and future directions. *BMC Med* 7:pp. 24, ISSN 1741-7015.

Solomon, R. J., M. K. Natarajan, S. Doucet, S. K. Sharma, C. S. Staniloae, R. E. Katholi, J. L. Gelormini, M. Labinaz, & A. E. Moreyra. (2007). Cardiac Angiography in Renally Impaired Patients (CARE) study: a randomized double-blind trial of contrast-induced nephropathy in patients with chronic kidney disease. *Circulation* 115 (25):pp. 3189-3196, ISSN 1524-4539.

Solomon, R. J., R. Mehran, M. K. Natarajan, S. Doucet, R. E. Katholi, C. S. Staniloae, S. K. Sharma, M. Labinaz, J. L. Gelormini, & B. J. Barrett. (2009). Contrast-induced nephropathy and long-term adverse events: cause and effect? *Clin J Am Soc Nephrol* 4 (7):pp. 1162-1169, ISSN 1555-905X.

Spargias, K., E. Alexopoulos, S. Kyrzopoulos, P. Iokovis, D. C. Greenwood, A. Manginas, V. Voudris, G. Pavlides, C. E. Buller, D. Kremastinos, & D. V. Cokkinos. (2004). Ascorbic acid prevents contrast-mediated nephropathy in patients with renal dysfunction undergoing coronary angiography or intervention. *Circulation* 110 (18):pp. 2837-2842, ISSN 1524-4539.

Staniloae, C. S., S. Doucet, S. K. Sharma, R. E. Katholi, K. R. Mody, J. T. Coppola, & R. Solomon. (2009). N-Acetylcysteine added to volume expansion with sodium bicarbonate does not further prevent contrast-induced nephropathy: results from the cardiac angiography in renally impaired patients study. *J Interv Cardiol* 22 (3):pp. 261-265, ISSN 1540-8183.

Toprak, O., M. Cirit, M. Yesil, D. W. Byrne, N. Postaci, S. Bayata, K. M. Majchrzak, & E. Esi. (2006). Metabolic syndrome as a risk factor for contrast-induced nephropathy in non-diabetic elderly patients with renal impairment. *Kidney and Blood Pressure Research* 29 (1):pp. 2-9, ISSN 1420-4096.

Vassallo, R., & J. J. Lipsky. (1998). Theophylline: recent advances in the understanding of its mode of action and uses in clinical practice. *Mayo Clinic Proceedings* 73 (4):pp. 346-354, ISSN 0025-6196.

Yoon, M. H., S. J. Tahk, H. M. Yang, J. S. Park, M. Zheng, H. S. Lim, B. J. Choi, S. Y. Choi, U. J. Choi, J. W. Hwang, S. J. Kang, G. S. Hwang, & J. H. Shin. (2009). Comparison of the intracoronary continuous infusion method using a microcatheter and the intravenous continuous adenosine infusion method for inducing maximal hyperemia for fractional flow reserve measurement. *American Heart Journal* 157 (6):pp. 1050-1056, ISSN 1097-6744.

Zoungas, S., A. Patel, J. Chalmers, B. E. de Galan, Q. Li, L. Billot, M. Woodward, T. Ninomiya, B. Neal, S. MacMahon, D. E. Grobbee, A. P. Kengne, M. Marre, & S. Heller. (2010). Severe hypoglycemia and risks of vascular events and death. *New England Journal of Medicine* 363 (15):pp. 1410-1418, ISSN 1533-4406.

14

Quantitative Coronary Angiography in the Interventional Cardiology

Salvatore Davide Tomasello[1], Luca Costanzo[2] and Alfredo Ruggero Galassi[1]
[1]*Department of Internal Medicine and Systemic Disease, Catheterization Laboratory and Cardiovascular Interventional Unit, Cannizzaro Hospital, University of Catania*
[2]*Department of Internal Medicine and Systemic Disease, Clinical Division of Cardiology, Ferrarotto Hospital, University of Catania*
Italy

1. Introduction

Coronary angiography through selective injection of radiopaque contrast agent into the coronary arteries is currently the gold standard for evaluating coronary artery disease (CAD). Subjective visual estimation of lesion severity has been shown to be inadequate due to high degrees of intraobserver and interobserver variability (Topol & Nissen, 1995). Since the late 1980s methods and algorithms for quantitative coronary angiography (QCA) have been developed in order to objectively quantify the extent of CAD (Serruys et al., 1984).
Furthermore, validation of specific QCA measurements associated with clinical outcomes has led to their incorporation into various scoring systems and trials endpoint.

2. Two-dimensional QCA

This technique is based on contrast coronary angiograms obtaining parameters that quantify objectively the coronary lumen measuring the significance of a coronary stenosis. Notably, a single coronary angiography image gives only a two-dimensional (2D) radiographic image while coronary arteries can be highly tortuous three-dimensional structures thus at least two projections orthogonal to each other and both perpendicular to the analyzed coronary segment are necessary to obtain the most complete data to avoid foreshortening or underestimation of stenosis severity.
Most of the systems available nowadays are based on vessel edge detection algorithms to designate the arterial lumen on conventional coronary angiograms providing, therefore, the assessment of the lesion in an operator-independent way exploiting specific and dedicated software. The earliest form of quantitative angiography was the application of calipers to visually estimate percent diameter stenosis. In 1971 Gensini and colleagues described an electronic caliper system in which the arterial borders of the lesion and normal segments are manually defined by moving cursors (Gensini et al., 1971). In the years several generations

of QCA systems have been developed based on edge detection algorithms to improve measurement accuracy. First-generation algorithms have been introduced at the beginning of the Eighties (Mancini et al., 1987; Reiber et al., 1985) improving the reliability of coronary measurements (Spears et al., 1983); the main pitfall of these first generation systems was the overestimation of the diameters of small vessels (Herrington et al., 1993a), an issue which was improved in the second generation systems (diameter approximation \1.2 mm) and producing more reliable results at the low end of the spectrum of vessel size (Hausleiter et al., 1997). In more recent years cardiovascular X-ray imaging systems are equipped with flat-panel (FP) detectors (Spahn et al., 2003) replacing the combination of image intensifier and charge-couple device camera providing better image quality and enabling further image enhancement. Novel QCA third-generation system which took advantage of digital flat-panel (FP) detectors instead of the conventional image intensifier systems were better able to determine smaller diameter vessels (Van Herck et al., 2004) and analyze complex lesion morphology with irregular borders (Van der Zwet & Reiber, 1994). However differences in results using FP systems compared with classic image intensifier-based imaging systems were shown to be clinically not significant (Tuinenburg et al., 2006). In the common clinical practice there are different computer systems for QCA that have been validated: among them the most commonly employed are CAAS (PIE Medical, Maastricht, The Netherlands) and QAngio XA (Medis, Leiden, The Netherlands) (Garrone et al., 2009).

3. Three-dimensional QCA

Currently, 2-dimensional (2D) QCA is the most commonly used and validated form of QCA. However, 2D angiography technology has limitations because of vessel overlap and vessel foreshortening during image acquisition. This is especially problematic in more complex lesions such as bifurcations. 3D angiography utilizes standard 2D angiographic images obtained at least 30 degrees apart and with minimal vessel overlap, and reconstructs 3D images. Several 3D QCA programs are now available: among them the most commonly employed are CardiOp-B (Paieon Medical Ltd. Park Afek, Israel) and CAAS 5 (Pie medical Imaging, Maastricht, The Netherlands, and Medis, Leiden, The Netherlands) (Ng & Lansky, 2011). In these systems, the user defines the area of interest by defining the proximal end, distal end and area of stenosis. However, the systems differ in their calibration methods. CardiOp-B requires the operator to input the size of the catheter in the image into the program, whereas the Medis and CAAS 5 systems automatically calibrates the images using DICOM (Digital Imaging and Communications in Medicine) information embedded in the angiographic images (Gradaus et al., 2006; Ramcharitar et al., 2008a). Once the image is created, operators can manipulate the images by zooming in or rotating the image. This allows the operator to have a better understanding of coronary anatomy and could also help the operator find an optimal angle to image of a vessel for an intervention (Dvir et al., 2005; Agostoni et al., 2008). An example of coronary after reconstructed with CardiOp-B system is shown in figure 1.

3D QCA programs have been validated (Schuurbiers et al., 2009; Tsuchida et al., 2007) and are now available to provide information of vessel size, percent diameter stenosis, minimal lumen diameter, bifurcation angle and other QCA values. It was thought that 3D QCA would have improved accuracy by resolving problems with vessel foreshortening and out of plane magnification. However, comparisons of 3D QCA programs to conventional 2D QCA programs have shown mixed results regarding the accuracy of this technology (Ramcharitar et al., 2008a; Dvir et al., 2005; Tsuchida et al., 2007; Meerkin et al., 2010; Wellnhofer et al., 1999; Tu et al., 2010). One small study has compared the two current 3D QCA programs using phantom models demonstrated that the CAAS 5 system may be more accurate than the CardiOp-B system (Ramcharitar et al., 2008a).

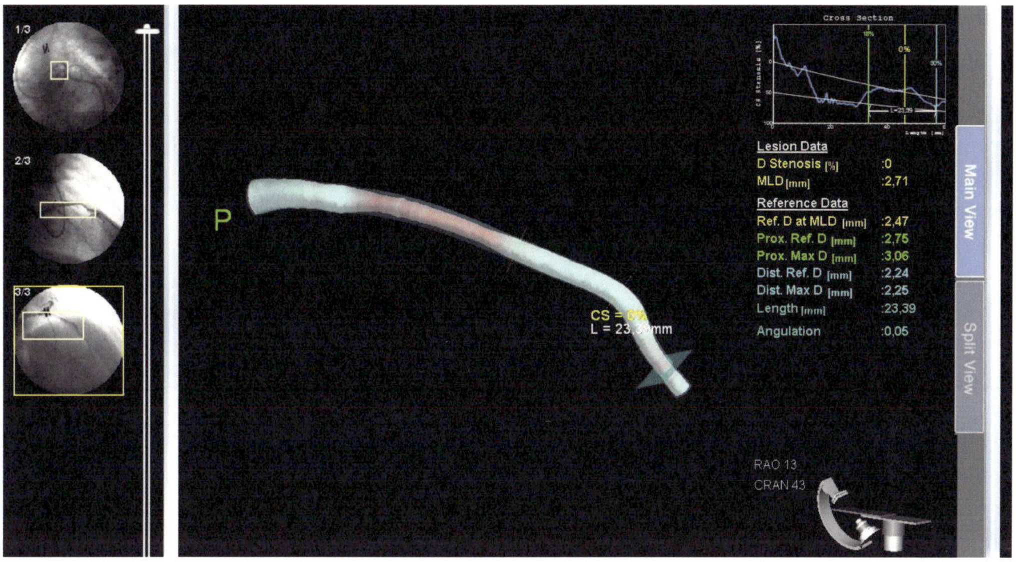

Fig. 1. Reconstruction with 3-D CardiOp-B system of proximal left anterior descending artery.

4. Materials and procedural details

The first step in order to perform a QCA analysis is to acquire high-quality angiographic images of the coronary artery segment of choice using a standard and reliable technique. Coronary angiography actually provides a two-dimensional luminogram of a three-dimensional structure, formed not only of the lumen itself but also of the vessel wall. Therefore, coronary angiography has important limitations that can have a significant impact on the results of QCA (Topol & Nissen, 1995). It is thus clear that coronary angiography cannot analyze coronary remodeling mechanisms, that is, the outward or inward changes in total vessel area that may not correspond to outward or inward changes in lumen area typical of atherosclerosis in an effective way (Glagov et al., 1987). Furthermore, to get coronary angiographic images that profile the exact coronary anatomy with as much details as possible and avoid foreshortening or underestimation of stenosis severity, it is necessary also that the C-arm tube is directly orthogonal to the coronary segment analysed, and it is advisable to get at least two projections orthogonal to each other and both perpendicular to the coronary segment in order to obtain the most complete data.

Selection of a coronary image for analysis depends on several factors linked to the limits of radiographic coronary images. The real issue is the choice of the sequence where the stenosis has the minimal foreshortening and the minimal overlap with other structures (e.g., other coronary arteries, bifurcation branches, catheters, or radiopaque surrounding structures such as a calcified mitral valve). The greater is the contrast between the radiopaque contrast-filled coronary artery and the radiotransparent background, the greater are the accuracy of QCA analysis and reliability of the algorithm for the automated detection and reconstruction of the lumen edges. That is why it is also important that the coronary images are obtained when the patient is in deep inspiration, which increases the radiotransparent lung fields surrounding the heart and thus the possibility that the stenosis is in front of this radiotransparent field. It is also important that the distal tip of the coronary angiography catheter is present in the sequence, at least in the initial frames.

Indeed, the tip of the catheter, whose diameter in French or millimeters is known, is the basic tool for calibration (i.e., to estimate the proportion between pixels in the digitalized images and mm of length). Finally, intracoronary nitroglycerine (e.g., 200 μg) might be administered to obtain coronary vasodilatation and avoid to mistakenly confounding vasospasm with atherosclerotic processes.

After choosing the appropriate run, a single static image (i.e., frame) is selected which should be chosen in end-diastole, when coronaries tend to "stretch" along their course on the released heart muscle without being subject to contraction or squeezing, even in the case of intra-myocardial course. Regardless of the type of software, the analysis proceeds similarly and the following steps consist in: *digitization*, *image calibration* and arterial *automatic contour detection*. Advances have been made to each of these steps over the last several decades. The process of *digitization* from cine film using cine video converter is obsolete and it has been replaced by digital systems with direct digital input to a video camera. The analogic video output signal is modified electronically and results in a greater contrast difference in the parts with high X-ray absorption and lower contrast differences in areas with low X-ray absorption, significantly improving image quality. *Image calibration* is often done with contrast-filled injection catheters (Figure 2), and can be problematic due to variable image quality and out-of-plane magnification that can be overcome by using biplane calibration.

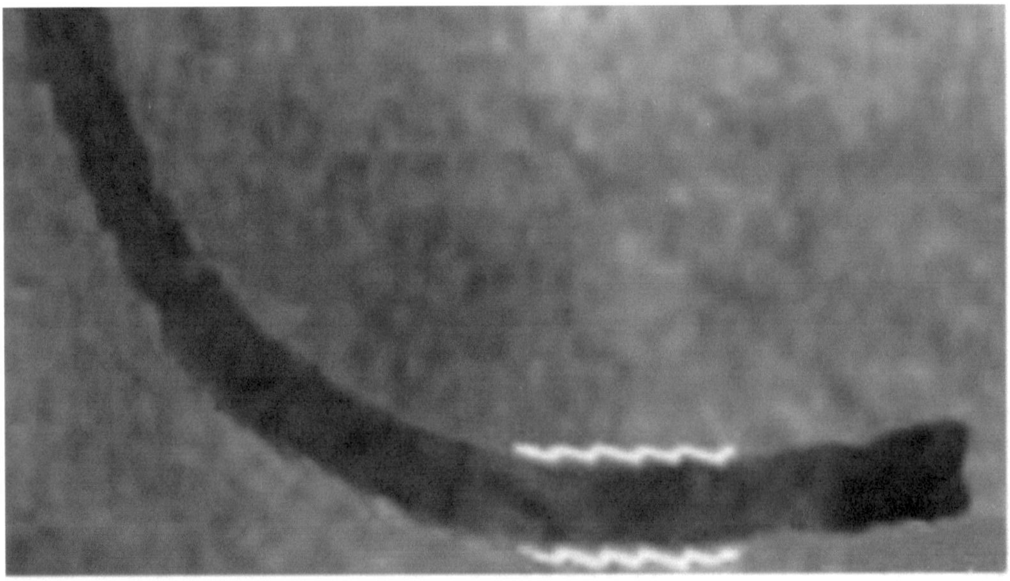

Fig. 2. Image calibration using contrast-filled injection catheter.

A central line is usually then drawn by hand along the stretch of the catheter tip and the software automatically recognizes its margins by using specific algorithms that, by means of digital images, recognize the change from radiopaque pixels (black or dark grey) to radio-transparent pixels (light grey or white) according to a densitometric analysis. The software then transforms every pixel into a square with sides characterized by known dimensions (mm). This parameter is then employed to measure the coronary segment of interest that must be focused on the stenosis or lesion undergoing treatment. The proximal and distal coronary segments should be relatively free of disease and are referred to as reference segments. Afterwards, a central line is traced manually and the software automatically recognizes the margins of the coronary segment under consideration taking advantage of the *automatic contour detection* .

This procedure determines the vessel edge based on the weighted sum of the first and second derivative functions of the brightness values of scanlines perpendicular to the centerline, which in turn undergoes an analysis that determines the optimal contour path along the segment (Figure 3).

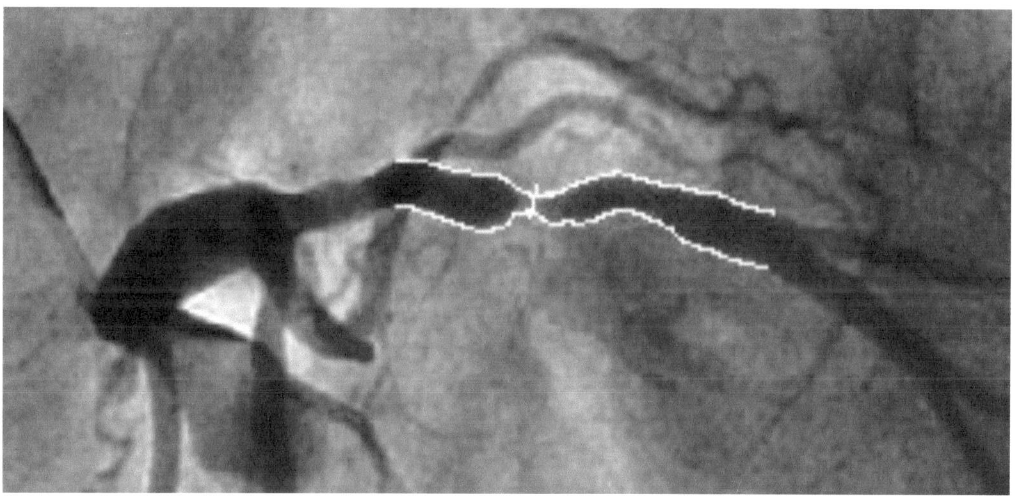

Fig. 3. After having traced a central line the software recognizes the margins elaborating automatically the contours.

A further step allows, always automatically, the reconstruction of the hypothetically normal coronary lumen. An algorithm then creates a line of the coronary margin that interpolates the coronary segment considered free from illness located proximally and distally to the region of interest with the ones of the region of interest. The algorithm then reconstructs the reference coronary segments (i.e., those apparently free from disease) (Figure 4).

This technique is essentially based on the calculation of a mean value of the diameters of the lumen in the segments of reference located upstream and downstream to the lesion. It appears thus clear the importance of including two coronary segments in the QCA analysis, one proximal and one distal to the target segment and both angiographically-free from significant disease. These steps produce different parameters, some measured directly and others derived with interpolation techniques.

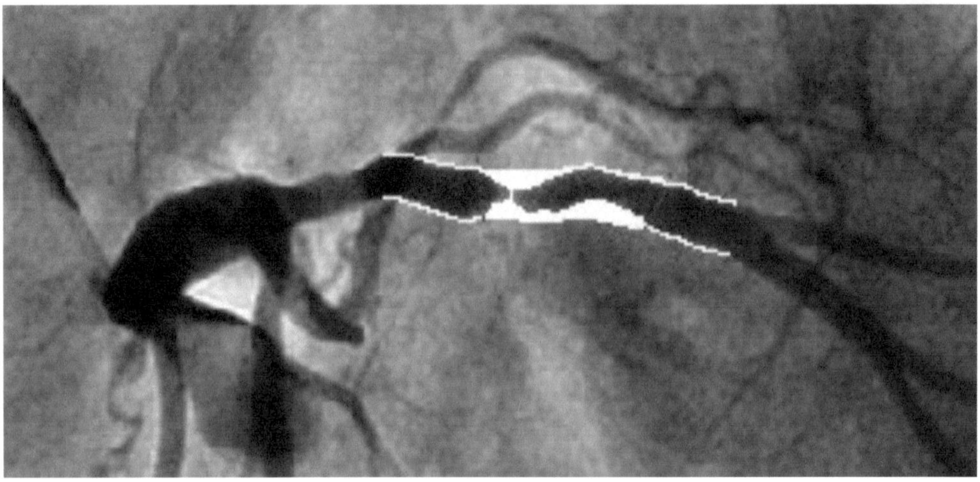

Fig. 4. Software algorithm reconstructs the reference coronary segment.

5. Parameters

Coronary lesions can be assessed qualitatively and quantitatively, in terms of severity of the lesion itself. The qualitative evaluation is based on the visual estimation of the lesion and it depends very much on the operator's experience. The quantitative evaluation, based on QCA, allows instead to obtain numeric parameters that are much more independent from the operator acquiring the images or the one performing the analyses. The coronary parameters of major interest are summarized in Table 1.

Parameter	**Range commonly used**	**Meaning**
Minimal Luminal Diameter (MLD)	0-6.00 mm	The smallest lumen diameter in the segment of interest
Reference Vessel Diameter (RVD)	1.5-6.0 mm	The averaged diameter of the coronary assumed without atherosclerotic disease
Lesion length	0-60.0 mm	Length of the stenosis as measured by 2 points where the coronary margins change direction, creating a shoulder between the angiographically normal subsegment and the diseased subsegment
Acute gain	0-4.0 mm	Post-procedural MLD - pre-procedural MLD
Late loss (LL)	0.10 to 3.00	Post-procedural MLD - MLD at follow-up
Diameter stenosis (DS)	0-100%	(RVD-MLD)/RVD
Binary restenosis (BR)	Yes or no	DS >50% at follow-up coronary angiography in the treated coronary segment

Table 1. Main parameters obtained with QCA (adapted from Garrone et al., 2009)

Additional tool of QCA are also available, indeed it is possible analysis of the stent edges after stent implantation. In fact, the radiopaque stent can generally be visualized during angiographic sequence when the contrast medium has not yet been injected in the coronary vessel. By comparing this image with the frame selected for the QCA analysis, it is possible to determine the two edges, proximal and distal, of the implanted stent. The software then enables to mark the edges with a line transversal to the vessel lumen in order to automatically calculate the segment where the stent has been implanted and to calculate the 5-mm segments that lie proximal and distal to the stent. Therefore, it is possible to determine MLD and DS for each one of the three segments considered.
Several angiographic phenomena can bias QCA and lead to overestimation or underestimation of QCA parameters such as acute or chronic thrombus, extensive calcium deposits, dissections, diffuse disease, and slow flow, therefore it is of paramount importance to add a qualitative analysis for lesion features to any QCA analysis (Garrone et al., 2009).

6. Applications

QCA can be employed in clinical practice during diagnostic coronary angiography (online), to have an objective and independent parameter for the assessment of stenosis severity as the human eye does not have the resolution capability of software. Usually, visual interpretation of the severity of a coronary stenosis is expressed in intervals of percentage of stenosis while QCAproduces a single specific measure for DS, improving the accuracy and reproducibility of the severity assessment (Kalbfleisch et al., 1990). It has been shown that the visual assessment tends to underestimate stenoses<50% and to overestimate those >50% (Fleming et al., 1991) therefore the online use of QCA assessing the lesion length and RVD might allow to obtain objective parameters to decide which specific measures (mainly diameter and length) of the device (e.g., balloon or stent) should be chosen.
In the field of clinical research QCA allows serial analysis of the same coronary segment over time in an indipendent way. In trials on coronary devices typically at least three QCA runs are performed, one before treatment, another immediately after treatment, and a final one at angiographic follow-up, after a respecified time.
In recent years late luminal loss and binary restenosis have taken an important role in several studies aimed at evaluating PCI devices, in particular, stents. These values, more specific and more prevalent of the clinically relevant end-point of target lesion revascularization (TLR), allow researchers to compare different types of devices in clinical trials, with greater statistical power, and thus with fewer patients. In fact, late luminal loss is a continuous parameter and is in itself statistically more powerful and precise, while binary restenosis, despite being a value present or absent as the TLR, occurs with an incidence roughly two times higher than the incidence of TLR. Therefore QCA can reduce the number of patients needed in a clinical trial to obtain significant differences between different devices.
Another interesting application is the study of plaque progression/regression that is based on at least two QCA runs made over a pre-specified interval of time, usually at least 1 year. The change in MLD of the coronary segments of interest is quantified after a given pharmacologic regimen that purports to act on the development or progression ofatherosclerotic disease.

7. Prediction of functional significance of a stenosis

2D-QCA systems have substantially improved reproducibility and accuracy of lesion dimension assessment, especially percent diameter stenosis, however its use for the prediction of functional significance of the lesion was shown to have only a modest correlation with the more accurate Flow Fractional Reserve (FFR) (Bartunek et al., 1995; Fischer et al., 2002). Conversely, 3D-QCA has shown reasonable accuracy in predicting FFR < 0.75 in patients with visually determined intermediate stenosis (Saad et al., 2009). Recently, Yong and co-workers investigated the accuracy of 3D-and 2D-QCA measurements in predicting both FFR <0.75 and ≤0.80, and compared the correlation of FFR with 3D- and 2D-QCA measurements in 63 coronary lesions (Yong et al., 2011). Interesting, the relationship between FFR and apparent stenosis severity was found to be curvilinear. Of all measurements of lesion severity obtained by 3D-QCA, MLA best correlated with FFR (R = 0.63, P < 0.001), and was the most accurate predictor of FFR < 0.75 (C statistic 0.86, P = 0.001). Of 2D-QCA measurements, MLD correlated best with FFR (R = 0.58, P < 0.001), and best predicted FFR <0.75 (C statistic 0.80, P < 0.001). Overall, 3D-QCA showed a non-significant trend towards more accurate prediction of FFR than 2D-QCA, especially in intermediate lesions. The authors then concluded that both 3D- and 2D-QCA were less accurate in intermediate lesions and in predicting FFR ≤0.80 than in predicting FFR < 0.75 (Yong et al., 2011).

8. Special coronary lesion subset: chronic total occlusion and bifurcations

8.1 QCA in chronic total occlusion

Chronic total occlusions (CTOs) of the coronary arteries are one of the most technically challenging lesion subsets for interventional cardiologists due to the most significant difficulty in crossing the lesion with guidewire compared with other lesions subset (Di Mario et al., 2007). This might be considered a failure of conventional 2D-angiography to properly represent stump morphology and true lesion geometry (Safian et al., 1988; Kinoshita et al., 1995). Moreover CTOs are often long lesions length, with severe calcifications and tortuosity (Di Mario et al., 2007), therefore the evaluation of these complex geometric factors is difficult with conventional 2D angiography, often leading to misjudgement of the potential and proper method of treatment (Herrington et al, 1993b).

Recently, Dvir and colleagues evaluated real-time 3D reconstruction of CTOs with CardiOp-B system in a series of 58 patients (61 CTOs) (Dvir et al., 2008). Authors reported a 3D reconstruction success rate of 83% with improved visualization of stump area and/or missing segment. Importantly, in 92% of the successful 3D reconstructions, the artery path in the lesion area could be delineated and in 95% of cases, in which post-stenting 3D reconstruction performed, the vessel path was similar to the lesion path suggested before stenting. Interestingly, the mean stenosis area was significantly smaller in the 3D reconstructions vs. 2D images (94 6 5.1% vs. 99 6 0.3%, P < 0.001) and the mean lesion length was significantly shorter (15.3 6 7.4 mm vs. 20.9 6 8 mm, P < 0.001). A possible explanation proposed by the Authors was that in these highly complex lesions, where lesion path was not visible, the 2D measurements were severely inaccurate. Thus 3D reconstructions may be considered as a useful tool in CTO procedures to improve assessment of CTO lesions characteristics (Dvir et al., 2008).

8.2 Bifurcations

With the expanding practice of stenting coronary bifurcation lesions worldwide , the need for reliable, standardized and reproducible quantitative bifurcation analyses became apparent. A fundamental challenge in assessing bifurcations using quantitative methods is in acquiring the entire bifurcation lesion without significant foreshortening or vessel and side branch overlap. While current QCA standards require a minimum of two orthogonal views more than 30° apart, optimal visualization of the bifurcation lesion (parent vessel and side branch) is typically available in one best single view. When QCA is applied using a standard operating procedure, i.e. by including in the analyzed segment the proximal main vessel (PMV) and distal main vessel (DMV), the RVD function takes an average of the "normal" segments of the proximal and distal vessel. Tapering, however, causes the proximal RD and thus the percentage diameter reduction of lesions proximal to the bifurcation to be underestimated, while the distal RD and %DS of lesions distal to the bifurcation will be overestimated. If on-line QCA is used for guidance during a procedure, this can lead to inappropriate balloon selection, with significant under sizing of balloons used for dilatation of the proximal segment and equally, over sizing of balloons used for the distal segment of the main vessel (MV). The operator must manually redraw the proximal segment within the MV and is forced to tediously correct for the contours of the lesion, a possible source of inaccuracy and subjectivity. Even with optimal angiographic views, the main issues of conventional QCA in the analysis of bifurcation lesions are: defining the true reference vessel size of both the parent vessel and its side branch; the assessment of side-branch (SB) stenoses when truly ostial. In the non-diseased state, the RD of the main vessel is reduced from proximal to distal relative to the side branch. It has been shown that the change in RD of the main vessel across the side branch is a function of the size of the PMV, the DMV and that of the SB. Murray was the first to describe the mother/daughter-vessel relations in vascular bifurcations, in terms of a cost function: i.e., the sum of function power loss and metabolic power dissipation proportional to blood flow. Murray described the optimal conditions for vascular bifurcation, known as Murray's law, which states that the cube of the radius of the mother vessel equals the sum of the cubes of the radii of the daughter vessels: $D_m^3=D_{d1}^3+D_{d2}^3$ (Murray, 1926). Afterwards, a simplified equation relating the size of the proximal and distal main vessel and the side branch, in the non-diseased state, has been described by a constant [$D_1= 0.687 (D_2 + D_3 + \ldots)$] (Kassab, 2006; Kamiya & Takahashi, 2007) such that the reference size of any one segment can always be derived if the two other segment sizes are known (Finet et al., 2007). Standard QCA algorithms are designed to detect vessel contours assuming minimal vessel tapering; thus, the reference vessel dimensions are inherently inaccurate when applied to bifurcation lesions. Several techniques have been used to attempt to overcome this limitation but remain problematic (Lansky et al., 2009).

8.2.1 Dedicated bifurcation QCA algorithms

Currently two dedicated bifurcation QCA software packages are commercially available (Medis medical imaging systems, Leiden and The Netherlands and Pie Medical, Maastricht, The Netherlands). The main issue for the application of QCA in bifurcating segments include:

- minimal user interaction in the selection and processing of the coronary segments to be analysed;

- minimal editing of the automatically determined results;
- short analysis time;
- providing highly accurate and precise results, with small systematic and random errors
- providing suitable reporting and data exchange mechanisms.

The Medis medical imaging systems. This system contains two bifurcation models: a T-shape bifurcation model (suitable for bifurcations with a standard side branch structure) (Figure 5 A) and a Y-shape bifurcation model (suitable for bifurcations with distal branches of equal size) (Figure 5 B).

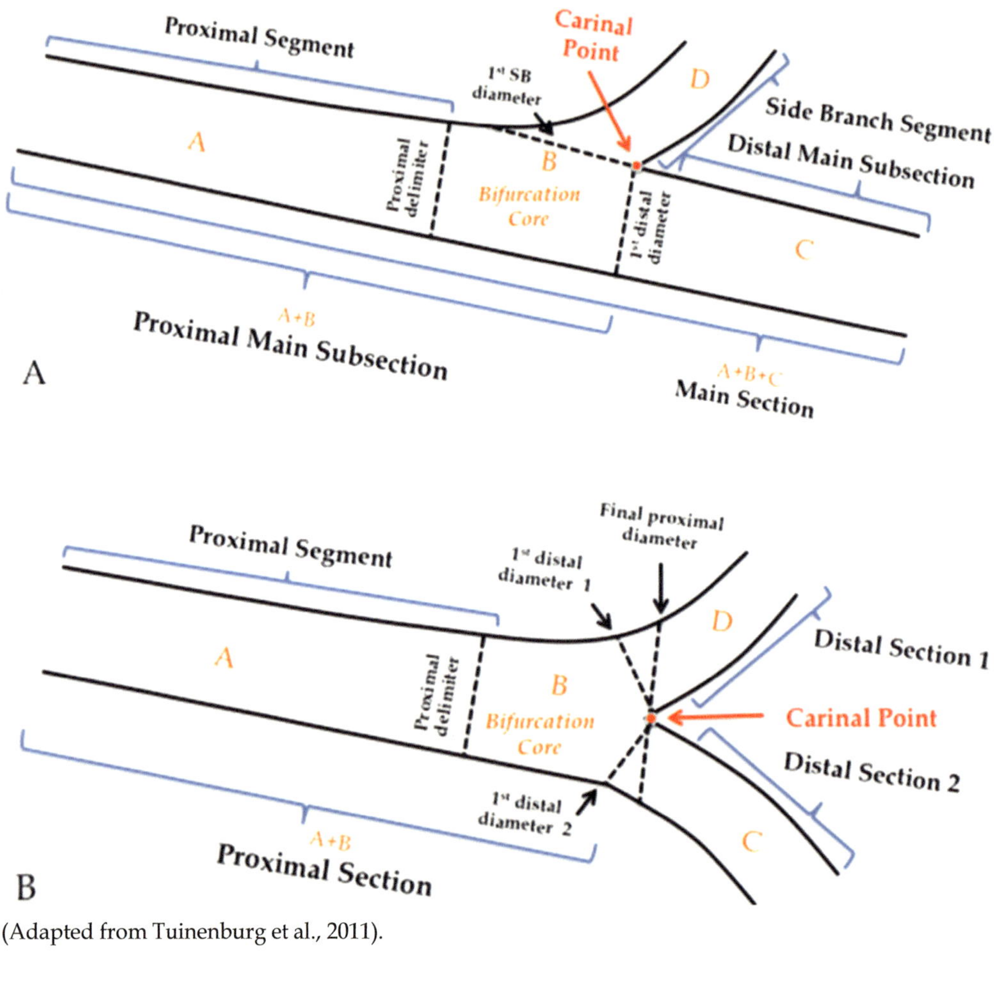

(Adapted from Tuinenburg et al., 2011).

Fig. 5. T-shape model (A) and Y-shape model (B) showing the segments, proximal delimiter, and sections terminology. For each model, the segment generated four segments that represent the building blocks of the models. A) Using the T-shape model, the arterial and reference diameters of the ostium of the side branch and the whole main section (including the transition within the bifurcation core) can be accurately determined. B) Using the Y-shape model, the arterial and reference diameters up to the carinal point and in the distal 1 and 2 sections can be determined accurately.

The particular advantage of these models is that they combine the proximal and two distal vessel segments with the bifurcation core, resulting in a total of two or three sections, all derived from one analysis procedure, such that each of these sections has its own diameter function and associated parameter data.

Step 1. *Contour detection.* Three path-line points have to be selected to define the arterial bifurcation segment: a start point in the proximal parent vessel (PV), and end points in the distal PV and the SB. From these points, two pathlines are constructed followed by the automated detection of the arterial contours of all three vessel segments using an algorithm.

Step 2. *Lesions analysis.* The bifurcation core is defined automatically as the area between the first diameter of the distal PV segment, and the interpolated contour between the proximal and distal PV segments.

In the T Bifurcation model, the proximal and distal PV and core segments are combined to define the first section and the SB segment forms the second section. For the entire PV section the arterial diameter function is calculated following the conventional Medis straight analysis approach, while for the SB section the Medis ostial analysis approach is followed.

For the Y bifurcation model, the core segment is defined as the area between the automatically determined proximal boundaries of the proximal segment and the carinal point. Excluding the core segment, three sections are defined with each arterial diameter functions calculated using the conventional straight analysis approach.

Step 3. *Result reporting.* The results of the bifurcation analysis are reported individually for the proximal segment (combining the proximal PV and core segments), the distal PV segment, the SB segment, and the "combined lesion" results (combined proximal, core, and distal PV). Conventional angiographic parameters will be reported including the obstruction, reference, minimum, maximum, and mean diameters and areas, the percent diameter and area stenosis, as well as the vessel and lesion lengths.

The Pie Medical Analysis Principles: CAAS 5 QCA bifurcation methodology. In this system the bifurcated vessel is considered to be a single entity, including the central bifurcation area divided in 10 segments when stented (Ramcharitar S, 2008) (Figure 6).

In this analysis, the segments 1, 4 and 6 are 5 mm beyond the stent edge. The main vessel stent is divided at the carina as that proximal and distal corresponding to segments 2 and 3 respectively, with the side branch stent confined to segment 5. The central portion, segment 7 is an independent region called the Polygon of Confluence (POC) that is unique to the bifurcation and represents a new quantification modality. Segment 8 is an ostial region of side branch including 5 mm distal from the end of bifurcation. The CAAS 5 quantitative analysis of bifurcations can be summarized in six steps:

1. *Contour detection,* that is performed in a semi-automated process employing either manually drawn initial pathline, or three user-defined points (one at the proximal side of the main vessel and two at both distal ends of the bifurcated branches). The algorithm automatically calculates path lines and the contours. The software assumes the bifurcated vessel is a single object delineated by a left, middle and right contour, specifically making no further assumptions.

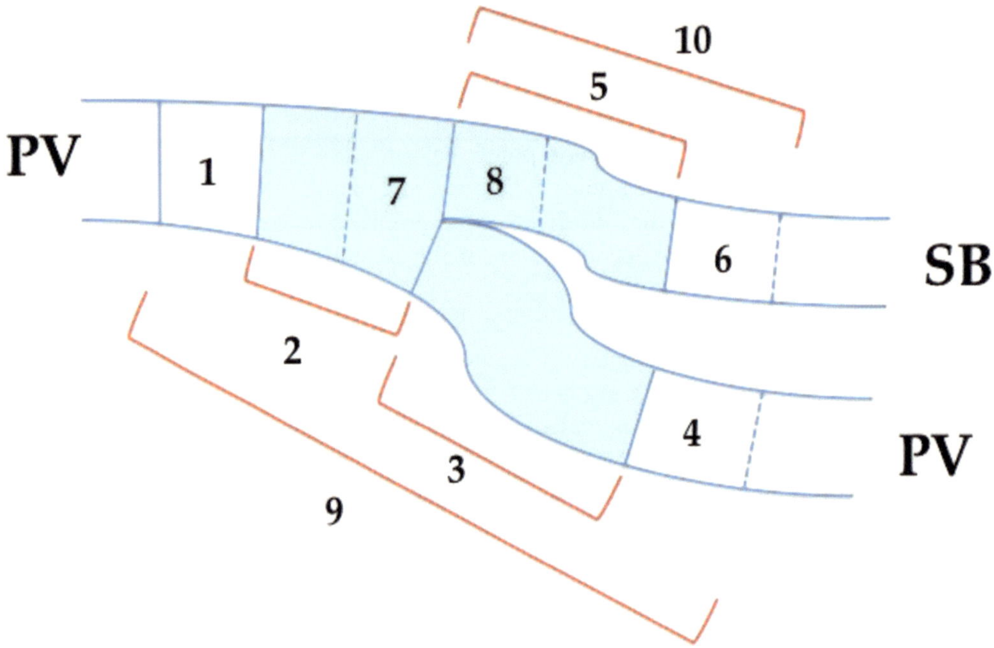

1 - Proximal Edge (5 mm)	6 - Distal Edge Side (5 mm)
2 - Proximal Main Stent	7 - Polygon of Confluence
3 - Distal Main Stent	8 - Ostium of the Side Branch (5 mm)
4 - Distal Edge Main (5 mm)	9 - MV Stent + Edges
5 - Side Branch Stent	10 - SB Stent + Distal Edge

Fig. 6. The 10 segments used in CAAS (Adapted from Ramcharitar et al., 2008b)

2. *Construction of the centreline and defining the Point of Bifurcation (POB).* The Point of Bifurcation (POB) is defined as the point where all the centrelines meet; the centrelines being the lines through the middle of the vessel. The POB is defined as the midpoint of the largest circle that can be fitted in the bifurcation area, touching all three contours. The intersections between this circle and the centrelines identify the start and end positions of the bifurcation region the boundaries of a new measurement entity the POC (Figure 7).
3. *Defining the POC.* The POC represents the smallest possible independent region that behaves differently from a single vessel segment. It is defined on the 2D radiographic image as the area or region that encompasses the start and the end of the bifurcation region. Regions outside of the POC behave similar to single vessels in classic QCA. The polygon shape is created by connecting begin and end boundaries of the POC by the luminal borders of the vessel. Depending on the type of bifurcation it can have different shapes, such as a pentagon. The plaque area can be evaluated against the actual luminal area or volume to give the percentage area or volume stenosis as a single value for the POC after reconstruction the vessel to its healthy situation. Furthermore the absolute POC area can be compared between pre-, post- and follow-up in clinical studies as a measure for procedural success (Figure 7).

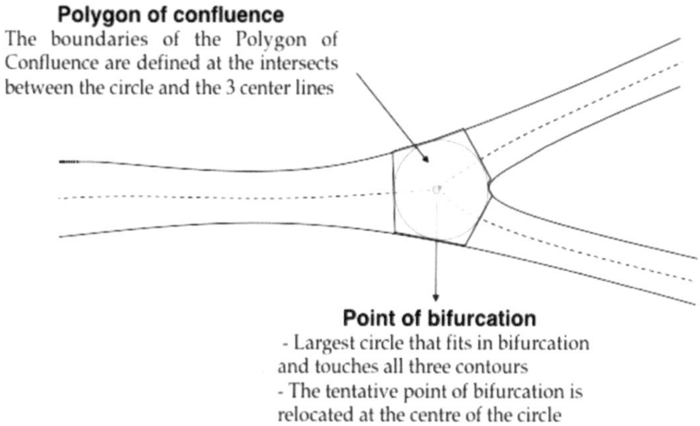

Fig. 7. Polygon of confluence and point of bifurcation in CAAS system (Adapted from Ramcharitar, 2008b)

4. *Determination diameter and reference values within the bifurcation.* Traditional diameter measurements can also be obtained. However, unlike the branches where the diameter measurements are determined by the distance between left and right border, it is not straightforward inside the POC. In order to derive such data within the POC the "Minimum Freedom" approach must be employed. In this approach shortest distances between a centreline point and the boundaries are determined, and the distance between these points used as best estimate for the diameter within the POC for that location along the centreline. The MLD at the bifurcation can be found using this approach by walking through points along the termini of the bifurcation to the centre point within the polygon of confluence. The reference diameter outside the POC is determined from the edges of the 'healthy' part of the vessel. It is based only on the characteristics of the branch itself as in the CAAS single vessel software.
5. *Determining the bifurcation angulation.* For the calculation of the angles between the arterial branches, a method that employs lines derived from the circle used for the definition of the "POC" can be used. The intersection positions of the circle with the centrelines are used as the centres for new circles. These new circles have the same radius as the circle within the "POC" and are not dependent on the mean vessel diameter of the specific branch.
6. *Report.* Different versions of the bifurcation analysis software are available for clinical and core lab use. Available analysis methods include automatic reference obstruction analysis, local reference analysis, user defined subsegments as well as the 10 segmental analysis method to analyse the stented bifurcations, post-procedure and at follow-up.

8.2.2 3D QCA in bifurcation

3D-QCA analysis is able to follow the complex arterial curvilinear structure of the bifurcation and to select the most appropriate view to avoid foreshortening in the region of interest. 3D-QCA, as compared to conventional two-dimensional QCA, allows a more appropriate imaging of bifurcation geometry, with chance of an online assessment of the bifurcation and deviation angle values, which may help the operator to choose the best strategy to approach each lesion (Galassi et al., 2010). Although there are multiple software programs dedicated for 3-dimensional QCA, only two software packages are dedicated for bifurcation analysis: The CardiOp-B system (Dvir et al., 2007; Galassi et al., 2010) and the recent CAAS 5 QCA 3D bifurcation software (Onuma et al., 2011).

CAAS 3-D QCA, while following the already described algorithm based on vessel size adjusted vectors, calculates BA values in 3-D space without overlap, therefore theoretically more precisely than 2-D QCA. On the other hand, in CardiOp-B angle values were computed between the weighted vectors of direction of the respective vessel segments. The weighted vector is calculated as the sum of two vectors, each of them connecting the bifurcation point with distal points along the vessel centre line, distant by 5 mm and 10 mm, respectively. This algorithm was employed in a recent substudy of the SYNTAX trial, the first ever to describe the 3-D angulation of the left main before and after intervention and its impact on 1-year clinical outcome (Girasis et al., 2010a). When it comes to the quantification of stenosis, CardiOp-B provides diameter-derived and cross-sectional (densitometric) data together with the lesion length; lesion markers can be manipulated, in order to relocate the region of interest across the main vessel or from the PMV into the SB. (Figure 8)

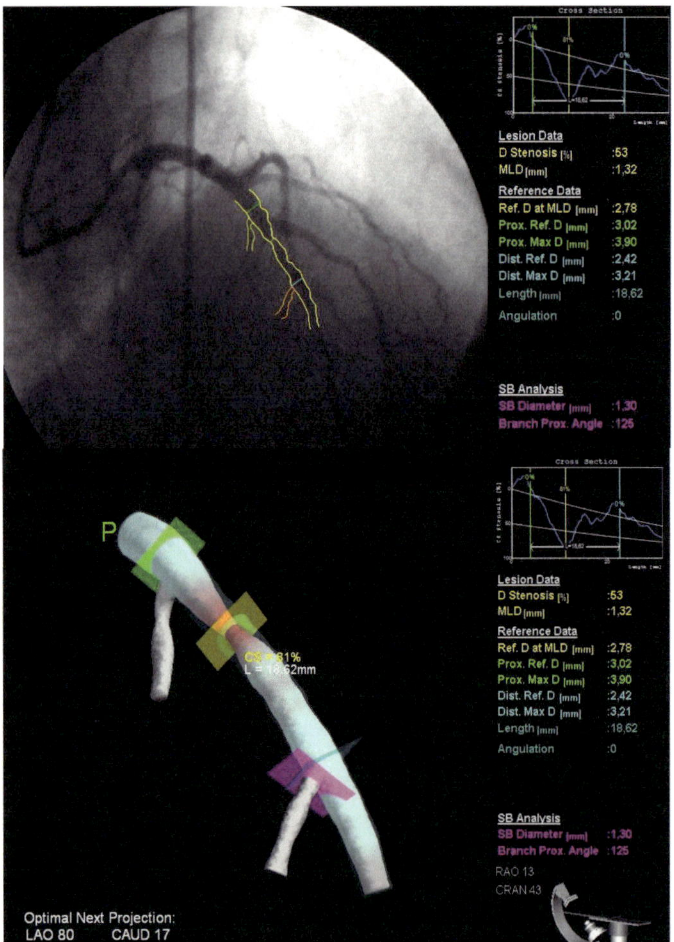

Fig. 8. An example of coronary bifurcation lesion reconstructed with 3D- CardiOp-B software.

In CAAS 5, a 3-D model of the central bifurcation area is constructed taking into account the fact that the contour information obtained from the 2-D projections may contain vessel overlap, since the bifurcated vessel might be partly obscured in at least one of the projections. To overcome this problem the 3-D cross-section shape is created using virtual vessel contours by virtue of information derived outside the bifurcation region (Onuma, 2011).

Cross-sectional area values are calculated on the assumption that the vessel has an elliptical cross section based on the luminal diameters from the two different 2-D projections; this elliptical cross-section is the primary measured parameter. The equivalent luminal diameter, minimum luminal diameter and maximal luminal diameter curves are calculated based on a circularity assumption. Reference vessel lines, up to the entrance of the POC and within the POC, are based on the 2-D approach adapted to 3-D.

So far, there is not direct comparison between these two QCA bifurcation software packages, both of which recostruct from two projections, thus the issue of overlapping vessels in tortuous bifurcation lesions may still be a problem. Particularly, there are two special challenging situations in QCA analysis: a diffusely diseased bifurcation region with no apparent healthy reference and an ostial stenosis in a short left main trunk (Girasis, 2010 b). Based on the scaling laws of Murray (Murray, 1926) and Finet (Finet, 2007), the size of any bifurcation vessel segment could be determined, if the reference of the other two vessel segments is known. This is not the case in a diffusely diseased bifurcation region; however, extrapolation of the reference of the PMV even on the basis of less accurate RVD values for the DMV and SB could avoid a gross underestimation of the PMV true size (Girasis, 2010 b).

In the case of an ostial stenosis in a short left main stem, both contour detection and sizing could be challenging. Manual contour corrections would not be unreasonable, especially if there is overlap with the angiographic catheter. For the RVD determination, either a user-defined reference outside the obstructions boundaries but within the left main, or a value back-calculated from the distal branches reference values can be chosen (Girasis, 2010 b).

Altough 3-D new techniques allow more extensive analyses for coronary bifurcations, there are several limitations such as reproducibility, accuracy and standard reference values for special lesion subsets that need further studies.

9. Conclusion

Although QCA was born more than 20 years ago and still burden well established limitations, it remains a useful tool in clinical research, whereas its role in clinical practice is mainly complementary to standard coronary angiography and other imaging techniques, such as computed tomography (CT), intravascular ultrasound (IVUS), virtual histology and optical coherence tomography. In recent years QCA has advanced to provide more accurate measurements and descriptions of the coronary vascular tree and still continues to evolve as 3D coronary angiographic techniques provide more detailed descriptions of complex lesions such as bifurcations, eccentric lesions and chronic total occlusions. However standard values in these lesions will need to be determined and validated.

10. References

Agostoni, P.; Biondi-Zoccai, G. & Van Langenhove, G. (2008). Comparison of assessment of native coronary arteries by standard versus three-dimensional coronary angiography. Am J Cardiol 102:272–279.

Bartunek, J.; Sys, S.U. & Heyndrickx, G.R.; (1995). Quantitative coronary angiography in predicting functional significance of stenoses in an unselected patient cohort. J Am Coll Cardiol 26:328–334.

Di Mario, C.; Werner, G.S. & Sianos, G. On behalf of the Euro CTO Club (2007). European perpective in the recanalizzation of Chronic Total Occlusion (CTO): consensus document from the Euro CTO Club. Eurointerv 3:30-43.

Dvir, D.; Marom, H. & Guetta, V. (2005). Three-dimensional coronary reconstruction from routine single plane coronary angiograms: in vivo quantitative validation. Int J Cardiovasc Intervent 7:141–145.

Dvir, D.; Marom, H. & Assali, A. (2007). Bifurcation lesions in the coronary arteries: early experience with a novel 3-dimensional imaging and quantitative analysis before and after stenting. EuroIntervention 3:95-9.

Dvir, D.; Assali, A. & Kornowski, R. (2008). Percutaneous coronary intervention for chronic total occlusion: novel 3-dimensional imaging and quantitative analysis. Catheter Cardiovasc Interv 71:784-789.

Fleming, R.M.; Kirkeeide, R.L. & Smalling, R.W. (1991). Patterns in visual interpretation of coronary arteriograms as detected by quantitative coronary arteriography. J Am Coll Cardiol 18:945–951.

Finet, G.G.M.; Perrenot, B. & Rioufol, G. (2007). Fractal geometry of arterial coronary bifurcations. A quantitative coronary angiography and intravascular ultrasound analysis. EuroInterv 3:490-498.

Fischer, J.J.; Samady, H. & McPherson, J.A. (2002). Comparison between visual assessment and quantitative angiography versus fractional flow reserve for native coronary narrowings of moderate severity. Am J Cardiol 90:210–215.

Galassi, A.R.; Tomasello, S.D. & Capodanno, D. (2010). A novel 3-d reconstruction system for the assessment of bifurcation lesions treated by the mini-crush technique. J Interv Cardiol 23:46-53.

Garrone, P.; Biondi-Zoccai, G. & Salvetti, I. (2009). Quantitative coronary angiography in the current era: principles and applications. J Interv Cardiol 22:527-536.

Gensini, G.G.; Kelly, A.E. & DaCosta, B.C.B. (1971). Quantitative angiography: The measurement of coronary vasomobility in the intact animal and man. Chest 60:522-530.

Girasis, C.; Serruys, P.W. & Onuma, Y. (2010a). 3-Dimensional Bifurcation Angle Analysis in Patients With Left Main Disease A Substudy of the SYNTAX Trial (SYNergy Between Percutaneous Coronary Intervention With TAXus and Cardiac Surgery). JACC Cardiovasc Interv 3:41-48.

Girasis, C.; van Jeuns, R.J. & Onuma, Y. (2010b). Essentials of quantitative angiography for bifurcation lesions. Eurontervention Supplement Vol. 6 (Supplement J) J36-J43.

Glagov, S.; Weisenberg, E. & Zarins, C.K. (1987). Compensatory enlargement of human atherosclerotic coronary arteries. N Engl J Med 316:1371–1375.

Gradaus, R.; Mathies, K.; Breithardt G, Bocker D (2006). Clinical assessment of a new real time 3D quantitative coronary angiography system: evaluation in stented vessel segments. Catheter Cardiovasc Interv 68:44–49.
Hausleiter, J.; Jost, S. & Nolte, C.W. (1997). Comparative in vitro validation of eight first- and second-generation quantitative coronary angiography systems. Coron Artery Dis 8:83–90.
Herrington, D.M.; Siebes, M. & Walford, G.D. (1993a). Sources of error in quantitative coronary angiography. Cathet Cardiovasc Diagn 29:314–321.
Herrington, D.M.; Siebes, M. & Sokol, D.K. (1993b). Variability in measures of coronary lumen dimensions using quantitative coronary angiography. J Am Coll Cardiol 22:1068–1074.
Kalbfleisch, S.J.; McGillem, M.J. & Pinto, I.M. (1990). Comparison of automated quantitative coronary angiography with caliper measurements of percent diameter stenosis. Am J Cardiol 65:1181–1184.
Kamiya, A. & Takahashi, T. (2007). Quantitative assessments of morphological and functional properties of biological trees based on their fractal nature. J Appl Physiol 102:2315–2323.
Kassab, G.S. (2006). Scaling laws of vascular trees: Of form and function. Am J Physiol Heart Circ Physiol 290:894–903.
Kinoshita, I.; Katoh, O. & Nariyama, J. (1995). Coronary angioplasty of chronic total occlusions with bridging collateral vessels: Immediate and follow-up outcome from a large single center experience. J Am Coll Cardiol 26:409–415.
Lansky, A.; Tuinenburg, J. & Costa, M. (2009). European Bifurcation Angiographic Sub-Committee. Quantitative Angiographic Methods for Bifurcation Lesions: A Consensus Statement from the European Bifurcation Group. Catheter Cardiovasc Interv 73:258-266.
Mancini, G.B.; Simon, S.B.; & McGillem, M.J. (1987). Automated quantitative coronary arteriography: morphologic and physiologic validation in vivo of a rapid digital angiographic method. Circulation 75:452–460.
Meerkin, D.; Marom, H. & Cohen-Biton, O. (2010). Three-dimensional vessel analyses provide more accurate length estimations than the gold standard QCA. J Interv Cardiol 23:152–159.
Murray, C.D. (1926) The physiological principle of minimum work. I. The vascular system and the cost of blood volume. Proc. Natl Acad. Sci. USA 12:207-214.
Ng, V.G. & Lansky, A.J (2011). Novel QCA methodologies and angiographic scores. Int J Cardiovasc Imaging 27:157-165.
Onuma, Y.; Girasis, C. & Aben, J.P. (2011). A novel dedicated 3-dimensional quantitative coronary analysis methodology for bifurcation lesions. Eurointervention [Ahead of Print].
Ramcharitar, S.; Daeman, J. & Patterson, M. (2008a). First direct in vivo comparison of two commercially available three-dimensional quantitative coronary angiography systems. Catheter Cardiovasc Interv 71:44–50.
Ramcharitar, S.; Onuma, Y. & Aben, J.P. (2008b). A novel dedicated qualitative coronary analysis methodology for bifurcation lesions. Eurointervention 3:553–557.

Reiber, J.H.; Serruys, P.W. & Kooijman, C.J. (1985). Assessment of short-, medium-, and long-term variations in arterial dimensions from computer-assisted quantitation of coronary cineangiograms. Circulation 71:280–288.

Saad, M.; Toelg, R. & Khattab, A.A. (2009). Determination of haemodynamic significance of intermediate coronary lesions using three-dimensional coronary reconstruction. Eurointervention 5:573–579.

Safian, R.D.; McCabe C.H. & Sipperly, M.E. (1988). Initial success and long-term follow-up of percutaneous transluminal coronary angioplasty in chronic total occlusions versus conventional stenoses. Am J Cardiol 61:23G–28G.

Schuurbiers, J.C.; Lopez, N.G. & Ligthart, J. (2009). In vivo validation of CAAS QCA-3D coronary reconstruction using fusion of angiography and intravascular ultrasound (ANGUS). Catheter Cardiovasc Interv 73:620–626.

Spahn, M.; Heer, V. & Freytag, R. (2003). Flat-panel detectors in X-ray systems. Radiologe 43:340–350.

Serruys, P.W.; Reiber, J.H.C. & Wijns, W (1984). Assessment of percutaneous transluminal coronary angioplasty by quantitative coronary angiography: Diameter versus densitometric area measurements. Am J Cardiol 54:482–488.

Spears, J.R.; Sandor, T. & Als, A.V. (1983). Computerized image analysis for quantitative measurement of vessel diameter from cineangiograms. Circulation 68:453–461.

Topol, E.J. & Nissen, S.E. (1995). Our preoccupation with coronary luminology. The dissociation between clinical and angiographic findings in ischemic heart disease. Circulation 92:2333–2342.

Tsuchida, K.; van der Giessen, W.J. & Patterson M (2007) In vivo validation of a novel three-dimensional quantitative coronary angiography system (CardiOp-B): comparison with a conventional two-dimensional system (CAAS II) and with special reference to optical coherence tomography. EuroIntervention 3:100–108.

Tu, S.; Koning, G. & Jukema, W. (2010). Assessment of obstruction length and optimal viewing angle from biplane X-ray angiograms. Int J Cardiovasc Imaging 26:5–17.

Tuinenburg, J.C.; Koning, G. & Seppenwoolde, Y. (2006). Is there an effect of flat-panel-based imaging systems on quantitative coronary and vascular angiography? Catheter Cardiovasc Interv 68:561-566.

Tuinenburg, J.C.; Koning, G. & Rareş, A. (2011). Dedicated bifurcation analysis: basic principles. Int J Cardiovasc Imaging 27:167-74.

Van der Zwet, P.M. & Reiber, J.H. (1994) A new approach for the quantification of complex lesion morphology: the gradient field transform; basic principles and validation results. J Am Coll Cardiol 24:216–224.

Van Herck, P.L.; Gavit, L. & Gorissen, P. (2004). Quantitative coronary arteriography on digital flat-panel system. Catheter Cardiovasc Interv 63:192–200.

Wellnhofer, E.; Wahle, A. & Mugaragu, I. (1999). Validation of an accurate method for three-dimensional reconstruction and quantitative assessment of volumes, lengths and diameters of coronary vascular branches and segments from biplane angiographic projections. Int J Card Imaging 15:339–353 discussion 355–356.

Yong, A.S.; Ng, A.C. & Brieger, D. (2011). Three-dimensional and two-dimensional quantitative coronary angiography, and their prediction of reduced fractional flow reserve. Eur Heart J 32:345-53.

15

Summarized Coronary Artery Caliber and Left Ventricle Mass for Scoring of Cardiac Ischemia: Diagnostic and Prognostic Value

Edvardas Vaicekavicius
Clinic of Radiology, Lithuanian University of Health Sciences
Lithuania

1. Introduction

1.1 Importance of methods for scoring coronary angiograms to reflect extent and severity of CAD

Despite advances in modern medicine, the early detection of patients with obstructive coronary lesions remains an unresolved problem due to frequently occurring atypical, painless, and asymptomatic clinical variants of ischemic heart disease. For example, 80 to 90% of sudden cardiac deaths occur with a background of significant coronary artery disease (Zipes, 1998) and sudden death is often the first presentation of the cardiac disease. It is estimated that sudden death occurs in 33% to 70% of cardiac disease patients (Davies, 2000). In addition, an acute myocardial infarction (MI) usually develops in patients with multi-vessel coronary disease (Goldstein et al., 2000), while angiographic studies have shown that an acute MI may develop in coronary segments having only slight or moderate stenosis. It is well known that a ruptured atheromatous plaque in the coronary artery can initiate intracoronary thrombosis and occlusion with the subsequent development of an acute MI. However, plaque rupture with platelet activation and thrombus formation are more recognized as the key events in the pathogenesis of acute coronary syndrome than are the extent and severity of the coronary artery disease (CAD). Additionally, the symptoms of myocardial ischemia may not be caused by obstructive lesions in the coronary arteries at all. Myocardial ischemia may occur not only due to decreased blood flow through epicardial coronary arteries, but also because of the increased oxygen demand in patients with myocardial hypertrophy or hyperfunction. Myocardial hypertrophy may be the cause of cardiac arrhythmias due to coronary insufficiency in hypertensive patients. However, even in the absence of obstructive CAD, hypertensive patients frequently have angina or may show electrocardiographic abnormalities suggestive of myocardial ischemia due to coronary insufficiency (Vogt et al., 1992).

In this era of great achievements in cardiology, we are still in need of a convenient and informative coronary arteries analysis system that would allow us to quantitatively estimate the size and severity of atherosclerotic CAD and myocardial ischemia burden.

1.2 Consecutive steps in development of coronary scoring methods

Initially, the purpose of creating methods to score coronary angiograms was to assess the severity of the underlying CAD and to determine whether the severity of angina and the degree of altered left ventricular function were closely correlated with the severity and extent of the underlying CAD. Multiple methods for evaluation and scoring of the coronary angiograms were created. However, there was no difference in the frequency of angina when the patients with the lowest coronary score were compared to patients with the highest coronary score (Leaman et al., 1981). Clinically, it is possible to have severe angina with one-vessel CAD or moderate angina with severe three-vessel CAD. Likewise, it is possible to have well-preserved left ventricular function with severe three-vessel CAD as well as to have severe left ventricular dysfunction with only one-vessel CAD.

Later, the coronary scores were used for risk stratification, because it was determined that the prognosis and outcomes in patients were in large part dependent on the extent (one-, two-, or three-vessel) and the severity of CAD (Ringqvist et al., 1983). This scoring system is still used today. Sullivan et al., (1990) developed a new angiographic scoring system for the extent of coronary disease (extent score). Therefore, the coronary scores seemed to be essential for the selection of a tailored therapeutic strategy. Subsequently, the coronary scores were used for the investigation of the relationship between the coronary lesion scores and the levels of serum lipoproteins (Hamsten et al., 1986; Jenkins et al., 1978). Eventually, a non-invasive coronary calcification scoring system became popular among investigators because coronary artery calcification strongly correlated with the severity of coronary atherosclerosis and the probability of obstructive disease (Kwon et al., 2011). The development of an invasive coronary scoring system would have to be much more effective in diagnosing and optimizing the treatment strategy, due to the fact that the non-invasive methods could not reflect the extent and severity of CAD.

In order to increase the value of the coronary scores in the selection of coronary patients for angioplasty, the American College of Cardiology/American Heart Association (ACC/AHA) in 1988 presented a system of classification of coronary lesions to predict the success and complications of balloon angioplasty (Krone et al., 2000). Although, the lesion type (A, B, or C) was not predictive of complications, specific lesion morphologies were predictive of adverse events and device use (Zaacks et al., 1998). Additionally, the type of lesion can impact the outcome of coronary bypass operations (Graham et al., 1999; Jalal, 2007). Thus, to choose an optimal revascularization strategy for patients with three-vessel and/or left-main-stem disease, there is one important requirement: to quantify the complexity of CAD while taking into account not only the number of significant lesions and their location, but also the complexity of each lesion independently. For this purpose, the SYNTAX scoring system was created (Garg et al., 2010; Sianos et al., 2005) The SYNTAX score was developed in order to characterize the coronary vasculature in terms of the number, functional impact, location, and complexity of the lesions.

However, in the myocardial infarction reperfusion era, it has become increasingly apparent that clinical outcomes are not only associated with coronary flow in the epicardial arteries but also with the quality of myocardial reperfusion. Quantitative angiographic indexes of coronary artery blood flow -- TIMI (thrombolysis in myocardial infarction) flow grades, corrected TIMI frame count, and TIMI myocardial perfusion grade -- gave new insights into the pathophysiology of acute coronary syndromes (Gibson et al., 1999, 2000, 2002; Korosoglou et al., 2007; Kunadian et al., 2009). Until recently, it was assumed that the blood flow in the non-culprit arteries in patients with acute coronary syndromes was normal. However, according to the data of Gibson et al., (2000) the coronary flow in the non-involved arteries in acute MI was, in fact, 40% slower than normal. It was also noted that the slower flow throughout all three arteries in acute MI could be associated not only with the extensive damage of microvasculature circulation but also might be the result of more extensive damage of non-culprit epicardial arteries. Greater lesion complexity might also be associated with poorer epicardial and myocardial perfusion.

1.3 The new challenges for coronary scoring

Because of these unresolved issues, it is imperative to extend the scope of investigations to include the impact of multi-vessel lesions in epicardial coronary arteries in order to elucidate the pathogenetic mechanism and prognosis of CAD. Therefore, we have created a completely new scoring system for the quantification of coronarography and ventriculography data. Using SYNTAX and other recent angiographic scoring methods, we often have no opportunity to assess the impact of myocardial mass and function on the myocardial ischemia and anginal severity. Hypertensive left ventricular hypertrophy is a powerful predictor of coronary events (Ghali et al., 1992; Koren et al., 1991) and develops due to impaired coronary blood flow autoregulation, decreased coronary reserve, increased minimal coronary vascular resistance, and carries an increased risk of cardiac death in the presence of coronary occlusion (Vogt et al., 1992). These events can be primarily dependent on the size and severity of the coronary lesions and on the functional and morphological status of the myocardium which requires a greater amount of blood for its nutrition. This new angiographic scoring system, which assesses the extent of coronary disease, myocardial mass, hypertrophy, and function, is simple to perform and it correlates better with the clinical symptoms of CAD.

2. Methods and patients

2.1 Different technical solutions in calculation of coronary scores

The exact quantification of total coronary artery damage is very complicated in clinical practice. Several different approaches have been proposed to determine the total coronary score: 1) the number of vessels diseased, 2) the number of proximal arterial segments diseased, 3) the proximal arterial segments score (Ringqvist et al., 1983), 4) the Friesinger index (Friesinger et al., 1970), 5) the modified Gensini index (Gensini et al., 1971), 6) the National heart and chest hospital (NHCH) index (Ringqvist et al., 1983), and 7) other methods. The most common problems with these methods were: 1) the interpretational differences in the estimation of the percentage of coronary artery narrowing due to differences in the selection of optimal reference diameter (Brown et al., 1977; Dodge et al., 1988), 2) the difficulties in the accurate assessment of the true hemodynamic value for each narrowing, 3) the difficulties in angiographic quantification of diffuse CAD (Graham et al., 1999; Jalal, 2007), and 4) the differences in techniques of measurements (Kalbfleisch et al., 1990). The hemodynamic value used by some authors is set only by the degree of narrowing. By other authors, the severity of luminal narrowing is weighted according to the usual flow to the left ventricle in each coronary vessel (Leaman et al., 1981) and according to the flow to muscle mass rather than to the actual volume of flow (Brandt et al., 1977; Gensini, 1983). However, it is difficult to accurately assess the coronary artery blood supply zones due to variable coronary artery dominance and multiple branching options. Still some authors tend to offset the impact of longevity of stenosis (Dodge et al., 1992) on myocardial blood flow.

However, the determined angiographic CAD scores in most cases had a poor correlation with the severity of angina pectoris and myocardial function. Therefore, the development of new coronary scoring methods needs a different approach from those which have been previously adopted for the accounting of coronary obstructions only.

2.2 Technique for determination of summarized caliber of coronary arteries and left ventricle mass

It is well established that the development and progression of CAD involves three processes: the reduction of the total caliber of coronary arteries, the increase in myocardium weight, and the deterioration of left ventricular pump function. Therefore, we have sought to create a specific coronary lesion scoring system which would avoid the subjectivity in the determination of degree of stenosis and in the selection of normal reference diameter which is highly variable and dependant on multiple variants in coronary dominance and branching.

The severity of the coronary lesion was expressed by the sum of residual calibers of all coronary arteries in the selected level. The extent of the coronary lesion was expressed by the calculation of the summarized caliber of three levels (Fig. 1). The narrowest diameters of the selected segments were used to calculate the coronary caliber expressed by coronary square area (CSA = $0.785 \times D^2$). The assessment of the SCCA at the first coronary branching level included the sum of the cross-sectional areas at the narrowest points of the 1st and 5th segments, at the second level - the areas of the 2nd, 6th, and 11th segments, and at the third level - the areas of the 3rd, 7th , 9th, 12th , and 13th segments. The average of the arterial calibers at each level was considered to be the SCCA.

The computer-assisted calculating algorithm for SCCA is very simple, and coronary diameters can be measured using a quantitative analysis program readily available in almost every modern angiographic unit. We measured the narrowest diameters of each coronary segment in at least two projections of video images. In cases of uncommon variants of coronary dominance or branching, we also measured and summed all segments of the trunk below its second bifurcation.

Contrasting of the left ventricle was performed while the patient was taking a deep breath at the right anterior oblique 30° body position. We performed a quantitative analysis of the ventriculographic data using the radial method (Fig. 2). We computed the end-systolic and diastolic volumes and estimated the myocardial mass by determining the wall thickness of the left ventricle. The end-systolic and end-diastolic volumes were calculated using the equation for spherical formations:

$$V = 4/3 \pi R_a^3 \times K \quad (1)$$

In the equation above, we used the following abbreviations: V – systolic or diastolic volume, R_a – average systolic or diastolic radius (cm), and K – a factor of correction.

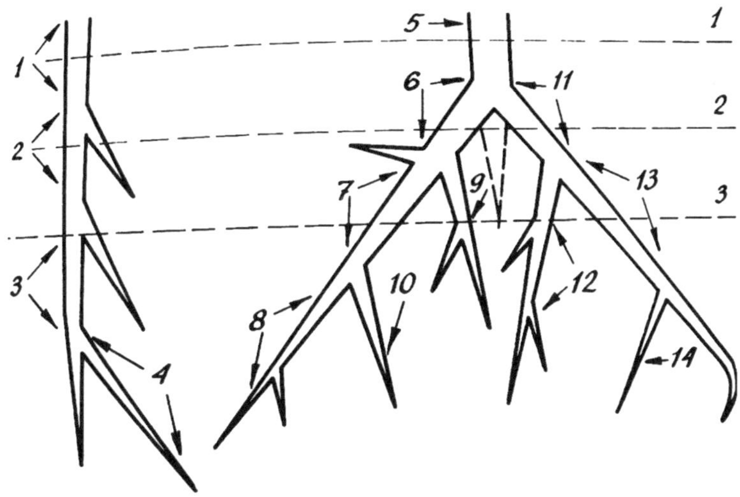

Fig. 1. A scheme of 15 segments of the coronary tree proposed by the American Heart Association which was used to calculate the summarized caliber of coronary arteries (SCCA). The cross-sectional areas in the narrowest points of the segments at each level were added together to represent the coronary caliber at one of the three coronary tree levels: above the first bifurcation, below the first bifurcation, or below the second bifurcation of the right and left coronary arteries. The average of the arterial calibers at the three levels was considered to be the average SCCA.

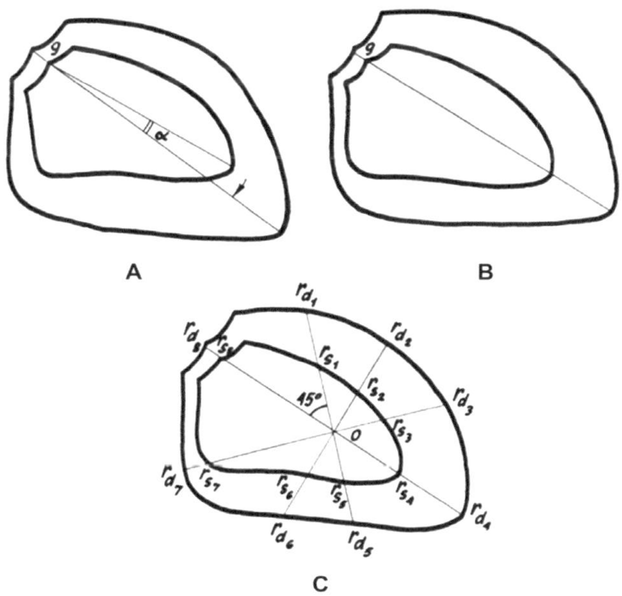

Fig. 2. Radial scheme used in the quantitative analysis of ventriculographic data: A -- superposed end-systolic and end-diastolic profiles of the left ventricle with the α angle of apex rotation; B -- superposed end-systolic and end-diastolic contours after the correction of apex rotation; C -- a scheme of radial delineation; we used the midpoint of the long axis of left ventricle (in diastole) to intersect the radial lines.

We calculated the left ventricular mass using the thickness (h) of the anterior wall of the left ventricle using the following equation:

$$LVM = (4/3 \pi \times (h + R_a)^3 \times K - 4/3 \pi R_a^3 \times K) \times 1.05 \quad (2)$$

In the equation above, we used the following abbreviations: LVM -- left ventricular mass, h -- thickness of the anterior wall of left ventricle (cm), R_a --average systolic or diastolic radius (cm), K – a factor of correction, and 1.05 – a comparative weight of the myocardium (g/cm^3). We measured the thickness of the anterior wall of the left ventricle at the midpoint between the aortic valve and the apex.

2.3 Creation of the angiographic characteristics of myocardial supply

2.3.1 Angiographic coronary index

Initially, the SCCA was indexed to the supplied left ventricular mass. This parameter was intended for the expression of the morphologic adequacy between the coronary artery tree and the supplied myocardial mass. This diagnostic criterion was entitled angiographic coronary index (ACI) and was calculated according the formula:

$$ACI = (SCCA/LVM) \times 10 \quad (3)$$

In the equation above, we used the following abbreviations: ACI -- angiographic coronary index, SCCA -- summarized caliber of coronary arteries (mm^2), LVM – mass of the left ventricle (g), and 10 -- normalization factor used to reduce the average value of the index to 1.
During the post-mortem examinations, we performed a post-mortem coronary angiography, an excision of coronary arteries by cutting them in intervals of 10 mm to analyze their luminal square areas by planimetry. An autopsy of both ventricles was performed with the separation of its masses with and without fatty tissues. We found that the patients without any cardiovascular disease had the SCCA-to-LVM ratio approximately equal to 1. The ratio was also almost the same as in the control group of patients who had no CAD symptoms.

2.3.2 Angiographic anginal index

Myocardial quantity (mass) does not represent the quality of myocardial tissue nor its viability or its demand for arterial supply; instead, the greater myocardial mass usually represents a lower functional status. To represent the functional status of the myocardium, we used a ratio between the angiographic coronary index (ACI) and the ejection fraction of the left ventricle (LVEF). We named the ratio an anginal index, because we noticed a very prominent negative correlation between this index and the intensity of angina. However, there was no correlation between the ACI and LVEF.
When the ACI exceeded 1.0 and the ACI was higher than the LVEF, the inadequacy between the blood supply and the demand was theoretically absent. In contrast, when the ACI was less than the LVEF, the inadequacy was present. The angiographic anginal index in these cases was less than 1.0. Therefore, the angiographic anginal index allowed us to express quantitatively the favorable conditions for myocardial ischemia.

2.3.3 Angiographic prognostic index

The complete characterization of the myocardial perfusion state and its prognostic impact on the follow-up results using only the ACI-to-LVEF ratio was not possible. For example, in patients with decreased SCCA and low LVEF (due to the presence of post-infarction myocardial scars) the ratio did not show the inadequacy between the blood supply and demand and masked the poor prognosis for these patients. Both the diminished SCCA and the lowered LVEF may equally increase risk in patients. Therefore, the compound of ACI and LVEF was labeled angiographic prognostic index (API). It was calculated using this equation:

$$API = ACI + LVEF = (SCCA / LVM) + LVEF \quad (4)$$

In the equation above, the API stands for the angiographic risk index, ACI -- angiographic coronary index, SCCA -- summarized caliber of coronary arteries (mm^2), LVM - mass of the left ventricle (g), and LVEF - ejection fraction of the left ventricle.

2.4 Patient groups

In this way, we have quantitatively analyzed coronarographic and ventriculographic data in 403 patients with different clinical forms of ischemic heart disease. All patients were divided into groups according to the size and severity of coronary obstructions and the left ventricular mass. There were 59 (14.6%) patients with normal coronary arteries, 165 (40.9%) patients with arteries narrowed up to 50% of diameter, and 179 (44.4%) patients with lesions which obstructed more than 50% of the coronary artery diameter. Among patients with coronary narrowing of up to 50%, 88 (24.8%) patients had a normal ventricular weight and 77 (19.1%) had an increased weight of the left ventricle. The patients with increased left myocardial weight were divided into two subgroups: the cardiomyopathy (obstructive and hypertrophic) subgroup and the secondary hypertrophy due to hypertension subgroup. The majority of patients (82 or 45.8%) with obstructions of more than 50% had coronary disease of a single branch, 67 (37.4%) patients had disease in two branches, and the remaining 30 (16.7%) patients had lesions in all three branches. Twenty six (14.5%) patients had left main coronary artery disease. The average age of patients was 47.8 ± 0.4 years. The dominant gender was male (95.5%). Additionally, patients were divided into groups according to clinical diagnosis (stable angina pectoris, post-infarction angina, hypertensive cardiopathy, and hypertrophic cardiomyopathy). The follow-up results after 2 to 7 years were analyzed in 136 patients with CAD (52 underwent surgery, and 84 were treated conservatively). Thirteen of these patients died after surgical intervention, and nineteen died after conservative treatment.

We performed 176 necropsy examinations with postmortem coronarography and epicardial excision of the coronary trunks. The trunks were cut in slices for morphologic analysis and the myocardium of the right and left ventricles was separated into three parts according to the supply zones of the anterior descending artery, the circumflex branch of the left coronary artery, and the right coronary artery. The majority (n = 146) of these patients died from CAD: 70 patients experienced sudden death and the rest died from different complications of CAD. Three control groups were formed from the remaining 30 patients who died from other, non-cardiac diseases: the 1st control group was comprised of patients who died younger than age 50, the second control group was comprised of patients who died older than age 50, and the third control group included patients of any age who died having signs of cardiac hypertrophy without any obstructions in the coronary arteries.

2.4.1 Statistical analysis

The study data was processed using STATISTICA 5 and SPSS 10 (Statistical Package for Social Science) software. All data were presented as mean values ± standard deviations. The following statistical methods of analysis were used: paired t-test for differences in groups, t-test for differences between two groups, ANOVA for differences between multiple groups, and chi-square (χ^2) - for categorical data. A p-value less than 0.05 was regarded as statistically significant.

3. Results

3.1 Calculation of angiographic coronary index using autopsy data

The necropsy study consisted of the following parts: 1) performance of the post-mortem coronary angiography (Fig. 3A); 2) the longitudinal excision of contrasted coronary artery trunks from the myocardial tissue and cutting them into 10 mm-long pieces for microscopic analysis, and 3) the division of the myocardial mass of both ventricles (with and without fatty tissues) into three parts according to the supply regions of the right coronary artery, the circumflex branch and the anterior descending artery (Fig. 3B).

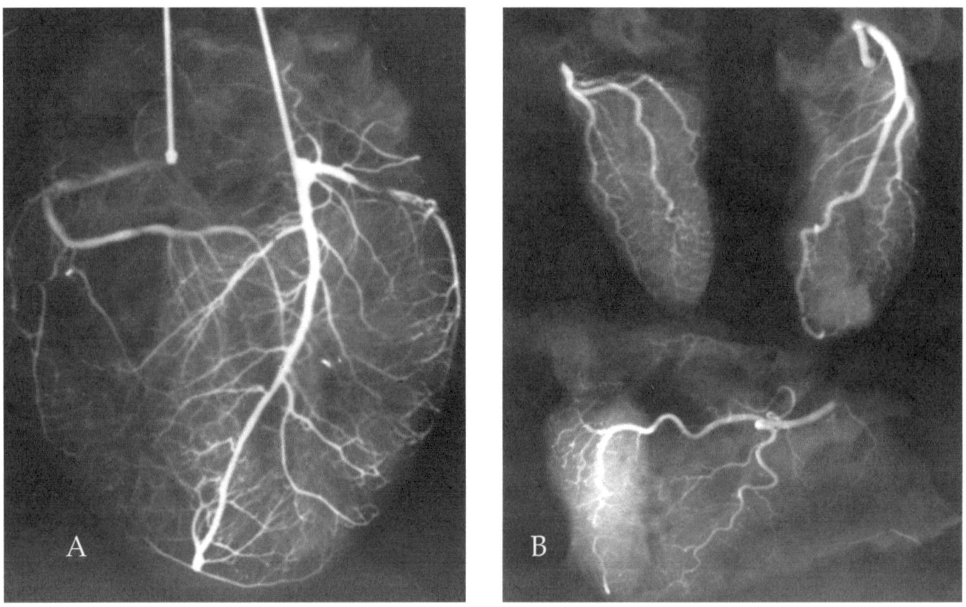

Fig. 3. The anteroposterior view of postmortem coronary angiography (A). Myocardial cutting into parts differing according to blood supply regions: in the upper left position is the part supplied by the circumflex branch, in the upper right is the part supplied by anterior descending artery, and in the bottom is the part supplied by the dominant right coronary artery (B).

The coronary arteries were contrasted with 40% solution of $BaSO_4$. The contrast material was injected using 120 mmHg pressure through a special cannula inserted and fixed into the orifice of the right and left coronary arteries (Fig. 3). The coronarograms were made after the stagnation of contrast material. The measurements of the coronary arteries were performed using the methodology for the determination of SCCA. The second step was supplemented by weighing the different parts of the myocardium, by calculation of the coronary caliber, and by the assessment of the three separate ACIs for each coronary artery.

The examination of the arterial cuts revealed the diffuse nature of the obstructive lesions in patients who died suddenly or died after complications of chronic heart disease. In the control group of younger patients, the slight narrowing (less than 50%) covered only 5.9 - 8.1% of the coronary artery length. In the second control group of older patients, the same lesions covered 9.8 to 13.3% of coronary artery length. However, in patients who died from CAD, the total length of the obstructed segments covered from 73.6% to 91.6% of coronary artery length; furthermore, one-half of the segments had less than 50% narrowing. This means that the quantitative estimation of the degree of stenosis using the referential normal adjacent segment for calculation may often be incorrect.

The assessment of the coronary artery diameter without the calculation of the degree of stenosis is more objective. The SCCA in control patients was almost the same at each level and there were no significant differences between the control groups. However, the difference between each level SCCA of the two groups of died patients, from one side, and of the three control groups, from other side, was noticed (Table 1). These findings are a consequence of differences in the size, location, and severity of obstruction in CAD patients. At the same time the decrease in SCCA with the simultaneous increase in myocardial weight was fixed in patients who died from sudden coronary death or from CAD complications (Table 2).

Patient groups	No. of pts.	SCCA of different levels, mm^2		
		1st level	2nd level	3rd level
1st control group (age 34.2 ± 10.2 yrs.)	12	27.1 ± 5.2	29.1 ± 1.5	24.8 ± 4.2
2nd control group (age 67.5 ± 9.7 yrs.)	9	25.2 ± 5.4	25.6 ± 6.0	25.0 ± 4.6
3rd control group (LV hypertrophy)	7	23.6 ± 7.2	25.6 ± 5.6	24.3 ± 4.5
4th group (sudden coronary death)	14	14.9 ± 6.8	7.58 ± 3.3	11.7 ± 4.2
5th group (death from CAD complications)	17	12.9 ± 7.4	10.3 ± 4.0	7.8 ± 4.7

Table 1. The summarized caliber of coronary arteries of three levels in different groups of died patients.

The post-mortem assessment of the ACI in the first and second control groups has shown that the value of the ACI slightly exceeded 1. Additional analysis showed that the ACI of the right coronary artery was lower than the ACI of the left coronary artery ($p < 0.03$). This distinction could be caused by functional peculiarities of both ventricles. Because the SCCA was almost the same in all three groups, the diminished ACI in the third group was associated with the increased weight of the myocardium. However, the SCCA in patients of the fourth and the fifth groups with CAD was significantly smaller, and the ACI was consequently low, also.

Patient groups	No. of pts.	SCCA, ACI, and myocardial mass		
		Average SCCA, mm^2	ACI	Myocardial mass without lipid tissue, g
1st control group (age 34.2 ± 10.2 yrs.)	12	27.2 ± 3.9	1.41 ± 3.90	226.4 ± 11.0
2nd control group (age 67.5 ± 9.7 yrs.)	9	25.3 ± 4.4	1.42 ± 0.16	209.9 ± 12.2
3rd control group (LV hypertrophy)	7	25.0 ± 4.4	0.84 ± 0.06	337.8 ± 4.90
4th group (sudden coronary death)	14	11.1 ± 3.2	0.14 ± 0.04	306.0 ± 17.6
5th group (death from CAD complications)	17	9.9 ± 4.5	0.22 ± 0.04	305.1 ± 12.7

Table 2. The SCCA, ACI, and myocardial mass in different groups of deceased patients.

Six sudden death patients in the fourth group had no obvious segmental obstructions in their coronary arteries; however, the ACI was significantly lower (0.62 ± 0.01) than the control values ($p < 0.001$). The lowered ACI was caused by increased left ventricular weight and lowered SCCA, compared to the control groups. The detailed analysis of the myocardium in these patients did not revealed any signs of myocardial infarction. We may assume that the relative insufficiency could be the starting mechanism for the expressed myocardial ischemia and for the possible life threatening arrhythmia. This background factor of inadequacy between the SCCA and the myocardial mass could be a cause of the sudden coronary death.

3.2 Assessment of angiographic characteristics of myocardial supply (ACMS) in clinical setting

Various authors have expressed difficulties in creating an unbiased angiographic coronary scoring system intended for researchers as well as for clinical practice. In particular, all the diagnostic and prognostic capabilities of angiographic coronary scoring remain undetermined.

3.2.1 Difficulties in assessment of angiographic coronary scores associated with the anatomical variability of coronary dominance and branching

Because only three types of anatomic variants of coronary dominance are commonly used in previous scoring systems and all possible coronary branching types are not taken into consideration, the hemodynamic value of each stenosis might be calculated inaccurately.

We have analyzed the impact of coronary dominance on the diameters of all fifteen coronary segments while using not three but six types of coronary dominance. The six types were determined using the ratio between the myocardial mass supplied by the right and the myocardial mass supplied by the left coronary arteries. Using a topographic scheme shown in Fig. 4, we have calculated the ratio by delineating myocardial zones supplied by the right and left coronary arteries. Coronarograms performed in the left and right anterior oblique 30° views are shown in the upper part of the figure. The views are most informative in understanding the branching peculiarities of both coronary arteries supplying the posterior and inferior walls of the left ventricle. A percept used to calculate the amount of myocardial tissue supplied by the right and left coronary arteries is shown in the lower part of the picture. This approach was chosen according the information obtained from post-mortem studies. The whole myocardial tissue (mass) was assigned 20 conceptual mass units. Five units were assigned to the right ventricle, another five to the septum (3 units to the anterior and 2 units to the posterior septum), and the remaining 10 units were assigned to the mass of the left ventricle divided into ten equal parts.

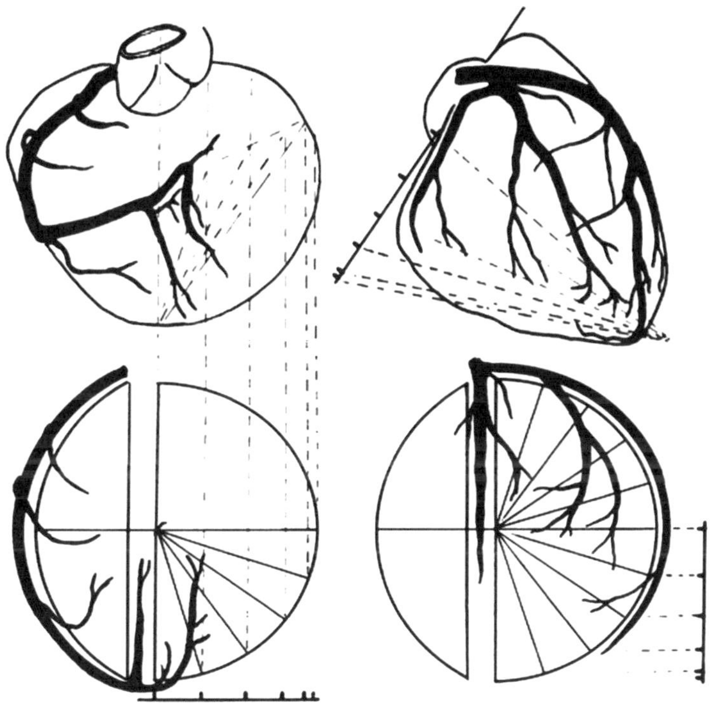

Fig. 4. Topographic schemes reflecting the delineation and calculation of myocardial zones and mass supplied by the right and left coronary arteries. The lines divide myocardial tissue of the left ventricle into 10 zones (units), each of similar mass. Using the same principle, the right ventricle was assigned 5 units, the anterior septum -- 3 units, and the posterior septum -- 2 units.

Using this technique we could quantitatively define all possible variants of coronary blood supply to the right and left myocardial masses. To indicate the type of coronary dominance we used the ratio between myocardial masses supplied by the right and left coronary arteries. We used the R:L notation (where R and L correspond to the number of mass units supplied by the right and left coronary arteries). For example, the 5:15 ratio would indicate that 5 units were assigned to the right, and 15 units to the left myocardial supply zone. We have encountered the six most common variants of coronary dominance -- 5:15 (potentially, the variant of the left dominance), 6:14; 7:13; 8:12; 9:11, and 10:10 (potentially, the variant of the right dominance).

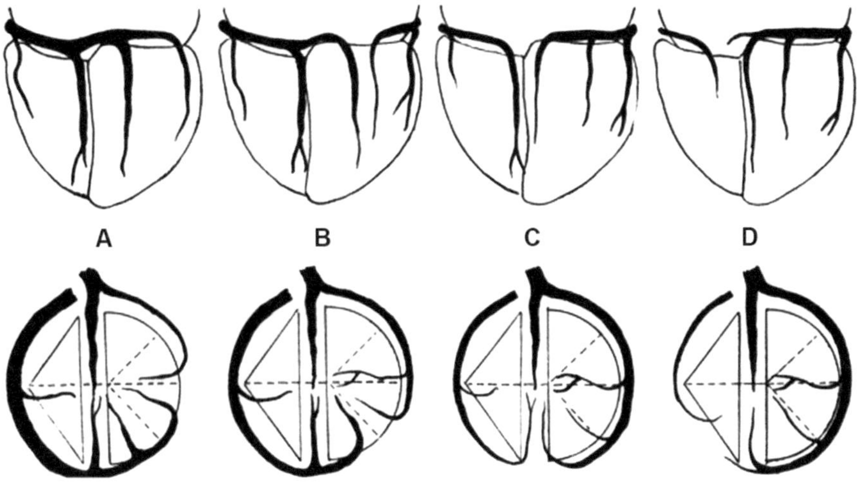

Fig. 5. The quantitative expression of coronary dominance: A, 12:8; B, 9:11; C, 6:14; D, 4:16.

The usage of the right-to-left myocardial mass ratio allowed us to define the coronary dominance variants more precisely (Fig. 5). Dividing control patients into the six groups (according to the most common coronary dominance variants) allowed us to obtain significant differences in segment diameters of the circumflex branch of the left coronary artery and the right coronary artery between all groups. However, there was no statistical difference between all groups according to the segments of the left anterior descending artery, because the caliber of these segments is more stable with respect to the variations in coronary dominance.

We have identified the four most frequent variants of coronary branching (Fig. 6) while using these topographic schemes for a more thorough analysis of the coronary supply zones. It is interesting to note that the following four variants of coronary branching had the exact same ratio of coronary dominance determined by the myocardial supply zones. However, the correlation between the caliber of the coronary segments and the size of their myocardial supply zones was found to be very high ($r = 0.96$) despite the variability of coronary dominance and branching. This finding shows the fundamental importance of assessing the contiguous segments to estimate the real degree of stenosis, because diameters of adjacent arterial segments usually visible in coronarograms may be diminished because of the diffuse obstructive changes in adjacent coronary arteries, and it becomes very difficult to decide whether the particular segment is damaged or not. Therefore, the assessment of the coronary lesion score using SCCA appears to be more objective; it does not require consideration of the coronary dominance and branching. At the same time, the location and degree of atherosclerotic obstructions may be detected automatically by measuring the diameter of the narrowest point in every segment at several levels. Therefore, to increase the accuracy of coronary scoring, it is important to calculate the SCCA in a higher number of levels.

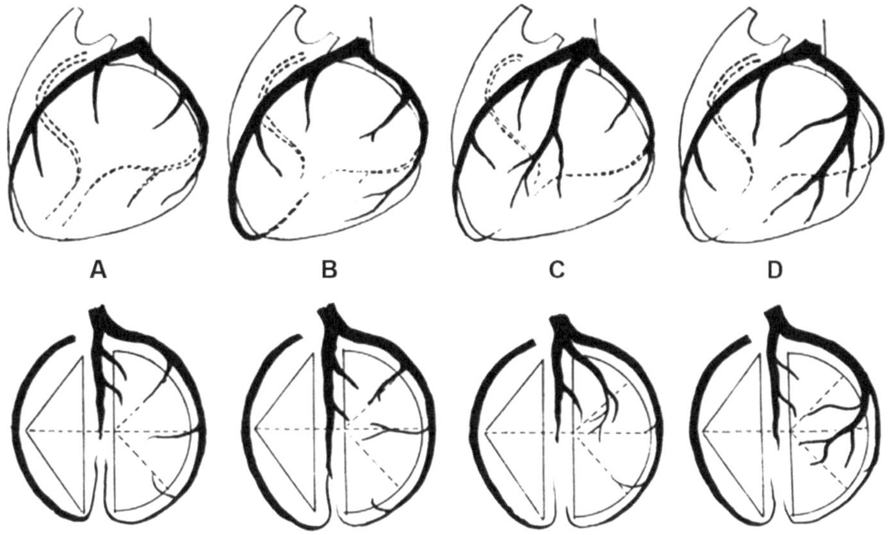

Fig. 6. The most frequent variants of coronary branching: A, common (6:14); B, left anterior descending dominance (6:14); C, trifurcation (6:14); and D, marginal (6:14).

3.2.2 Correlation between summarized caliber of coronary arteries and different angiographic coronary scores

We have analyzed the correlation between the data obtained by SCCA and by other coronary scores. The diagnostic features of the Friesinger, Leaman, and Gensini scores or indexes dedicated for the quantitative expression of the extent and severity of CAD were compared with each other and with SCCA.

The Friesinger index ranges from 0 to 15. Each of the three main coronary arteries is scored separately from zero to five. The scores are: 0 -- no arteriographic abnormalities; 1 - a trivial luminal narrowing less than 29%; 2 - a localized 30 to 68% luminal narrowing; 3 -- multiple 30 to 68% luminal narrowing; 4 -- 69 to 100% luminal narrowing without 100% occlusion of proximal segments; and 5 -- total obstruction of a proximal segment.

The Leaman index has another weighting system. If the vessel was totally occluded, the coronary artery segment value was multiplied by 5.0. If there was a 90 to 99% occlusion, it was multiplied by 3.0. For a 70 to 89% obstruction, it was multiplied by 1.0. The segmental scores were then added to derive the total coronary score.

The modified Gensini index assigns a heavier weight to the more severe luminal narrowing (Gensini, 1983). Weights are also assigned to each segment depending on vessel size and importance; segments serving larger regions of myocardium are more heavily weighted. For example, the left main coronary artery receives the heaviest weight. Each arterial segment is weighted by a value from 0.5 to 5.0. (The weight for segments 1 through 4 is changed to 0.5 if the system is left dominant.) The stenosis is weighted from 2 to 64. The product of these two weights is the total weight for each arterial segment. The modified Gensini index is the sum of the total weights for each segment. For each segment the two weights are multiplied. The sum of the products is the modified Gensini score.

So, we have compared fundamentally different angiographic coronary scoring methods taking into account: 1) the degree of stenosis regarding the diameters of adjacent segments,

2) the degree (weight) of stenosis for each segment regarding the three types of coronary dominancy, and 3) the average SCCA. The comparative analysis of different scoring methods showed that the lowest correlation was observed between the methods that were based on different coronary scoring principles. For example, Friesinger index has only moderate correlation with ACI (r = -0.45). The correlation between Gensini index and ACI was only insignificantly better (r = -0.54). However, the correlation between Friesinger and Gensini indexes was high (r = 0.84).

3.3 Value of angiographic characteristics of myocardial supply in diagnostic improvements

Primarily, we investigated the relationship between angiographic characteristics of myocardial supply (ACMS), on the one hand, and clinical symptoms of myocardial ischemia and clinical forms of ischemic heart disease, on the other hand. For the expression of myocardial supply features by angiographic characteristics, we have chosen what we consider the three most important summarized indices of all angiographic indices, namely, the angiographic coronary index (ACI), the angiographic anginal index (AAI), and the angiographic prognostic index (API).

3.3.1 Interrelation between clinical symptoms of CAD and the angiographic characteristics of myocardial supply

The dependence of ACMS from the functional class of angina pectoris determined according to the classification of Canadian Cardiovascular Society is shown in Table 3. The data show that there is a very well defined relationship between all ACMS and the clinical severity of anginal symptoms. In addition, we have analyzed the relationship between the ACMS and the character of anginal pain (Table 4). Patients were divided into 3 groups: the 1st group consisted of patients with atypical prolonged anginal pain, the 2nd group -- of patients with typical anginal symptoms, and the 3rd group -- of patients who had typical pain but after an effective treatment of acute MI the anginal symptoms disappeared.

Class of Angina Pectoris	No. of pts.	SCCA, mm^2	ACI (SCCA / LV mass)	AAI (ACI / LVEF)	API (ACI+EF)
1°	49	23.4 ±1.0	0.68 ± 0.03	1.0 ± 0.06	0.78 ± 0.07
2°	21	18.0 ± 1.1	0.49 ± 0.04	0.8 ± 0.08	0.45 ± 0.08
3°	22	13.2 ± 0.7*	0.39 ± 0.05	0.6 ± 0.03	0.23.9 ± 0.14
P	1 vs. 2	0.001	0.001	0.019	0.006
	1 vs. 3	0.001	0.013	0.007	0.007
	2 vs. 3	0.005	0.009	0.05	0.05

Table 3. ACMS in patients with different functional class of angina pectoris.

All angiographic characteristics were worse in patients with typical angina (2nd group) compared to patients with atypical chest pain (1st group). Similar significant differences were discovered between the 1st and 3rd groups of patients who did not have the post-infarction angina. The patients who did not have the post-infarction angina also had worse average SCCA, ACI, and anginal index. It is interesting that there were no differences in ACMS between patients in the 2nd (typical angina) and 3rd groups (no post-MI angina).

Character of anginal pain	No. of pts.	Average SCCA, mm^2	ACI (SCCA / LV mass)	AAI (ACI /LVEF)	API (ACI+EF)
1° atypical AP	49	27.3 ± 1.2	71.1 ± 4.1	1.0 ± 0.05	0.71 ± 0.07
2° typical AP	21	20.8 ± 1.2	57.2 ± 2.9	0.83 ± 0.06	0.48 ± 0.05
3° disappeared post-MI AP	22	22.9 ± 2.2	48.7 ± 4.4	1.33 ± 0.1	0.63 ± 0.1
P	1 vs. 2	0.001	0.009	0.05	0.05
	1 vs. 3	0.05	0.001	0.05	
	2 vs. 3			0.004	

Table 4. Angiographic characteristics of myocardial supply in patients with different character of anginal pain. The statistical significance of the differences in angiographic characteristics between the three different characters of anginal pain is shown in the lower part of the table.

However, the difference in the angiographic anginal index between these three groups existed not because of the difference in SCCA but because of the difference in left-ventricular ejection fraction that was evidently lower in post-MI patients. Furthermore, there was no inadequacy between the diminished SCCA and the diminished left-ventricular ejection fraction in post-infarction patients.

3.3.2 Interrelation between clinical forms of coronary artery disease and angiographic characteristics of myocardial supply

We have studied the levels of ACMS in patients divided into groups according to the different clinical forms of ischemic heart disease. The values of different ACMS obtained from patients with different clinical diagnoses of ischemic heart disease are shown in Table 5. The SCCA was highest in control patients and lowest in patients with multivessel CAD. The SCCA of all patients groups with CAD was lower compared with the groups without CAD. This consistent pattern was observed in the comparison of patients according to ACI, except that the ACI was the same in patients with one vessel disease and in patients with myocardial hypertrophy. The same regularity was noted between groups compared according to AAI and API. The anginal syndrome was expressed mostly in patients with multi-vessel disease. The AAI and API were equally expressed between patients with one-vessel disease and patients with myocardial hypertrophy.

The various ACMS in patients with different clinical forms of myocardial infarction are shown in table 6. The 1st group included patients with myocardial infarction without ST segment elevation (NSTEMI). The 2nd group included patients with ST elevation myocardial infarction (STEMI).

After comparing both groups of patients, we noticed that NSTEMI and STEMI were significantly different according to AAI and API only. The SCCA and ACI differed insignificantly. The API was worse in NSTEMI patients. Similar findings confirm the studies of other authors.

Diagnosis	No. of pts.	SCCA, mm^2	ACI (SCCA / LV mass)	AAI (ACI /LVEF)	API (ACI+EF)
Stable AP in patients with one-vessel disease	101	18.9 ± 0.66^1	57.2 ± 2.32^2	0.82 ± 0.04^3	128.4 ± 2.75^4
Stable AP in patients with multi-vessel disease	34	12.6 ± 1.40	30.3 ± 3.47	0.50 ± 0.07	93.7 ± 5.06
Stable post-infarction AP	96	18.7 ± 0.83^1	49.2 ± 2.41	1.04 ± 0.07	101.9 ± 3.40
Stable AP with myocardial hypertrophy & insignificant CAD	110	23.7 ± 0.64	56.0 ± 1.36^2	0.82 ± 0.024^3	127.2 ± 2.09^4
Controls without CAD and AP	35	32.8 ± 1.23	95.2 ± 4.44	1.5 ± 0.091	163.2 ± 6.0

Table 5. ACMS in different groups of patients with ischemic heart disease. Statistically significant differences ($P < 0.01$) were found between all groups of patients, except the groups shown in superscript.

MI in anamnesis	No. of pts.	SCCA, mm^2	ACI (SCCA / LV mass)	AAI (ACI /LVEF)	API (ACI+EF)
NSTEMI (1st group)	21	18.1 ± 1.0	51.7 ± 3.2	0.93 ± 0.08	0.45 ± 0.05
STEMI (2nd group)	22	21.3 ± 1.1	55.1 ± 5.5	0.75 ± 0.04	0.79 ± 0.08
P value	2 vs. 3			0.001	0.008

Table 6. ACMS in groups of patients with different clinical forms of myocardial infarction.

3.4 Evaluation of angiographic characteristics of myocardial supply in predicting of outcomes

Death of cardiac origin has occurred in only 32 out of 136 patients analyzed during the seven-year follow-up period. We did not notice any progression of disease after 3 to 7 years in 40 patients with CAD who had a slightly lower ACI and left-ventricular ejection fraction but normal prognostic index. We performed a detailed analysis of ACMS indices in patients who died within three years (Table 7).

Myocardial infarction in anamnesis	No. of pts.	SCCA, mm^2	LVEF	ACI (SCCA / LV mass)	AAI (ACI / LVEF)	API (ACI+EF)
Death during the 3rd year (1st group)	7	20.7 ± 8.2	0.53 ± 0.03	0.51 ± 0.04	0.98 ± 0.03	1.04 ± 0.05
Death during the 2nd year (2nd group)	5	22.7 ± 6.6	0.29 ± 0.03	0.31 ± 0.05	1.07 ± 0.05	0.60 ± 0.08
Death during the 1st year (3rd group)	6	14.3 ± 0.1	0.67 ± 0.04	0.36 ± 0.06	0.53 ± 0.06	1.03 ± 0.09
P	1 vs. 2		0.001	0.05		0.001
	1 vs. 3				0.001	
	2 vs. 3		0.001		0.001	0.01

Table 7. ACMS in patients who died within three years.

All 18 patients were divided into 3 groups: the 1st group ($n = 7$) consisted of patients who died during the third year of investigation, the 2nd group ($n = 5$) of patients who died during the second year of investigation, and the 3rd group ($n = 6$) of patients who died during the first year of investigation. Patients who died during the first year after coronarography had the most diminished average SCCA, but their left-ventricular ejection fraction was normal. These patients usually experienced a sudden coronary death. However, the patients who died later, during the 2nd year after investigation, had not only a lower ACI but also a lower left-ventricular ejection fraction. They usually died from heart failure. It is interesting to point out that these patients had a worse API and a normal AAI. They did not have typical anginal symptoms. The patients with a lower ACI and a decreased LVEF lived slightly longer despite the fact that they had clinical symptoms of heart failure but they were treated more intensively. It is very important to emphasize that inadequacy between ACI and ejection fraction, when left ventricular hypertrophy has developed, increases the risk for sudden cardiac death. This is a consequence of expressed multi-vessel CAD in patients with viable myocardial hypertrophy. In patients who survived three years, the left-ventricular ejection fraction, ACI and API were better. Therefore, we believe that the survival and death of patients with CAD can be better predicted with the help of ACMS. The product of both angiographic criteria (the ACI expressing the supply adequacy to the myocardial mass and the anginal index expressing the adequacy of supply to the functional requirements) could be the most informative prognostic index of survival in CAD. The product of ACI and ACI/EF could be named the angiographic outcome index (AOI). Mathematically, it can be calculated using the following equation:

$$AOI = ACI \times (ACI / EF) = (SCCA / LVM) \times (SCCA / LVM) / EF = SCCA^2 / LVM^2 \times EF \quad (5)$$

In the equation above the ACI stands for the angiographic coronary index, AOI – angiographic outcome index, SCCA -- summarized caliber of coronary arteries (mm^2), LVM – mass of the left ventricle (g), and EF – ejection fraction of the left ventricle. The AOI was statistically different in all three groups of patients who died during the 1st, 2nd, or 3rd year after intervention. It was subsequently 0.1 ± 0.03, 0.33 ± 0.02, and 0.5 ± 0.02 ($p < 0.009$, $p < 0.001$, and $p < 0.007$).

4. Discussion

The quantification of coronary stenosis is an important practice in cardiology from both a clinical and a research standpoint. In the recent past, there have been several imaging methods which could differently characterize the size and severity of obstructive CAD: coronary angiography, computed tomography, magnetic resonance imaging, and intravascular ultrasound. Various techniques with differing degrees of sophistication were used to measure the amount of luminal narrowing. Each method has provided new opportunities for a more thorough understanding of the pathogenesis of ischemic heart disease and variability of clinical picture. Angiography, performed with the use of digital techniques, has been shown to have significant advantages over the above-listed techniques due to its excellent reproducibility and accuracy (Funabaschi et al., 2003; Kalbfleisch et al., 1990; Molloi et al., 2001). However, for the effective computerized assessment of coronary lesion scores, we need to develop programs which can help to determine the size and severity of CAD more accurately. To achieve this aim, the proposed SCCA assessment system could be useful both theoretically and practically. Let us compare this innovative system to other methods of analysis.

All scoring systems have been based on percentage of stenosis evaluation using the "normal" diameter in the adjacent coronary segment. The validity of this reference is in question because coronary atherosclerosis is often diffuse and the adjacent segment could also be narrowed (Marcus et al., 1983; Seiler et al., 1992). In addition, serial segmental narrowing representing a type of diffuse disease is not taken into account because of the absence of a true normal reference segment. To assess the severity of diffuse CAD (with or without segmental narrowing) it is necessary to know what the normal arterial lumen size would be at each segment in the absence of coronary atherosclerosis. Various authors have attempted to solve this problem in different ways (Kucher et al., 2001; Seiler et al., 1992). Kucher et al. (2001) showed that in a population without cardiac disease, women have smaller coronary artery size even after normalization for left ventricular mass. The existence of a gender difference in coronary artery size remains controversial.

Our search for a "normal" diameter at each segment showed that the successful solution to this problem is impossible due to high variability in coronary dominance and branching. However, our experience and several other experimental and clinical reports (Dodge et al., 1992; Roberts C & Roberts W, 1980; Seiler et al., 1992) have shown a direct relationship between the coronary artery lumen size and the myocardial mass supplied by this artery. Therefore, the variability in coronary diameter and its direct relationship to myocardial mass have led us to propose a methodology which could be used to assess the degree and cause of any imbalance between residual coronary diameter and the supplied myocardial mass.

An analysis of patients with intact coronary arteries and increased myocardial mass showed that the SCCA can increase along with the degree of myocardial hypertrophy, especially if this process takes place at a young age. This phenomenon does not disturb the balance between SCCA and left ventricular mass. Therefore, the ratio remains normal. In cases of myocardial hypertrophy in older populations where the process of atherosclerosis has begun, the SCCA does not increase in conjunction with myocardial mass. This relative discrepancy is well illustrated by the lowering of the angiographic coronary index. Similar findings have been described by Marcus et al., (1983). Myocardial ischemia is frequently observed in patients with cardiac hypertrophy even when the conduit coronary arteries are normal (Fig. 7.2 and 7.3). Recent studies indicate that impaired coronary reserve in hypertrophied hearts probably occurs because the growth of the coronary bed does not keep pace with increase of cardiac mass (Fig. 7.4). The imbalance between vascular proliferation and muscle growth is probably most severe when the cardiac hypertrophy is caused by pressure overload or atherosclerotic infiltration (Fig. 7.5). These observations suggest that abnormalities in the coronary microcirculation which accompany cardiac hypertrophy play a significant role in the pathogenesis of the complications associated with cardiac hypertrophy.

The diminishing ACI in people without blockage of epicardial coronary arteries usually is associated with the onset of typical or atypical anginal symptoms. Syndrome X can be associated with chest pain and chest discomfort in people who do not show signs of obstruction in the larger coronary arteries. No one knows exactly what causes Syndrome X and it is unlikely to have a single cause. Today, we speculate that Syndrome X may be caused by microvascular dysfunction. A large majority of women have typical anginal symptoms which are not associated with the presence of atherosclerotic plaques. Scientists speculate that the blood vessels in these women are diffusely abnormal and smaller than in males (Kucher et al., 2001). It is possible that the diminishing ACI is a causative factor in the development of Syndrome X.

Additionally, the relationship between the angiographic coronary index and the functional status of the left ventricle expressed by ejection fraction may specify the adequacy of myocardial supply to myocardial functional demands. First, the inadequacy of myocardial supply with the inadequacy of myocardial nutritional requirements may lead to the occurrence of ischemic pain and its severity. The relationship between the angiographic coronary index and the ejection fraction we named the angiographic anginal index, because we found a strong negative correlation between this index and the intensity of angina.

Recent techniques have revealed new characteristics and expanded our understanding of painless or silent myocardial ischemia. These techniques include treadmill exercise testing; radioisotope techniques, including ejection fraction studies, stress thallium scintigraphy, and tomographic imaging. These new noninvasive tests should be used to detect transient ischemia, estimate its severity, and measure patient's risk for adverse coronary events especially in patients with painless or silent myocardial ischemia (Selwyn, 1990). Usage of anginal angiographic index in clinical practice can facilitate the selection of such high-risk patients with silent ischemia. Patients with diabetes, chronic renal insufficiency and other coexisting diseases have an increased prevalence of coronary artery disease with silent myocardial ischemia, complex ventricular arrhythmias, atrial fibrillation, and left ventricular hypertrophy (Das et al., 2006; Chipkin et al., 1987). These risk factors for cardiovascular morbidity and mortality contribute to the increased incidence of cardiovascular morbidity and mortality seen in patients with the above mentioned concomitant diseases (Selwyn, 1990). It is also important to stress that the energy needs of the left ventricle are not always proportional to the ejection fraction. LVEF can be permanently reduced due to post-infarction scar development, but the LVEF may temporarily decrease due to inadequate blood supply to the heart muscle. This phenomenon is known as myocardial hibernation (Camici et al., 2008). In both situations with the disappearance of anginal pain the occurrence of symptomatic heart failure can manifest with the clinical symptoms of ischemic cardiomyopathy (Felker et al., 2002).

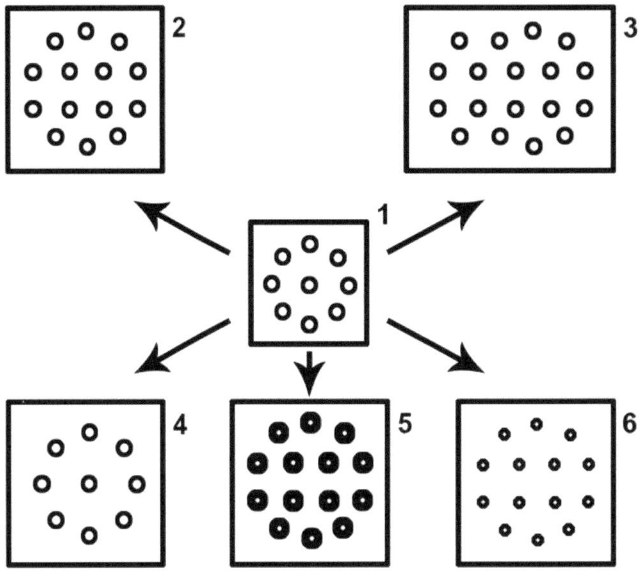

Fig. 7. Changes occurring in the coronary angiogenesis during development of myocardial hypertrophy. The size of the square indicates the presence of myocardial hypertrophy and its degree. The number and size of vessels are shown in each shape: 1, normal number of vessels in non-hypertrophied myocardium; 2 and 3, increased number of normal vessels in hypertrophied myocardium; 4, the non-increased number of normal vessels in hypertrophied myocardium; 5, increased number of atherosclerotic thickened-wall vessels in hypertrophied myocardium; and 6, increased number of spastic vessels in hypertrophied myocardium.

The diagnostic value of angiographic anginal index can be confirmed by the fact that during the development of myocardial hibernation or ischemic cardiomyopathy anginal pain reduces and can disappear completely. During the last decade, the existence of totally asymptomatic myocardial ischemia has been conclusively established. We would like to emphasize that the severity of angina depends upon the inadequacy between myocardial nutrition and functional demand, and this was shown by the angiographic anginal index. This index reflecting the adequacy between myocardial supply and demand cannot express the real degree of coronary and myocardial damage, because there may be a supply-demand adequacy in patients with equally expressed damage in the coronary arteries and the myocardium. Knowing the limited prognostic capabilities of the angiographic anginal index, we have created the angiographic outcome index for outcome prediction, and the angiographic prognostic indexes.

The prognostic capabilities of different coronary scores were confirmed by several authors (Friesinger et al., 1970; Graham et al., 1999; Korosoglou et al., 2007; Ringqvist 1983). The complex angiographic coronary index, anginal index, and left-ventricular ejection fraction are more informative for predicting CAD outcomes. It was shown that only an increase in LV mass in initially healthy persons with essential hypertension resulted in more complications and deaths (Koren et al., 1991). Differently determined left ventricular hypertrophy is an important prognostic marker in patients with or without coronary artery disease (Ghali et al., 1992). It was shown that only reduced LVEF has a clear predictive value in patients without known obstructive CAD. Reduced LVEF was related to sudden death from the absolute presence of CAD as well as the increased number of vessels with obstruction (Min et al., 2010).

4.1 Limitations

We have measured the lumen areas of different segments at their narrowest points on coronarograms in this study. Very small measurements sometimes cannot be done without interpretative errors; however, the margin of error is not high. The possibility of underestimating the impact of a single expressed lesion on the diminishing SCCA could be a limitation of this method. It is well known that such single-culprit lesions may cause the development of acute myocardial infarction. However, the main goal of this quantitative analysis system is to assess the total real size and severity of the epicardial coronary lesion using the SCCA as a coronary score.

5. Conclusion

The most important advantage of this SCCA calculation system is that it provides an easier and more objective assessment of an angiographic coronary lesion score in patients with a wide spectrum of CAD, ranging from a minimal stenosis to extensive diffuse involvement of the coronary arteries. The SCCA as a coronary lesion score is simple and easily interpreted; it gives no reason for interpretative differences. First, the estimation of the average SCCA does not require a precise assessment of stenosis degree, coronary dominance, or branching peculiarities. Second, it provides the possibility to analyze the relationship between coronary score and myocardial function what implies a correlation between myocardial supply and demand. In addition, this quantitative analysis system can give more diagnostic and prognostic information about the real mechanisms of myocardial ischemia, the character of angina pectoris, and the possible risk for occurrence of life threatening complications. Furthermore, the technique for interpretation of angiographic data and computation of quantitative characteristics has been considerably facilitated.

6. Acknowledgment

I would like to thank the staff of the Department of Clinical Pathology, Lithuanian University of Health Sciences for their valuable assistance in performing post-mortem examinations.

7. References

Brandt, P.; Partridge, J. & Wattie, W. (1977). Coronary arteriography: method of presentation of the arteriogram report and a scoring system. *Clin Radiol*, Vol. 28, pp. 361-365, ISSN 0009-9260

Brown, B.; Bolson, E.; Frimer, M. & Dodge, H. (1977). Quantitative coronary arteriography: estimation of dimensions, hemodynamic resistance, and atheroma mass of coronary artery lesions using the arteriogram and digital computation. *Circulation*, Vol. 55, pp. 329-337, ISSN 0009-7322

Camici, P.; Prasad, S. & Rimoldi, O. (2008). Stunning, hibernation, and assessment of myocardial viability. *Circulation*, Vol. 117, pp. 103-114, ISSN 1524-4539

Chipkin, S.; Frid, D.; Alpert, J.; Baker, S.; Dalen, J. & Aronin, N. (1987). Frequency of painless myocardial ischemia during exercise tolerance testing in patients with and without diabetes mellitus. *Am J Cardiol*, Vol. 59, pp. 61-55, ISSN 0002-9149

Das, M.; Aronow, W.; McClung, J. & Belkin, R. (2006). Increased prevalence of coronary artery disease, silent myocardial ischemia, complex ventricular arrhythmias, atrial fibrillation, left ventricular hypertrophy, mitral annular calcium, and aortic valve calcium in patients with chronic renal insufficiency. *Cardiol Rev*, Vol. 14, pp. 14-17, ISSN 1061-5377

Davies, M. (2000). The pathophysiology of acute coronary syndromes. *Heart*, Vol. 83, pp. 361-366, ISSN 1355-6037

Dodge, J.; Brown, B.; Bolson, E. & Dodge, H. (1988). Intrathoracic spatial location of specified coronary segments on the normal human heart. Applications in quantitative arteriography, assessment of regional risk and contraction, and anatomic display. *Circulation*, Vol. 78, pp. 1167-1180, ISSN 0009-7322

Dodge, J., Brown, B.; Bolson, E. & Dodge, H. (1992). Lumen diameter of normal human coronary arteries. Influence of age, sex, anatomic variation, and left ventricular hypertrophy or dilation. *Circulation*, Vol. 86, pp. 232-246, ISSN 0009-7322

Felker , G.; Shaw, L. & O'Connor, C. (2002). A standardized definition of ischemic cardiomyopathy for use in clinical research. *J Am Coll Cardiol*, Vol. 39 pp. 210-218, ISSN 0735-1097

Friesinger, G.; Page, E. & Ross, R. (1970). Prognostic significance of coronary arteriography. *Trans Assoc Am Physicians*, Vol. 83, pp. 78-92. ISSN 0066-9458

Funabashi, N.; Kobayashi, Y.; Perlroth, M. & Rubin, G. (2003). Coronary artery: quantitative evaluation of normal diameter determined with electron-beam CT compared with cine coronary angiography initial experience. *Radiology*, Vol. 226, pp. 263-271, ISSN 0033-8419

Garg, S.; Sarno, G.; Garcia-Garcia, H.; Girasis, C.; Wykrzykowska, J.; Dawkins, K.; et al. (2010). A new tool for the risk stratification of patients with complex coronary artery disease: the Clinical SYNTAX Score. *Circ Cardiovasc Interv*, Vol. 3, pp. 317-326, ISSN 1941-7632

Gensini, G.; Kelly, A.; Da Costa, B. & Huntington, P. (1971). Quantitative angiography: the measurement of coronary vasomobility in the intact animal and man. *Chest*, Vol. 60, pp. 522-530, ISSN 0002-9149

Gensini G. (1983). A more meaningful scoring system for determining the severity of coronary heart disease. *Am J Cardiol*, Vol. 51, p. 606, ISSN 0012-3692

Ghali, J.; Liao, Y.; Simmons, B.; Castaner, A.; Cao, G. & Cooper, R. (1992). The prognostic role of left ventricular hypertrophy in patients with or without coronary artery disease. *Ann Intern Med*, Vol. 117, pp. 831-836, ISSN 0003-4819

Gibson, C.; Cannon, C.; Murphy, S.; Marble, S.; Barron, H. & Braunwald, E. (2002). Relationship of the TIMI myocardial perfusion grades, flow grades, frame count, and percutaneous coronary intervention to long-term outcomes after thrombolytic administration in acute myocardial infarction. *Circulation*, Vol. 105, pp. 1909-1913, ISSN 1524-4539 (Electronic)

Gibson, C.; Goel, M.; Murphy, S.; Dotani, I.; Marble, S.; Deckelbaum, L. et al. (2000). Global impairment of coronary blood flow in the setting of acute coronary syndromes (a RESTORE substudy). Randomized efficacy Study of Tirofiban for Outcomes and Restenosis. *Am J Cardiol*, Vol. 86, pp. 1375-1377, A5, ISSN 0002-9149

Gibson, C.; Murphy, S.; Rizzo, M.; Ryan, K.; Marble, S.; McCabe, C.; et al. (1999). Relationship between TIMI frame count and clinical outcomes after thrombolytic administration. Thrombolysis in Myocardial Infarction (TIMI) Study Group. *Circulation*, Vol. 99, pp. 1945-1950, ISSN 1524-4539 (Electronic)

Goldstein, J.; Demetriou, D.; Grines, C.; Pica, M.; Shoukfeh, M. & O'Neill, W. (2000). Multiple complex coronary plaques in patients with acute myocardial infarction. *N Engl J Med*, Vol. 343, pp. 915-922, ISSN 0028-4793

Graham, M.; Chambers, R. & Davies, R. (1999). Angiographic quantification of diffuse coronary artery disease: reliability and prognostic value for bypass operations. *J Thorac Cardiovasc Surg*, Vol. 118, pp. 618-627, ISSN 0022-5223

Hamsten, A.; Walldius, G.; Szamosi, A.; Dahlen, G. & de Faire, U. (1986). Relationship of angiographically defined coronary artery disease to serum lipoproteins and apolipoproteins in young survivors of myocardial infarction. *Circulation*, Vol. 73, pp. 1097-1110, ISSN 0009-7322

Jalal A. (2007). An objective method for grading of distal disease in the grafted coronary arteries. *Interact Cardiovasc Thorac Surg*, Vol. 6, pp. 451-455, ISSN 1569-9285 (Electronic)

Jenkins, P.; Harper, R. & Nestel, P. (1978). Severity of coronary atherosclerosis related to lipoprotein concentration. *Br Med J*, Vol. 2, pp. 388-391, ISSN 0007-1447

Kalbfleisch, S.; McGillem, M.; Pinto, I.; Kavanaugh, K.; DeBoe, S. & Mancini, G. (1990). Comparison of automated quantitative coronary angiography with caliper measurements of percent diameter stenosis. *Am J Cardiol*, Vol. 65, pp. 1181-1184, ISSN 0002-9149

Koren, M.; Devereux, R.; Casale, P.; Savage, D. & Laragh, J. (1991). Relation of left ventricular mass and geometry to morbidity and mortality in uncomplicated essential hypertension. *Ann Intern Med*, Vol. 114, pp. 345-352, ISSN 0003-4819

Korosoglou, G.; Haars, A.; Michael, G.; Erbacher, M.; Hardt , S.; Giannitsis, E. et al. (2007). Quantitative evaluation of myocardial blush to assess tissue level reperfusion in patients with acute ST-elevation myocardial infarction: incremental prognostic value compared with visual assessment. *Am Heart J*, Vol. 153, pp. 612-620, ISSN 1097-6744 (Electronic)

Krone, R.; Laskey, W.; Johnson, C.; Kimmel, S.; Klein, L.; Weiner, B. et al. (2000). A simplified lesion classification for predicting success and complications of coronary angioplasty. Registry Committee of the Society for Cardiac Angiography and Intervention. *Am J Cardiol*, Vol. 85, pp. 1179-1184, ISSN 0002-9149

Kucher, N.; Lipp, E.; Schwerzmann, M.; Zimmerli, M.; Allemann Y. & Seiler, C. (2001). Gender differences in coronary artery size per 100 g of left ventricular mass in a population without cardiac disease. *Swiss Med Wkly*, Vol. 131, pp. 610-615, ISSN 1424-7860

Kunadian, V.; Harrigan, C.; Zorkun, C.; Palmer, A.; Ogando, K.; Biller, L. et al. (2009). Use of the TIMI frame count in the assessment of coronary artery blood flow and microvascular function over the past 15 years. *J Thromb Thrombolysis*, Vol. 27, pp. 316-328, ISSN 1573-742X (Electronic)

Kwon, S.; Kim, Y.; Shim, J.; Sung, J.; Han, M.; Kang, D. et al. (2011). Coronary artery calcium scoring does not add prognostic value to standard 64-section CT angiography protocol in low-risk patients suspected of having coronary artery disease. *Radiology*, Vol. 259, pp. 92-99, ISSN 1527-1315 (Electronic)

Leaman, D.; Brower, R.; Meester, G.; Serruys, P.; van den Brand M. (1981). Coronary artery atherosclerosis: severity of the disease, severity of angina pectoris and compromised left ventricular function. *Circulation*, Vol. 63, pp. 285-299, ISSN 0009-7322

Marcus, M.; Koyanagi, S.; Harrison, D.; Doty, D.; Hiratzka, L. & Eastham, C. (1983). Abnormalities in the coronary circulation that occur as a consequence of cardiac hypertrophy. *Am J Med*, Vol. 75, pp. 62-66, ISSN 0002-9343

Min, J.; Lin, F.; Dunning, A.; Delago, A.; Egan, J.; Shaw, L. et al. (2010). Incremental prognostic significance of left ventricular dysfunction to coronary artery disease detection by 64-detector row coronary computed tomographic angiography for the prediction of all-cause mortality: results from a two-centre study of 5330 patients. *Eur Heart J*, Vol. 31, pp. 1212-1219, ISSN 1522-9645 (Electronic)

Molloi, S.; Kassab, G. & Zhou, Y. (2001). Quantification of coronary artery lumen volume by digital angiography: in vivo validation. *Circulation*, Vol. 104, pp. 2351-2357, ISSN 1522-9645 (Electronic)

Ringqvist, I.; Fisher, L.; Mock, M.; Davis, K.; Wedel, H.; Chaitman, B. et al. (1983). Prognostic value of angiographic indices of coronary artery disease from the Coronary Artery Surgery Study (CASS). *J Clin Invest*, Vol. 71, pp. 1854-1866, ISSN 0021-9738 (Linking)

Roberts, C. & Roberts, W. (1980). Cross-sectional area of the proximal portions of the three major epicardial coronary arteries in 98 necropsy patients with different coronary events. Relationship to heart weight, age and sex. *Circulation*, Vol. 62, pp. 953-959, ISSN 0009-7322

Seiler, C.; Kirkeeide, R. & Gould, K. (1992). Basic structure-function relations of the epicardial coronary vascular tree. Basis of quantitative coronary arteriography for diffuse coronary artery disease. *Circulation*, Vol. 85, pp. 1987-2003, ISSN 0009-7322

Selwyn, AP. (1990). Current technology in assessing painless and painful ischemia. *Am Heart J*, Vol. 120, pp. 722-725, ISSN 0002-8703

Sianos, G.; Morel, M.; Kappetein, A.; Morice, M.; Colombo, A.; Dawkins, K. et al. (2005). The SYNTAX Score: an angiographic tool grading the complexity of coronary artery disease. *EuroIntervention*, Vol. 1, pp. 219-227, ISSN 1774-024X

Sullivan, D.; Marwick, T. & Freedman, S. (1990). A new method of scoring coronary angiograms to reflect extent of coronary atherosclerosis and improve correlation with major risk factors. *Am Heart J*, Vol. 119, pp. 1262-1267, ISSN 0002-8703

Vogt, M.; Motz, W. & Strauer, B. (1992). Coronary haemodynamics in hypertensive heart disease. *Eur Heart J*, Vol. 13 Suppl D, pp. 44-49, ISSN 0195-668X

Zaacks, S.; Allen, J.; Calvin, J.; Schaer, G.; Palvas, B.; Parrillo, J. et al. (1998). Value of the American College of Cardiology/American Heart Association stenosis morphology classification for coronary interventions in the late 1990s. *Am J Cardiol*, Vol. 82, pp. 3-9, ISSN 0002-9149

Zipes, D. &Wellens, H. (1998). Sudden cardiac death. *Circulation*, Vol. 98, pp. 2334-2351, ISSN 0009-7322

16

Woven Coronary Artery

Ayşe Yıldırım[1] and A. Deniz Oğuz[2]
[1]Kosuyolu Heart and Research Hospital, Pediatric Cardiology, Istanbul
[2]Gazi University Medical Faculty Pediatric Cardiology, Ankara
Turkey

1. Introduction

In this chapter we will discuss the woven coronary artery which is one of the most interesting coronary arterial anomalies. Although it is difficult to estimate the real incidence of coronary artery anomalies due to the difficulty in specific identification, it is approximately %0.3 - %1.3. The main reasons of underestimation of coronary artery anomalies may be that, in many individuals; don't lead to symptoms, morbidity, or mortality (Friedman & Silverman, 2010).

2. Woven coronary artery

Woven coronary artery is an extremely rare congenital malformation characterized by the division of epicardial coronary artery into thin channels which then reanastomose with the distal part of the abnormal coronary artery. Generally this anomalous segment of the coronary artery is limited to several centimeters long. By means of several angiographic studies it has been shown that the blood flow is completely normal in all segments of the woven coronary artery. This is a totally benign malformation which doesn't lead to any pathologic cardiac event.

Woven coronary artery was first described by Sane et al. in 1988, during the coronary angiography performed on a 55 year old woman with congestive heart failure seven years after from her aortic valve replacement and mitral valve commissurotomy (Sane, 1986). He defined this branching and reanastomosing structure as ''figure 8''pattern and named this congenital anomaly as ''woven coronary artery''.

Approximately nine adult and only one pediatric patient with woven coronary artery have been reported since then. Most of these patients were males diagnosed accidentally at the coronary angiography performed due to chest pain, after acute myocardial infarction or due to the suspicion of left coronary artery aneurysm in Kawasaki disease. Although the pathology is mostly seen in the right coronary artery, woven structures have also been demonstrated in left coronary arteries or in circumflex artery. These are listed in Table 1.

	No: 10	Age	Gender	Previous history	Cause of coronary angiography	Coronary Angiography	Stres test	Procedure
Sane et al.	1 patient	55 Y	F	AVR + MVC	CHF	Woven RCA		
Berman Et al	1 patient							
Gregorini et al.	3 patients	60Y 62Y 45Y	M F	- - -	Angina pectoris Angina after AMI AMI	Woven LCA LAD stenosis Woven LCXA Distal LAD plaque, Woven LCA	positive	- Mid LAD coronary angiooplasty -
Martuscelli et al.	1 patient	42 Y	M	Hypercholesterolemia	Angina	LAD stenosis Woven RCA		LAD coronary angioplasty
Kursaklıoglu et al.	1 patient	48Y	M	No	Exertional chest pain	RCA Mid stenosis, Woven mid CX	positive	RCA stenting
Kaya et al.	1 patient	56Y		LAD coronary angioplasty	Dyspnea after AMI	Wowen RCA		Medical treatment
Yıldırım et al.	1 patient	9 moths	M	Kawasaki disease	Aneurysmatic LCA	Aneurysmatic LCA, Woven RCA	-	Medical treatment
Iyisoy et al.	1 patient	58Y	M	Smoking	Exertional chest pain.	Mid LAD stenosis, Woven RCA	positive	LAD stenting

AVR: aortic valve replacement, MVC: mitral valve commissurotomy, CHF: Congestive heart failure, LAD: left anterior descending artery, RCA: right coronary artery, LCA: left coronary artery, AMI: acute miyocardial infarction, LCXA: Left circumflex artery

Table 1. The summary of the demographic and clinical data of the patients with woven coronary artery in the literature.

2.1 Embryology of coronary artery

As there are very few number of woven coronary artery cases, the embryological development of this rare coronary artery anomaly has not been explained yet. However, there are two models of explanation for the embryologic development of normal coronary arteries. Previously it had been thought that the cells of the myocardium nourished from the blood in the ventricular cavity thicken and become close to the ventricular cavity by means of multiple trabeculations. These trabeculations then develop into sinusoids which were the forerunners of the coronary vascular system (Tomanek et al, 1996). The new model of coronary arterial development suggests that the cells of the primordial liver form a proepicardial protrusion. These cells establish the proepicardium and the epicardial cells then migrate over the surface of the heart. The epicardial cells invade the subepicardial matrix and form the coronary vascular plexus. By an undefined mechanism, probably involving multiple growth factors, the epicardial cells undergo epithelial mesenchymal transformation and form mature vessels. These small vessels on the surface of the heart fuse and grow inward to penetrate the aorta fusing with the coronary vessels. The new experimental data on the development of the coronary system suggests that beside multiple growth factors, several adhesion molecules and chemotactic factors play role in this complicated coordinated migration and transformation of cells to form coronary vessels. The presence of congenital anomalies of coronary arteries may be due to abnormalities in these signaling pathways or alterations in local factors that direct coronary vessel development. (Matherne & Lim, 2008)

2.2 Etiology of woven coronary artery

The number of case studies published about woven coronary artery is so limited that the etiology of this rarely encountered anomaly has not been clearly understood yet. The reported cases on this anomaly are mostly adult patients. Recently a case report about an infant nine- months-old with woven coronary artery has been published (Yıldırım et al., 2010). Therefore it is now suspected that woven coronary artery may be a congenital malformation and advanced studies are needed to lighten this issue

2.3 Incidence of woven coronary artery

The real incidence of woven CA is not known. The diagnosis of the patients in the literature have been made accidentally so far. A remarkably high number of woven CA cases might have been misdiagnosed as coronary artery thrombus, stenosis or dissection. It can be claimed that the frequency of this anomaly could have been higher if woven coronary artery anomaly had not been misinterpreted in this way.

3. Clinical features of woven coronary artery

As mentioned above "woven coronary artery" is accepted as a benign condition. Most of the woven coronary artery patients in the literature are the cases diagnosed unexpectedly during the coronary angiography made upon acute myocardial infarction or angina pectoris. In the case report of İyisoy at al., (2010) severe stenosis in the middle segment of left anterior descending coronary artery and multiple thin channels in the right coronary artery were demonstrated during the same coronary angiography session, however stenosis was accused to be responsible from the myocardial ischemia. Another coronary angiography performed on a patient with positive stress test by Kursaklıoğlu et al. (2006) revealed stenosis in the mid-segment of the right coronary artery and the division of arterial lumen into multiple thin channels in the mid-segment of the circumflex artery. They thought that the severe stenosis in the right coronary artery was the most possible reason of the positive stress test in this patient rather than the woven coronary anomaly. In the cases reported by Martuscelli et al.(2000), Kursaklıoglu et al.(2006) and Yıldırım et al.(2010) no adverse coronary events occurred during 4 to 5 year follow-up periods. Repeated control coronary angiograms of the patients with coronary arterial stenting or cardiac surgery have revealed no structural change in woven coronary arteries. This finding suggests that the cause of chest pain, angina pectoris, acute myocardial infarction or positive stress test is not dependent on woven coronary artery anomaly.

4. Diagnosis of woven coronary artery

Although there is an anatomically abnormal coronary artery, the blood flow and the myocardial contraction is normal. Therefore the physical examination, laboratory findings, chest x-rays, electrocardiographic and echocardiographic investigations of the woven coronary artery patients are completely normal. The echocardiography is not helpful for the diagnosis. The gold standard for the diagnosis of woven coronary artery is coronary angiography. There is no angiographic uniform image of woven coronary arteries however the most important angiographic criteria is definite intraluminal globular filling defects in repeated angiographic views.

4.1 Cardiac catheterization

In the coronary angiography it is seen that the arterial lumen is divided into multiple thin channels at the proximal segment of affected coronary arteries or their branches; subsequently, these channels proceed distally with a slightly twisting route and then fuse again. Distal to this woven segment, the downstream blood flow is absolutely normal (Figures 1A, B and C).

During the coronary angiography division of coronary artery may be misdiagnosed as a complicated plaque with thrombus formation instead of coronary artery malformation. In addition, coronary artery stenosis, spontaneous coronary artery dissection, intracoronary thrombosis or recanalization of a thrombus may mimic this woven structure. These mimicking pathologies have lead to the misdiagnosis of woven coronary artery (Martuscelli et al., 2000; Kaya et al., 2006). However for an accurate explanation of the etiology, more detailed information about the characteristics and the development of this malformation is needed.

5. Differential diagnosis

In differential diagnosis of woven coronary artery the important criteria is the absence of coronary artery disease history of the patient with normal stress tests such as treadmill, echocardiography and myocardial scintigraphy. The patient with a woven coronary artery anomaly usually demonstrates normal coronary reserve during stress test.

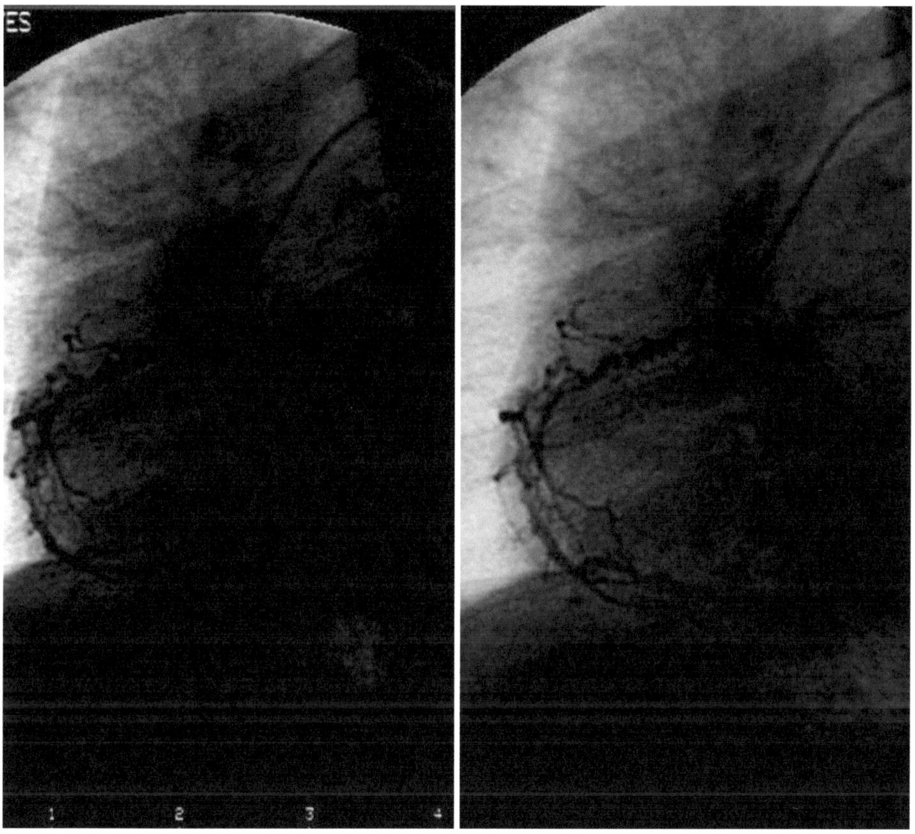

Fig. 1A. and B. Right coronary angiography showed proximal thin channels and distal reanastomosis

This is dependent on normal blood flow distal to the anomalous segment (Kursaklıoglu et al., 2006; Yıldırım et al., 2010; İyisoy et al., 2010). In woven coronary artery anomaly, normal blood flow can be maintained distal to the anomalous segment, therefore coronary blood reserve is not disturbed with stress tests, especially myocardial perfusion imaging (İyisoy et al., 2101). Even if there is clinical evidence of myocardial infarction or angina pectoris in a patient with woven coronary artery, coronary angiography should be repeated to eliminate other coronary artery pathologies. Radiologically, the examination and the interpretation of the angiographic image are crucial to prevent misdiagnosis of the woven coronary arteries. In this coronary anomaly, although the filling is defective, flow is normal; which differentiates this structure from other pathologies such as intracoronary thrombus, stenosis or dissection.

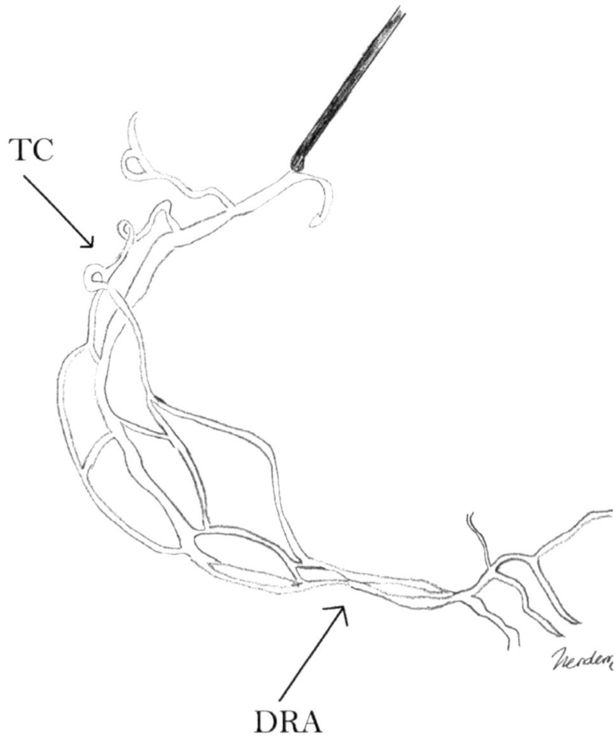

Fig. 1C. Diagram of the right woven coronary artery showing proximal thin channels (TC) and distal reanastomosis (DRA)

6. Associated diseases

Up to now, woven coronary artery cases have only been reported as isolated coronary artery anomaly (Sane et al., 1988; Berman et al.1990; Gregorini et al., 1995; Martuscelli et al., 2000; Kursaklıoglu et al., 2006; Kaya et al., 2006; İyisoy et al., 2010). Only in the case report of Yıldırım et al., (2010) the woven coronary artery was described as the part of a systemic disease, Kawasaki disease, in an infant patient of nine months old. In this patient, routine echocardiographic evaluation of coronary arteries revealed aneurysm of the left coronary artery, leading to an angiographic study in which a woven right coronary artery was detected coincidentally. In fact there is also a tendency for the development of thrombus in Kawasaki disease and this condition should not be confused with woven coronary artery (Yıldırım et al., 2010). For this reason, the pediatric and adult cardiologists should be aware that woven coronary artery may accompany Kawasaki Disease and they should perform coronary angiography to distinguish real thrombus from this coronary anomaly.

7. Treatment

Woven coronary artery is an anatomic abnormality and it doesn't disturb cardiac functions at all. Therefore it is not necessary to treat this anomaly. However other coronary artery pathologies such as coronary artery stenosis, thrombosis, dissection or myocardial infarction should be carefully distinguished from woven coronary artery. This point is crucial to prevent misdiagnosis and treatment of woven coronary artery unnecessarily.

8. Conclusion

Angiographic examination of the patients with suspected coronary artery pathologies should be performed carefully to make differential diagnosis of dissection, thrombosis stenosis and woven coronary artery. The catheter angiography scenes should be evaluated repeatedly not to misinterpret the coronary artery pathologies. Such a detailed evaluation and definitive diagnosis is important to reduce the risk of unnecessary percutaneous coronary interventions, which expose the patients to several complications. Woven coronary artery does not need treatment but follow-up is required as there are only a few reports about the progress of this rare event. Advanced studies are needed on this unknown entity to demonstrate its detailed pathology. Even though this anomaly appears to be a benign coronary anomaly without any major adverse cardiovascular events, we need more data to figure out its exact natural history.

9. Acknowledgment

As the current collected data about the woven coronary arteries has been provided from a very limited number of cases, we believe that the embryology, pathophysiology, clinical feature and the prognosis of this rare coronary anomaly will be explained better with advanced studies.

10. References

Berman AD, Kim D, Baim DS.(1990) "Woven" right coronary artery: case report and therapeutic implications. *Cathet Cardiovasc Diagn* ; 21:258–259.

Gregorini L, Perondi R, Pomidossi G, Saino A, Bossi IM, Zanchetti A. (1995). Woven left coronary artery disease. *Am J Cardiol* ;75(4): 311-2.

Friedman AH and Silverman NH. Congenital anomalies of the coronary artery. (2010) *Pediatric Cardiology* In Anderson RH, Baker EJ, Penny D, Redington, AN, Rigby ML, Wernovsky G. (third edition), Churchill Livingstone and Elsevier, Philadelphia pp:933-943

Iyisoy A, Celik T, Yuksel UC, Isik E. Woven right coronary artery: a case report and review of the literature. *Clin Cardiol. 2010;33:43-45.*

Kaya D, Kilit C, Onrat E. (2006)An uncommon congenital anomaly of coronary arteries misdiagnosed as intracoronary thrombus: woven coronary artery disease. *Anadolu Kardiol Derg*. 6:383-384.

Kursaklioglu H, Iyisoy A, Celik T. (2006) Woven coronary artery: a case report and review of literature. *Int J Cardiol* 113(1) 121-3.

Martuscelli E, Romeo F, Giovannini M, Nigri A. (2000) Woven coronary artery: differential diagnosis with diffuse intracoronary thrombosis. *Ital Heart J*. 1(4):306-7.

Matherne GP and Lim DS. Congenital anomalies of the coronary vessels and the aortic root (2008). Moss and Adams' Heart Disease in Infant, Children and Adolescents including the Fetus and Young Adult. In Allen HD, Driscoll DJ, Shaddy Re, Feltes TE. (seventh edition) Lippincott Williams & Wilkins, Philadelphia. Pp:702-715.

Sane DC, Vidaillet JH Jr. (1988) Woven right coronary artery: a previously undescribed congenital anomaly. *Am J Cardiol* 61(13):1158.

Tomanek RJ.(1996) Formation of the coronary vasculature: A brief review. *Cardiovasc Res* 31 Spec No: E46-51

Tomanek RJ. (2005) Formation of the coronary vasculature during development. *Angiogenesis* 8:273-284

Yıldırım A, Oğuz D, Olguntürk R (2010). Woven Right and Aneurysmatic Left Coronary Artery Associated with Kawasaki Disease in a 9-month-old Patient. *Cardiol Young* 20:342-344.

17

Image Post-Processing and Interpretation

Masahiro Jinzaki, Minoru Yamada and Sachio Kuribayashi
Dept. of Diagnostic Radiology, Keio University School of Medicine
Japan

1. Introduction

Image post-processing is defined as the process of integrating a series of axial images into a form that is often easier to interpret than the sections themselves. The source transverse section is a fundamental image for interpretation. However, because of the complexity of coronary anatomy, interpreters must review coronary CT angiography interactively on workstations capable of 3-dimensional (3D) displays. The 3D data set can be reformatted according to the needs of the investigator using several types of post-processing algorithms. Coronary artery interpretation includes assessment of calcium scoring on non-contrast image and coronary angiography on enhanced image. Non-coronary cardiovascular findings and extra-cardiac findings should be reviewed in addition to recognize primary and secondary comorbid pathology and to identify findings that lead to alternative non-cardiovascular diagnoses. The ultimate objective of post-processing and interpretation is to convey diagnostic information to the treating physician with as much clarity and accuracy as possible. Interpretation times vary, usually depending on the image quality and the user's experience and knowledge of cardiac CT and the individual workstation. Normally, experienced users usually spend no more than 10 minutes segmenting and interpreting cardiac CT studies.

2. Post-processing technique

The source transverse sections are the primary tools for interpretation of coronary CT angiography examinations. Post-processing imaging is performed from reconstructed axial images and is useful in allowing clinically relevant information to be extracted from large number of axial images. In addition, the diagnostic accuracy of axial images (86% sensitive and 78% accurate) for the detection of coronary stenosis is low compared with combination of post-processing techniques (98% sensitive and 94% accurate) (Jinzaki et al, 2009). Thus, the review of 3D displays is necessary for the coronary artery interpretation due to the complexity of coronary anatomy. These include volume rendering, multiplanar reformation, thin-slab maximum intensity projection, curved multiplanar reformation, angiographic view, and plaque-loaded angiographic view. A post-processing image which enables the evaluation of coronary artery disease with fewer images and one that is understandable to the third person is preferable.

2.1 Multiplanar reformation (MPR)

MPR is a high-resolution reconstruction format that allows display of planar images at any angular section through the acquisition volume, which permits visualization in not only the axial plane but also in orthogonal (coronal and sagittal) or oblique planes that better follow the arterial course in the thorax. The slice thickness can be modified, and a thick slab may be helpful in visualizing tortuous coronary artery. MPR is a simple algorithm which can be rendered quickly and accurately on any image-processing workstations. The distance measurements in MPR are accurate. Different structures in MPR are accurate and do not overlap. There is no loss of voxel value information due to threshold.

MPRs are best suited for evaluation of the individual cardiac chambers, aorta (Fig. 1), and pulmonary vasculature with cardiac CT. MPRs are also well suited for selective evaluation of a coronary short segment. If a narrowing is suspected on axial views, display in coronal or sagittal orientations can confirm the presence of a stenosis (Fig. 2).

The disadvantage of MPR is that only short segments can be analyzed at a time due to the nonlinear pathway of the coronary arteries. Thus, MPR requires the creation of numerous images in different planes at every suspected location of coronary stenosis. Furthermore, it is less suited for displaying the length of an artery. Grading of a stenosis is not advisable with coronal, sagittal, or oblique reconstructions alone, because of partial averaging (Johnson et al, 2010).

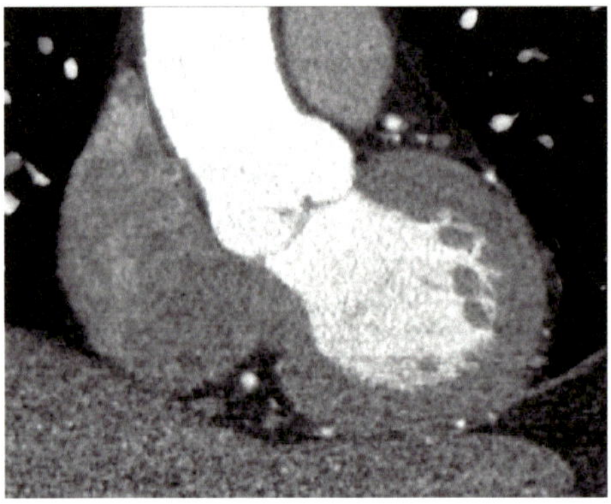

Fig. 1. Multiplanar reformation of cardiac structure

Oblique coronal image orientate better the planes of the geometrical orientations of cardiac structure (left chamber and aorta).

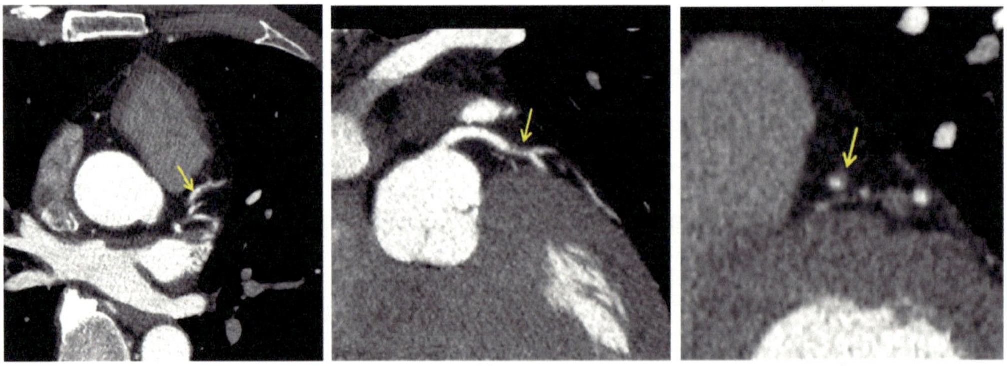

a) b) c)

Fig. 2. Multiplanar reconstruction of coronary stenosis

When a narrowing (arrow) is suspected on axial views (a), multiplanar reformation can be used to set the planes (b, c) in an orientation that matches one of the coronary short segments.

2.2 Thin-slab maximum intensity projection (Thin-slab MIP)

In both thin-slab MIP and MPR, orthogonal or oblique planes can be reviewed interactively. MIP is a projection technique, in which only the highest density pixel in the projection direction is displayed to reconstruct the two-dimensional images. MIP image allows the differentiation between enhanced vascular structures and non-vascular structures, because the result is a projection of the highest density. In practice, MIP is usually performed interactively with a sliding slab, enabling the radiologist to adjust the window, select the optimal orientation to display each artery, and modify the slab thickness (Fishman et al, 2006).

The advantage of thin-slab MIP is the creation of a vascular map quickly without modification of several parameters (Fig. 3). In addition, MIP is better for displaying small-caliber segments: the minimum vessel diameter seen with MIP was 0.7 mm versus 1.5 mm for volume rendering (VR) (Zhang et al, 2004). This is because MIP is designed to selectively demonstrate the arterial vasculature, which involves selection of the highest attenuation voxels along rays projected through the volume. It is controversial whether thin-slab MIP can be used for the diagnosis of coronary artery stenosis. One study compared interpretation of 3 sets of orthogonally oriented thin-slab MIPs with axial sections with 16-slice CT (Choi et al, 2006). For all three radiologists, the Az (area under the ROC curve) values from the MIP images were higher than those Az values from the transaxial images, however, the difference was significant for only one reader.

MIP has a tendency to overestimate stenosis. Heavily calcified arteries cannot be evaluated with MIP. Thus, thin-slab MIP cannot be used for the quantity evaluation of plaque, including the determination of grading of a stenosis. In addition, numerous images in different planes are required for the evaluation of the whole coronary arteries. Thin-slab MIP is useful as an adjunct to VR. However, it should not be the sole technique used for interpretation.

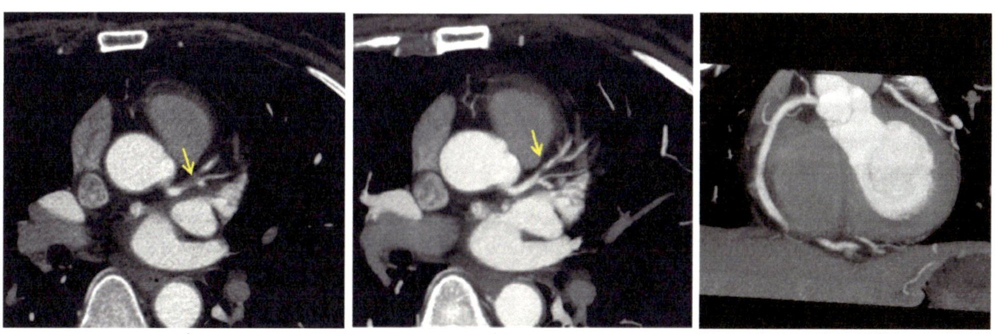

a) b) c)

Fig. 3. Thin-slab maximum intensity projection of coronary stenosis

When a narrowing (arrow) is suspected on axial views (a), the use of thin-slab maximum intensity projection (b) increases the overview of each coronary artery. Thin-slab maximum intensity projection enables creation of a vascular map (c) quickly without modification of several parameters.

2.3 Curved multiplanar reformation (curved MPR)

The development of curved MPR format made it possible for the interpreter to follow the course of a tortuous vessel for longer distances as it changes direction (Fig. 4) (Ferencik et al., 2007). The artery can be displayed as a straight line (Fig. 5). This method enables one entire coronary artery to be followed and displayed in one reconstruction, and reduces the number of planar images needed, compared with MPR. An automated program is possible to track the coronary arteries using placement of a single point in any portion of each artery or ascending aorta, the computer can trace a given coronary vessel departing proximally and distally from the point chosen, and extract the images in seconds. Other automated program tracks the path of the coronary artery, when the operator selects two points: one at the beginning and one at the end of the vessel. These applications also provide MPRs that are orthogonal to the vessel centerline, thus creating cross-sectional cuts of each coronary arterial segment (Fig. 5). All other surrounding structures are automatically eliminated that are any distance from this centerpoint, possibly decreasing problems seen with other reconstruction methods from tortuosity and overlap.

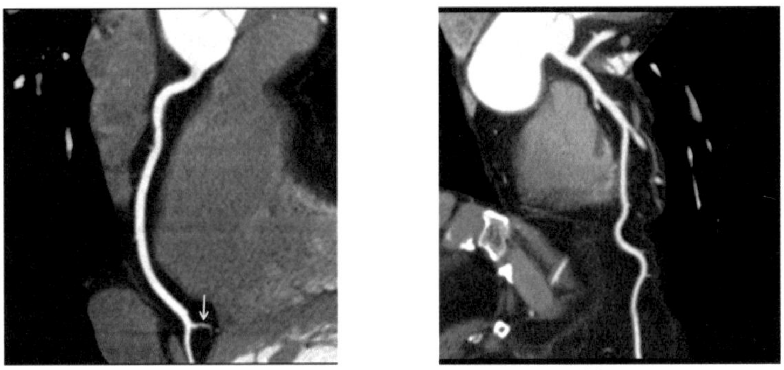

a) b)

Fig. 4. Curved multiplanar reformation of the coronary arteries.

The vessel can be seen in a long length with this technique. Fig. 4a demonstrates a multiplanar reformation of the entire right coronary artery, including a segment of posterolateral marginal branch. The atrio ventricular node artery (arrow) would require a second reconstruction to follow that artery. The left anterior descending (b), with multiple diagonal branches, often needs multiple reconstructions to demonstrate its entire course.

Curved MPR with coronary CT angiography has been reported with high sensitivity and specificity (Achenbach et al., 1998). Significant stenosis and occlusions of the coronary arteries can be visualized with an accuracy that exceeds 90%, since the CT value is preserved, making it fairly easy to delineate calcifications from the lumen. Recognition of calcifications with either higher or lower density than inner lumen contrast is very difficult with VR, somewhat better with MIP, and best with MPR. In addition, curved MPR is used to identify and quantify the degree of stenosis without being hindered by partial averaging (Fig. 5). This method is also useful in delineating the morphology of plaque and its effect on the lumen and adjacent vessel wall. Furthermore, the distance measurements in the curved MPR images represent the true distance. Overall, curved MPR, because they can be rendered quickly and convey all the information about the different CT densities within the vessel, is an extremely useful tool to evaluate contrast-enhanced CT angiography data.

The drawback of curved MPR is that only one vessel can be visualized in one image and that side branches are not depicted unless separate reconstructions are rendered for every side branch (Achenbach et al., 1998). Angiographic view is better in evaluating multiple branches. Furthermore, accurate assessment for stenosis requires correct centerline placement. Since the quality and ability of the computer workstation for tracking the vessel depends on border definition and overall image quality, off-axis centerline placement may happen, which result in misinterpretation of stenosis. Thus, curved MPR requires some editing in most cases. This commonly occurs in the presence of heavy arterial calcification and at the site of origin of branch.

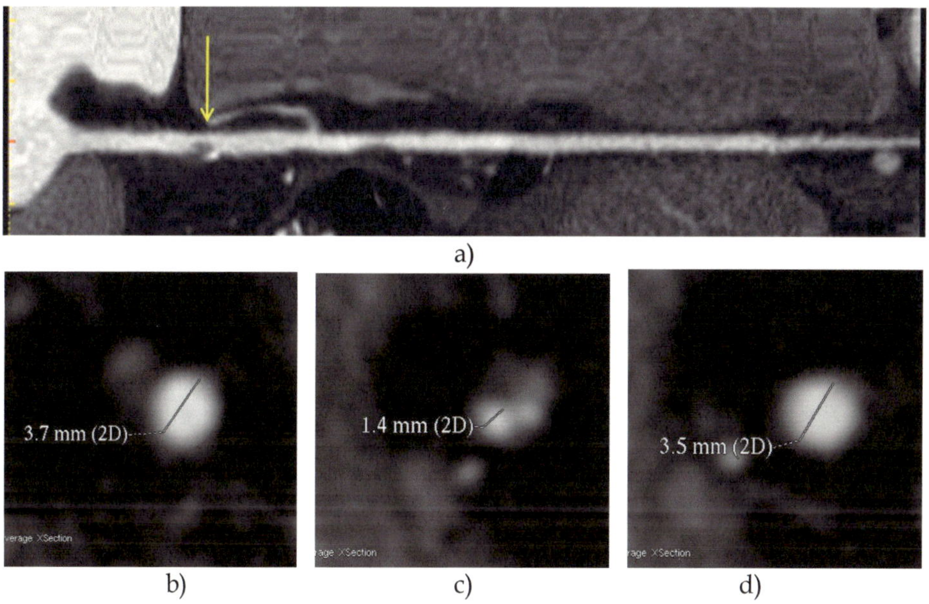

Fig. 5. Curved multiplanar reformation for coronary artery stenosis

Coronary stenosis (arrow) is demonstrated in the proximal segment of the right coronary artery. The observer can always create a plane orthogonal to the direction of the vessel, which allows the evaluation of the configuration of plaque and grading of a stenosis. The three orthogonal planes are at the level of a proximal normal lumen (b), a significant stenosis (c), and a distal normal lumen (d), respectively.

2.4 Volume rendering (VR)

Rendering is a term taken from computer graphics and represents the process of generating a 3D model from a 2D image. Opacity and color are assigned to each CT value interval via transfer function, which is selectable and interactively modifiable (Calhoun et al., 1999). For example, normal soft tissue is assigned high transparency, enhanced vascular structures slight opaqueness and bone strong opaqueness. The sum of all CT values along each search ray from the observer through the 3D data volume, weighted by the transfer function, is displayed. In addition, color is used in most cases, with the color intensity decreasing with increasing distance to the observer in order to generate depth information and a 3D impression. The image can be rotated to different views, allowing the interpreter some flexibility in seeing the segment from multiple angles (Fig. 6).

VR provides an excellent overview of the cardiac and vascular anatomy, such as defining the course of coronary anomalies (Fig. 7a), the presence and course of coronary bypass grafts (Fig. 7b), the analysis of thoracic cardiovascular anatomy and congenital heart disease (Fig. 7c). Because VR creates volumetric 3D representations with the illusion of spatial integrity, it is helpful for surgeons to understand the anatomic complexity before surgery, and for teaching purposes and as illustrations for patients.

It is controversial whether VR can be used for the assessment of coronary stenosis. One study using 16 slice CT compared 3D VRs with combination of techniques including axial images, MPRs, and curved MPRs and MIPs. Sensitivity (63% vs 74%), specificity (80% vs 76%), and accuracy (78% vs 75%) were not significantly different between VR and the combination of techniques, respectively (Cordeiro et al., 2006). However, the diameter of vessels and the apparent thickness of the vessel lumen are dependent on threshold or transparency settings and the computer algorithm that is used to subtract non-vascular structures with VR (Ferencik et al., 2007) (Fig. 8). Furthermore, the overlap of cardiac veins on coronary arteries often hinders the coronary artery stenosis at the overlapped segment on VR (Fig. 9). Another disadvantage of VR is that due to its use of threshold or transparency setting which obscure the lower attenuation structures, the visualization of smaller vessel may be inferior compared with other displaying methods (Johnson et al, 2010). VR also requires several angles to evaluate the entire coronary artery (Fig. 6).

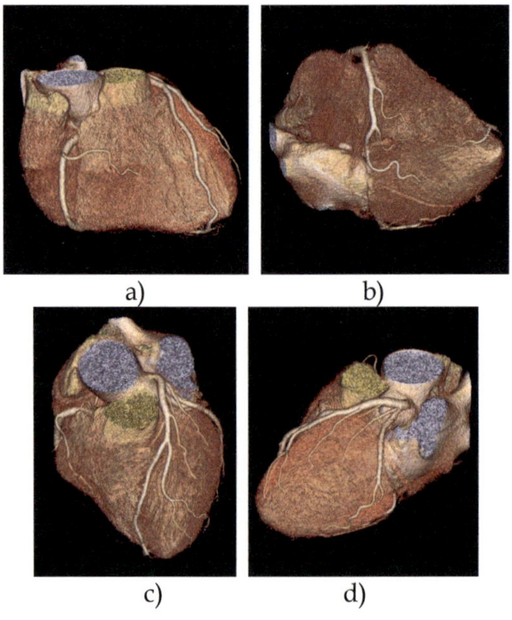

Fig. 6. Volume rendering of the coronary arteries.

Volume rendering provides an excellent overview of coronary anomalies, the course of coronary bypass grafts, and congenital heart disease

a. Coronary anomalies: both coronary arteries originate from left coronary cusp (stent is placed in the proximal segment of left descending artery).
b. Bypass grafts: right internal thoracic artery (RITA) graft communicate with the left descending artery and left internal thoracic artery (LITA) graft communicate with obtuse marginal branch.

c. Major aortopulmonary collateral artery in patients with Tetralogy of Fallot (red: aortic arch, yellow: right pulmonary artery arising from aorta, green: left pulmonary arteries arising from ductus arteriosus).

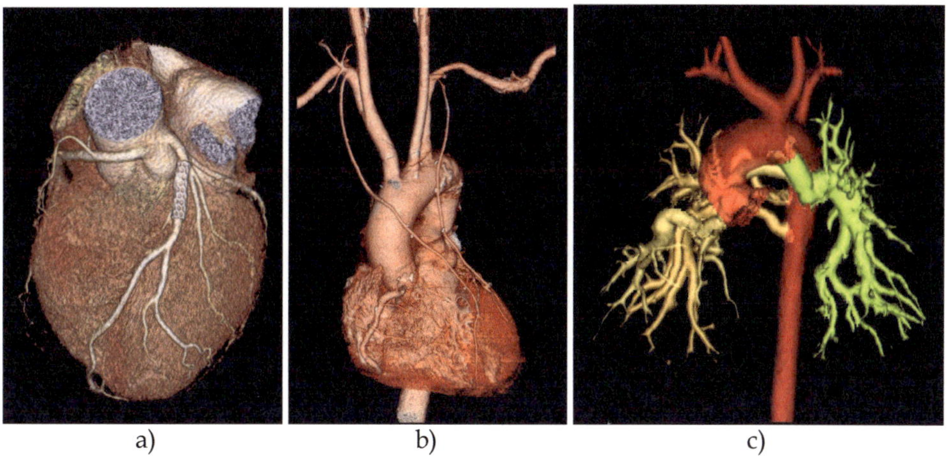

Fig. 7. Volume rendering of cardiac and vascular anatomy

Volume rendering allows an easy overview of coronary artery anatomy. It assists significantly in understanding the topography of coronary vessels and position of the lesion in coronary tree. Dedicated projections for each of the three main vessels are performed. The proximal and middle segment of the RCA is visualized in a view from the right side (a). The distal segment of the RCA is visualized in a right caudal view (b). The left anterior descending artery is visualized in a left anterior view (c). The left circumflex artery is visualized in a left cranial view and a left view (d).

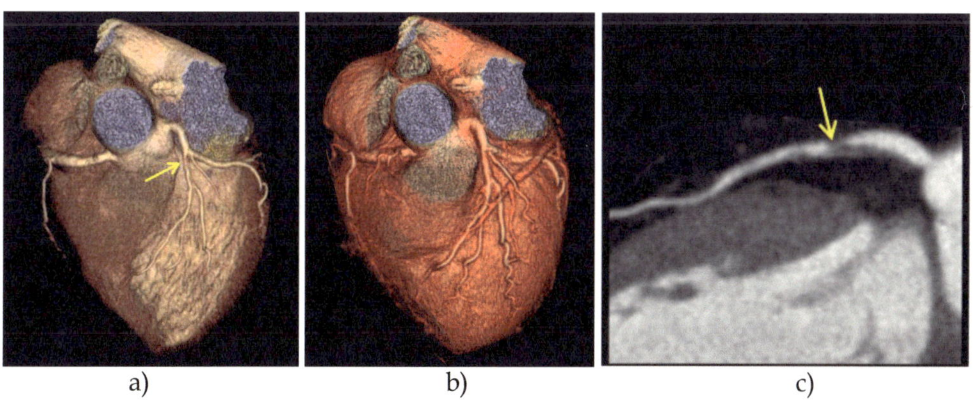

Fig. 8. The affect of modifying threshold and opacity setting on volume rendering

Coronary stenosis (arrow) is suspected in the proximal segment of left descending artery in the image with high opacity setting (a), while it is difficult to detect coronary stenosis in the image with low opacity setting (b). Significant coronary stenosis (c: arrow) is seen in curved MPR at the same location suspected in volume rendering with high opacity setting. The diameter of coronary artery is also modified by changing the threshold and opacity setting.

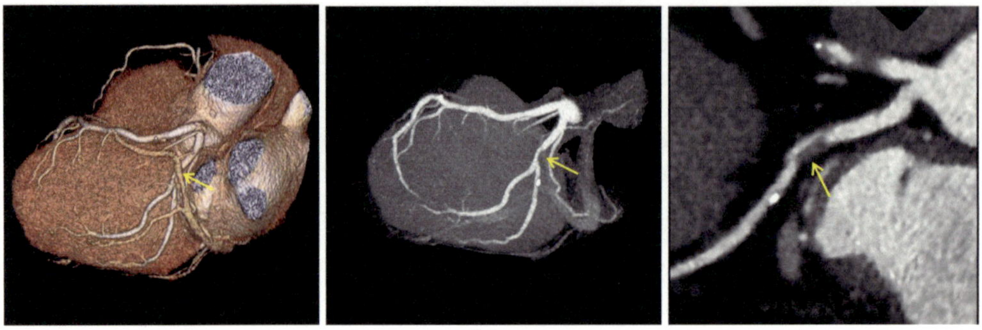

a) b) c)

Fig. 9. Overlapped coronary vein on volume rendering

Coronary stenosis in the proximal left circumflex artery (arrow) is hindered by overlapped great cardiac vein on volume rendering (a), while it is well visualized on angiographic view (b: arrow) and curved MPR (c: arrow).

2.5 Angiographic view (AGV)

AGV is an whole heart MIP image in which contrast media of the ventricles is eliminated (Fig.10). This image is similar to that from invasive conventional coronary angiography (CAG). In our institute, AGV images divided into right and left coronary artery were rendered interactively from at least three angles for right coronary artery and six angles for left coronary artery (Fig. 11). If necessary, reconstructions were rendered from additional angles to visualize the entire coronary tree. AGV was originally automatically created only in GE workstation, but is available in many other workstations. It can be created in 3 steps after VR of cardiac CT is created in the usual method (Jinzaki et al., 2006). First, the origins of the right and left coronary arteries are separated from the ascending aorta. Second, the image of the ascending aorta and left ventricle is selected and singled out by clicking any area of the ascending aorta. Third, this image is subtracted from the original cardiac image, which leaves only the image of the coronary artery. Similar images can be created by tracking and extracting the coronary artery itself; however, tracking or extracting requires the threshold of CT attenuation, so the images can vary depending on the threshold and the ability of the workstation being used. AGV keeps the coronary artery untouched, and thus AGV does not vary among workstations.

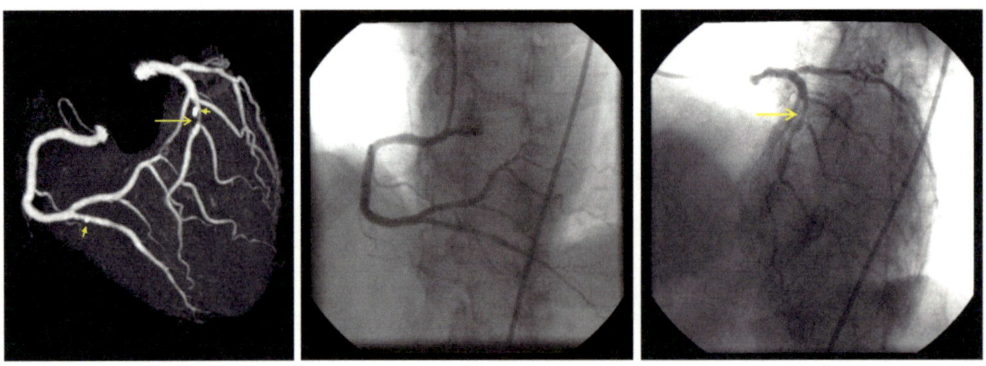

a) b) c)

Fig. 10. Angiographic view

Angiographic view image clearly demonstrates the distribution of coronary artery stenosis (long arrow) and coronary calcifications (short arrows) in one image. This resembles the images of coronary angiography and is understandable by third parties. Angiographic view image (a) and coronary angiography (b, c) shows considerable consistency in the detection of coronary artery stenosis (long arrows).

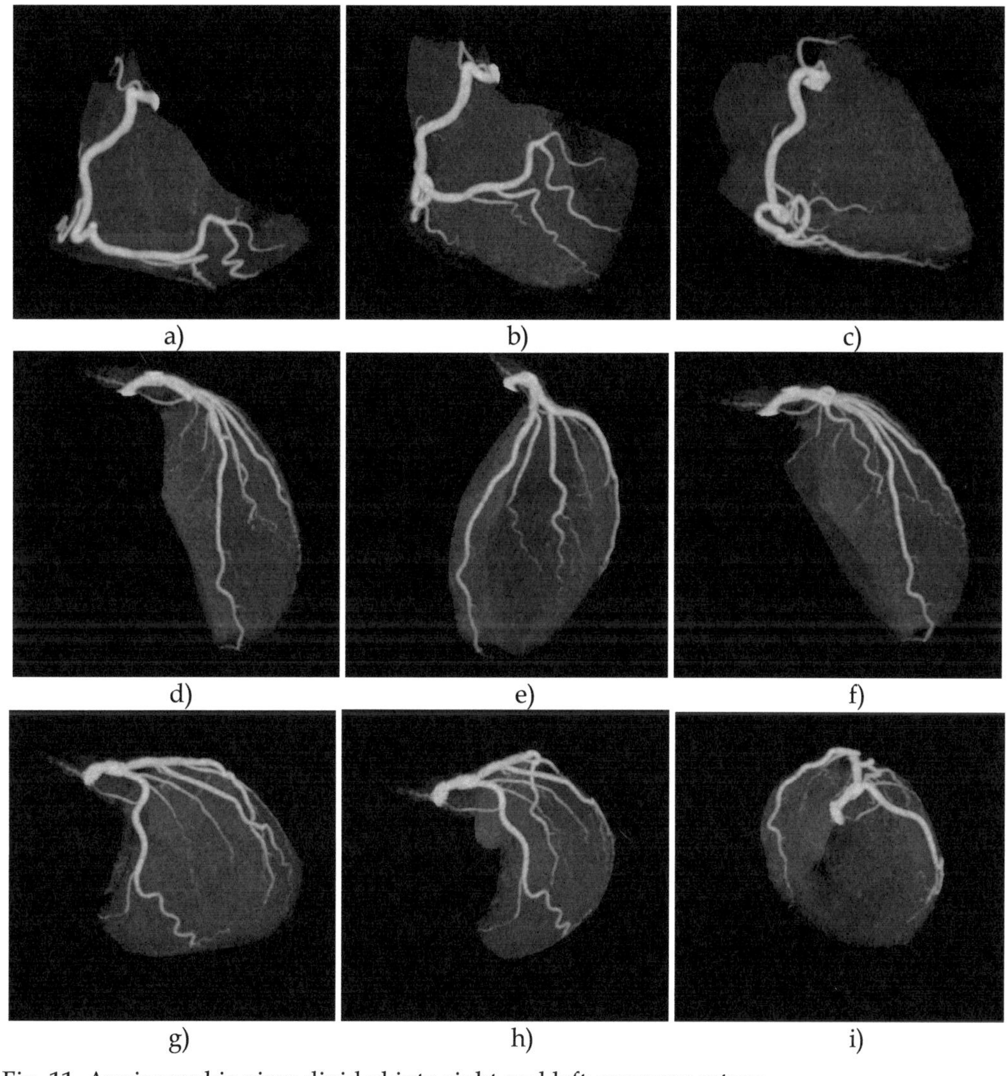

Fig. 11. Angiographic view divided into right and left coronary artery

Angiographic view image divided into right and left coronary artery enables viewing the coronary arteries with the same angle as CAG. We create three directions in RCA [a: left anterior oblique (LAO) 45 and cranial angulations (CRA) 0, b: LAO 20 and CRA 30, c: right anterior oblique (RAO) 30 and CRA 0) and 6 directions in LCA (d: LAO 0 and CRA 30, e: LAO 45 and CRA 25, f: RAO 20 and CRA 40, g: RAO 30 and caudal angulations (CAU) 30, h: RAO 0 and CAU 30, i: LAO 50 and CAU 30].

The advantage of AGV image is that it clearly demonstrates the distribution of high-density lesions, such as coronary calcifications and stents, and coronary artery stenosis in a single image, making it easier to be understood when viewed by any third party. Because the structures are displayed based upon their brightness, calcium and metal are easily distinguished from the contrast-enhanced lumen. For the detection of coronary stenosis, AGV was equally sensitive (98%) and accurate (91%) to a combination of conventional techniques, including interactive MIP and MPR as well as preset curved MPRs (98%sensitive, 94% accurate) (Jinzaki et al., 2009). AGV is also better for displaying small-caliber segments as described in thin-slab MIP. Furthermore, AGV divided into right and left coronary artery enables viewing the lesion with the same angle as CAG, and the detection of best angle of the lesion prior to PCI (Fig. 12). Collateral arteries are also well visualized in AGV. The whole collateral arteries are demonstrated with AGV in less images than volume rendering, since AGV is a projection image (Fig. 13). Thus, AGV would be useful for explaining the severity of disease to the patient, as a guide for the reading due to its high diagnostic accuracy, and in the discussion of the treatment strategy in conference.

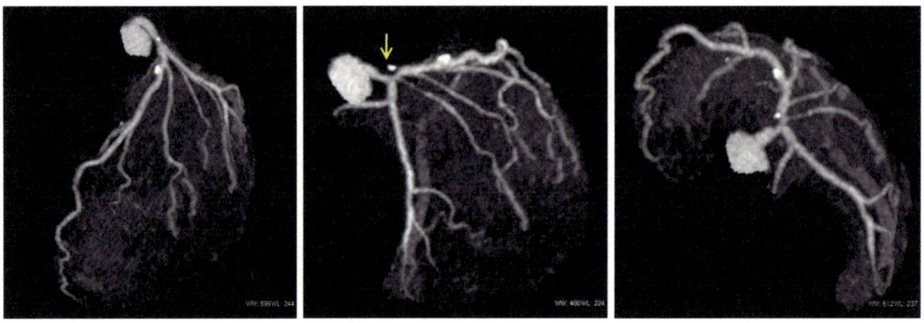

Fig. 12. The detection of best angle of the lesion prior to PCI

The coronary stenosis (arrow) is best visualized in the view of RAO 30 and CAU 30 (middle). This information will help cardiologists in discussing treatment strategy and reduce the number of CAG image acquisitions.

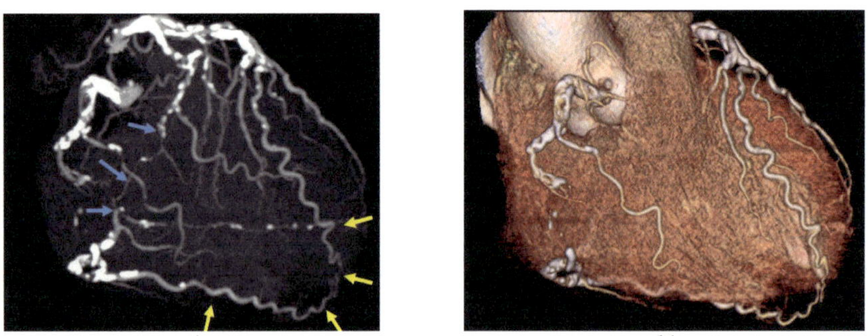

a) b)

Fig. 13. Angiographic view in case with collateral vessels

In patients with chronic total occlusion of RCA, collateral vessels are seen between left descending artery and posterior descending artery (yellow arrows), left circumflex artery and posterolateral artery (blue arrows). These collateral vessels are well demonstrated in one image with angiographic view (a), while the whole collateral arteries are not visualized in one image with volume rendering (b).

A disadvantage of AGV is that since it is a 2D display, it requires review of multiple rotated images to understand 3D relationships. MIP does not provide in-depth information or attenuation detail within the slice, because overlapped higher-density structures obscure the lower-density structures of interest. Static MIP images can be misleading, by incorrect placement of arteries. Another disadvantage is that MIP algorithm is prone to artifacts. One well-known pitfall is the "string of beads" appearance, because a normal small vessel passing obliquely through a volume is only partially represented by voxels along its length (Calhoun et al., 1999). Because MIP selects the highest density voxels along a ray projected through the volume, adequate contrast enhancement is imperative. MIP has a tendency to overestimate the stenosis, especially in case with calcification (Rubin et al., 1994). Non-calcified plaque may be overlooked unless it creates significant luminal narrowing, because of its low attenuation value.

2.6 Plaque-loaded angiographic view (PLAG)

So far, there is no post-processing technique that can display an overview image of the lumen and vessel wall of a whole heart in one image (Fig. 14). PLAG is the image in which the non-calcified plaque image is merged with the AGV (Jinzaki et al., 2008). As a result, PLAG allows the noninvasive visualization of the whole coronary lumen and the vessel wall in one image. PLAG is now available in GE workstation and some other workstations. If this is not available in your workstation, it can be generated as follows: First, the color-coded plaque image of each coronary artery is created (Fig 14a). The CT attenuation of the coronary lumen is usually larger than 250HU, while that of non-calcified plaque is typically less than 120HU. Setting the color code range at less than 120 HU can generate a "plaque image", in which only the vessel wall and the non-calcified plaques are color-coded. Second, AGV image of the entire coronary artery (Fig 14b), which is similar to that shown by a CAG is separately generated, which displays the distribution of calcified plaques as well as the lumen in more detail. Third, the color-coded "plaque image" in curved MPR is re-formatted into a MIP image to merge with AGV image. Finally, loading the MIP "plaque image" onto AGV image completes the process (Figs 14c). The critical factors in PLAG are that the merged images are both in MIP format, and taking advantage of a relatively large CT attenuation discrepancy between the lumen and non-calcified plaque allows color-coding, which helps to better visualize plaques when loaded onto AGV.

PLAG will provide comprehensive information for coronary CT angiography in discussing the treatment strategy of both coronary stenosis and non-stenotic non-calcified plaques. This image also enables the overview of the tortuous vessel in the chronic total occlusion (CTO), which would be useful for the percutaneous revascularization of CTO (Fig.15).

In future, with the further improvement of temporal and spatial resolution of MDCT, and with enhanced accuracy of plaque volume quantification is enhanced, this image could also be useful in evaluating and demonstrating the therapeutic effect of anti-atherosclerotic drugs in patients with multiple soft plaques in coronary arteries (the so-called vulnerable patients) on one image.

The characteristics of each post-processing

For the effective use of the various post-processing techniques, knowledge of the characteristics of each post-processing method is mandatory. The strengths and weaknesses of the available post-processing technique are summarized in Table 1.

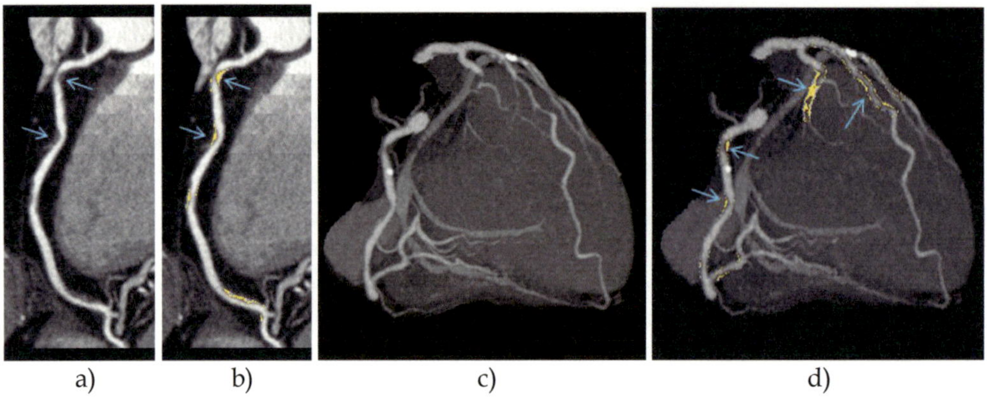

Fig. 14. Plaque-loaded Angiographic View of multiple non-calcified plaques

Curved MPR of the right coronary artery (a) demonstrates the non-stenotic non-calcified plaques (arrows), which are assigned blue in color-coded image (b). The angiographic view image (c) demonstrates the lumen of the entire coronary artery. The color-coded image in curved MPR is re-formatted into a MIP image and merged with the Angiographic View image. The Plaque-loaded Angiographic View image (d) demonstrates the lumen and multiple plaques (arrows) of coronary arteries in one image.

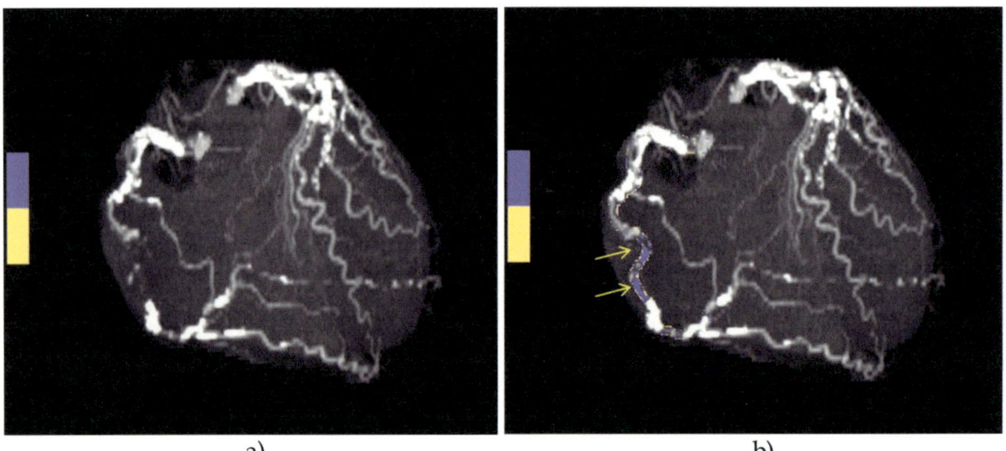

Fig. 15. Plaque-loaded Angiographic View of chronic totally occlusion
An angiographic view image (a) could not provide the information of the occluded lesion. The Plaque-loaded Angiographic View image (b) demonstrates the overview of the tortuous vessel (arrows) in the occluded lesion.

3. Image interpretation

At the beginning of interpretation, an overview of the data set should be performed to detect artifacts, gross abnormalities and the presence of non-coronary cardiac or extra-cardiac abnormalities. Coronary artery interpretation is then performed using post-processing images

Type of technique	Advantage	Disadvantage
Segment evaluation		
Axial image	true data	numerous images required for overview
	anatomical overview	improper for coronary stenosis evaluation
	quick review	
MPR	true data	numerous images required for overview
	anatomical overview	improper for coronary stenosis evaluation
	accurate distance measurements	
	quick review	
Thin-slab MIP	partial overview of the interested vessel	many images required for overview
	high visualization of small vessel	overestimation of coronary stenosis
	quick review	
The entire artery and segment evaluation		
Curved MPR	overview of one entire coronary artery	many images for branch evaluation
	accurate distance measurements	manual editing
	coronary stenosis evaluation	
Whole image		
VR	anatomical overview	user dependent (threshold and transparency setting)
		improper for coronary stenosis evaluation
		low visualization of small vessel
AGV	overview of coronary stenosis	no in-depth information
	high visualization of small vessel	prone to artifact
		low visualization of non-stenotic plaque (non-calcified)
PLAG	overview of stenosis and	no in-depth information
	non-stenotic plaque	prone to artifact
	high visualization of small vessel	Not yet accurate for quantity evaluation of plaque volume

Table 1. Comparison of post-processing techniques

3.1 Examination of image quality

It is imperative that an interpreter spend the first minute making sure the dataset is adequate. Artifacts due to motion, calcification, and metallic densities; image noise; and poor contrast enhancement may degrade the quality of the study as well as simulate or obscure coronary stenoses (Achenbach et al., 2003, Ferencik et al, 2003). To evaluate the image quality, the axial CT source images, multiplanar reformatted images, and also three-dimensional images were analyzed. The reader should specifically state if an artery or artery segment is not interpretable and why.

3.1.1 Artifact

"Artifact" can be defined as any discrepancy between the reconstructed Hounsfield values in the image and the true attenuation coefficients of the object in such a way that these discrepancies are clinically significant or relevant as judged by the radiologist (Hsieh, J., 2003). Artifacts of coronary CT angiography were classified into three categories (Table 2). The first is cardiac motion-related artifact (Choi et al., 2004). This is caused by many factors, including a heart rate greater than 70–75 beats per minute during imaging acquisition, variations in heart rate during breath holding (Fig 16), arrhythmia, and inappropriate selection of pitch or reconstruction window. Artifacts are classified into two patterns: motion blurring or stepladder effects. Blurring occurs when movement in the cardiac structure of interest exceeds the temporal resolution of scanning, either because of a fast heart rate or because of an inappropriate selection of the reconstruction window for the particular coronary artery. Stepladder artifacts are due to motion occurring between reconstruction of sequential heartbeats. The easiest way of reducing cardiac motion artifacts is to lower the heart rate by the prior administration of-blocker. Customized reconstructions at a different cardiac phase may be successful by either adjusting the phase of reconstruction or removing data from undesirable beats.

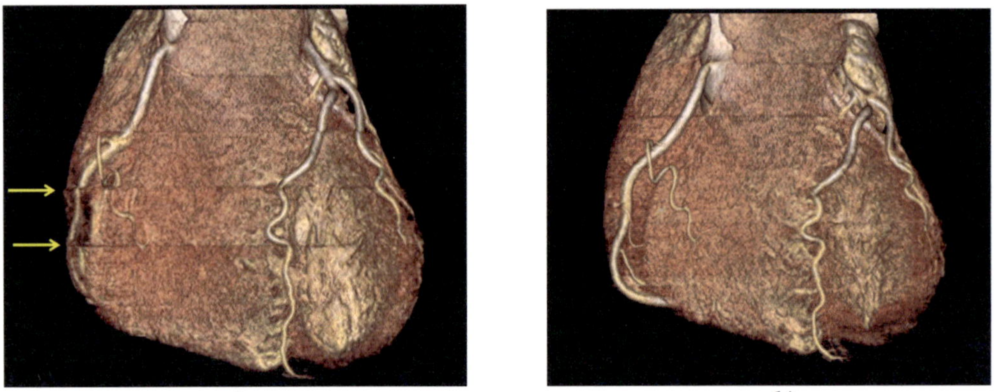

a) b)

Fig. 16. Stepladder artifact due to changing heart rate during CT acquisition. Volume-rendered image (a) shows a severe motion-related artifact (arrows) caused by acceleration in heart rate toward the end of the breath hold. Selection of an optimal reconstruction window reduced the artifact (b).

The second is voluntary motion that is generally preventable with careful instruction of the patient (Choi et al., 2004). Artifacts due to breathing (Fig 17) or body motion are distinctive because they affect the bones of the anterior or lateral chest wall in addition to the coronary arteries; these are less likely to be correctable by additional reconstructions. Oxygen supplementation may help dyspneic patients hold their breaths for a longer period.

The third is high-attenuating artifact (Choi et al., 2004). High-attenuating artifact includes, blooming artifacts, beam hardening artifacts and streaking artifacts. Blooming artifact is a result of partial-volume effects, causing the status that small high-contrast objects appear larger than they are. These artifacts commonly make calcified plaque (Fig 18a) and stents appear to narrow the lumen more than they actually do. Use of appropriate reconstruction filters may reduce these artifacts. Beam hardening presents as dark banding between dense objects. These are also seen in calcified plaque and stents (Fig 18b). Streaking artifact is a kind of reconstruction artifact due to undersampling, photon starvation, motion, beam hardening, or scatter. In coronary CT angiography, these are usually caused by metallic objects such as clips, markers, and wires used in coronary artery bypass surgery, and often called as metal artifact (Fig 18c).

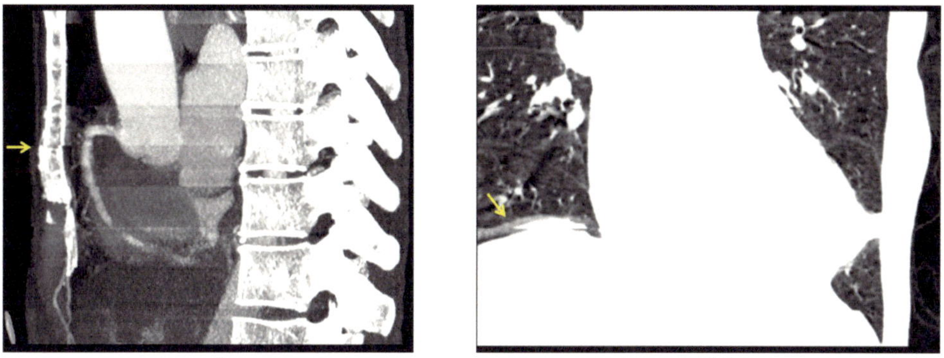

a) b)

Fig. 17. Stepladder artifact due to breathing

Sagittal maximum intensity projection image (a) and coronal MPR image (b) show a severe respiration-related artifact in the anterior chest wall (arrow) and at the diaphragm (arrow).

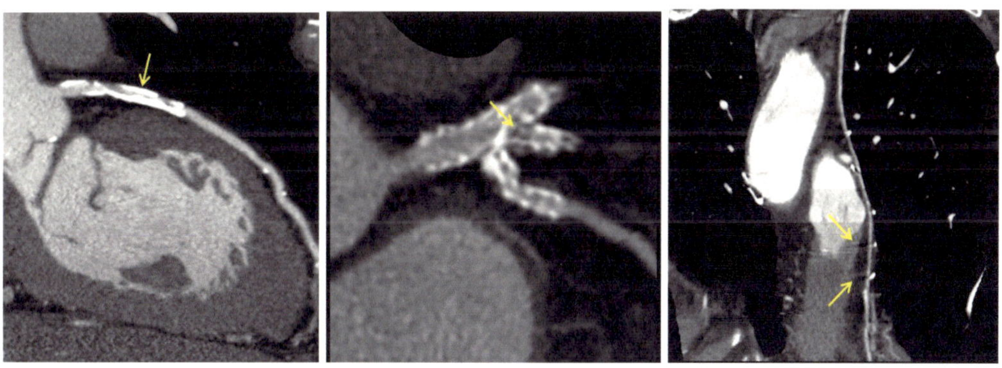

a) b) c)

Fig. 18. High-attenuating artifacts

a. Blooming artifact caused by severe coronary calcifications that interfere with the evaluation of luminal stenosis.
b. Beam hardening artifacts caused by coronary stent that prevents accurate evaluation of the stent lumen.
c. Metal artifacts caused by surgical clips.

3.1.2 Image noise

Improper scan parameter (low tube output for a given body size) causes poor signal-to-noise (Fig 19). This is mainly due to obesity. Improper reconstruction during a part of the cardiac cycle with reduced tube current from EKG-guided tube modulation also results in low image quality.

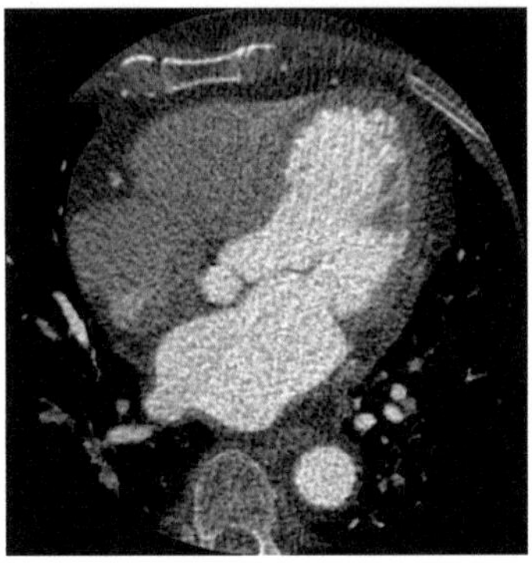

Fig. 19. Low image quality due to improper scan parameters.

Poor signal-to-noise is caused by low tube output for a given body size

3.1.3 Low contrast enhancement

The methods of reconstruction rely on Hounsfield units (HU) to make images. Values of 250 HU and above are ideal, and current protocols generally yield mean enhancement levels in the range of 300 to 350 HU for right and left coronary arteries (Johnson et al., 2009, Husmann et al., 2009). Low contrast attenuation may be secondary to improper image acquisition timing or slow contrast injection.

Artifact	Cause	Manifestation	Solution
Cardiac motion	High heart rate	Blur	Prior administration of beta-blocker
	Heart rate change	Stepladder artifact	Selection of appropriate reconstruction Window
	Premature contraction	Stepladder artifact	Removing data from undesirable beats
	Inappropriate reconstruction window	Blur	Selection of appropriate reconstruction window
Voluntary motion	Respiration	Blur & stepladder artifact Careful instruction to patient	Oxygen supplementation;
	Body motion	Blur &Stepladder artifact	Minimization of anatomic coverage Careful instruction to patient
High-attenuating	Metallic object (Surgical clip, marker, or wire)	Beam hardening Streaking artifact	Use of nonmetallic materials
	Coronary stent	Blooming artifact Beam hardening	Use of appropriate image filters
	Calcification	Blooming artifact Beam hardening	Use of appropriate image filters

Table 2. Various artifacts in coronary CT angiography

3.2 Non-coronary cardiac findings

Non-coronary cardiovascular structures include the pericardium, cardiac chambers, interatrial septum, interventricular septum, atrioventricular valves, ventriculo-arterial valves, pulmonary arteries, pulmonary veins, thoracic aorta, imaged aortic branch arteries, and central systemic veins. The axial images or MPRs is useful for a general understanding of the spatial relationship of these structures and abnormality. Left ventricular and left atrial myocardial walls and chamber cavities should be examined for hypertrophy, dilation, thinning (Fig. 20a), hypodense enhancement, thrombus (Fig 20b), masses, and congenital anomalies. These structures should be reviewed within the cardiac field-of-view and any abnormalities described.

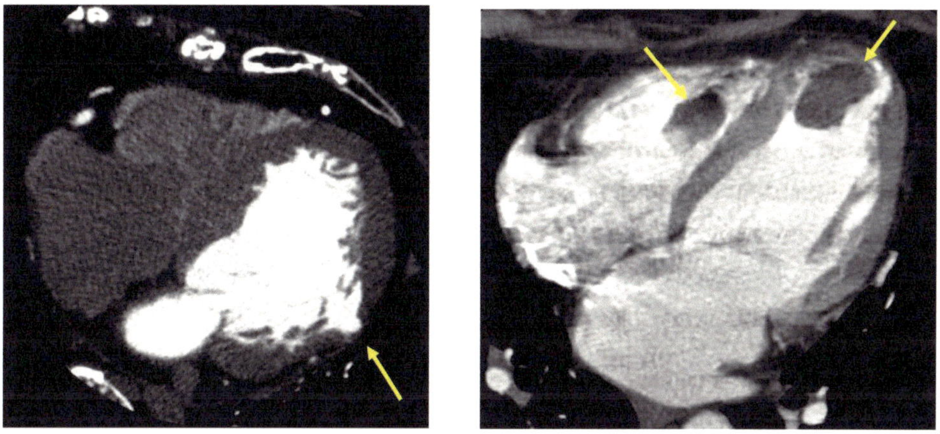

a) b)

Fig. 20. Non-coronary cardiac findings

a. Focal thinning of myocardial wall due to ventricular diverticula (arrow)
b. Thrombus in ventricular chamber (arrow)

3.3 Extra-cardiac structures

Extra-cardiac structures within the field of view of routine coronary CT angiography include the mediastinum, hilum, trachea and bronchi, lung parenchyma, pleura, chest wall, esophagus, stomach, liver, spleen, and colon. Interpretation of the axial images or MPR provides a general understanding of the anatomic relationships of the heart and coronary arteries with surrounding extra-cardiac structures. Review of all visible non-cardiovascular structures is important for two principal reasons: (1) recognition of primary and secondary comorbid pathology and (2) identification of findings that lead to alternative non-cardiovascular diagnoses.

3.4 Coronary artery interpretation

In analyzing coronary arteries, a systematic approach using axial images and post-processing images should be followed. Realizing from the outset that no single method of analysis is without limitations, the incorporative review of the 2D images and the different 3D renderings is necessary. However, how to use the various available post-processing techniques remains a matter of personal experience and may differ among various operators.

3.4.1 Interpretation of axial images

The axial image evaluation is a fundamental and essential step, because information from the original data set (axial images) can be lost as a consequence of processing the images for advanced postprocessing methods. Scrolling through the axial images in the cranio-caudal direction allows interpretation of the anatomy and gross abnormality of coronary arteries. Myocardial bridge of coronary artery is often easily noticed in axial images than post-processing images (Fig 21a). However, following each segment on each level (over 50-80contiguous images) may be difficult, and the evaluation of coronary stenosis is often more difficult compared with the post-processing methods (Jinzaki et al., 2009) (Fig 21b). For example, correct diagnosis of coronary stenosis is difficult with the axial images in the lesions located in the segment running horizontal to the axial section. Diffuse concentric plaque with positive remodeling also has a tendency to be incorrectly viewed as stenotic on axial images, possibly because the reference diameter (vessel diameter in non-diseased artery immediately proximal to the lesion) of these lesions is not measurable on the axial image. The post-processing image is better suited for evaluation of these types of lesions.

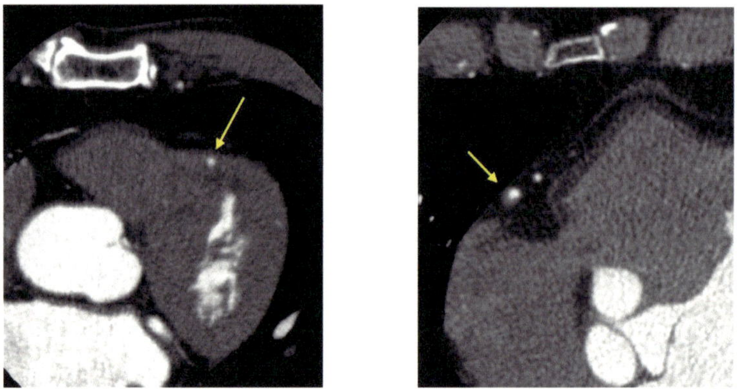

a) b)

Fig. 21. Interpretation of axial images

Myocardial bridge of coronary artery (a: arrow) is often easily noticed in axial images. The diagnosis of coronary stenosis is easy in the lesions located in the segment running the cranio-caudal direction (b: arrow), however difficult in the lesions located in the segment running horizontal to the axial section.

3.4.2 The use of post-processing images

After the interpretation of axial images, the readers should shift to post-processing images. VR provide an overview of the coronary tree. Also, more complex anatomy (such as congenital heart disease or bypass grafts) is easily seen. For coronary artery evaluation, the combination of several types of post-processing algorithms such as thin-slab MIP, MPR and curved MPR is usually used. However, these methods require numerous images to evaluate the whole coronary artery, while AGV would be easy to overview the distribution of coronary lesion. Thus, as an initial guide for the interpretation, we recommend first to use AGV. Furthermore, in the comparison of the AGV image and combination of several types of post-processing, sensitivity was the same (98%) and there was no significant difference in accuracy (Jinzaki et al., 2009). If coronary artery stenosis is detected on AGV, the lesion should be evaluated further for vessel wall morphology and composition using curved MPR. Further evaluation could be omitted in branch vessels with no stenotic lesions on AGV, since the negative predictive value of AGV is very high (99%) and evaluating multiple diagonal branches or obtuse marginal branches is time-consuming with curved MPR or other methods. However, even if stenotic lesion is not detected in three main arteries on AGV, we recommend reconstructing curved MPR of these arteries to evaluate non-stenotic non-calcified plaque, which may be missed on AGV. This is because acute myocardial infarction is frequently related to a segment that was not significantly stenosed at previous angiography (Littele, et al., 1988, Giroud et al., 1992). Acute coronary occlusions leading to myocardial infarction tend to cluster in predictable "hot spots" within the proximal third of the coronary arteries (Wang et al., 2004). Identification of low attenuation plaques in these high-risk zones for acute coronary occlusions will be important for potentially locally directed preventive strategies.

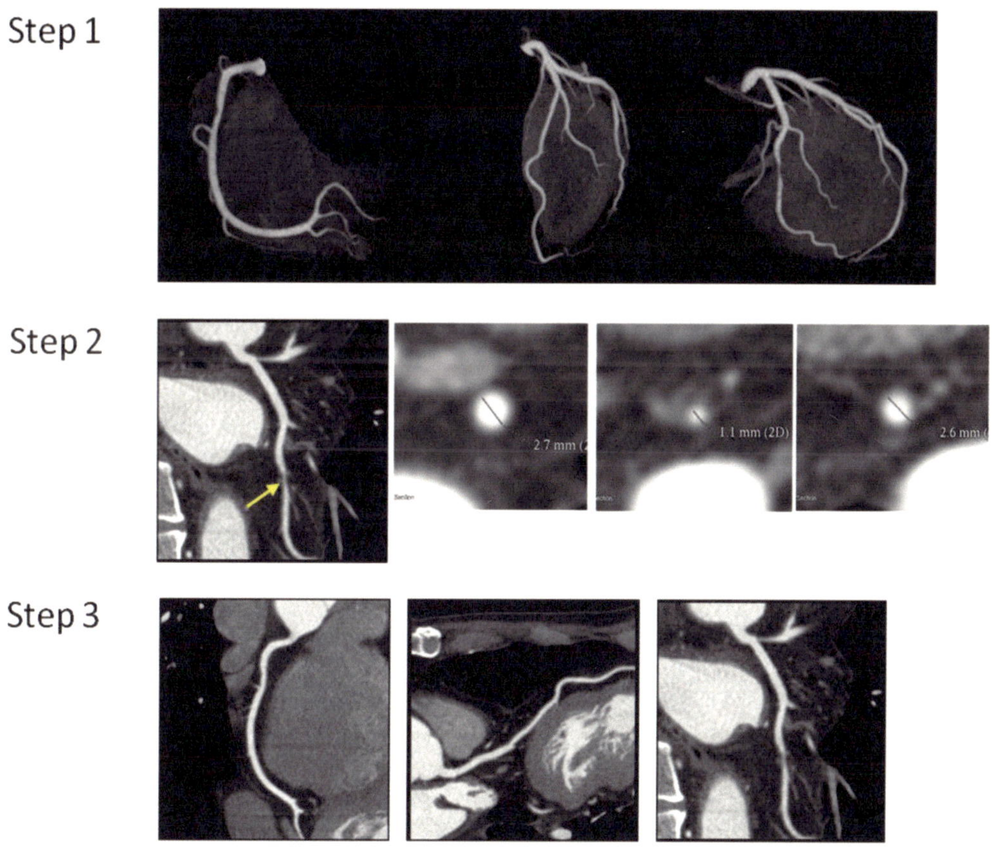

Fig. 22. Workflow of post-processing and interpretation for coronary artery evaluation

Step 1. Overview of coronary artery on angiographic view
Step 2. Quantitative evaluation of coronary lesions detected on angiographic view
Step 3. Evaluation of three main arteries using curved MPR and no further evaluation in branch vessels without stenotic lesions on angiographic view

3.4.3 The guiding principles of interpretation

To analyze coronary arteries a systemic approach should be followed. It is recommended that the coronary segments are evaluated in a sequential order from segment 1 to segment 15 following the standard report of the American Heart Association. The interpretation of coronary arteries include (1) assessment of stenosis severity, (2) vessel wall morphology and composition, (3) total occlusions, and (4) bypass graft and stent.

a. Assessment of stenosis severity

The description of luminal stenosis grading and plaque length is important in the interpretation. The degree of coronary stenosis is manually calculated by subtracting vessel diameter at the site of maximal stenosis from the mean of the vessel reference segment diameters (proximal and distal references) and then dividing the difference by the mean of the vessel reference segment diameters on curved MPR and cross-sectional image (Fig 22). Recent cardiac- vessel analysis packages enables calculating percent stenosis automatically when the user selects the area of maximum narrowing and normal vessel proximal and distal to the stenosis (Busch et al., 2007). However, current spatial resolution of CT has not demonstrated sufficient reproducibility or accuracy in predicting findings of CAG to make such measurements a routine requirement. Thus, at the present time, Society of Cardiovascular Computed Tomography guideline recommends that arterial segments be described within broad stenosis ranges (Cheng et al., 2008, Raff et al., 2009) (Table 3), although future technical developments may improve the precision of stenosis quantification.

0 Normal: Absence of plaque and no luminal stenosis
1 Minimal: Plaque with <25% stenosis
2 Mild: 25%–49% stenosis
3 Moderate: 50%–69% stenosis
4 Severe: 70%–99% stenosis
5 Occluded

Table 3. Quantitative Stenosis Grading

b. Vessel wall morphology and composition

Vessel wall morphology and composition are important information of coronary CT angiography, since these are not available on CAG. coronary CT angiography can visualize intramural presence of positively remodeled plaque and differentiate calcific, non-calcific, and mixed plaque. Society of Cardiovascular Computed Tomography recommends that the description of plaques as "non-calcific" is preferable to "soft" or "lipid-rich" since low CT density (in Hounsfield units) levels do not necessarily correlate closely with anatomic pathology or biochemistry (Raff et al., 2009). Recent studies revealed that the CT characteristics of plaques associated with ACS include positive vascular remodeling, low plaque density<30HU, and spotty calcification (Motoyama et al., 2009) (Fig. 23). Thus, the description of these features will assist interpretation. The vascular remodeling index is defined as lesion diameter/reference diameter, and is reported as positive when the diameter at the plaque site was at least 10% larger than the reference segment. Spotty calcification was defined when the calcification is <3 mm in size. Features of plaque morphology such as ulceration, dissection, and fissuring are also noted when image quality is sufficient.

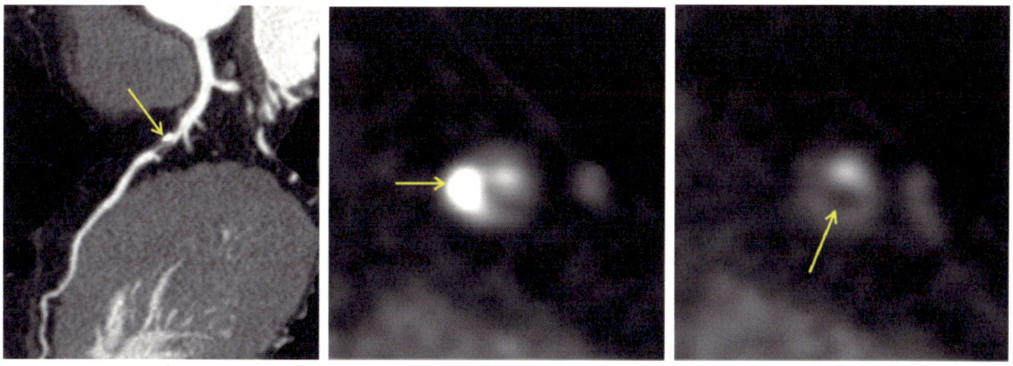

a) b) c)

Fig. 23. Low attenuation plaque and spotty calcification

Curved MPR demonstrates significant stenosis in left descending artery (a: arrow). The lesion is accompanied with spotty calcification (b: arrow) and area < 30HU (c: arrow).

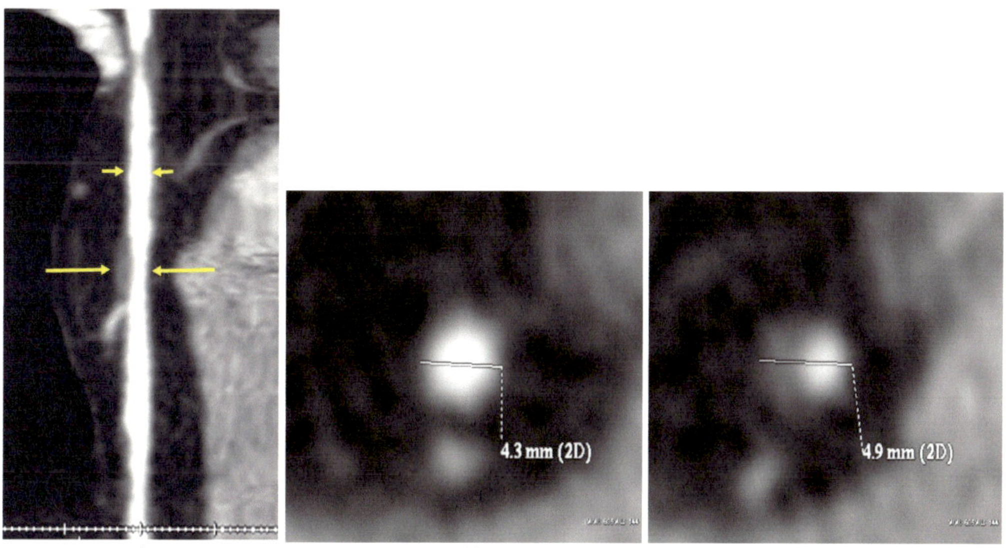

a) b) c)

Fig. 24. Positive remodeling

Non-calcified plaque (a: long arrows) in right coronary artery is positively remodeled as compared with the normal coronary segment proximal to the lesion (short arrows). The diameter was 4.3 mm in normal segment (b) and 4.9 mm in the lesion (c). Remodeling index was 1.14.

c. Total occlusions

PCI of CTO has a lower success rate than PCI of non-occluded coronary stenosis. Failure of guide-wire crossing the occluded lesion is the main cause of unsuccessful PCI of CTO. Coronary CT angiography may provide useful information for selecting patients suitable for PCI of CTO (Soon et al., 2007). It can show the collateral supply in the distal vessel beyond the occlusion (Fig. 13). The proximal and distal ends of an occluded segment can be distinctively seen on coronary CT angiography. Therefore, the occlusion length can be measured on CCTA (Fig. 24). Mollet et al. also reported that CTO lesion length > 15 mm measured on CT was associated with higher failure rate of PCI (Mollet et al., 2005). Heavy calcification of CTO has been reported to be an independent predictor of failed PCI of CTO (Noguchi et al., 2000). The exact location of calcified plaque on the image of coronary CT angiography may help the interventionist to steer the guide wire away from the calcified lesion that is not well seen on conventional angiography. PLAG images are able to demonstrate the overview of occluded lesion, which are helpful in providing the roadmap for interventionists during the process of wiring the occluded vessel (Fig. 15).

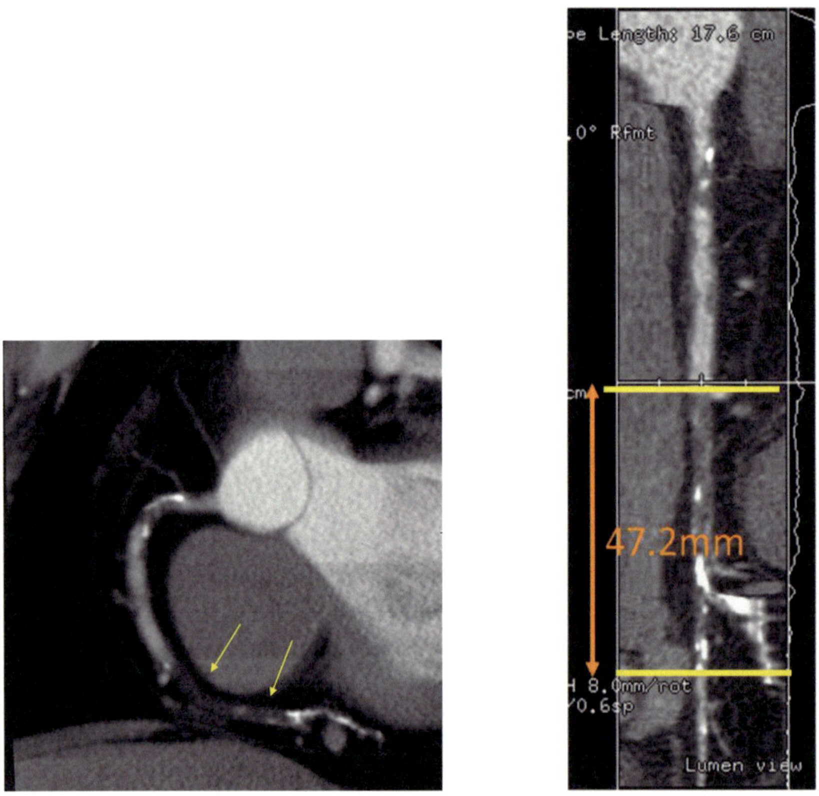

a) b)

Fig. 25. CT evaluation of chronic total occlusion

The total occlusion is seen in the distal segment of right coronary artery on thin-slab MIP images (a: arrows). The occlusion length can be measured on stretched MPR (b). Calcified plaque is also well visualized.

d. Bypass grafts, stents

The evaluation of coronary bypass grafts by coronary CT angiography is highly accurate in predicting the findings on invasive coronary angiography (Meyer et al., 2007). The location and anastomoses of bypass grafts should be described in addition to the location and severity of stenoses. The evaluation of stents by MDCT is often difficult due to blooming artifact and beam hardening effects. The evaluation of in-stent stenosis depends highly on stent size and composition. Stents 3.0 mm or larger (85%) were judged assessable; 26% of stents smaller than 3 mm were judged assessable (Schroeder et al., 2008). Different stent compositions and structures appeared to be associated with variations in the extent of residual artifact. The use of special reconstruction algorithms improved visualization of the stent lumen and reduced blooming artifact with a drawback of a modest increase in noise in the images (Maintz et al., 2006).

4. Conclusion

Many post-processing images are available for the evaluation of coronary artery. The interpreter should know the advantage and disadvantage of each post-processing image, and perform the incorporative review of the 2D images and the different 3D renderings.

5. References

Achenbach, S., Moshage, W., Ropers, D., & Bachmann, K. (1998). Curved multiplanar reconstructions for the evaluation of contrast-enhanced electron beam CT of the coronary arteries. *AJR Am J Roentgenol*, Vol.170, No.4, (Apr 1998), pp. 895-899.

Achenbach, S., Giesler, T., Ropers, D., Ulzheimer, S., Anders, K., Wenkel, E., Pohle, K., Kachelriess, M., Derlien, H., Kalender, WA., Daniel, WG., Bautz, W., & Baum, U. (2003). Comparison of image quality in contrast-enhanced coronary-artery visualization by electron beam tomography and retrospectively electrocardiogram-gated multislice spiral computed tomography. *Invest Radiol*, Vol.38, No.2, (Feb 2003), pp. 119–128.

Busch, S., Johnson, TR., Nikolaou, K., von Ziegler, F., Knez, A., Reiser, MF., & Becker, CR. (2007). Visual and automatic grading of coronary artery stenoses with 64-slice CT angiography in reference to invasive angiography. *Eur Radio*l, Vol.17, No. 6, (Jun 2007), pp.1445-1451.

Cademartiri, F; Mollet, NR & Nieman, K. (2005). Image post-processing, In *Computed Tomography of the Coronary Arteries*, Feyter PJ & Krestin GP, (ed.), 27-46, Taylor & Francis, New York

Calhoun, PS., Kuszyk, BS., Heath, DG., Carley, JC., & Fishman, EK. (1999). Three-dimensional volume rendering of spiral CT data: theory and method. *Radiographics*, Vol.19, No.3, (May-Jun 1999), pp. 745-764.

Cheng, V., Gutstein, A., Wolak, A., Suzuki, Y., Dey, D., Gransar, H., Thomson, LEJ., Hayes, SW., Friedman, JD., & Berman, DS. (2008). Moving beyond binary grading of coronary arterial stenoses on coronary computed tomographic angiography: insights for the imager and referring clinician. *J Am Coll Cardiol Imaging*, Vol.1, No. 4, (Jul 2008), pp. 460-471.

Choi, HS., Choi, BW., Choe, KO., Cho,i D., Yoo, KJ., Kim, MI., & Kim, J. (2004). Pitfalls, artifacts, and remedies in multi- detector row CT coronary angiography. *Radiographics,* Vol.24, No.3, (May-Jun 2004), pp. 787-800.

Choi, JW., Seo, JB., Do, KH., Choi, SI., Lee, W., Ko, SM., Lee, SH., Lee, JS., Song, JW., Song, KS., & Lim, TH. (2006). Comparison of transaxial source images and 3-plane, thin-slab maximal intensity projection images for the diagnosis of coronary artery stenosis with using ECG-gated cardiac CT. *Korean J Radio,l* Vol.7, No.1, (Jan-Mar 2006), pp. 20-27.

Cordeiro, MA., Lardo, AC., Brito, MS., Rosário Neto, MA., Siqueira, MH., Parga, JR., Avila, LF., Ramires, JA., Lima, JA., & Rochitte, CE. (2006). CT angiography in highly calcified arteries: 2D manual vs. modified automated 3D approach to identify coronary stenoses. *Int J Cardiovasc Imaging,* Vol.22, No.3-4, (Jun-Aug 2006), pp.507-516.

Ferencik, M., Moselewski, F., Ropers, D., Hoffmann, U., Baum, U., Anders, K., Pomerantsev, EV., Abbara, S., Brady, TJ., & Achenbach, S.(2003). Quantitative parameters of image quality in multidetector spiral computed tomographic coronary imaging with submillimeter collimation. *Am J Cardiol,* Vol.92, No.11, (Dec 2003), pp. 1257–1262.

Ferencik, M., Ropers, D., Abbara, S., Cury, RC., Hoffmann, U., Nieman, K., Brady, TJ., Moselewski, F., Daniel, WG., & Achenbach, S. (2007). Diagnostic accuracy of image postprocessing methods for the detection of coronary artery stenoses by using multidetector CT. *Radiology,* Vol.243, No.3, (Jun 2007), pp. 696–702.

Fishman, EK., Ney, DR., Heath, DG., Corl, FM., Horton, KM., & Johnson, PT. (2006). Volume rendering versus maximum intensity projection in CT angiography: what works best, when, and why. *Radiographics,* Vol.26, No.3, (May-Jun 2006), pp. 905-922.

Giroud, D., Li, JM., Urban, P., Meier, B., Rutishauer, W. (1992). Relation of the site of acute myocardial infarction to the most severe coronary arterial stenosis at prior angiography. *Am J Cardiol,* Vol.69, No.8, (Mar 1992), pp. 729-732.

Hsieh, J. (2003). Image artifacts: appearances, causes, and corrections. In *Computed tomography: principles, design, artifacts, and recent advance,* Hsieh, J, (Ed.), 167–240, SPIE Press, Bellingham, USA

Husmann, L., Gaemperl,i O., Valenta, I., Schepis, T., Scheffel, H., Stolzmann, P., Leschka, S., Desbiolles, L., Marincek, B., Alkadhi, H., & Kaufmann, PA. (2009). Impact of vessel attenuation on quantitative coronary angiography with 64-slice CT. *Br J Radil,* Vol.82, No.980, (Aug 2009), pp. 649-653.

Jinzaki, M., Sato, K., Tanami, Y., Yamada, M., Kuribayashi, S., Anzai, T., Asakura, Y., & Ogawa, S. (2006). Novel method of displaying coronary CT angiography -Angiographic view-. *Circ J,* Vol.70, No.12, (Dec 2006), pp. 1661-662.

Jinzaki, M., Sato, K., Tanami, Y., Yamada, M., Anzai, T., Kawamura, A., Ueno, K., & Kuribayashi, S. (2009). Diagnostic accuracy of angiographic view image for the detection of coronary artery stenoses by 64-detector row CT: a pilot study comparison with conventional post-processing methods and axial images alone. *Circ J,* Vol.73, No.4, (Apr 2009), pp. 691-698.

Jinzaki, M., Yamada, M., Sato, K., Tanami, Y., Anzai, T., Sasaki, K., & Kuribayashi, S. (2008). Overview Image of the Lumen and Vessel Wall in Coronary CT

Angiography -The Plaque-Loaded Angiographic View-. *Circ J*, Vol.72, No.4, (Apr 2008), pp. 671-673.

Johnson, PT., Pannu, HK., & Fishman, EK. (2009). IV contrast infusion for coronary artery CT angiography: literature review and results of a nationwide survey. *AJR Am J Roentgenol* Vol.192, No.5, (May 2009), pp.W214–221.

Johnson, PT., & Fishman, EK. (2010). Postprocessing techniques for cardiac computed tomographic angiography. *Radiol Clin North Am*, Vol.48, No.4, (Jul 2010), pp. 687-700.

Little, WC., Constantinescu, M., Applegate, RJ., Kutcher, MA., Burrows, MT., Kahl, FR., Santamore, WP. (1988). Can coronary angiography predict the site of a subsequent myocardial infarction in patients with mild-to-moderate coronary artery disease? *Circulation*, Vol.78, No.5, (Nov 1988), pp. 1157-1166.

Maintz, D., Seifarth, H., Raupach, R., Flohr, T., Rink, M., Sommer, T., Ozgün, M., Heindel, W., & Fischbach, R.(2006). 64-slice multidetector coronary CT angiography: in vitro evaluation of 68 different stents. *Eur Radiol*, Vol.16, No. 4, (Apr 2006), pp. 818-826.

Meyer, TS., Martinoff, S., Hadamitzky, M., Will, A., Kastrati, A., Schomig, A., & Hausleiter, J. (2007). Improved noninvasive assessment of coronary artery bypass grafts with 64-slice computed tomographic angiography in an unselected patient population. *J Am Coll Cardiol*, Vol.49, No. 9, (Mar 2007), pp. 946-950.

Mollet, NR., Hoye, A., Lemos, PA., Cademartiri, F., Sianos, G., McFadden, EP., Krestin, GP., Serruys, PW., & de Feyter, PJ.(2005). Value of preprocedure multislice computed tomographic coronary angiography to predict the outcome of percutaneous recanalization of chronic total occlusions. *Am J Cardiol*, Vol.95, No. 2, (Jan 2005), pp. 240–243.

Motoyama, S., Sarai, M., Harigaya, H., Anno, H., Inoue, K., Hara, T., Naruse, H., Ishii, J., Hishida, H., Wong, ND., Virmani, R., Kondo, T., Ozaki, Y., & Narula, J. (2009). Computed tomographic angiography characteristics of atherosclerotic plaques subsequently resulting in acute coronary syndrome. *J Am Coll Cardiol*, Vol.54, No. 1, (Jun 2009), pp. 49-57.

Noguchi, T., Miyazaki, MD S., Morii, I., Daikoku, S., Goto, Y., & Nonogi, H. (2000). Percutaneous transluminal coronary angioplasty of chronic total occlusions. Determinants of primary success and long-term clinical outcome, *Catheter Cardiovasc Interv* Vol.49, No. 3, (Mar 2000), pp. 258–264.

Raff, GL., Abidov, A., Achenbach, S., Berman, DS., Boxt, LM., Budoff, MJ., Cheng, V., DeFrance, T., Hellinger, JC., Karlsberg, RP., & Society of Cardiovascular Computed Tomography. (2006). SCCT guidelines for the interpretation and reporting of coronary computed tomographic angiography. *J Cardiovasc Comput Tomogr*, Vol.3, No. 2, (Mar-Apr 2006), pp.122-136.

Rubin, GD., Dake, MD., Napel, S., Jeffrey, RB Jr., McDonnell, CH., Sommer, FG., Wexler, L., & Williams, DM. (1994). Spiral CT of renal artery stenosis: Comparison of three-dimensional rendering techniques. *Radiology*, Vol.190, No.1, (Jan 1994), pp. 181–189.

Schroeder, S., Achenbach, S., Bengel, F., Burgstahler, C., Cademartiri, F., de Feyter, P., George, R., Kaufmann, P., Kopp, AF., Knuuti, J., Ropers, D., Schuijf, J., Tops, LF., & Bax, JJ.; Working Group Nuclear Cardiology and Cardiac CT; European

Society of Cardiology; European Council of Nuclear Cardiology. (2008). Cardiac computed tomography: indications, applications, limitations, and training requirements: report of a Writing Group deployed by the Working Group Nuclear Cardiology and Cardiac CT of the European Society of Cardiology and the European Council of Nuclear Cardiology. *Eur Heart J,* Vol.29, No. 4, (Feb 2008), pp. 531-556.

Soon, KH., Selvanayagam, JB., Cox, N., Kelly, AM., Bell, KW., & Lim, YL. (2007). Percutaneous revascularization of chronic total occlusions: review of the role of invasive and non-invasive imaging modalities. *Int J Cardiol,* Vol.116, No. 1, (Mar 2007), pp. 1-6.

Wang, JC., Normand, SL., Mauri, L., & Kuntz, RE. (2004). Coronary artery spatial distribution of acute myocardial infarction occlusions. *Circulation,* Vol.110, No.3, (Jul 2004), pp. 278-284.

Zhang, ZH., Jin, ZY., Li, DJ., Lin, SB., Zhang, SY., Kong, LY., Wang, Y., Wang, LH., Zhao, WM., Mou, WB., Zhang, LR., Zhu, WL., Ni, C., Ren, H., Yu, HQ., Miao, Q., & Fang, Q. (2004). Non-invasive imaging of coronary artery with 16-slice spiral computed tomography. *Chin Med Sci J,* Vol.19, No.3, (Sep 2004), pp. 174-179.

18

Novel Insights Into Stenosis on Coronary Angiography–Outline of Functional Assessment of Stable Angina Patients with Angiographic Stenosis

Shinichiro Tanaka
The Second Department of Internal Medicine,
Gifu University Graduate School of Medicine, Gifu
The Department of Cardiology,
Gifu Prefectural General Medical Center,Gifu
Japan

1. Introduction

Coronary angiography is an invasive technique for imaging the coronary artery lumen and remains one of the most accurate methods for diagnosing coronary artery disease. Furthermore, this invasive technique is the standard method for guiding revascularization procedures such as percutaneous coronary intervention (PCI) and coronary-artery bypass graft (CABG), as well as for guiding stent placement during PCI. However, the degree of coronary stenosis is usually decided by visual estimation of the percentage diameter narrowing using the proximal assumed normal arterial as a reference. There is 20% variation among readings of experienced angiographers, and the same angiographer may even render a different interpretation at a time remote from the first reading. Borderline stenosis, or angiographic narrowing of 40 to 70%, does not always correspond to abnormal physiology and myocardial ischemia (1,2). For such lesions, noninvasive or direct physiological measurements of impaired flow validate the decision to initiate revascularization therapy. Though quantitative coronary angiography can be reproduced for assessment of coronary stenosis, the inability to determine the functional severity of coronary stenosis remains a limitation of coronary angiography.

Intracoronary physiological parameters have been introduced to assess functional coronary lesion severity during cardiac catheterization. Measurement of coronary flow reserve (CFR; coronary flow velocity response to adenosine) and fractional flow reserve (FFRmyo; coronary pressure-derived with adenosine) provide information about functional severity (3). Furthermore, FFRmyo, which is calculated from coronary pressure measurements, is an invasive index used to identify a stenosis responsible for reversible ischemia (4,5,6).

For most patients with stable angina, the goal of treatment is complete, or nearly complete elimination of anginal chest pain and return to normal activities with a functional capacity corresponding to Canadian Cardiovascular Society (CCS) class I angina. This goal should be accomplished with minimal side effects, as well as with a reduced risk of mortality (7). The topics of this chapter encompass the activities of daily life and functional stenosis in patients with angiographically demonstrated stenosis.

2. Functional severity

For coronary angiographic assessment employing cardiac catheterization, it should be noted that the stenotic lumen is compared to a nearby angiographically normal lumen, which may still show diffuse atherosclerotic disease. Furthermore, lesions containing diffuse, concentric, symmetrical disease, remodeling, or dissection, will be underestimated when disease severity is assessed (Fig.1). CFR and FFRmyo, which provide information about functional severity, can be performed during cardiac catheterization.

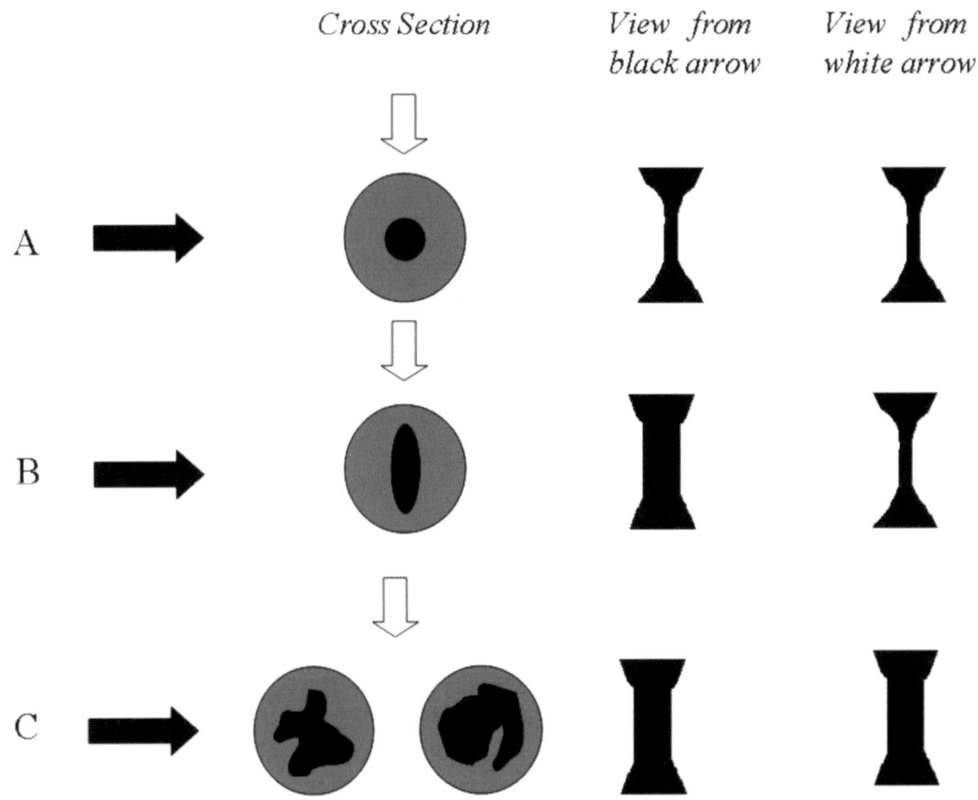

(A) Stenosis can be visualized from multiple angles. (B) Stenosis can be viewed as indicated by the white arrow, but is normally visualized as indicated by the black arrow. Stricture necessitates changing the angle. (C) Vascular conduits appear normal at all angles despite the existence of stenosis.

Fig. 1. Angiographic images and vascular conduits

CFR reflects both epicaudal and microvascular disease but does not identify these entities by itself (8,9). Intra-coronary flow velocity can be measured with a 0.014-inch doppler guide wire during baseline measurements and maximum hyperemia which is induced by administering adenosine. CFR was calculated as the ratio of hyperemic to baseline of the average peak velocity (10,11). CFR can also be measured with a temperature sensor-tipped guidewire, as the ratio of the inverse mean transit times obtained by thermodilution curves at baseline and during hyperemia (12,13,14). The parameters of CFR show agreement at a cut-off value of 2.0 (11,15).

On the other hand, FFRmyo is an accurate functional index of epicaudal stenosis (4,5). Intra-coronary pressure can be measured with a 0.014-inch pressure-monitoring guidewire, which was first calibrated, then set to be equal with the aortic pressure in the guiding catheter, and finally positioned distal to the coronary lesion. Mean aortic and distal pressures were obtained during baseline measurements, and FFRmyo was calculated as the ratio of the mean distal pressure to the mean aortic pressure during maximum hyperemia (3,4,5). Although a previous report emphasized the importance of combining pressure and flow velocity measurements to evaluate coronary lesion severity and microvascular involvement (11), FFRmyo is a reliable index of the functional severity of coronary stenosis, and an FFRmyo value of 0.75 distinguishes stenoses associated with inducible ischemia from those that are not. Indeed, in patients with stable chest pain, the most important prognostic factor is the occurrence of myocardial ischemia reflected by an FFRmyo of < 0.75 (5,6, Fig.2).

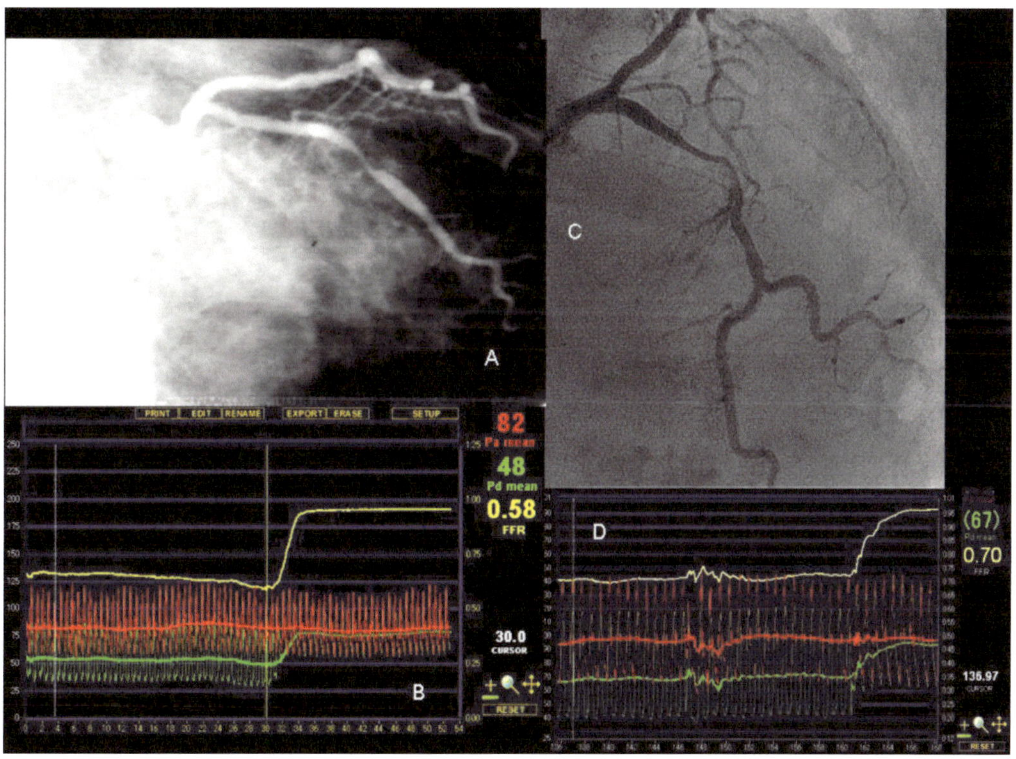

In the case on the left, angiographic stenosis was 56% in the left circumflex branch (LCX) by quantitave coronary angiography (A). During adenosine infusion, the wire was pulled back to track coronary pressure from the far distal LCX to the catheter, and after crossing the lesion produced a change in coronary pressure (FFRmyo = 0.58).

Likewise, in the case shown on the right, angiographic stenosis was 46% in left anterior descending branch (LAD) by quantitative coronary angiography (C), and FFRmyo = 0.70 (D)

Fig. 2. Representative case of FFRmyo

Even when treated with PCI, the clinical outcomes of these patients are significantly worse than those of patients with functionally insignificant stenoses (FFRmyo ≥ 0.75) (16,17). When FFRmyo was used to divide patients into a group in which stenosis was most likely to be physiologically significant (FFRmyo < 0.75) and a group in which it was not, the overlap between the 2 groups in terms of angiographic severity was so large that it suggested angiography (16,17) could not be used to predict the absence or presence of inducible ischemia in individual patients (4,18, Fig.3). In fact, however, in patients with multivessel coronary artery disease undergoing PCI with drug eluting stents, routine measurement of FFR in addition to angiographic guidance, as compared with PCI guided by angiography alone, results in a significant reduction in major adverse events (19).

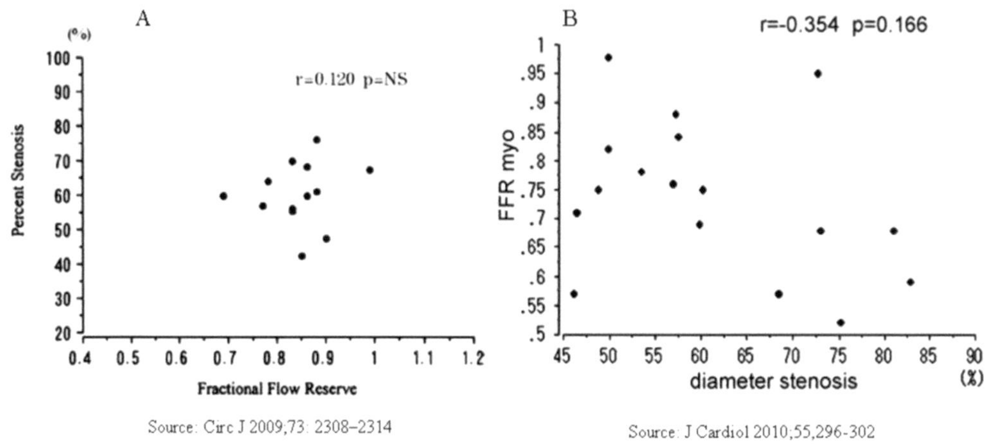

(A) The percent stenosis is likely to be physiological; FFRmyo. (B) The overlap between stenosis and FFRmyo was large.

Fig. 3. Variations in percent stenosis on coronary angiography and FFRmyo

3. Functional capacity

The factors contributing to impaired exercise capacity appear to be multifactorial and include increasing age, sedentary lifestyle, depression, obesity and other comorbidities as well as impaired cardiovascular function. Poor exercise capacity is generally considered to be a predictor of mortality in patients with ischemic heart disease as well as all cause mortality (20,21). Traditional exercise tests such as the treadmill test or walking distance in 6 minutes are well-known methods for measurement of exercise capacity.

Additionally, self-assessed questionnaires, such as the Duke Activity Status INDEX (DASI) (22), the Specific Activity Questionnaire (SAQ) (23) and the Veterans Specific Activity Questionnaire (VSAQ) (24), can also measure exercise capacity as a well validated measure of functional capacity that can be expressed as metabolic equivalents (METs) and have been shown to correlate with adverse outcomes. Self-assessed questionnaires can be a simple and easy tool that contributes to the global risk assessment (10).

The cardiopulmonary exercise test (CPX) is useful for measurement of excise capacity employing various parameters at each stage in a series of exercises (Fig.4). A symptom-limited incremental exercise test is usually performed using an upright, electromagnetically braked cycle ergometer or treadmill with measurement of breath-by-breath VO2, carbon dioxide production (VCO2) and minute ventilation (VE). This evaluates peak VO2, oxygen uptake at the anaerobic threshold (AT) and so on. A 12-lead electrocardiogram (ECG) and heart rate were continuously monitored throughout the test, and cuff blood pressure was measured every minute using an automatic manometer. CPX testing is more useful than self-assessed health status, which is subjective and can vary among patients depending upon symptom complexity and the unique perceptions, expectations and preferences of individuals (7).

CPX report

SEX	female	AGE	58	Temperature	26.9 °C
WEIGHT	62.8 kg	MODE	Ramp	Pressure	759 mmHg
HEIGHT	158 cm	The Number of Data	290	Humidity	30.8 %

		Rest	Warm Up	AT-1min	AT	Rc	Peak
Real Time	Min:Sec	00:09	04:15	08:54	09:54	13:09	13:09
Start/End	Min:Sec	04:15	07:15				
Exec Time	Min:Sec			01:54	02:54	06:09	06:09
VO2	ml/min	235	415	475	528	832	832
VCO2	ml/min	215	374	444	471	851	851
R		0.92	0.90	0.93	0.89	1.02	1.02
HR	beat/min	59	73	77	78	98	98
VO2/W	ml/kg/min	3.7	6.6	7.6	8.4	13.3	13.3
METS		1.07	1.89	2.16	2.40	3.79	3.79
RR	n/min	16.9	20.6	24.0	21.0	25.7	25.7
VE	l/min	9.7	15.3	18.5	18.0	30.1	30.1
LOAD	Watt	0	10	27	37	70	70
RPM	rpm	1	52	51	50	48	48

		DATA	(%)	Normal
Peak VO2/W	ml/kg/min	13.3	55	23.9
Peak HR	beat/min	98	60	162
minimum VD/VT		0.34		
AT trend VO2/W	ml/kg/min	8.4	52	16.2

		DATA	(%)	Normal
minimum VE/VCO2	ml/ml	35.4	126	28.0
Peak VO2/HR		8.5	91	9.3
VE-VCO2 Slope		29.5	108	27.3
AT V-Slope VO2/W	ml/kg/min	8.7	55	15.9

		DATA	(%)	Normal	regression equation
ΔVCO2/ΔVO2VsU		1.24			Y= 1.24X -192 R= 0.997
ΔVCO2/ΔVO2VsD		0.686			Y= 0.686X +112 R= 0.979
ΔVO2/ΔLOAD		6.87	67	10.3	Y= 6.87X +312 R= 0.971

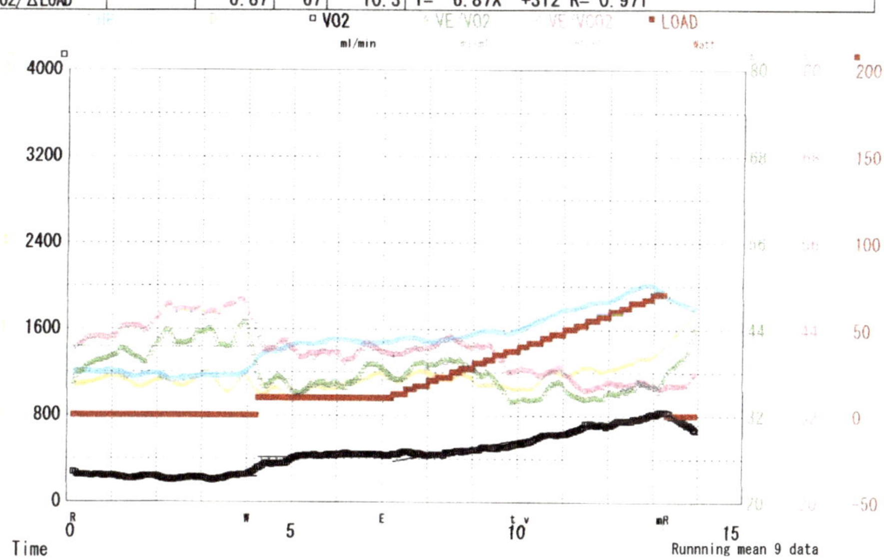

Fig. 4. Representative case of CPX

4. Functional severity and exercise capacity in patients with angiographic stenosis

Coronary angiography employing cardiac catheterization has an important role in revascularization procedures such as PCI, and PCI has become a common initial management strategy for patients with stable angiographic stenosis. However, at present, the initial management strategy of patients with stenosis on coronary angiography should be to reduce not only the risks for major cardiac events but also to eliminate angina and allow a return to normal activities. Previous studies have shown that PCI does not reduce the long-term rates of death, myocardial infarction or other major cardiovascular events with compared to optimal medical therapy alone (25). PCI can provide an incremental benefit in quality of life compared with that provided by optimal medical therapy alone among patients with chronic coronary artery disease for approximately 24 months (26). Another previous study showed that in patients with stable coronary artery disease and an angiographically documented stenosis treatable by PCI, a 12-month exercise-training program resulted in a higher event-free survival rate and higher exercise capacity than standard PCI (27). Additionally, PCI significantly increased exercise capacity values such as AT and peak VO2 in patients with peak VO2 < 15 ml/kg/min, whereas it yielded no significant improvement in those with peak VO2 ≥ 15 ml/kg/min (28). Based on these observations, the existence of stenosis on coronary angiography is an insufficient indication for revascularization. It has been reported that an increase in functional capacity as indicated by self-assessed questionnaire is associated with an increase in CFR, although 86% of subjects did not have significant stenosis on coronary angiography (10). Impaired overall functional capacity is independently associated with coronary microvascular dysfunction or endothelial dysfunction, among the most important determinants of myocardial ischemia. On the other hand, routine FFRmyo measurement with angiographic guidance resulted in a significant reduction in major adverse cardiac effects, even when patients underwent PCI with drug-eluting stents (19). Furthermore, FFRmyo is associated with inducible ischemia which other measures are not, thereby providing higher accuracy than for any other invasive or noninvasive test. According to the aforementioned reports, it seemed that the existence of stenosis on coronary angiography is a notwell validated measure of stable angina. FFRmyo and functional capacity should be determined in stable angina patients with angiographic stenosis. Previously, we assessed the relationship between FFRmyo and CPX values (4).

Our study subjects were 15 males (65.8+/-8.9 years old) with stable angina and 75% angiographic stenosis in one coronary artery. Eligible patients had no evidence of acute coronary syndromes, prior myocardial infarction, significant valvular heart disease, diabetes mellitus treated with insulin, smoking; or occupational, orthopedic and other conditions that precluded exercise. Neither did they have left main coronary artery stenosis > 25% or high-grade proximal left anterior descending artery stenosis with significant stenosis (> 75%) of other vessels, nor left ventricular angiography-based detection of abnormal wall motions such as asynergy or diffuse hypokinesis, or reduced left ventricular function (ejection fraction < 55%). The %diameter stenosis (%DS) was determined to be 61.7+/-9.1% based on quantitative coronary angiography. Mean FFRmyo was 0.84+/-0.66, peak VO2 was 17.1+/-3.2ml/kg/min and AT was 11.1+/-2.0ml/kg/min. There was no significant correlation between %DS and FFRmyo ($r = 0.12$, p = ns, Fig.3A), peak VO2 ($r = -0.051$, p = ns) or AT ($r = -0.013$, p = ns). By contrast, there was a significant positive correlation (Fig.5) between FFRmyo and peak VO2 ($r = 0.534$, $p < 0.05$) and between FFRmyo and AT (r =

0.542, $p < 0.05$). A previous study showed stable angina patients with impaired functional capacity as assessed by a CPX test to likely have reduced FFRmyo. The present study also showed that an FFRmyo value of 0.75 reflects stenoses associated with inducible ischemia and hence appears to correspond to a peak VO2 value of 15.0. A cut-off value of FFRmyo of 0.75 nearly matched the exercise capacity value (peak VO2; 15 ml/kg/min) improvement with PCI. As noted above, exercise capacity in patients with stable angina reflects functional rather than angiographic stenosis. Exercise training can improve myocardial perfusion, as revealed by myocardial scintigraphy, as well as maximal exercise capacity (27). Therefore, that study suggested that it may be possible to improve FFRmyo by increasing exercise capacity through training.

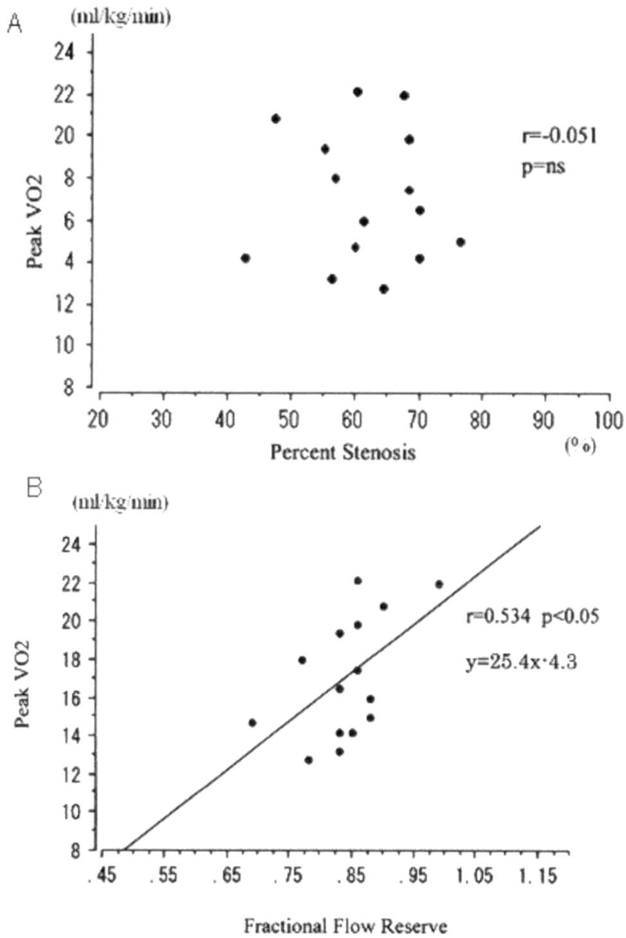

(A) There is no correlation between angiographic stenosis and peak VO2. However, there is a positive correlation between FFRmyo and peak VO2 (B). (Source: Circ J 2009;73: 2308–2314)

Fig. 5. Relationship between exercise capacity and stenosis.

4.1 Case report

This is a representative case showing improvement in functional capacity despite the existence of angiographic stenosis.

A 58-year-old woman presented with unstable angina. Coronary angiography revealed 99% stenosis of the right coronary artery (RCA#3), and 75% stenosis (#11) and 90% stenosis (#12) of the left circumflex branch (LCX). She received stent implantation to #3 in the emergent stage (Fig.6). Thallium-201 scintigraphy with adenosine revealed ischemia in the LCX area (Fig.7A). PCI was recommended, but the patient refused because the condition was asymptomatic in her daily life. This patient did not wish to undergo revascularization of the LCX and continue to receive cardiac rehabilitation (physical training at AT level). Peak VO2 increased from13.3 ml/kg/min (Fig.4) to 16.8 ml/kg/min. Thallium-201 scintigraphy (Fig.7B) with adenosine documented improved myocardial perfusion distal to the LCX. (Ischemia area reduced from 13.7% to 8.75%)

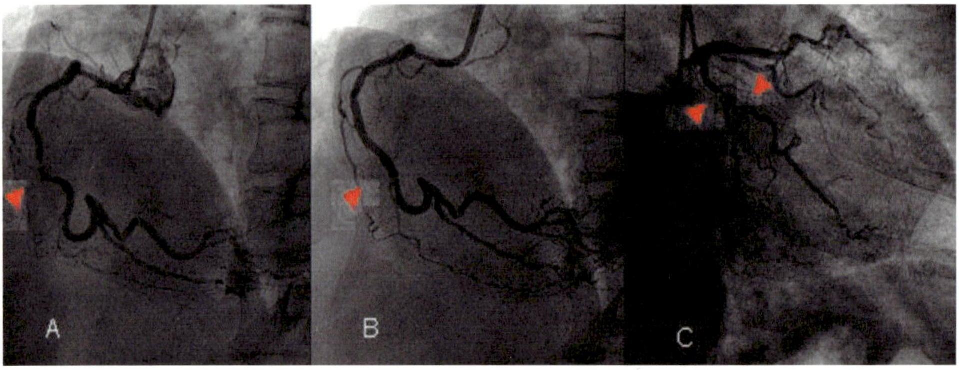

There was (A) 99% stenosis of the right coronary artery (RCA #3) and a (B) stent was implanted. Left coronary angiongraphy revealed 75% stenosis (#11) and 90% stenosis (#12) of the left circumflex branch (LCX).

Fig. 6. Coronary angiographies of case repor

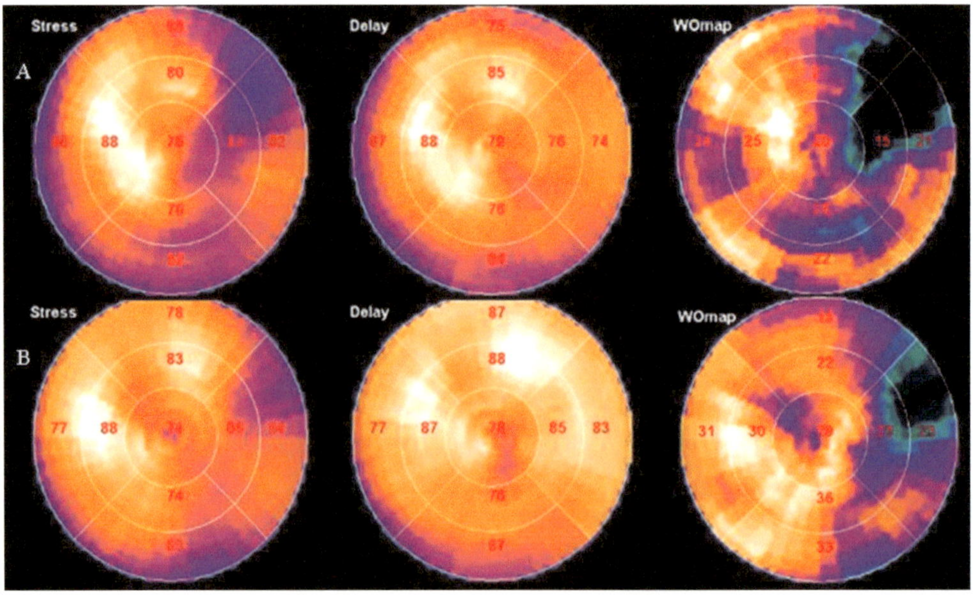

Fig. 7. Bull's eye image from thallium-201 single-photon emission computed tomography (A) pre-training (ischemic area 13.7%), and (B) post-training (ischemic area 8.75%)

5. Functional severity, exercise capacity and tissue characterization

Acute coronary syndrome is triggered by microscopic ulcerations of vulnerable atherosclerotic plaques. The majority of vulnerable plaques appear "angiographically insignificant" before their rupture (less than 75% diameter stenosis). In contrast, most of the "significant" plaques (greater than 75% stenosis) visualized at angiography are at low risk for plaque rupture (29).
Intravascular ultrasound (IVUS) allows cross-sectional imaging of coronary arteries and provides a more comprehensive assessment of the atherosclerotic plaques in vivo (30, Fig 8). Studies using IVUS have indicated that coronary atherosclerosis is underestimated when visually analyzing angiographic results owing to coronary compensatory remodeling and the diffuse nature of coronary atherosclerosis, which frequently makes the reference vessel appear normal angiographically (31).

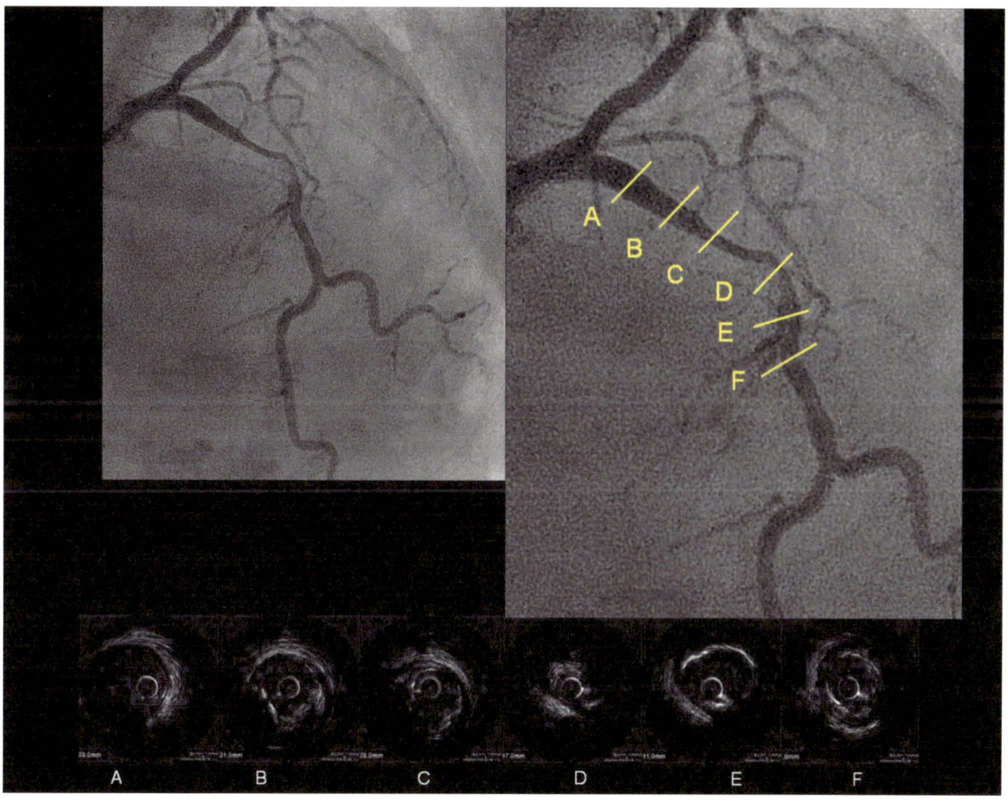

Intravascular ultrasound provides an image of an atheroma in a normal segment (B,E) as well as a stenotic lesion (C,D) on angiography

Fig. 8. Representative angiographic and IVUS images

An integrated backscatter intravascular ultrasound (IB-IVUS) system has been developed in which two-dimensional color-coded maps allowing plaque tissue characterization in coronary arteries can be constructed by computer (32,33). A computer equipped with IB-IVUS software is connected to the IVUS imaging system to obtain radio frequency signal output, signal trigger output, and video image output. IB is calculated as the average power of the ultrasound backscattered signal from a small volume of tissue using fast Fourier transform measured in decibels (dB) (32). IB-IVUS is a useful method for analyzing coronary plaque tissue (Fig.9), which accurately and quantitatively differentiates among calcification, dense fibrosis, fibrosis and lipid components (33). IB-IVUS results previously suggested that classifying plaques as vulnerable or stable using this technique is an effective means of predicting acute coronary syndrome. When evaluated using IB-IVUS, plaques are deemed vulnerable when the lipid area is > 65% and the fibrotic area is < 25% (30). Thus, functional stenosis and tissue characterization may be linked to clinical outcome. Previously, we assessed the relationship between functional stenosis and the characterization of plaque tissue using FFRmyo and IB-IVUS (18).

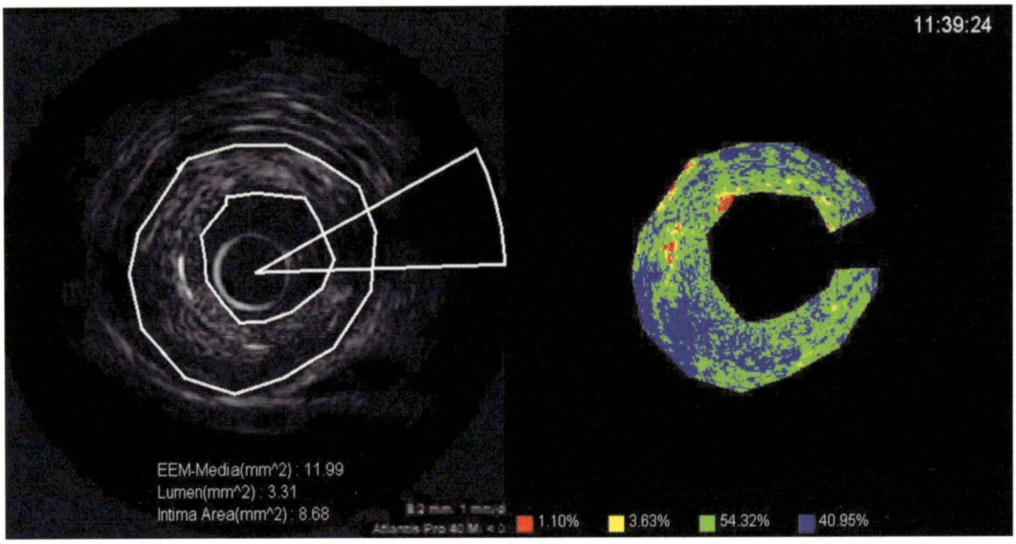

The initial image was constructed by tracing the lumen and the external elastic membrane. In the color-coded map, red is calcification, yellow and green are fibrosis, and blue represents the lipid pool.

Fig. 9. Representative IB-IVUS images

We studied 17 lesions showing 75%-stenosis visually by coronary angiography in 17 stable angina patients (64.2+/-9.1 years old, 11 males). We found no correlation between FFRmyo and %DS ($r = -0.354$, $p = 0.166$, Fig.3B). Nor was there a correlation between FFRmyo and plaque burden ($r = -0.241$, $p = 0.359$, Fig.1B), or between FFRmyo and minimum lumen cross-sectional area ($r = -0.002$, $p = 0.995$). Likewise, neither %DS nor plaque burden correlated with the tissue characterization values (Figs.10A). There was no correlation between FFRmyo and %CA (calcification area) ($r = -0.068$, $p = 0.799$). By contrast, we observed a significant positive correlation between FFRmyo and %F ($r = 0.620$ $p = 0.0067$), and a significant negative correlation between FFRmyo and %LP (lipid pool area) ($r = -0.524$, $p = 0.0293$) (Fig.10B).

Our previous findings indicate that the tissue characteristics of coronary plaques in intermediate lesions affect functional stenosis. Fibrous tissue and FFRmyo also correlate positively. Lipid pool and FFRmyo correlate negatively. The apparently contradictory results obtained in this study might be explained by the progression of human atherosclerotic lesions leading to increasing fibrosis and stenosis. Distal pressure, additionally, decreases with the severity of coronary narrowing in the epicardial arteries, contributing to the progression of atherosclerosis. However, intermediate or moderate lesions remain distinct in terms of functional and angiographic severity. The increase in fibrous tissue is likely an adaptive response to this distal pressure aimed at redistributing and modulating the mechanical stress (34). The increased fibrosis may also be an adaptive response to reduced elasticity of the arterial wall in the area of the lesion. An earlier in vivo study showed that elasticity in the area of stenosis can exacerbate the pressure drop across the lesion, thereby reducing flow (35).

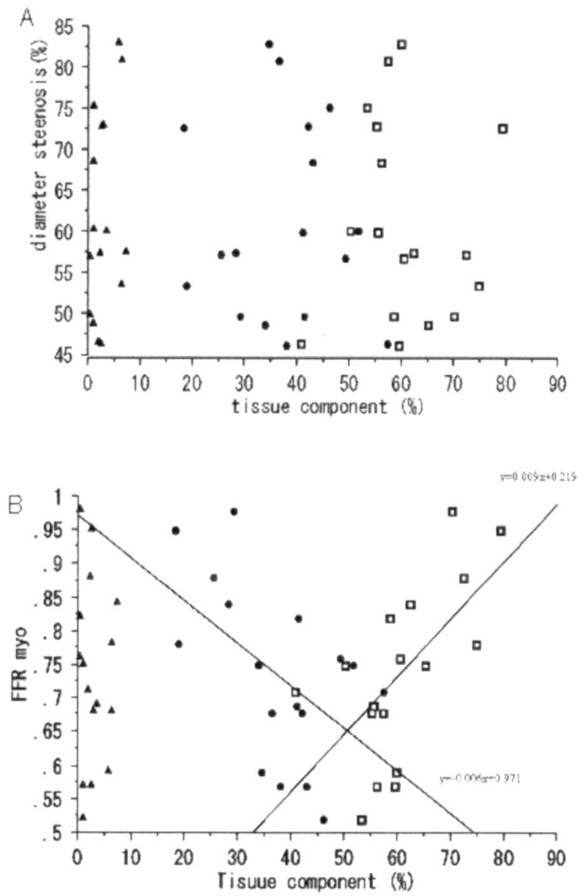

(A) There was no correlation between angiographic stenosis and tissue characterization (B). There was a significant positive correlation between FFRmyo and fibrosis, and a significant negative correlation between FFRmyo and the lipid pool: ▲, %CA = percent calcification area; □, %F = percent fibrotic area; ●, %LP = percent lipid pool area. (Source: J. Cardiol; 2010 ;55,296 – 302)

Fig. 10. Relationship between stenosis and tissue characterization

Our studies showed that angina patients with reduced FFRmyo are likely to have reduced functional capacity, and that the tissue characteristics of coronary plaques in intermediate lesions affect functional stenosis. According to these studies, high exercise capacity in patients with stable angiographic stenosis is linked to the stability of coronary plaques. Another report on coronary computed tomographic angiography indicated that coronary plaque characteristics were identified in patients with progressively reduced exercise times, and that functional ischemia was more severe in those with mixed plaque. (36)

Thus, though coronary angiography is one of the most accurate methods for diagnosing coronary artery disease, comprehensive assessment of health status is necessary for stable angina patients with angiographic stenosis.

6. References

[1] Zir LM, Miller SW, Dinsmore RE, Gilbert JP, Harthorne JW. Interobserver variability in coronary angiography. Circulation. 1976;53:627-32.

[2] DeRouen TA, Murray JA, Owen W. Variability in the analysis of coronary arteriograms. Circulation. 1977;55:324-8.

[3] Kern MJ, de Bruyne B, Pijls NH. From research to clinical practice: current role of intracoronary physiologically based decision making in the cardiac catheterization laboratory. J Am Coll Cardiol. 1997;30:613-20.

[4] Tanaka S, Noda T, Segawa T, Minagawa T, Watanabe S, Minatoguchi S. Relationship between functional exercise capacity and functional stenosis in patients with stable angina and intermediate coronary stenosis. Circ J. 2009 ;73:2308-14.

[5] Pijls NH, De Bruyne B, Peels K, Van Der Voort PH, Bonnier HJ, Bartunek J Koolen JJ, Koolen JJ. Measurement of fractional flow reserve to assess the functional severity of coronary-artery stenoses. N Engl J Med. 1996;334:1703-8.

[6] Pijls NH, Van Gelder B, Van der Voort P, Peels K, Bracke FA, Bonnier HJ, el Gamal MI. Fractional flow reserve. A useful index to evaluate the influence of an epicardial coronary stenosis on myocardial blood flow; Circulation. 1995;92:3183-93.

[7] Tanaka S, Yokoyama C, Kawamura I, Takasugi N, Kubota T, Ushikoshi H, Aoyama T, Kawasaki M, Nishigaki K, Takemura G, Minatoguchi S. Conservative medication follow-up for over 20 years of a patient with ischemic heart disease after diagnosis of chronic total occlusion of the 3 main coronary arteries. Circ J. 2008;72:1205-9.

[8] Albertal M, Regar E, Van Langenhove G, Carlier SG, Serrano P, Boersma E, Bruyne B, Di Mario C, Piek J, Serruys PW; DEBATE Investigators. Flow velocity and predictors of a suboptimal coronary flow velocity reserve after coronary balloon angioplasty. Eur Heart J. 2002;23:133-8.

[9] Albertal M, Voskuil M, Piek JJ, de Bruyne B, Van Langenhove G, Kay PI, Costa MA, Boersma E, Beijsterveldt T, Sousa JE, Belardi JA, Serruys PW; Doppler Endpoints Balloon Angioplasty Trial Europe (DEBATE) II Study Group. Coronary flow velocity reserve after percutaneous interventions is predictive of periprocedural outcome. Circulation. 2002;105:1573-8.

[10] Handberg E, Johnson BD, Arant CB, Wessel TR, Kerensky RA, von Mering G, Olson MB, Reis SE, Shaw L, Bairey Merz CN, Sharaf BL, Sopko G, Pepine CJ. Impaired coronary vascular reactivity and functional capacity in women: results from the NHLBI Women's Ischemia Syndrome Evaluation (WISE) Study;J Am Coll Cardiol. 2006 7;47: S44-9.

[11] Meuwissen M, Chamuleau SA, Siebes M, Schotborgh CE, Koch KT, de Winter RJ, Bax M, de Jong A, Spaan JA, Piek JJ. Role of variability in microvascular resistance on fractional flow reserve and coronary blood flow velocity reserve in intermediate coronary lesions. Circulation. 2001;103:184-7.

[12] Matsuo H, Watanabe S, Yasuda S, Hirose T, Iwama M, Tanaka S, Yamaki T, Ono K, Takahashi H, Segawa T, Matsuno Y, Minatoguchi S, Fujiwara H. Myocardial perfusion during transient slow-flow in the patient with old vein graft intervention: assessment by

serial measurement of pressure-derived fractional flow reserve and thermodilution-derived coronary flow reserve. Catheter Cardiovasc Interv. 2003;60:392-8.
[13] De Bruyne B, Pijls NH, Smith L, Wievegg M, Heyndrickx GR. Coronary thermodilution to assess flow reserve: experimental validation. Circulation. 2001;104:2003-6.
[14] Pijls NH, De Bruyne B, Smith L, Aarnoudse W, Barbato E, Bartunek J, Bech GJ, Van De Vosse F. Coronary thermodilution to assess flow reserve: validation in humans. Circulation. 2002;105:2482-6.
[15] Miller DD, Donohue TJ, Younis LT, Bach RG, Aguirre FV, Wittry MD, Goodgold HM, Chaitman BR, Kern MJ. Correlation of pharmacological 99mTc-sestamibi myocardial perfusion imaging with poststenotic coronary flow reserve in patients with angiographically intermediate coronary artery stenoses. Circulation. 1994;89:2150-60.
[16] Bech GJ, De Bruyne B, Pijls NH, de Muinck ED, Hoorntje JC, Escaned J, Stella PR, Boersma E, Bartunek J, Koolen JJ, Wijns W. Fractional flow reserve to determine the appropriateness of angioplasty in moderate coronary stenosis: a randomized trial;Circulation. 2001;103:2928-34.
[17] Pijls NH, van Schaardenburgh P, Manoharan G, Boersma E, Bech JW, van't Veer M, Bär F, Hoorntje J, Koolen J, Wijns W, de Bruyne B. Percutaneous coronary intervention of functionally nonsignificant stenosis: 5-year follow-up of the DEFER Study;J Am Coll Cardiol. 2007;49:2105-11.
[18] Tanaka S, Noda T, Segawa T, Iwama M, Minagawa T, Watanabe S, Minatoguchi S. Relation between functional stenosis and tissue characterization of intermediate coronary plaques in patients with stable coronary heart disease. J Cardiol. 2010;55:296-302.
[19] Tonino PA, De Bruyne B, Pijls NH, Siebert U, Ikeno F, van' t Veer M, Klauss V, Manoharan G, Engstrøm T, Oldroyd KG, Ver Lee PN, MacCarthy PA, Fearon WF; FAME Study Investigators. Fractional flow reserve versus angiography for guiding percutaneous coronary intervention. N Engl J Med. 2009 15;360:213-24.
[20] Gulati M, Pandey DK, Arnsdorf MF, Lauderdale DS, Thisted RA, Wicklund RH, Al-Hani AJ, Black HR. Exercise capacity and the risk of death in women: the St James Women Take Heart Project. Circulation. 2003;108:1554-9.
[21] Mora S, Redberg RF, Cui Y, Whiteman MK, Flaws JA, Sharrett AR, Blumenthal RS. Ability of exercise testing to predict cardiovascular and all-cause death in asymptomatic women: a 20-year follow-up of the lipid research clinics prevalence study. JAMA. 2003;290:1600-7.
[22] Hlatky MA, Boineau RE, Higginbotham MB, Lee KL, Mark DB, Califf RM, Cobb FR, Pryor DB. A brief self-administered questionnaire to determine functional capacity (the Duke Activity Status Index). A brief self-administered questionnaire to determine functional capacity (the Duke Activity Status Index). Am J Cardiol. 1989;64:651-4.
[23] Rankin SL, Briffa TG, Morton AR, Hung J. A specific activity questionnaire to measure the functional capacity of cardiac patients. Am J Cardiol. 1996;77:1220-3.
[24] Myers J, Bader D, Madhavan R, Froelicher V. Validation of a specific activity questionnaire to estimate exercise tolerance in patients referred for exercise testing. Am Heart J. 2001;142:1041-6.
[25] Boden WE, O'Rourke RA, Teo KK, Hartigan PM, Maron DJ, Kostuk WJ, Knudtson M, Dada M, Casperson P, Harris CL, Chaitman BR, Shaw L, Gosselin G, Nawaz S, Title LM, Gau G, Blaustein AS, Booth DC, Bates ER, Spertus JA, Berman DS, Mancini GB, Weintraub WS; COURAGE Trial Research Group. Optimal medical therapy with or without PCI for stable coronary disease. N Engl J Med. 2007;356:1503-16.
[26] Weintraub WS, Spertus JA, Kolm P, Maron DJ, Zhang Z, Jurkovitz C, Zhang W, Hartigan PM, Lewis C, Veledar E, Bowen J, Dunbar SB, Deaton C, Kaufman S,

O'Rourke RA, Goeree R, Barnett PG, Teo KK, Boden WE; COURAGE Trial Research Group, Mancini GB. Effect of PCI on quality of life in patients with stable coronary disease;N Engl J Med. 2008;359:677-87.
[27] Hambrecht R, Walther C, Möbius-Winkler S, Gielen S, Linke A, Conradi K, Erbs S, Kluge R, Kendziorra K, Sabri O, Sick P, Schuler G. Percutaneous coronary angioplasty compared with exercise training in patients with stable coronary artery disease: a randomized trial.Circulation. 2004;109:1371-8.
[28] Barmeyer A, Meinertz T. Anaerobic threshold and maximal oxygen uptake in patients with coronary artery disease and stable angina before and after percutaneous transluminal coronary angioplasty;Cardiology. 2002;98: 127-31.
[29] Fraker TD Jr, Fihn SD; 2002 Chronic Stable Angina Writing Committee; American College of Cardiology; American Heart Association, Gibbons RJ, Abrams J, Chatterjee K, Daley J, Deedwania PC, Douglas JS, Ferguson TB Jr, Gardin JM, O'Rourke RA, Williams SV, Smith SC Jr, Jacobs AK, Adams CD, Anderson JL, Buller CE, Creager MA, Ettinger SM, Halperin JL, Hunt SA, Krumholz HM, Kushner FG, Lytle BW, Nishimura R, Page RL, Riegel B, Tarkington LG, Yancy CW. 2007 chronic angina focused update of the ACC/AHA 2002 guidelines for the management of patients with chronic stable angina: a report of the American College of Cardiology/American Heart Association Task Force on Practice Guidelines Writing Group to develop the focused update of the 2002 guidelines for the management of patients with chronic stable angina.J Am Coll Cardiol. 2007;50:2264-74.
[30] Sano K, Kawasaki M, Ishihara Y, Okubo M, Tsuchiya K, Nishigaki K, Zhou X, Minatoguchi S, Fujita H, Fujiwara H. Assessment of vulnerable plaques causing acute coronary syndrome using integrated backscatter intravascular ultrasound. J Am Coll Cardiol. 2006;47:734-41.
[31] Nissen SE, Yock P. Intravascular ultrasound: novel pathophysiological insights and current clinical applications. Circulation. 2001;103:604-16.
[32] Kawasaki M, Takatsu H, Noda T, Sano K, Ito Y, Hayakawa K, Tsuchiya K, Arai M, Nishigaki K, Takemura G, Minatoguchi S, Fujiwara T, Fujiwara H. In vivo quantitative tissue characterization of human coronary arterial plaques by use of integrated backscatter intravascular ultrasound and comparison with angioscopic findings. Circulation. 2002;105:2487-92
[33] Okubo M, Kawasaki M, Ishihara Y, Takeyama U, Kubota T, Yamaki T, Ojio S, Nishigaki K, Takemura G, Saio M, Takami T, Minatoguchi S, Fujiwara H. Development of integrated backscatter intravascular ultrasound for tissue characterization of coronary plaques. Ultrasound Med Biol. 2008;34:655-63.
[34] Stary HC, Chandler AB, Dinsmore RE, Fuster V, Glagov S, Insull W Jr, Rosenfeld ME, Schwartz CJ, Wagner WD, Wissler RW. A definition of advanced types of atherosclerotic lesions and a histological classification of atherosclerosis. A report from the Committee on Vascular Lesions of the Council on Arteriosclerosis, American Heart Association. Circulation. 1995;92:1355–1374.
[35] Siebes M, Campbell CS, D'Argenio DZ. Fluid dynamics of a partially collapsible stenosis in a flow model of the coronary circulation. J Biomech Eng. 1996 ;118:489-97
[36] Lin FY, Saba S, Weinsaft JW, Wong FJ, Szulc M, Kligfeld P, Okin PM, Berman DS, Shaw LJ, Min JK. Relation of plaque characteristics defined by coronary computed tomographic angiography to ST-segment depression and impaired functional capacity during exercise treadmill testing in patients suspected of having coronary heart disease.Am J Cardiol. 2009 ;103:50-8.

19

Optimization of Radiation Dose and Image Quality in Cardiac Catheterization Laboratories

Octavian Dragusin[1], Christina Bokou[1],
Daniel Wagner[2] and Jean Beissel[2]
[1]*Entente des Hôpitaux Luxembourgeois*
[2]*Institut National de Chirurgie Cardiaque et de Cardiologie Interventionnelle*
Luxembourg

1. Introduction

Radiation exposure is a concern for those who participate in the practice of interventional cardiology. However, many cardiologists are unaware that they may be exposing patients to relatively high levels of radiation during cardiac catheterization procedures. Interventional cardiology techniques are highly appreciated for its less invasive character than surgery. A wide range of interventions, from diagnosis to treatment of heart and coronary specific disorders are performed in both adults and children. Interventional cardiology procedures can involve significant radiation exposure. Therefore, it is essential to reduce the radiation dose as far as possible, by keeping an adequate image quality for diagnostic and therapeutic purposes. Over the last years, introduction of new technologies like flat-panel detectors have revolutionized fluoroscopy imaging. Most of the digital detectors can potentially be used at lower doses. In practice, technical optimization studies are rarely reported (especially for cardiac catheterization laboratories), notwithstanding the fact that optimal settings could be very different from the optimal settings with the traditional image intensifier systems.

This chapter is structured in three parts. The first part focuses on background notions concerning X-ray production, radiation quantities and units, personal health risks and concepts of radiation protection. The second part reviews the radiation exposure in cardiovascular practice. The last part presents optimization strategies of image quality and radiation dose and recommendations for limiting radiation exposures.

2. Radiation dose related to interventional cardiology

X-rays are special types of electromagnetic radiation which can ionize matter. The interaction of radiation with tissue is dependent on the spectral distribution of the radiation as well as on the thickness, density, and atomic composition of the matter. Cardiac imaging systems use two forms of dynamic X-ray imaging: fluoroscopy and cineangiography. Fluoroscopy mode uses relatively low radiation dose levels and aids in the guidance and positioning of medical devices within the patient. Cineangiography mode (shortly cine mode) is the acquisition of a series of high definition dynamic images. It is mainly used to image vessels injected with contrast media. The necessity of obtaining high contrast and sharp edge definition with low noise images requires higher radiation dose rates. The basic components of a fluoroscopic imaging chain are shown in Figure 1. The chain is composed by an X-ray tube and generator, which are capable to produce a stable X-ray output over long exposure times, a detector mounted opposite the X-ray tube, capable of dynamic imaging, digital image processing and storage facilities, and a display system capable for viewing real-time or recorded digital image series.

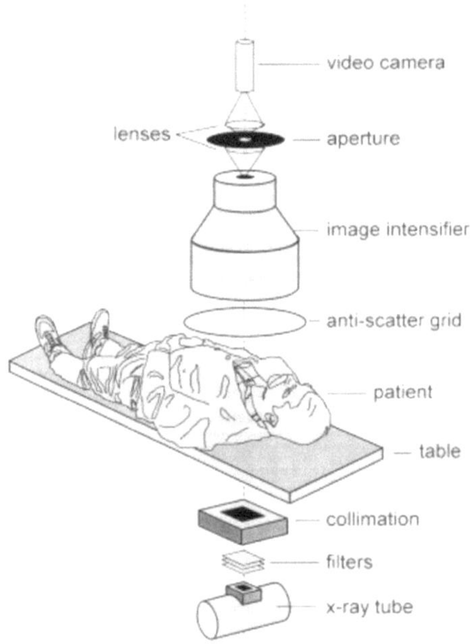

Fig. 1. Example of a fluoroscopic imaging chain equipped with image intensifier

X-ray detector is a significant component of the overall imaging chain. Two generations of detector technology are present in the catheterization laboratories: image intensifier (II) connected to a charged coupled device camera and flat-panel detectors (FD), also known as active-matrix flat-panel imagers. Briefly, for II-based fluoroscopy systems, X-ray photons exiting the patient are incident on the II's input surface. The photons strike the CsI input phosphor, absorbed and produce a large number of light photons. Then electrons are produced from visible light photons and accelerated until they hit the output screen. From the collision with output screen results light photons that are recorded by a video or cine camera. Charges coupled device camera is used for direct digitalization of the image. The process is illustrated in Figure 2, left. The FD detectors are classified into indirect and direct detectors. Indirect detectors use a phosphor (scintillator) material that absorbs X-rays and produces a proportionate number of light photons that subsequently interact with a photodiode electrode on the TFT array (thin film transistor). A typical indirect FD detector is shown in Figure 2, right. Direct FDs use a semiconductor material sandwiched between two electrodes to absorb and convert the X-ray energy directly into ion pairs. Currently, amorphous selenium (a-Se) is the only clinical choice.

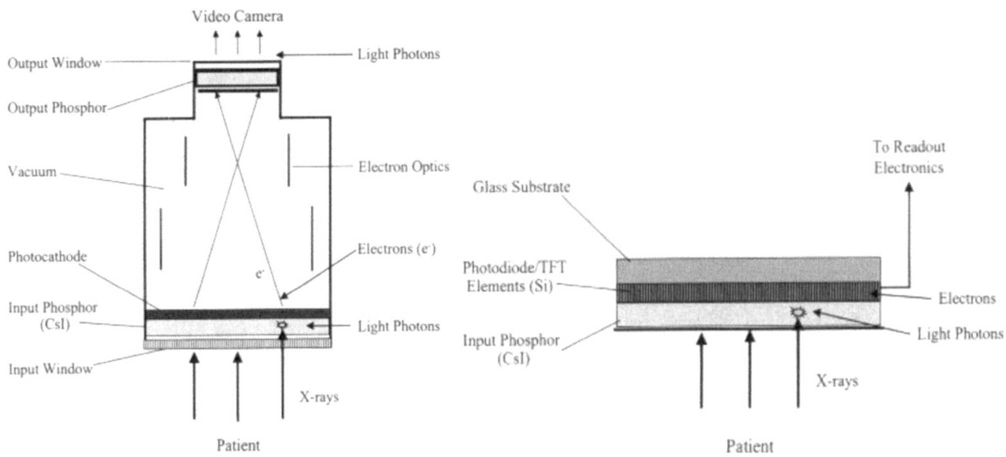

Fig. 2. X-ray detector technology. On the left, image intensifier (II) technology. On the right, flat-panel indirect detector (FD) technology.

There is a common consensus that FDs provides advantages in terms of image quality and dose efficiency comparing with II technology. Advantages include image uniformity, no geometrical distortions, no veiling glare and vignetting, wider dynamic range and better ergonomics for patient accessibility. On the other hand, for FDs, system noise remains a limiting factor and performance is rather limited for low exposure levels. (Holmes et at., 2004; Seibert, 2006; Davies et al., 2007).

2.1 Radiation quantities and units

Quantities describing patient dose from radiation exposures have been defined by the International Commission on Radiation Protection (ICRP, Publication 60, 1990 and ICRP, Publication 103, 2007) and by the International Commission on Radiation Units and Measurements (ICRU, Report 74, 2005). To make it simple, we will focus only on dose quantities and radiation units that are often used in interventional cardiology. We propose to divide them in three categories: dose quantities outside the patient's body, dose quantities to estimate risks of skin injuries and effects that have threshold and dose quantities to estimate stochastic risks.

Radiation quantities outside the patient's body are used to describe the beam of X-rays. These quantities can express total amount of radiation or can express radiation at a specific point. The X-ray beam is emitted from a small source (point) from the tube and is constantly spreading out as it moves away from the source. Absorbed dose, D, is the mean energy imparted per unit mass by ionizing radiation. The SI unit of D is the Gray (Gy), where 1 Gy = 1 J/Kg. The Kerma (Kinetic Energy Released in a MAterial) is the sum of the initial kinetic energies of all charged ionizing particles liberated by uncharged particles in a material of a specific mass. The SI unit is also Gray (Gy). To make it simply, in diagnostic radiology, absorbed dose D and Kerma are equal. It is possible to calculate the absorbed dose in a material if the exposure is known, by using a conversion coefficient depending on medium. Absorbed dose or air kerma in X-ray field can be measured with dosimeters. A practical quantity that gives an indication of the absorbed dose is dose-area product (DAP) or kerma-area product (KAP). It is the product of dose to air (air kerma) and the area of the X-ray beam, and it is expressed in units Gy*cm^2. The use of DAP-meter provides a complete

measurement of the total exposure of the patient. The DAP-meter is a flat large-area ionization chamber mounted at the exit window of the X-ray tube and intercepts the entire useful beam. In interventional cardiology, we work also with other quantities that influence radiation dose. One of them is fluoroscopy time, which can be adopted as starting unit in a quality assurance program (for comparison between operators, centers, procedures, for the evaluation of protocols, and for the evaluation of operator skills). Other quantity is the number of acquired cineangiographic images or number of series.
Entrance skin dose (ESD) includes the scatter from the patient. ESD = D*BF, where backscatter factor ranges from 1.2-1.4 as a function of field size. The SI unit for ESD is the Gray (Gy). Values of absorbed dose to tissue, compared with to air, will vary by a few percent depending on the exact composition of the medium that is taken to represent soft tissue. To evaluate the dose inside the patient's body, we use the mean absorbed dose in a tissue or organ, D_T, in fact the energy deposited in the organ divided by the mass of that organ. Organ doses cannot be measured on real patients. They can be measured in anthropomorphic phantoms simulating examinations or by dedicated software tools that simulates the interaction of X-rays on mathematical or realistic phantoms.

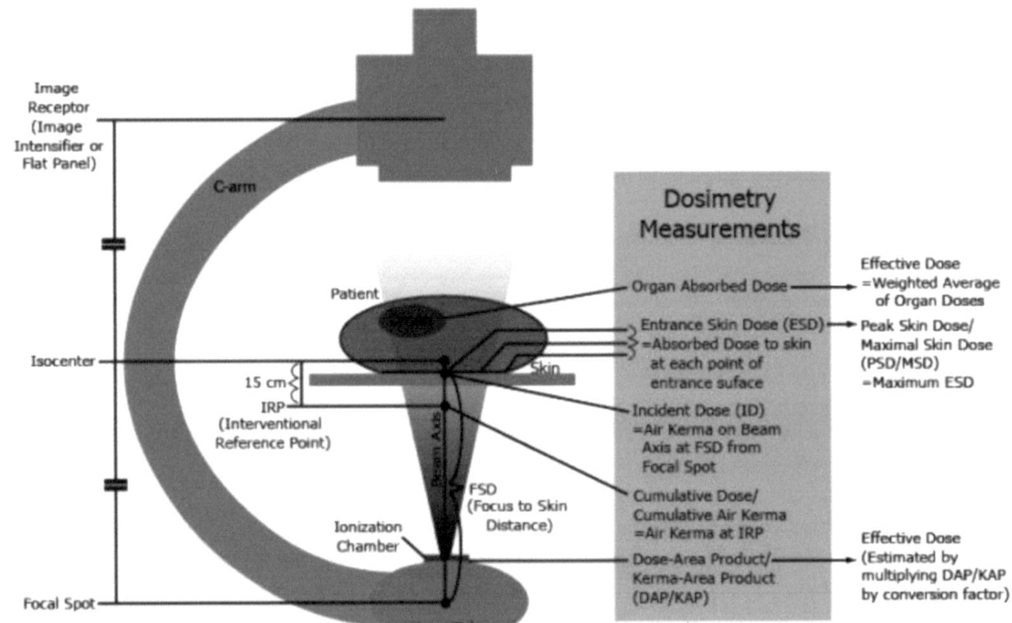

Fig. 3. Dosimetry terminology used in interventional cardiology (Adapted from ICRP Publication 85).

A second category of dose quantities are the ones related to estimate risks of skin injuries and effects that have threshold. Approximate entrance dose thresholds have been determined for various skin changes, ranging from early transient erythema at 2 Gy to painful dermal necrosis of about 18 Gy. For interventional procedures, maximal skin dose (MSD) can be assessed with different methodologies: (a) by direct calculation, with off or on-line techniques, (b) by direct measurements on the patient with point detectors (thermoluminescent detectors, TLDs, or other solid state detectors), (c) by direct measurements on the patient with large area detectors (films and TLDs array), and (d) by portal monitoring with area or point/area detectors. The new cardiac X-ray systems are able to display on the monitors dosimetric parameters at the interventional reference point (IRP). The IRP is the reference point intended to be representative of the position of the patient's skin at the entrance site of the X-ray beam during an interventional procedure. For fluoroscopic systems with an isocentre, the IRP is located along the central ray of the X-ray beam at a distance of 15 cm from the isocentre in the direction of the focal spot (Figure 3).

Radiation exposure of the different organs and tissues in the body results in different probabilities of harm and different severity. The combination of probability and severity of harm is called detriment. For instance in young patients, organ doses may significantly increase the risk of radiation-induced cancer in later life. The equivalent dose (H) is the absorbed dose multiplied by a dimensionless radiation weighting factor, w_R, which expresses the biological effectiveness of a given type of radiation. $H = D \times w_R$. The SI unit of H is the Sievert (Sv). For X-rays, the w_R is 1 so H is equal to D. The mean equivalent dose in a tissue or organ H_T is the energy deposited in the organ divided by the mass of that organ. To reflect the detriment from stochastic effects due to the equivalent doses in the different organs and tissues of the body, the equivalent dose is multiplied by a tissue weighting factor, w_T. The equivalent doses to organs and tissues weighted by the relative w_T are summed over the whole body to give the effective dose, E. The SI unit of E is also the Sievert (Sv). $E = \sum_T w_T \times H_T$. Till 2007 the tissue weighting factors of ICRP Publication 60 were used. A recent estimation of those factors was published in ICRP report 103. Main differences between publications for tissue weighting factors, w_T are presented in Table 1. Stochastic risk is calculated multiplying effective dose by a risk factor specific for sex and age at the exposure.

Figure 3 illustrates the dosimetry terminology used in interventional cardiology. To summarize, the biological effects and risks from ionizing radiation are divided into deterministic and stochastic effects. Deterministic effects have a dose threshold, and the intensity of the effect increases with increasing dose. Stochastic effects include cancer and genetic risk. Probability of stochastic risks increases with increasing dose, but the intensity of the effect is not a function of the absorbed dose. For personnel working in cardiac catetherization laboratories, the major worries about radiation exposure are the potential risk of cancer, cataracts, and genetic birth defects of pregnant staff if the appropriate protective measures are not used. For patients, deterministic effects can be produced by high doses of fluoroscopic X-rays. In addition, stochastic effects can appear on patients with repeated interventional cardiac procedures, especially if are performed in young population.

Risks of exposure to ionizing radiation are contra balanced by the need for and potential benefit for a patient to have a cardiac interventional procedure. In fact medical use of radiation is a unique situation in which patients are intentionally irradiated. The risk should be minimised by utilizing techniques and procedures that keep exposure to a level *As Low As Reasonably Achievable* (ALARA principle). The principle of ALARA is the axiom for all radiation workers. Its successful implementation in catheterization laboratory require understanding of factors responsible for levels of radiation exposure and applying optimized procedures to obtain the medical diagnostic or therapeutic goal with minimum radiation risks.

ICRP Report 60 (1990)		ICRP Report 103 (2007)	
Tissue	Tissue weighting factor, w_T	Tissue	Tissue weighting factor, w_T
Lung	0.12	Lung	0.12
Stomach		Stomach	
Colon		Colon	
Bone Marrow		Bone Marrow	
		Breast	
		Remainder	
Gonads	0.20	Gonads	0.08
Thyroid	0.05	Thyroid	0.04
Oesophagus		Oesophagus	
Bladder		Bladder	
Liver		Liver	
Breast			
Remainder			
Bone surface		Bone surface	
Skin		Skin	
		Brain	
		Salivary glands	

Table 1. Differences between w_T tissue weighting factors in ICRP Publication 60 and Publication 103.

3. Literature review of patient and staff doses in clinical practice

Interventional cardiology procedures are usually fluoroscopy guided diagnostic and therapeutic interventions. Therapeutic interventions are often complex procedures and sometimes procedures are repeated for the same patient. In these situations patient high radiation dose levels occur. The specialized literature presents a series of case reports describing deterministic effects with growing incidence and more concern than stochastic long term risks. International Commission on Radiological Protection and World Health Organisation has requested attention to the skin dose problems of complicated radiological interventions. In this context, patient dosimetry approaches are an important issue. Many published dose data are expressed in terms of not particularly well defined dose quantities and without clear objective for the measurements performed. This section of the work aims to report and compare dosimetry approaches and eventually propose a classification of the different dosimetry objectives. Patient dosimetry methods currently used in interventional cardiology may be divided in three categories according to their purposes: (1) dosimetry for quality assurance; (2) dosimetry for stochastic risk evaluation, (3) dosimetry for deterministic effects evaluation.

Dosimetry for quality assurance is used to compare performance of equipment, operator skills or radiological practice among different teams or centers, to evaluate the optimization process or to establish diagnostic reference levels (DRL) for routine examinations. Useful dose quantity is the dose - area product, DAP. For cardiac procedures, usually the total DAP for whole procedure is documented. Sometimes, the DAP for the fluoroscopy part (DAP_{fluoro}) and the DAP for the cineangiography part of a procedure (DAP_{cine}) are indicated. Some authors propose additional technical quantities like the total fluoroscopy time of a procedure, the total number of acquired images, the number of series of acquired images, the mean number of images per series in a procedure. **Dosimetry quantities for stochastic risk evaluation** are organ equivalent doses to organ/tissue and effective dose. These quantities are indicators of overall exposure in the assessment of stochastic effects of radiation exposure for population. Use of these quantities allows us to compare exposures from different types of procedure, radiation type, and radiation quality, and irradiation geometry. From effective dose, using correct risk coefficients (ICRP Report 103), we can estimate the detriment of individuals or population from medical exposure. **Dosimetry for deterministic effects** focuses on skin dose assessment. For complex interventional cardiology procedures, the knowledge of irradiated skin area is important with respect to the potential for deterministic effects of radiation exposure. Different methodologies are used to express the maximal skin dose (MSD): off-line or on-line calculation, direct measurements on the patient with point detectors (TLDs or solid state detectors), direct measurements on the patient with the area detectors (TLD array and film) or by portal monitoring with point or area detectors. Unfortunately not all methods are feasible for routine work, specially the on-line ones. An alternative approach on two levels can be used. The first level able to prevent deterministic effects is using a threshold. This can be fluoroscopy time or a measurable quantity like DAP, able to alert the operator that a certain value of skin dose, corresponding to a threshold for deterministic effects can be reached. The second level to assess MSD requires specific methods. In case of electrophysiology procedures where stationary fields are used, electronic point detectors or computational methods able to assess skin dose distribution can be employed.

We will present a summary of published patient doses in interventional cardiology. Any attempt to compare published studies must be performed with circumspection due to the lack of standardization of data acquisition and the uncontrolled variables (equipment differences, radiographic technique, complexity of procedure, patient characteristics (size, age, sex).

3.1 Patient radiation doses during diagnostic and interventional cardiac catheterization

The most frequent procedures in adults are coronary angiography (CA) for diagnostic and percutaneous coronary intervention (PCI) for therapeutic examinations. Consequently, there are a large number of articles that review the patient radiation doses. For CA procedures, some authors report data for subcategories of procedures like CA with left ventricular angiography, or/and cardiac catheterization. PCIs are more complicated to classify because of the large number of technical factors, like number of lesions treated, the wire technique, simple, ostial or bifurcation stenting, flow and pressure wire or any other special devices. The most common quantities used were: DAP, fluoroscopy time, cine frames, cine time (dosimetry for quality assurance), effective dose (dosimetry for stochastic risks), and skin dose (dosimetry for deterministic risks). Published results are presented in Table 2 for CA and in Table 3 for PCI procedures. The studies presented are a little part of the literature survey. We present only median values and, where available, the range. We looked for studies from different time periods. It is evident from the tabulated data that the reported values for interventional cardiology procedures vary considerably. This can be attributed to procedural complexity, examination technique, use of radiation-reducing techniques, operator experience, workload, and catheterization laboratory examination. For example, Broadhead et al, 1997 compared patient dosimetry between single intensifier system and biplane image intensifier system, and found that the biplane system provides greater imaging capability but with increased dose. DAP for CA is 47.7 vs. 23.4 Gycm² (biplane vs. single system), and for PCI is 72.2 vs. 51.6 Gycm².

Study	Sample (number cases)	DAP (Gycm²)	Fluoroscopy time (min)	Cine frames (images)	Maximum skin dose (mGy)	Effective dose (mSv)
		Median (Range min - max)				
Zorzetto, 1997		52.5	4.9	1350		
Broadhead, 1997	2174	58.8				9.4
van de Putte, 2000		56.8 (max 144)			412 - 725	
Eftathopoulos, 2003	20	29				5
Kuon, 2003	509	23.6	3.4	339		
Dragusin, 2005	78	25.6 (9 -115)	4 (1 - 25)	767 (318 - 1331)		
Karambatsakiou, 2005	20	(18 -107)				
Vijakalakshmi, 2007	3752	19.1				4.8
D'Helft, 2008		13.6 - 231	0.22 - 27.6			
Tsapaki, 2008	549	31 (1 - 135)	4 (0.8-57)	688 (62 -2206)		
Bogaert, 2008	200					7.3
Dragusin, 2010	122	11.6	3	506		
Samara, 2010		55 (max 235)	3.1 (max 65)			

Table 2. Short review of patient doses during coronary angiography (CA) examinations

Bernardi et al., 2000 and Padovani et al., 2001 investigated the effect of complexity of PCI interventions, by separating the procedures in "simple", "medium" and "complex" procedure, based on a set of technical and clinical factors. (Median DAP values 66.7,96.4 and 132.7 Gycm²). Sandborg et al, 2003 compared the radial arterial approach to the femoral approach in term of radiation dose. They found that radial approach yielded significant higher doses (51 and 75 Gycm² for CA, respectively PCI), compared with femoral approach (38 and 47 Gycm²). Tsapaki et al. 2004 and Trianni et al., 2005a compared the patient doses of flat-panel systems (FD) to image intensifier (II) systems. Despite of the potential of FD to produce images of higher quality with lower entrance detector dose rates, in clinical practice and terms of patient dose could give opposite results. Trianni et al., 2005a reported 33.4 Gycm² (for FD) and 31,1 Gycm² (for II) during CA examinations and 66.9 Gycm² (for FD) and 52 Gycm² (for II) during PCI examinations. Some publications presented patient dosimetry in term of contribution of fluoroscopy and image acquisition to the total DAP

(Efstathopoulos et al., 2003, Kuon et al., 2004). Mean DAP for fluoroscopy and image acquisition calculated from the values reported in these studies are 18% DAP fluoroscopy and 81% DAP image acquisition for CA procedures. For PCIs, DAP is 41% from fluoroscopy and 59% from image acquisition. The patient radiation doses vary widely among published studies. These differences are related to patient, procedure, X-ray equipment and physician.

Study	Sample (number cases)	DAP ($Gycm^2$)	Fluoroscopy time (min)	Cine frames (images)	Maximum skin dose (mGy)	Effective dose (mSv)
		Median (Range min - max)				
Zorzetto, 1997		82.6	12.2	1500		
Broadhead, 1997	214	77.9				14.2
van de Putte, 2000		108 - 131				
Eftathopoulos, 2003	20	75				14
Kuon, 2003	233	22.2	9.7	208		
Dragusin, 2005	23	9 - 148.4	1.4 -44.5	206 -1524		
Karambatsakiou, 2005	10	16 - 115				
Vijakalakshmi, 2007	646	35				9.3
D'Helft, 2008		47.5 - 413	2-98			
Tsapaki, 2008	549	62	10.4 (3.2-53)	1257 (398-5940)	799 (320-1660)	
Bogaert, 2008	118					11.6
Dragusin, 2010	91	32.7	12.6	938		
Samara, 2010		144	9.1 (max 52)			

Table 3. Short review of patient doses during percutaneous coronary intervention (PCI) examinations

3.2 Patient radiation doses radiation doses during electrophysiology studies and pacemaker implantations

Cardiac electrophysiology is a subdiscipline of interventional cardiology that is focused on elucidating, diagnosing, and treating the electrical problems of the heart. The procedures are performed by invasive intracardiac catheter recordings of spontaneous activity as well as of cardiac responses to programmed electrical stimulation. These studies are performed to evaluate abnormal electrocardiograms and to assess complex arrhythmias. Typically therapeutic procedures are radiofrequency catheter ablations (RFCA). Patient doses are also influenced by the type of procedures. Diagnostic electrophysiological study (EPS) relies mainly on fluoroscopy. For therapeutic procedures, we can find different categories: RFCA without angiographic images using contrast medium, RFCA with angiographic images using contrast medium and RFCA of atrial fibrillation (AF) (Dragusin et al., 2005). The dosimetric data of this study is presented in Table 4. In the case of therapeutic examinations, the radiation doses varied according to the location of the tachycardia. Ablations in which contrast medium is used to take images need more radiation exposure. RFCA of atrial fibrillation had longer examination times and yielded the maximum radiation doses.

Parameter	Type of procedure (number cases)	Range	Mean ± SD	Median	Third quartile
DAP ($Gycm^2$)	EFO (72)	0.5 - 77.5	13.8 ± 16	7.2	17.3
	RFCA without contrast (85)	1.5 - 93.2	21.9 ± 20.5	14.3	27.9
	RFCA with contrast (52)	1.5 - 102.1	34.3 ± 26	32.1	47.6
	AF (36)	33.6 - 440.2	156.3 ± 99.4	129.6	183.6
Fluoroscopy time (min)	EFO (72)	1.6 - 39	11.2±8.6	8	13.8
	RFCA without contrast (85)	4.4 - 48.8	23.7±11.2	20.7	30.3
	RFCA with contrast (52)	10 - 61.3	26.5±11.2	22.9	31.2
	AF (36)	27.6 - 130	67.6±24.7	66.4	85.5

Table 4. Summary of patient radiation data for electrophysiological procedures (Dragusin et al., 2005)

Trianni et al., 2005b collected patient skin doses from 90 electrophysiological procedures. Mean maximum local skin doses were 0.03 Gy for pacemaker insertion, 0.17 Gy for RFCA for nodal tachycardia and 0.22 Gy for atrial fibrillation. Ector et al., 2007 investigated the effect of body mass index on radiation doses in patients undergoing pulmonary vein isolation for atrial fibrillation. 85 patients undergoing AF ablation guided by biplane low-frequency pulsed fluoroscopy (3 frames/s). Mean DAP values per hour of fluoroscopy were 58, 110 and 184 $Gycm^2$ in normal, overweight, and obese patients. The corresponding effective dose for AF ablation procedures were 15.2, 26.7, and 39 mSv.

3.3 Patient radiation doses radiation doses during pediatric cardiovascular procedures

According to the Euratom Directive 97/43, exposures of children and procedures involving high doses to the patient, such as interventional radiology, should be given special attention. Both criteria apply to the pediatric cardiac catheterization laboratories, so patient dose evaluations should thus be established with priority. On pediatric patients both diagnostic and therapeutic procedures are performed. Diagnostic examinations study complex congenital heart diseases. Therapeutic procedures mainly involve dilatation of stenotic vessels or valves and occlusion of abnormal communications. The main therapeutic procedures are balloon dilatation of the pulmonary valve, balloon dilatation of peripheral pulmonary stenosis, balloon dilatation for coarctation of the aorta, stent implantation, occlusion of patent ductus anteriosus, closure of atrial septal defect and closure of ventricular septal defect. We will discuss the results of a study regarding pediatric radiation doses performed in a catheterization laboratory equipped with a biplane FD system (Dragusin et al., 2008a). In this study, the population was divided in six age groups (0-30 days, 1-12 months, 1-3 years, 3-5 years, 5-10 years and 10-15 years). Data from 273 patients are presented in terms of DAP, fluoroscopy time and number of image acquisition series. For diagnostic procedures the median values per age group are 2.7, 2.5, 5.1, 5.8, 7.1, 9.9 $Gycm^2$, 11, 6, 10, 8, 8, 5 minutes, and 8, 6, 6, 10, 8, 6 acquisition series. For therapeutic procedures the median values per age group are 4.8, 5.9, 7.5, 9.5, 17.1, 46.8 $Gycm^2$ for DAP,

16.5, 12, 16, 18, 21, 20 minutes for fluoroscopy time and 9, 14, 12, 18, 22, 19 acquisition series. The effective doses for each patient were estimated using PCXMC software (STUK, Finland). The 25th, 50th and 75th percentile per each age group for diagnostic procedure is presented in Figure 4 and for therapeutic procedures is presented in Figure 5.

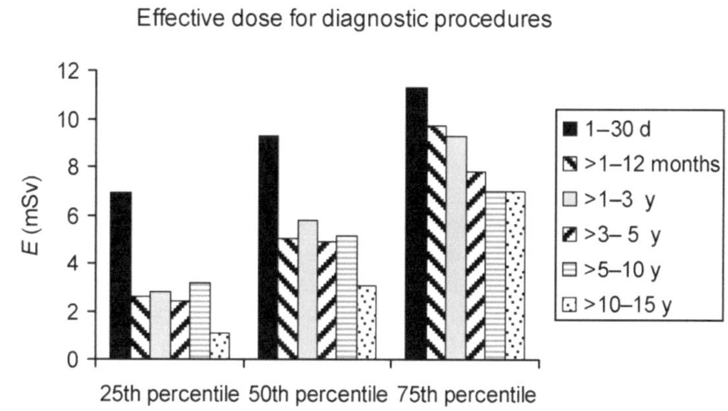

Fig. 4. Estimated effective doses for diagnostic procedures in pediatric interventional cardiology (Dragusin et al., 2008a)

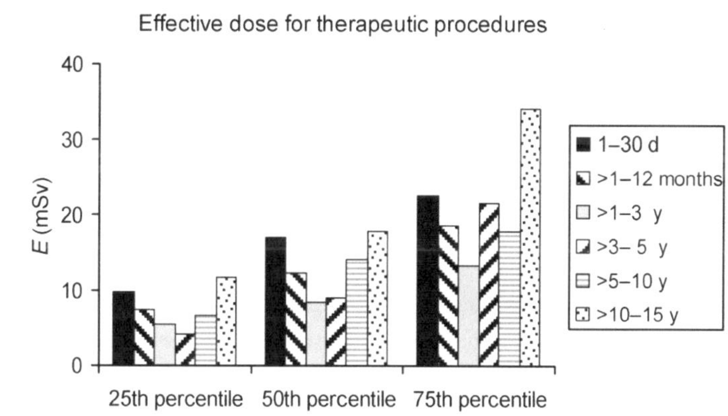

Fig. 5. Estimated effective doses for therapeutic procedures in pediatric interventional cardiology (Dragusin et al., 2008a)

Other study reported DAP values as 75th percentile of 6.2, 6.1, 9, 10, 15, 20, 27 and 36 Gycm² for 2114 patients divided in eight age groups from newborns to 21 y (Rassow et al.,2000). This study included diagnostic, therapeutic and myocardial biopsy procedures. Bacher et al., 2005 studied 60 patients of which 28 underwent diagnostic imaging. Patients age ranged from new born to 10 y. The DAP range for diagnostic was 0.96-14.6 Gycm2 and for therapeutic 0.4-20.4 Gycm2. Onnasch et al.,2007 expressed the results of dose data of a large population as DAP/body weight (Gycm²/kg) rather than DAPs for age groups. Using the 90th percentiles, he suggested as diagnostic reference level values of 0.81 Gycm²/kg for diagnostic procedures, and 1.16 Gycm²/kg for therapeutic interventions. Effective doses of 0.6 to 23.2 mSv for diagnostic procedures and from 1 to 37 mSv for therapeutic procedures were estimated by Bacher et al., 2005.

A number of specific conditions, such as higher heart rates, smaller cardiovascular structures, smaller body size, and wider variety of unusual anatomic variants with the potential need for relatively lengthy and complex studies, result in relatively high radiation doses to the patient. The improved survival of patients with complex anatomy (e.g., palliated single ventricle anatomies) implies that many such children with chronic cardiac disease require frequent catheterizations within the first few years of life. These factors, coupled with the increased radiosensitivity of children and a longer lifespan ahead of them in which to possibly develop radiation-related sequels, converge to create potentially unpleasant consequences.

3.4 Staff dosimetry

Occupational doses in interventional procedures guided by fluoroscopy are the highest doses registered among medical staff using X-rays. Interventional cardiologists experience radiation exposure with the patient, as they are close to the radiological source. Interventional cardiologists working in high-volume cardiac catheterization laboratories are exposed to significant occupational radiation risks of developing certain diseases, including hematopoietic cancers, thyroid diseases, skin diseases, cataracts, or upper respiratory disease (Venneri et al., 2009). Consequently, monitoring personnel exposure is compulsory and regulated for individual workers. Occupational doses limits apply, i.e a limit on effective dose of 20 mSv/year, averaged over 5 years. The equivalent dose should not exceed 150 mSv for lens of the eye, 500 mSv for the skin (average dose over 1 cm^2 of the most highly irradiated area of the skin) and 500 mSv for the hands and feet. Wraparound two-piece aprons, thyroid shields and eye protection are important personnel shields. Personnel dosimetry monitors include those using X-ray films (film badges) or thermoluminescent dosimeters (TLDs). Both detectors are placed in holders and the monitors are typically worn for one month before being submitted for processing. The laboratory readout the detectors and estimate the effective dose. For interventional cardiologists, it is recommended to wear two badges. One is worn outside the apron at the neck and one is worn under the apron at the waist. The second badge monitors the effectiveness of the lead apron. For other staff in the catheterization laboratory, a single badge is worn and it is usually placed outside the apron at collar level. The mean collar-level exposure per case for cardiologist who performs CA and PCI has been reported to be 0.04 to 0.16 mSv (Hujkens & Hummel, 1995, Zorzetto et al., 1997). Certain publications focus on the estimation of personnel doses for different anatomical locations by placing TLDs for each procedure. For example, Efstathopoulos et al, 2003 measured doses with five TLDs placed on the left branch of eyeglasses, the chest over and underneath the lead apron, the left hand and knee. The results of dose/procedure for cardiologists were 6 μGy (eyes), 0 μGy (chest under apron), 5.75 μGy (chest over apron), 22.5 μGy (left hand), 16.75 μGy (left knee). The assisting operator received less dose/procedure: 5.5 μGy (eyes), 0 μGy (chest under apron), 4 μGy (chest over apron), 17.5 μGy (left hand), 3.5 μGy (left knee). An interesting survey was performed by Vano et al, 2006, that evaluated the occupational doses of cardiologist for a period of 15 years (1989 to 2004). The mean values in mSv/year decreased from 11.6 (1989-1992) to 1.6 (1993-1998) and to 1.2 (1999-2004). The success of reduction in the effective dose by a factor of 10 is explained mainly by the training in radiation protection, optimization of procedures and improved performance of X-ray systems.

In conclusion, accumulation of radiation doses to interventional cardiologists has the potential of increasing risk of stochastic effects. To prevent radiation–associated diseases, radiation exposure to cardiologists should be reduced by using new generation cardiac X-ray systems, performing diagnostic and interventional procedures with shorter fluoroscopic times, and using effective shielding to protect from radiation.

4. Optimization strategies of image quality and radiation dose

In cardiac catheterization laboratory, the goal of the ALARA (As Low As Reasonably Achievable) principle is to provide maximal diagnostic and therapeutic outcome while requiring the lowest possible radiation dose. The following discussion focuses on the compromise between radiation dose and image quality. There are few directions to follow. First element on the equation of the dose-image quality is the cardiac catheterization laboratory equipment. Taking into account the advances in technology, today modern cardiac catheterization systems are equipped with reliable X-ray generation tubes and flat panel detectors. If most of the laboratories are equipped with mono plane systems, for electrophysiology or pediatric applications biplane equipments are probably more appropriate. This choice depends on the cardiology practice. The imaging chain has an important feature, the Automatic Exposure Control (AEC) that ensures relatively constant image brightness. The AEC works as a feedback mechanism from the digital video processor to the X-ray generator. As mentioned before, the cardiac X-ray system is capable of different imaging modalities. Fluoroscopy mode is used for live, real-time viewing and provides sufficient image quality to visualize the catheters. For permanent storage and review, images of higher image quality are acquired in cineangiography mode. Nowadays, all systems are delivered with pulsed fluoroscopy, with a range of pulse rate from 30 to 3 pulses/second. Note that the lower the pulse frequency the less radiation dose, at the expense of a jerkier motion. The systems have the capability to store the last fluoroscopic images as film (option "fluoro store" or "hold last image"). Cineangiography mode rates vary from 60 to 15 or 30 frames/second. Most of adult angiograms are performed at 15 frames/second, but faster frame rates are necessary for pediatric patients to view rapidly moving structures throughout the cardiac cycle.

Optimization of new cardiac equipment with flat panel detector consists of finding the adapted configuration that offers an acceptable image quality with relatively low dose. The detector entrance dose is known to influence the image quality, at least in the clinically used dose range. In practice, various settings of the system lead to different patient dose levels. The spectrum of the beam can be influenced by the kV, added Cu filtration, thickness of the patient and the presence or absence of the grid. Dragusin et al., 2008b investigated influence on image quality of three factors: detector entrance dose, effect of antiscatter grid and patient thickness using two contrast phantoms (Leeds TO10 and CDRAD). These phantoms were imaged in fluoroscopy and cineangiography mode. For cineangiography mode six levels of detector entrance dose were used: 100, 120, 140, 170, 200 and 240 nGy/frame for a rate of 15 frames/second. For fluoroscopy mode, three levels: low (10 pulses/second, detector entrance dose 32 nGy/pulse), medium (15 pulses/second, 45 nGy/pulse) and high (15 pulses/second, 65 nGy/pulse). The average fitted contrast-detail curve for CDRAD phantom for different entrance detector doses is presented in Figure 6. The variation of the contrast-detail curve with patient thickness (9 cm, 13 cm, 17 cm and 21 cm equivalent plexiglass material) is presented in Figure 7. The configuration of X-ray system corresponds to the acquisition mode 15 frames/second and 170 nGy/frame detector entrance dose. When looking at graphically representation of contrast-detail curves, it should be noted that improved image quality makes the curve to shift to the lower part of the graph. In Figure 6, it is evident that the poorest image quality corresponds to the fluoroscopy mode and the better image quality corresponds to acquisition mode with maximum detector entrance dose (240 nGy/frame).

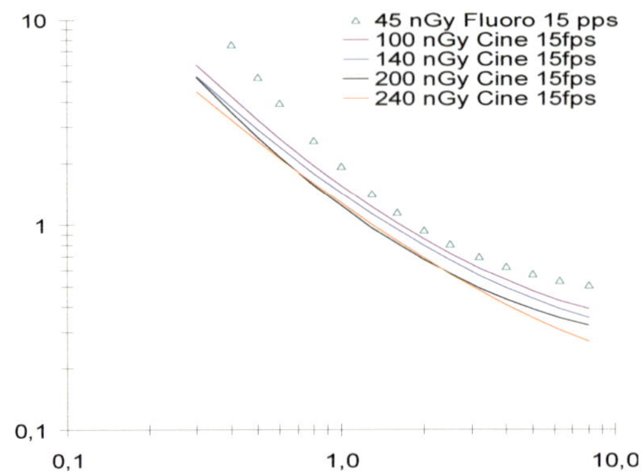

Fig. 6. Contrast-detail curves for CDRAD phantom for fluoroscopy mode and cine mode for different detector entrance doses.

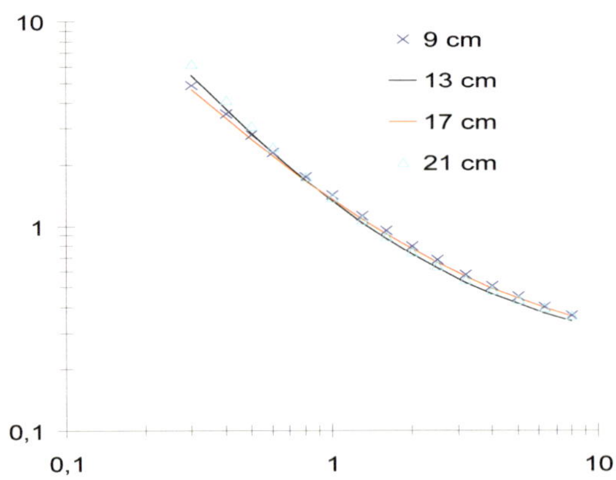

Fig. 7. Contrast-detail curves for CDRAD phantom for cine mode (15 frames/second; 170 nGy/frame) and different simulated patient thicknesses.

The improvement in image quality between settings is not very clearly visible because of the small changes in detector dose levels. Differences between detector dose settings are not significan (a factor of 2.4 between the minimum 100 nGy and maximum 240 nGy). This implies a little change in threshold contrast. Despite of the limitation of this study, the authors observed that just a simple change of the detector entrance dose from a superior to a next inferior setting (i.e. from 170 nGy/frame to 140 nGy/frame) will not dramatically change image quality. This simple action would potentially reduce the patient skin dose between 14-19% depending of the size of the patient. The limitation of the use of contrast detail phantoms consists of the difficulty to link with clinical image quality requirements. In particular for interventional cardiology, visualization of moving structures, visualization and grading of subtle lesions or anatomical structures during the passage of a contrast agent and the tracing of small catheters on the moving heart, implies the use of test objects that simulates this environment. To visualize moving structures in cardiovascular fluoroscopy systems, some dynamic phantoms have been created. Guibelalde et al., 2001 have constructed the Patient Movement Simulation Test Object (PAMOSITO), a 2D motor-controlled test object holder to simulate clinical situations in which patient movement could be a cause of image degradation. The Society for Cardiac Angiography and Interventions (SCA&I) and the National Electrical Manufacturers Association (NEMA) developed a phantom that allows visualizing moving structures. The device is a rotating spoke that contains five steel wires of different diameters. Two lead dots are used to evaluate lag and recursive filtering (Balter et al.,2001). Both dynamic phantoms have the disadvantage that they do not incorporate details or features that are directly linked with critical issues in clinical cardiac images (i.e., circulation of contrast agent, anatomical background, lesions or pulsating arteries).

Dragusin et al., 2008c used a phantom that models the human anatomy from the knee to the neck. The modular design of the phantom contains also the heart (dimensions 15 cm (atria/apex) x 10 cm wide x 9 cm (anterior/posterior). The arterial tree model is fabricated in transparent polyurethane. Calcifications can be inserted into main arteries. Medical devices like catheters can be inserted into the model, positioned in a particular arterial branch and visualized on X-ray images. A pump circulates flow through the vasculature of the phantom. The contrast agent boluses are injected in the circuit via femoral catheters (Figure 8).

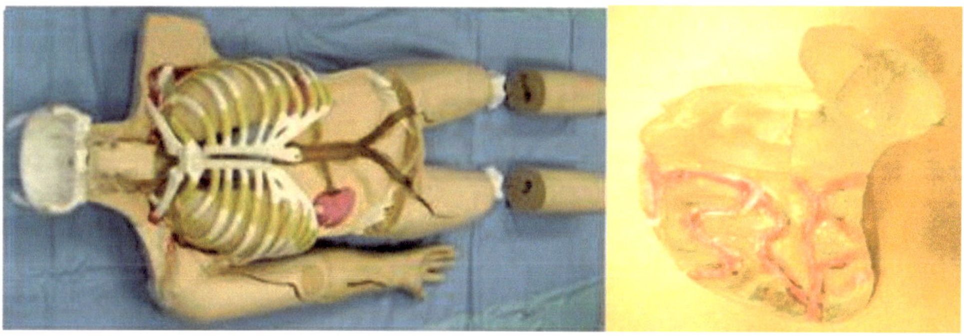

Fig. 8. (Left) Synthetic Arterial Model (SAM) integrated into phantom body. (Right) Close-up view of the heart model with coronary grooves highlighted

In this experiment were studied the effect of four technical variable of the X-ray equipment with an anticipated influence on image quality: tube voltage (kV), additional Copper filtration (mm Cu), detector entrance dose and dynamic density optimization (DDO). The last variable is particular to Siemens cardiac catheterization systems equipped with flat panel detector and is a image quality (post processing) parameter that works in real-time by harmonizing the distribution of gray steps in the image. The X-ray filming of the phantom allows the cardiologist to track the contrast agent circulation, to identify coronary lesions and evaluate their visibility in rapport with anatomical structures. In this study four calcified structures in the coronary arteries were used to simulate stenotic lesions. The first lesion was located on the proximal left anterior descending (LAD) segment, the second on the mid LAD segment, the third on the proximal circumflex segment (Cx) and the fourth on the distal Cx segment. Typical radiographic images, with indication of the lesions, are presented in Figure 9.

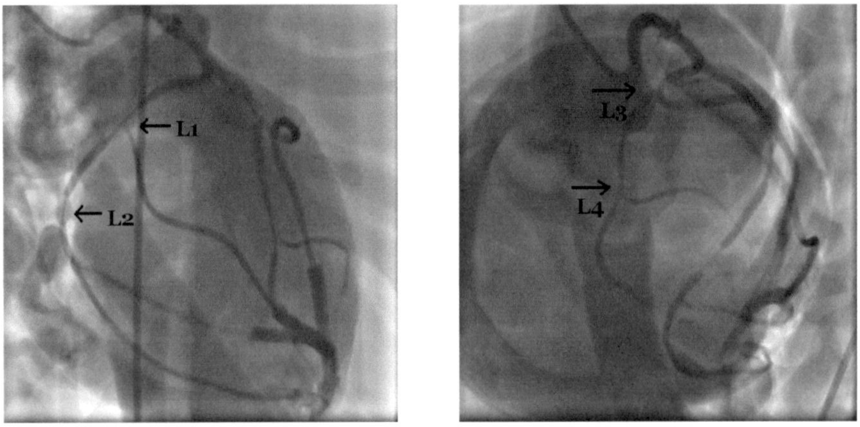

Fig. 9. X-ray images of the heart phantom under different experimental conditions. L1 to L4 indicate the location of simulated lesions.

The contrast media (Iodine) was injected in the phantom using the hand technique and a 6F catheter. 15 to 20 ml of iodine was used at the same flow rates and the image sequence is started a few seconds after the injection. For full characterization of the lesions, sets of two coronary angiograms from two viewing angle were recorded: RAO 30° and LAO 40°/CAUD20° (where RAO the right anterior oblique view, LAO the left anterior oblique direction and CAUD the caudal inclination). The duration of the angiograms was 5 seconds and was acquired at a rate of 15 frames/second. The angiograms were presented in a random order to eight interventional cardiologists (4 experienced interventional cardiologist and 4 residents). The observers were asked to subjectively assess the visibility of each simulated lesion and to give an overall score for each angiogram by using a five-point scale: 1 = not visible; 2 = poor visibility; 3 = acceptable visibility; 4 = good visibility and 5 = very good visibility. The evaluation of angiograms is presented in terms of image quality (IQ) scores. For every angiogram entrance skin dose was measured and an effective dose was estimated. Mean IQ scores ranged from 1.68 to 4.88. The highest IQ scores were obtained for the angiograms acquired with tube potential 80 kV, no added Cu filters, DDO 60%, RAO and LAO views and the highest entrance detector dose that has been used in the present study, namely 170 nGy/frame. Radiation doses (entrance skin dose approximately 40 mGy and effective dose of 1 mSv) were estimated for angiograms acquired at 15 frames/second, detector field-of-view 20 cm, and a length of 5 s. The following parameters improved the IQ factor significantly: a change in tube potential from 96 to 80 kV, detector entrance dose from 100 nGy/frame to 170 nGy/frame, the absence of Copper filtration. DDO variable which is a post-processing parameter should be carefully evaluated because it alters the quality of the images independently of radiation exposure settings. The SAM anthropomorphic phantom has the advantage of visualization of stenotic lesions during the injection of a contrast agent and using an anatomical background. In the future, this phantom could potentially bridge the gap between physics tests and the clinical reality in the catheterization laboratory. Future generation of phantoms should simulate the beating heart.

Optimization of X-ray equipment settings through experimental measurements is necessary, mainly when it involves new equipment or technology. The acceptance of optimized settings that affects image quality and radiation dose has to be accompanied by the training of the user. Authors of this work have experience in this area. In our center in Luxembourg

(Institut National de Chirurgie Cardiaque et de Cardiologie Interventionnelle), we perform continuously an internal audit related to radiation protection in clinical practice. Some results of our experience were already published (Bokou et al., 2008; Dragusin et al., 2010). All interventional cardiologists have taken part of two days continuous education course in radiation protection. The course was practically a discussion forum between cardiologists, radiation protection advisors and application specialist of X-ray equipment manufacturer, with theoretical and practical sessions demonstrating the different factors influencing patient and staff radiation doses. Before and after the course, a patient doses survey was performed. During that period the catheterization laboratories were equipped with image intensifiers. Later, the X-ray systems were upgraded and image intensifiers were replaced with new flat-panel detectors. The effects of education in radiation protection and new technology are visible on patient radiation doses (Figure 10). A decrease of 22% and 23% is noted for CA and, combined CA and PCI procedures. With FD system, the interventional procedures are performed with 6 pulses/second for fluoroscopy, compared with 15 pulses/second used on II system. For FD system, the entrance detector dose is 29 nGy/pulse for fluoroscopy, and 100 nGy/frame for cineangiography mode (lowest option available in our systems).

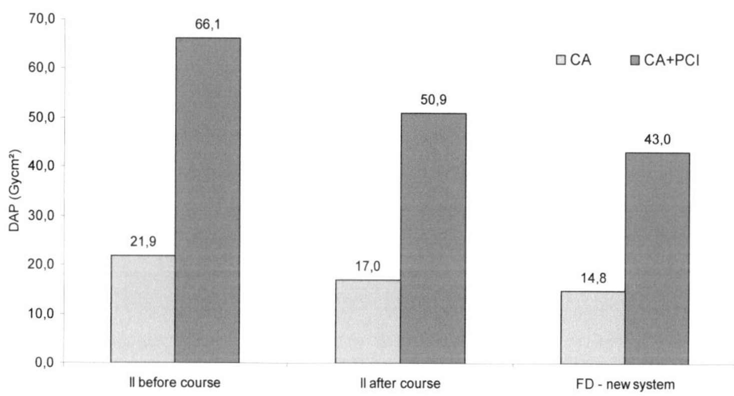

Fig. 10. Mean DAP patient values with II before and after training course and with FD for CA and PCI examinations.

Based on the survey of patient doses, we were able to establish reference levels (RL) for common interventional procedures. These indicators are DAP, fluoroscopy time and number of images, and give to the operator somehow the guideline of good and normal practice. Of course, higher doses might occur if the clinical status of the patient justifies the corresponding exposures to ionizing radiations. The goal to use RL is to control the level of optimization of the procedures. Once the dose indicators are collected, the RL are established as third quartile (75% percentile) of the distribution of observed data. In our center, INCCI Luxembourg, local RL values for CA procedures are: 23 Gycm^2 for DAP, 5 minutes for fluoroscopy time and 617 images. For PCI procedures, the RL values are 44 Gycm^2 for DAP, 15.5 minutes for fluoroscopy time and 1163 images. Our values were compared with reference levels at European level proposed by the SENTINEL consortium (Padovani et al., 2008). The data was collected from nine European centers, 672 CA and 662 PCI procedures. Comparison of our local reference values with the European values are shown in Figure 11 for CA procedures and in Figure 12 for PCI procedures.

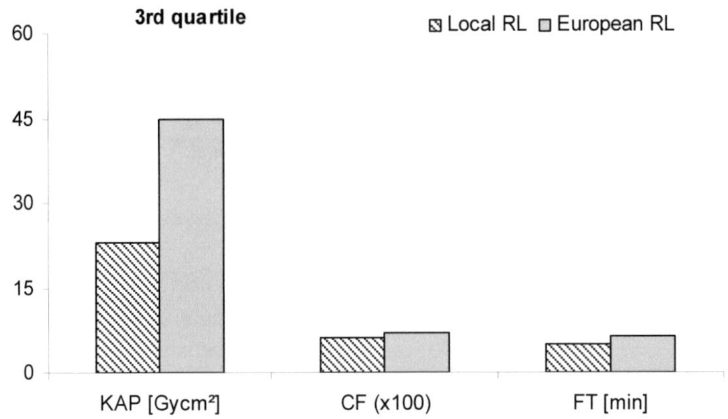

Fig. 11. Comparison of diagnostic reference levels for CA procedures between INCCI (local RL) and European study

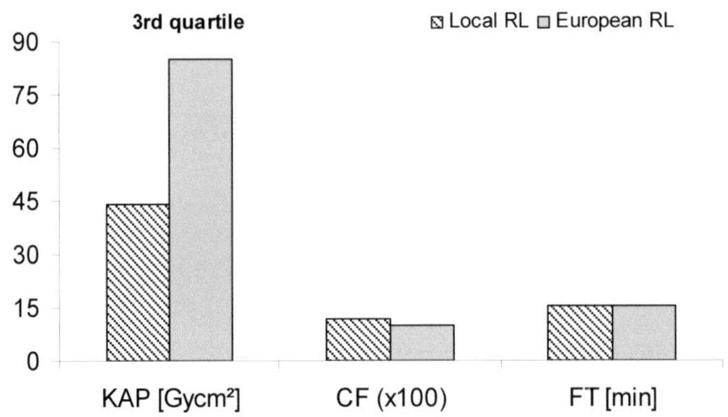

Fig. 12. Comparison of diagnostic reference levels for PCI procedures between INCCI (local RL) and European study

Strictly comparison between both studies is difficult to perform, because we do not have complete information about how the X-ray cardiac systems in the European study were configured. Also, we do not know if the cardiologist's experience and training education in radiation protection is uniform between centers.

Probably one of the factors that explain the difference is the configuration of the X-ray equipment for fluoroscopy mode. In our center the pulse rate is 6 pulses/s (low dose mode), where in European study, centers that submitted data work usually with 12.5 frames/s (for II systems) and 15 pulses/s (for FD systems). Our clinical experience shows that there is possible to optimize protocols when using new technology with little compromise on image quality but with benefit in reducing radiation dose levels to the patient.

5. Conclusion

Optimization of radiation dose - image quality and implementation of ALARA principle in catheterization laboratories are tasks that involve all actors: interventional cardiologists, auxiliary staff, medical physicist, and applications specialists. However, in daily practice some tactics for radiation dose reduction and image quality improvement should be known by all interventional cardiologists. We create a list of little steps that have an impact in radiation safety in daily practice.

Use the lowest acceptable clinical protocols during fluoroscopy and cineangiography. Pulsed fluoroscopy and cineangiography at lowest radiation level should be used. If the equipment allows, different protocols must be created and used in function on the type of structure that is being imaged (venous vs. arterial, fast-moving vs. slow-moving).

Correct placement of the patient in the isocenter on the table. Having the patient correct positioned in the isocenter facilitates keeping the heart at the center of the X-ray field. In this way there is no need of prolonged fluoroscopy to adjust the patient's position with each change in angiographic projection.

Avoid the use of fluoroscopy to make changes to the patient position or collimators. Fluoroscopy should be used very briefly to check the patient position. Movements to the correct position should be avoided by using fluoroscopy constantly. Modern units have "virtual" markers that enable the positioning of the collimators. The correct position of collimators should be checked by brief fluoroscopy rather then constant visualization.

Remove unnecessary instruments and body parts from the X-ray field. Presence of the patient's arm, operator's hands or any external instruments should never be visible on a cardiac study. These structures or objects result in an overall increase in radiation dose to the patient because of the demand of AEC system to compensate with increased radiation output.

Minimize the number of angiograms. Limit the number of projections to provide an overview of the status of the coronary arterial tree and indentify the ideal projections to be used for coronary angioplasty. Always performs test injection of a small amount of contrast material using fluoroscopy prior to acquiring an angiogram. This approach prevents the wasted angiogram that is taken with the catheter inadvertently wedged deeply in a vessel. Also fluoroscopy of test injection can aid in determining the correct magnification mode. Keep in mind that few seconds of fluoroscopy and little quantity of contrast material are less irradiating the patient than a full wasted angiogram. During complicated interventions, limit the use of magnification, because of the substantial increase in radiation dose.

Keep the detector (II or FD) as close to the patient as possible. The X-ray tube should be as far away as possible. If the detector is far from patient, the input doses will be higher and the scatter radiation increases.

Decrease beam on time. This is probably one of the most important rules. Fluoroscopy must not be applied when discussing or doing other manoeuvre. If the eye is not on the screen, the foot should not be on the fluoroscopic pedal. Use stored images rather than live images for studying the case.

Use angiographic projections that reduce operator exposure whenever possible. For right oblique projections, the X-ray tube moves away from the operator, while for left anterior oblique projection moves it closer. Kuon et al., 2004 published an interesting paper focused on identification of less-irradiation tube angulations in invasive cardiology. Di Mario & Sutaria, 2005 published a review of techniques to obtain optimal views of all segments of the coronary arterial system.

Remove anti-scatter grid when imaging small children. New cardiac X-ray systems have possibility to remove the grid. In pediatric patients a significant reduction in radiation dose is possible without compromising image quality.

Know your own cardiac X-ray equipment and its features. Work with radiation physicist, the manufacturer to regularly test and maintain the equipment in optimal working conditions.

Ensure protection of laboratory staff. Before starting fluoroscopy, ensure that everyone in the room use radiation protection shielding. Ask of laboratory staff to keep distance during cine angiography. Remember the inverse square law: doubling the distance from a point source reduces the radiation exposure to one-quarter. Keep the proper use and storage of lead aprons. Aprons that are not proper storage might develop cracks, compromising their effectiveness. Always use personal dosimeters.

Technology of X-ray cardiac system is continuously adapting and optimization of radiation doses with less compromise on image quality is possible. On the other side, activity in cardiac catheterization laboratories increases and more complex procedures are performed. All the actors involved in catheterization laboratory should be trained and familiar with the basic principles of radiation safety. Developing a radiation safety culture should be a priority. Attention to the simple rules of radiation safety and the planning of an interventional procedure should enable the interventional cardiologist to produce high quality images at low radiation level to the patient.

6. References

Bacher ,K; Bogaert, E; Lapere, R; De Wolf, D, &Thierens, H. (2005). Patient-specific dose and radiation risk estimation in pediatric cardiac catheterization. *Circulation.*Vol 111, pp.83-9.

Bernardi, G; Padovani, R; Morocutti, G; Vaño, E; Malisan, M.R; Rinuncini, M; Spedicato, L; &Fioretti, P.M. (2000). Clinical and technical determinants of the complexity of percutaneous transluminal coronary angioplasty procedures: analysis in relation to radiation exposure parameters.*Catheter Cardiovascular Interventional.* Vol 1, pp.121-9

Bogaert, E; Bacher, K & Thierens, H (2008) A large-scale multicentre study in Belgium of dose area product values and effective doses interventional cardiology using contemporary X-ray equipment. *Radiation Protection Dosimetry.* Vol.128, pp.312-323

Broadhead, DA; Chapple, CL; Faulkner, K; Davies, ML; &McCallum, H;(1997). The impact of cardiology on the collective effective dose in the North of England. *British Journal of Radiology,* Vol 70, pp.492-7

Davies, G.A.; Cowen, A.R.; Kengyelics, S.M.; Moore, J. & Sivananthan, M.U. (2007). Do flat detector cardiac X-ray systems convey advantages over image-intensifier-based systems? Study comparing X-ray dose and image quality. European *Radiology,* Vol.17, pp.1787-1794

D'Helft, C; McGee, A; Rainford, L; McFadden, S; Winder, J; Hughes, C; & Brennan, PC. (2008) Proposed preliminary diagnostic reference levels for three common interventional cardiology procedures in Ireland. *Radiation Protection Dosimetry.* Vol.129, pp.63-6

Di Mario, C & Sutaria, N. (2005). Coronary angiography in the angioplasty era: projections with a meaning. *Heart.* Vol. 91, pp. 968-976

Dragusin, O; Desmet , W ; Heidbuchel, H; Padovani, R; & Bosmans, H. (2005). Radiation dose levels during interventional cardiology procedures in a tertiary care hospital. *Radiation Protection Dosimetry.* Vol.117, pp.231-5.

Dragusin, O; Gewillig, W; Desmet, W; Smans, K; Struelens, L & Bosmans, H (2008a). Radiation dose survey in a paediatric cardiac catheterization laboratory equipped with flat-panel detectors *Radiation Protection Dosimetry,* Vol.129, pp.91-95

Dragusin, O; Smans, K; Jacobs, J; Inal, T & Bosmans, H (2008b). Evaluation of the contrast-detail response of a cardiovascular angiography system and the influence of equipment variables on image quality. *Proceedings SPIE Medical Imaging,* Vol.6913, San Diego, USA, March 2008

Dragusin, O; Bosmans, H; Pappas, C & Desmet, W. (2008c). An investigation of flat panel equipment variables on image quality with a dedicated cardiac phantom, *Physics in Medicine and Biology,* Vol.53, 4927-4940

Dragusin, O; Breisch, R; Bokou, C; & Beissel, J (2010). Does a flat panel detector reduce the patient radiation dose in interventional cardiology? *Radiation Protection Dosimetry,* Vol.139, pp.266-270

Ector, J; Dragusin, O; Adriaenssens, B; Huybrechts, W; Willems, R; Ector, H; & Heidbuchel, H. (2007). Obesity is a major determinant of radiation dose in patients undergoing pulmonary vein isolation for atrial fibrillation. *Journal of the American College of Cardiology.* Vol 50, pp.234-242.

Efstathopoulos, EP; Makrygiannis, SS; Kottou, S; Karvouni, E; Giazitzoglou, E; Korovesis, S; Tzanalaridou, E; Raptou, P.D; &Katritsis, D.G.(2003). Medical personnel and patient dosimetry during coronary angiography and intervention. *Physics in Medecine and Biology,*Vol 18, pp.3059-68.

Holmes, D.R.Jr.; Laskey, W.K.; Wondrow, M.A. & Cusma, J.T. (2004). Flat-panel detectors in cardiac catheterization laboratory: revolution or evolution - what are the issues? *Catheterization and Cardiovascular Interventions,* Vol.63, pp.324-330

Huyskens, CJ & Hummel, WA (1995). Data analysis on patient exposures in cardiac angiography. *Radiation Protection Dosimetry.* Vol 57, pp. 475-480.

ICRP, 1990 *Recommendations of the International Commission on Radiological Protection. Publication 60.* Ann. ICRP, Oxford, UK: Pergamon Press, 1991, 21(1-3)

ICRP, *Avoidance of Radiation Injuries from Medical Interventional Procedures. Publication 85.* Ann. ICRP, Oxford, UK: Pergamon Press, 2000, 30

ICRP,*The 2007 Recommendations of the International Commission on Radiological Protection. Publication 103.* Ann. ICRP, Oxford, UK: Pergamon Press, 2007, 37(2-4)

ICRU, International Commission on Radiation Units and Measurements. *Patient dosimetry for X-rays used in medical imaging.* ICRU Report 74, 2005, Journal of ICRU, Vol.5, No.2

Karambatsakidou, A; Tornvall, P; Saleh ,N; Chouliaras, T; Löfberg, PO;& Fransson A.(2005). Skin dose alarm levels in cardiac angiography procedures: is a single DAP value sufficient? *British Journal of Radiology,*Vol 78,pp.803-9.

Kuon, E ; Glaser, C ; & Dahm, JB.(2003). Effective techniques for reduction of radiation dosage to patients undergoing invasive cardiac procedures.*British Journal of Radiology.*Vol 76, pp.406-13.

Kuon, E; Empen, K; Rohde, D; & Dahm, JB.(2004a). Radiation exposure to patients undergoing percutaneous coronary interventions: are current reference values too high? *Herz,*Vol 2, pp.208-17.

Kuon, E; Dahm, J; Empen, K; Robinson, D; Reuter, G & Wucherer, M. (2004b). Identification of less-irradiation tube angulations in invasive cardiology. *Journal of American College of Cardiology.* ,Vol 44, pp.1420-1428.

Onnasch, D. G. W.; Schroder, F. K.; Fischer, G; & Kramer, H. M. (2007). Diagnostic reference levels and effective dose in paediatric cardiac catheterization. *British Journal of Radiology.* Vol80, pp.185-177.

Padovani, R; Bernardi, G; Malisan, M.R; Vañó, E; Morocutti, G, &Fioretti, P.M.(2001). Patient dose related to the complexity of interventional cardiology procedures.*Radiation Protection Radiology*.Vol 94, pp.189-92

Padovani, R; Vano, E; Trianni, A; Bokou, C; Bosmans, H; Bor, D; Jankowski, J; Torbica, P; Kepler, K; Dowling, A; Milu, C; Tsapaki, V; Salat, D; Vassileva, J & Faulkner, K. (2008). Reference levels at European level for cardiac interventional procedures. *Radiation Protection Dosimetry*. Vol 129,pp. 104-107

Rassow, J; Schmaltz, A. Hentrich, F; & Streffer, C. (2000). Effective dose to patients from paediatric cardiac catheterization. *British Journal of Radiology*.Vol 73,pp. 183-172.

Samara, TE; Aroua, A; Stauffer, JC; Bochud, F & Verdun, FR. (2010) Fluoroscopy-guided procedures in cardiology:is patient exposure being reduced over time? *Radiation Protection Dosimetry*, Vol.139, pp.271-274

Sandborg , M; Fransson, SG; & Pettersson, H. (2003). Evaluation of patient-absorbed doses during coronary angiography and intervention by femoral and radial artery access. *European Journal of Radiology*.Vol 4, pp.653-8.

Seibert, J.A. (2006). Flat-panel detectors: how much better are they? *Pediatric Radiology*, Vol.36, pp.173-181

Trianni, A; Bernardi, G; & Padovani, R.(2005a). Are new technologies always reducing patient doses in cardiac procedures? *Radiation Protection Radiology*.Vol 117, pp.101-97.

Trianni, A; Chizzola, G; Toh, H; Quai, E; Cragnolini, E; Bernardi, G; Proclemer, A & Padovani, R.(2005b). Patient skin dosimetry in haemodynamic and electrophysiology interventional cardiology. *Radiation Protection Radiology*.Vol 117, pp.241-6.

Tsapaki, V; Kottou, S; Kollaros, N; Dafnomili, P; Kyriakidis, Z; &Neofotistou ,V.(2004). Dose performance evaluation of a charge coupled device and a flat-panel digital fluoroscopy system recently installed in an interventional cardiology laboratory. *Radiation Protection Radiology*,Vol 3,pp.297-304.

Tsapaki, V; Patsilinakos, S; Voudris, V; Magginas,A; Pavlidis, S; Maounis, T; Theodorakis, G; Koutelou, M; Vrantza, T; Nearchou, M; Nikolaki, N; Kollaros, N; Kyrozi, E; Kottou, S; Karaiskos, P; Neofotistou, E; & Cokkinos, D. (2008) Level of patient and operator dose in the largest cardiac centre in Greece. *Radiation Protection Dosimetry*. Vol.129, pp.71-3

Van de Putte, S; Verhaegen, F; Taeymans ,Y; &Thierens, H.(2000). Correlation of patient skin doses in cardiac interventional radiology with dose-area product. *British Journal of Radiology*, Vol 73, pp. 504-13.

Vano, E; Gonzalez, L; Fernandez, JM; Alfonso, F & Macaya, C. (2006). Occupational radiation doses in interventional cardiology. *British Journal of Radiology*. Vol 79,pp. 383-8.

Venneri, L; Rossi, F; Botto, N; Grazia, M ; Salcone, N ; Emad, A ; Lazzeri, M ; Gori, C ; Vano, E & Picano, E (2009). Cancer risk from professional exposure in staff working in cardiac catheterization laboratory: Insights from the National Research Council's Biological Effects of Ionizing Radiation VII Report. *The American Heart Journal*. Vol 157, pp. 118-127.

Vijayalakshmi, K; Kelly, D ; Chapple, C.L; Williams, D ,Wright, R; Stewart, M.J; Hall, J.A; Sutton, A;Davis, A; Haywood, J; & Belder, M.A.(2007).Cardiac catheterization: radiation doses and lifetime risk of malignancy. Heart. Vol371, pp.370-371.

Zorzetto, M; Bernardi, G; Morocutti, G & Fontanelli, A. (1997) Radiation exposure to patients and operators during diagnostic catheterization and coronary angioplasty, *Catheterization and cardiovascular diagnosis*. Vol 40, pp. 348-51

20

Protection of the Patient and the Staff from Radiation Exposure During Fluoroscopy-Guided Procedures in Cardiology

Verdun Francis R., Aroua Abbas, Samara Eleni,
Bochud François and Stauffer Jean-François
Lausanne University Hospital
Switzerland

1. Introduction

The volume of diagnostic or therapeutic procedures in cardiology that require the use of ionizing radiation is increasing constantly. Currently, technological developments offer the possibility of exploring not only the cardiac function (measurement of ejection fraction, for example) but also the state of coronary and great vessels. In fact, the management of patients with heart disease often requires the use of investigative techniques using X-rays. For example 3.85 million cardiac catheterizations were performed in the United States in 2002 (Einstein et al., 2007). In Switzerland the last national survey on the exposure of the population by medical radiology revealed that nearly 34 000 coronary angiographies and more than 18 000 coronary dilatations were performed in 2008. They are associated to 65% of the collective dose related to interventional radiology and 8% to that related to all medical X-rays (Samara et al. 2011).

The increase in radiological examinations using ionizing radiation has been mentioned for several years not only in medical journals for professionals but also in the press addressing the general public. For example, in its edition of 17 June, 2007, the *New York Times* questioned the public opinion about the justification of the increasing number of CT examinations.

While most examinations deliver relatively low doses and thus add only a low risk to the procedure itself, there are situations where doses exceed the dose level where an excess risk of death from cancer has been demonstrated. In addition, some complex procedures may result in the occurrence of deterministic effects such as burns to the skin.

The substantial increase of fluoroscopy-guided procedures in cardiology over the past few years has been accompanied by a parallel growth in concern for patient radiation safety and for the safety of the operators who perform these procedures. Thus, radiation safety has become a major issue in radiology departments.

The aim of this chapter is:

- to recall the effects of ionizing radiation on the human body and the radiological risks;
- to introduce the dosimetric quantities (basic and operational) commonly used to quantify those risks;
- to briefly present the principles of radiation protection;
- to provide the tools (actions and means) necessary for operational radiation protection.

2. Radiation effects and dose

The aim of this section is to recall the effects of ionizing radiation on the human body and the radiological risks

2.1 Radiation effects

Effects associated with exposure to radiation are divided into two categories: stochastic and deterministic.

2.1.1 Stochastic effects of radiations

The major risks associated with a radiological procedure using ionizing radiation are due to stochastic effects. They induce a minimal genetic risk on offspring and especially add to the natural risk of developing cancer an additional risk. They strongly depend on age and are three to four times higher in children than in adults. One of the problems related to stochastic effects is that they are considered to be without threshold. It is therefore necessary to justify an examination using ionizing radiation and to be sure that the patient will benefit from the radiological procedure exceeds the associated risk. In addition, when the procedure is justified, the management of the patient dose must be optimized.

2.1.2 Deterministic effects of radiations

Deterministic effects include cataract, skin erythema, epilation, and skin burns at different stages depending on the degree of irradiation of the skin. Unlike the stochastic effects, deterministic effects present a threshold and appear only beyond a certain level of exposure of the skin to radiation. They occur only a few days or months after irradiation and the higher the dose to the skin is, the higher deterministic effects are severe as shown in table 1. Deterministic effects are generally not expected to result from purely diagnostic cardiac investigations, but are sometimes reported with the management of critical cases in particular after some complex interventional procedures such as the dilatation of the coronary arteries (PTCA), recanalizations or thermal ablations. They are certainly rare but they do exist (Suzuki et al., 2008).

Effect	Threshold dose (Gy)	Onset
Early transient erythema	2	Few hours
Temporary epilation	3	3 weeks
Main erythema	6	10 days
Permanent epilation	7	3 weeks
Dry desquamation	10	4 weeks
Dermal atrophy	11	> 14 weeks
Telangiectasia	12	> 52 weeks
Moist desquamation	15	4 weeks
Late erythema	15	6 to 10 weeks
Necrosis	18	> 10 weeks

Table 1. Deterministic effects to the skin

2.2 Basic dosimetric quantities

There are several dosimetric quantities that have been introduced to assess risks and control the exposure of the patient and the staff. This section will briefly describe the fundamental quantities.

2.2.1 Absorbed dose, D

X-rays or gamma rays are indirectly ionizing radiation because energy is released into the tissue through the electrons set in motion by the X-rays or gamma rays, which in turn will make a very large number of ionizations. The energy that these electrons deposit per unit mass of tissue, T, or organ is called the absorbed dose and is denoted D_T. This is the basic physical quantity used to measure the biological effects expected. It has the dimension of one joule per kilogram ($J\ kg^{-1}$) and is expressed in gray (Gy). This quantity is used to control the deterministic effects with a threshold of 0.5 Gy.

2.2.2 Equivalent dose, H

To reflect the fact that all types of radiation for a given absorbed dose, do not produce the same effect in humans the concept of dose equivalent in a tissue, T, or organ, denoted H_T was introduced. It is the product of D_T and a weighting factor, w_R, which depends on the type of radiation and expresses its effectiveness.

$$H_T = \Sigma_R\, w_R \,.\, D_{T,R}$$

H_T has the same dimension as D_T ($J\ kg^{-1}$), but is expressed in sievert (Sv).
As shown in table 2, X-rays or gamma rays are taken as reference radiation and w_R is therefore equal to unity. Thus, an adsorbed dose of 1 mGy is equivalent to a dose equivalent of 1 mSv

Radiation type	w_R ($ICRP_{60}$)	w_R ($ICRP_{103}$)
• Photons, electrons, muons	1	1
• Protons, charged particles	5	2
• Alpha particles, heavy nuclei, fission fragments	20	20
• Neutrons	5/10/20, depending on energy	A continuous function of neutron energy

Table 2. Radiation weighting factors according to $ICRP_{60}$ and $ICRP_{103}$

2.2.3 Effective dose, E

The effective dose (E) was firstly proposed by Jacobi in C). The aim of the E was to define a quantity that could be directly related to the probability of a detriment from low-dose exposure to ionizing radiation where only stochastic effects occur. The E concept was adopted by ICRP in 1977 (ICRP26, 1977) and further developed in its Recommendations ICRP60 (ICRP90, 1990) and ICRP103 (ICRP, 2007).
E is defined by the weighed sum of mean tissue and organ doses with radiation weighting factors taking into account a) the different radio-biological effectiveness of various radiations and b) the different sensitivity of tissue and organs with respect to stochastic effects. E is defined as:

$$E = \Sigma_T w_T . H_T = \Sigma_{T,R} w_T . w_R . D_{T,R}$$

where w_T is the tissue weighting factor (see table 3).

Organ/Tissue	$ICRP_{60}$	$ICRP_{103}$	$ICRP_{103}/ICRP_{60}$
Gonads	0.20	0.08	0.4
Colon	0.12	0.12	1.0
Lungs	0.12	0.12	1.0
Red bone marrow	0.12	0.12	1.0
Stomach	0.12	0.12	1.0
Bladder	0.05	0.04	0.8
Breast	0.05	0.12	2.4
Liver	0.05	0.04	0.8
Oesophagus	0.05	0.04	0.8
Thyroid	0.05	0.04	0.8
Bone surface	0.01	0.01	1.0
Skin	0.01	0.01	1.0
Brain		0.01	
Salivary glands		0.01	
Remainder	0.05*	0.01+	

* ICRP60 remainder tissues/organs: adrenals, brain, kidneys, muscle, pancreas, small intestine, large intestine, spleen, thymus, uterus.
+ ICRP103 remainder tissues/organs: adrenals, extrathoracic tissue, gall bladder, heart, kidneys, lymphatic nodes, muscle, oral mucosa, pancreas, prostate, small intestine, spleen, thymus, uterus/cervix.

Table 3. Tissue weighting factors

2.3 Operational dosimetric quantities

As above indicated to account for stochastic effects the effective dose (E) has to be determined. To estimate E associated with a radiological examination various operational quantities, easy to measure, are used. They are also listed at the end of the examination on the console of the X-ray unit

2.3.1 Entrance dose and dose area product

For radiographic examinations, the operational quantity used is called absorbed dose at the surface at the entrance of the beam in the patient and abbreviated as ESD. The ESD is expressed in mGy and is converted into effective dose, in mSv, by multiplying it by a factor which is for example 0.2 for a chest radiograph.
For fluoroscopy procedures the operational quantity used is called dose-area product and abbreviated as DAP. The unit commonly used is $Gy.cm^2$. Some manufacturers also express the DAP in $cGy.cm^2$ or $\mu Gy.m^2$. To convert the DAP in $Gy.cm^2$ into E in mSv, it has to be multiplied by a converting factor equal to 0.2 in the case of the exposure of the chest region (when $Gy.cm^2$ is used).
Table 4 shows the operational quantity and the effective dose associated with a series of routine examinations in diagnostic radiology.

•	Examination	Operational quantity	Typical values	Effective dose (mSv)
•	Bite-Wing (dental)	ESD (mGy)	2	0.01
•	OPG (dental)	ESD (mGy)	0.7	0.06
•	Chest PA	ESD (mGy)	0.1	0.02
•	Hip AP	ESD (mGy)	6	0.7
•	Abdomen PA	ESD (mGy)	3	1.2
•	Coronarography	DAP (Gy.cm^2)	60	12
•	PCI	DAP (Gy.cm^2)	80	16
•	RFCA	DAP (Gy.cm^2)	130	26
•	CTCA	DLP (Gy.cm)	1500	25

Table 4. Operational dose quantity and effective dose for a number of X-ray examinations

2.3.2 Skin accumulated dose

The estimation of absorbed dose at the surface of the skin by fluoroscopy, to account for deterministic effects, is a difficult task since the examination is conducted with changing regularly the incidence X-ray beam. However, it is possible to have an idea of the dose to the skin using a particular operational quantity, called the cumulative dose. This quantity estimates the dose that would have received the skin if the geometry was kept unchanged throughout the procedure. It may be considered that the cumulative dose indicated by the facility in cardiology overestimates the dose to the skin by a factor of 2-3 since several tube-detector incidences are used that distributes the exposure of the skin. If this operational quantity is not available, the skin dose could be estimated from the DAP knowing that we will be much less accurate. To estimate the skin dose in Gy, in a situation where the tube does not rotated around the patient during the procedure one can divide the DAP (Gy.cm^2) by 100 for a well collimated X-ray beam (100 cm^2 : area of the X-ray beam at the entrance of the patient).

2.3.3 Ambient dose equivalent

Another operational quantity used to assess the effective dose delivered to the operator is the ambient dose equivalent, H*(10), at the point of interest in the actual radiation field. It is defined (ICRU, 1992) as the dose equivalent which would be generated in the associated oriented and expanded radiation field at a depth of 10 mm on the radius of the ICRU sphere which is oriented opposite to the direction of incident radiation. This quantity is normalized traceable. It is representative of the effective dose the staff receives.

3. Principle of radiation protection

Radiation protection is assured by respecting three general principles which are: the justification of the practice, the optimisation of the protection and the individual dose limits. The justification of the practice is due to the fact that exposure to ionising radiation has deleterious effects on health. The principle of optimisation is introduced since some of these effects are considered as non-threshold's ones, and thus one has to reduce exposure to levels. The principle of individual limits is introduced as a safeguard to prevent situations where the respect of the two first principles would not be sufficient to protect individuals.

3.1 Justification

The first principle of radiation protection is justification. No exposure is acceptable unless its usefulness is demonstrated. In the medical practice any radiological modality or procedure has to be justified. It should be properly indicated to the diagnostic or therapeutic case. In other words it should be demonstrated that no other non-irradiating non invasive modality can give the same diagnostic or therapeutic results. In order to implement the justification principle, learned society in several countries (USA, UK, France, Switzerland and others) worked out referral guides in order to indicate which radiological modality/examination is suited to which diagnostic or therapeutic case.

3.2 Optimization

The second principle of radiation protection is optimization. When the exposure to radiation is justified, an effort must be engaged in order to keep the radiation dose delivered as low as reasonably achievable (ALARA principle). If justification reflects the will "to do the right thing", optimisation reflects the will "to do it right". In the medical practice the principle of optimization is implemented in different ways contributing together to lower the radiation doses to the patients and to the staff. The quality control of the X-ray unit is important to make sure the optimal settings are used. The auditing of the protocols used for each radiological procedure allows producing the quantity and quality of images sufficient to the diagnostic or therapeutic goal, with an optimum trade-off between image quality and radiation dose, and no unnecessary irradiation of the patient and staff. The use of protecting means contribute to cut down the radiation (direct or scattered) that is not useful in the imaging process. Training, informing, using diagnostic reference levels, all this helps spread a culture of optimization.

3.3 Limitation

The third principle of radiation protection is dose limitation in order to avoid excessive exposure of an individual. The ICRP recommends a set of dose limits for the general public and for people exposed in the course of their occupation (ICRP 103, 2007). The principle of dose limitation applies to health professionals (physicians, radiographers, medical physicists, etc.) but it does not apply to the patient. The sound benefit (diagnostic or therapeutic) from X-rays use implies that higher doses of radiation are tolerated as long as the radiological procedure is justified and optimized.

4. Operational radiation protection

Near a radiological room radiation protection of workers and of public is ensured by the limitation of the weekly ambient equivalent dose through the shielding of the rooms. Surveys have shown that doses to public and workers in such an environment are very low. However there is not ambient equivalent dose limitation near the X-ray imaging unit. Thus, it is mandatory to wear a lead apron when being near a running X-ray imaging device. Many professionals that use fluoroscopy units receive low dose of radiation since they only use these unit a few minutes (or less) per patient. Unfortunately, this is often not the case for cardiologists who can handle very complex procedures that not only expose the patient but also expose the staff present in the suite. Thus an effort to improve the radiation protection should get a high priority.

It is worth mentioning that the exposure of staff is not due to X-ray leakage from the X-ray tube of the fluoroscopy unit. Exposure to the staff is due to the X-ray scatter that is produced when the X-ray beam interacts with the tissues of the patient. Thus, the higher the dose to the skin of the patient the higher the amount of scattered radiation produced. From this, patient and staff exposure are interlinked. One should always remember that the patient is the main source of exposure of the staff. Therefore optimizing the patient dose will improve the staff radiation protection.

4.1 Patient

Patient dose can be quite high but deterministic effects should never be a surprise to the operator. Avoiding as much as possible the appearance of deterministic effects (short term radiological complications) the operator should also minimize the stochastic effects (long term radiological complications).

4.1.1 Patient positioning

The first thing to know is: where the source of radiation and the image detector are. The patient needs to be as far as possible from the source of radiation (X-ray tube). The patient needs to be as close as possible to the image detector.

4.1.2 X-ray tube orientation

The number of X-ray is reduced by a factor of two every 2 to 3 cm of tissue. Nevertheless, the number of photons required to obtain an image remains constant. Thus, the thicker is the patient the higher is the skin rate. Skin dose rate might be also very high when using oblique incidence and one should try to restrict as much as possible incidences where the path of the X-ray in the patient are long.

4.1.3 Image quality level

Fluoroscopy units provide the user with several image quality levels during fluoroscopy and cine runs. There is no free lunch, the better the image quality the higher the patient exposure. The cardiologist should be aware that he/she has control over the image quality level and he/she should avoid any waste of radiation. The temporal resolution (frame rate) should also be chosen according the requirement of the procedure.

4.1.4 Image magnification

Geometric magnification should never be used (see §4.1.1). Electronic or digital magnification requires in general an increase of the skin dose rate. Thus, magnification should be used with parsimony.

4.1.5 Introduction of an "intervention" level

During long procedures the threshold of the deterministic effects might be reached. Since the severity of the lesion is dose dependent one should define a DAP level (for example 100 $Gy.cm^2$) after which a particular care on patient exposure is exercised. One could try for example to change incidences to distribute the dose. A DAP threshold where the patient should be recalled to check for skin lesion should also be defined (for example 500 $Gy.cm^2$).

4.1.6 Patient dose record

The dose indicators (DAP and skin accumulated dose) of the procedure should be recorded in the file of the patient. Moreover dose survey should be organised and the results should be compared with published value to estimated one's practice.

4.2 Personnel

The X-ray beam enters the patient and interacts with the tissue. Some radiation will be absorbed in the patient and thus deposit energy to that patient. The transmitted radiation will impinge the image amplifier to produce images. Unfortunately, the X-ray interaction within the patient will also create scattered radiation emitted all around the patient which will expose the staff to ionizing radiations.

The dose the staff might receive when being at one meter from the patient is approximately 0.1% of the skin dose delivered to that patient when the size of the X-ray beam is large (typically 400 cm^2). For example if the skin dose rate is equal to 40 $mGy.min^{-1}$, ambient dose rate at one meter from the patient can be estimated to 2.5 $mSv.h^{-1}$ (natural background of 0.0001-0.0002 $mSv.h^{-1}$). During cine runs the skin dose rate can reach 1 $Gy.min^{-1}$ which implies a higher dose rate to the staff during this type of acquisition. The ratio between patient skin dose and staff dose is dependent on the size of the X-ray beam. The larger the field size the higher the ratio. It is thus important to always reduce the size of the X-ray beam to its strict minimum. Expressed in terms of DAP one can take 0.3% of the DAP (DAP expressed in $Gy.cm^2$ and E in mSv). Thus when a cardiologist has delivered a DAP of 60 $Gy.cm^2$ he might have received over his/her lead apron a dose of 0.2 mSv.

4.2.1 Shielding

Shielding allows the staff to be isolated from scattered radiation produced by the X-ray interaction in the patient. Barriers used for shielding may be fixed to the unit, movable or worn by individuals. The amount of radiation attenuated by a material depends on the elemental composition of the material, its thickness and the energy of the radiation passing through it. As an example, the transmission through 0.5 mm of lead is 3.2% at 100kV and 0.36% at 70 kV (Yaffe & Mawdsley, 1991).

To reduce the operator exposure, one should begin by creating a sort of booth with shielding devices around him or herself. To do so, an articulated ceiling leaded screen lengthened by a leaded flap beside the table, or a mobile barrier as the one shown in Figure 1, together with a longitudinal protection adjacent to the table can be used (Kuon et al. 2002). Each shield should be at least 0.5 mm lead equivalent. The operator has then to complete his or her protection by wearing a lead apron, which should be adjusted to his or her size. Concerning the lead equivalent content, most of the aprons are either 0.5 or 0.35 mm lead equivalent. The use of a 0.35 mm instead of a 0.5 mm lead equivalent reduces weight by about 30%, but increases the transmission of scattered radiation of almost a factor of 2 at 90 kV. However, Marshall in an experimental study showed that at 90 kV, wearing a 0.35 mm lead equivalent apron with an additional 0.35 mm lead equivalent thyroid shield resulted in a factor 2 greater reduction in effective dose than can be achieved by wearing a 0.55 mm lead equivalent apron alone (Marshall & Faulkner, 1993). Some aprons are made of composite materials which offers equivalent shielding properties but which are significantly less heavy than aprons containing lead as shield material (Yaffe & Mawdsley, 1991).

Figure 1 presents one way the operator can insulate himself from the scatter produced by the patient when the examination is performed in the chest area with a femoral access. One should always remember that it is at the surface where the X-ray beam enters the patient that the scatter dose rate is at its highest level. One should shield himself from that particular spot.

Figure 2 summarizes the efficiency of the shielding devices presented in Figure 1 for various tube-image amplifier orientations. It can be seen that an operator can significantly decrease his or her exposure when a shielding device is placed in such a way that the operator is as much as possible shielded from scattered radiation (Kuon et al., 2002). Unfortunately this is not always possible, as in the case of biliary drainage for example. In such a case, staff exposure is mainly controlled by the optimisation of patient exposure, the distance from the scatter source and personal shielding (Williams, 1997).

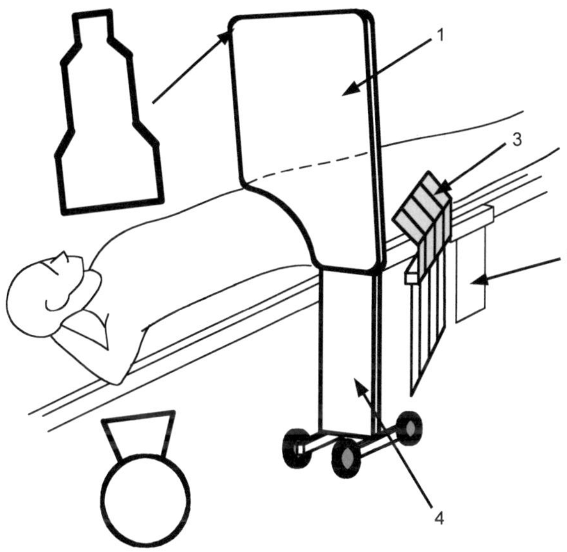

Fig. 1. Example of operator shielding with various devices (1 leaded glass, 2 and 3 leaded curtains, 4 leaded wall; 1 and 4 being on a mobile barrier)

To improve protection against cataract (which is a deterministic effect of ionising radiation), a 0.5 mm lead equivalent eyeglass should be used to reduce exposure to the lens by 10% to 65% (Nicholson, 1995). Finally, gloves made of composite material and offering the same tactile perception than regular chirurgical ones are available. Unfortunately, they offer a limited protection since they usually reduce dose by a factor less than 2 (Vaño & Guibelalde, 1997; Balter, 2001).

4.2.2 Effect of the examination geometry

Backscattered radiation is the radiation that is scattered back from the surface at the beam entrance. It is of high intensity because the entrance surface of the primary beam into the patient has not been attenuated. Thus, ambient dose rate will always be significantly higher when the operator is close to the x-ray tube, than when it is at the image amplifier side. Shielding of the operator should be performed considering these parameters (see Figure 3) (Brateman, 1999).

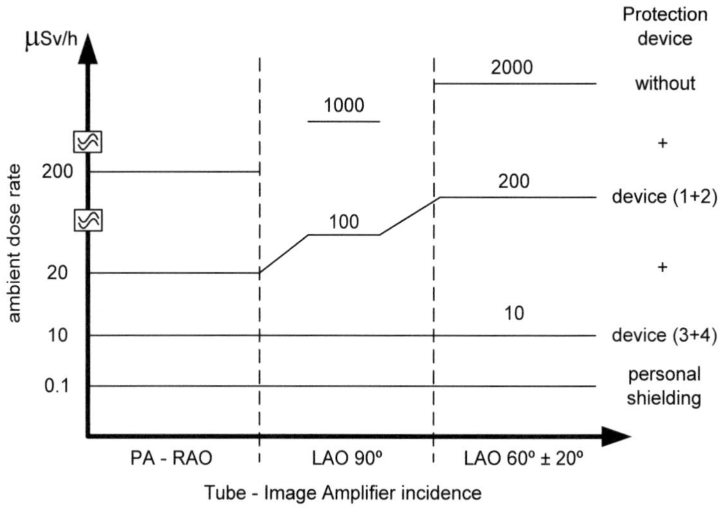

Fig. 2. Mean ambient dose rate to the operator (µSv.h^{-1}) for different tube-image amplifier orientations. The dose rate corresponds to an examination in the cardiac area of a Rando phantom, representative of a 70 kg standard patient, the operator being at about 1 m from the central beam impinging the phantom (situation presented in Figure 1). Without any radiation protection device, the dose rate is in the range of 2 to 0.2 mSv.h^{-1}. As expected, the LAO angulations are the ones which potentially deliver the highest dose to the operator. The addition of the protection devices 1 and 2 allows a reduction of the ambient dose rate at operator's level by a factor of 10. A further reduction is obtained by completing the shielding with devices 3 and 4. Finally, the use of personal shielding devices (i.e. lead apron, thyroid shield and leaded glasses) reduces the ambient dose rate to about 0.1 µSv.h^{-1} (adapted from Kuon et al., 2002).

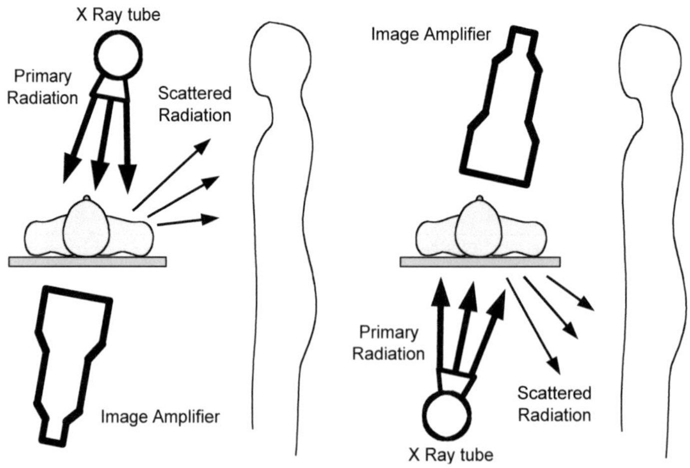

Fig. 3. The schematics show the influence of the tube-image amplifier orientation on the operator's exposure. When the tube is below the table, exposure to the legs and the lower part of the abdomen is the highest. When the tube is above the table, exposure to the face, neck and chest is the highest.

4.2.3 Inverse square law

The exposure rate from a point source of radiation decreases as the distance from the source squared. This inverse square law is the results of the geometric relationship between the surface area, A, and the radius, r, of a sphere: $A = 4 \pi r^2$. As an example, for a field size of the primary beam impinging the patient of about 100 cm^2, the ambient dose rate at 90° to the incident beam decreases from 1.2 $mGy.h^{-1}$ to 0.3 $mGy.h^{-1}$ when moving from 50 cm to 1m from the patient (i.e. a dose rate reduction as a function of $1/r^2$) (Bushberg et al., 2002). Unfortunately, when the size of the field impinging the patient is large, the dose reduction is slightly less efficient since dose rate reduction is no more as a function of r^{-2} but only as a function of r^{-1}. Nevertheless, backing away from the primary beam is a very efficient way to reduce staff exposure.

5. Conclusion

Several recently published studies showed that there is a high potential to reduce radiation doses to the patient and subsequently to enhance radiation safety for the staff. The aim of this chapter was to introduce the effects of ionizing radiation and the radiological risks, and to present various methods that may be used to reduce patient and personnel exposure during fluoroscopy-guided procedures in cardiology, such as the reduction of patient exposure, the increase of the distance from the source of scatter, and the shielding.

Every effort needs to be made in order to reduce patient and staff exposure as much as possible, not for legal purposes but simply for workers health. This applies in particular in the field of interventional radiology where exposure to the staff is potentially very high. Dose reduction to the staff can be reduced by the optimisation of patient exposure. Thus the introduction of the diagnostic reference levels (DRL) will certainly improve the control of staff exposure. Moreover, the application of simple rules, such as the ones mentioned in this contribution, allow radiologists to use fluoroscopy units minimising their exposure as much as possible. The respect of these rules allow also to improve the protection of other medical staff present near the patient and who are less familiar with radiation protection.

6. References

Einstein, A.J.; Moser, K.W., Thompson R.C., Cerqueira M.D., Henzlova M.J. (2007). Radiation dose to patients from cardiac diagnostic imaging. Circulation, 116:1290-1305

Samara, E.; Aroua, A., Vader, J.-P., Trueb, Ph., Bochud, F., Verdun, F.R. (2011). Exposure of the Swiss Population by Radiodiagnostics: 2008 Review. Health Physics, submitted

Suzuki, S.; Furui, S., Isshiki, T. (2008). Patients' skin dose during percutaneous coronary intervention for chronic total occlusion. Catheter Cardiovasc Interv, 71:160-164

Jacobi, W.; (1975). The concept of effective dose - a proposal for the combination of organ doses Radiat Environ Biophys, 12:101-109

ICRP 26 (1977). International Commission on Radiological Protection: The recommendations of the international commission on radiological protection. ICRP Publication 26, Elsevier

ICRP 90 (1990). International Commission on Radiological Protection: The recommendations of the international commission on radiological protection. ICRP Publication 90, Elsevier

ICRP 103 (1007). International Commission on Radiological Protection: The recommendations of the international commission on radiological protection. ICRP Publication 103, Elsevier

ICRU 47 (1992). International Commission on Radiation Units and Measurements. ICRU Report 47, ICRU, Bethesda, Maryland, USA (1992).

Yaffe, M.J. & Mawdsley, G.E. (1991). Composite materials for x-ray protection. Health Phys 60:661-664

Kuon, E.; Schmitt, M. & Dahm, J.B. (2002). Significant reduction of radiation exposure to operator and staff during cardiac interventions by analysis of radiation leakage and improved lead shielding. Am J Cardiol 89: 44-49

Marshall, N.W. & Faulkner, K. (1993). Optimization of personnel shielding in interventional radiology. Proceedings of the Radiation Protection Committee of the BIR (British Institute of Radiology) and of the Commission of the European Communities (CEC). London

Williams; J.R.; (1997). The interdependence of staff and patient doses in interventional radiology. Br J radiol 70: 498-503

Vaño, E. & Guibelalde, E. (1997). Proceedings of the European radiation protection education and training ERPET course - Radiation protection in interventional radiology. Madrid 12-14 May 1997, European Commission DG XII, Brussels

Balter, S.; (2001). Stray radiation in the cardiac catheterisation laboratory. Radiat Prot Dosim 94(1-2): 183-188

Brateman, L.; (1999) The AAPM/RSNA Physics tutorial for residents - Radiation safety considerations for diagnostic radiology personnel. Radiographics 19:1037-1055

Bushberg, J.T.; Seibert, J.A., Leidholdt, E.M., Boone, J.M. (2002). The essential physics of medical imaging. Lippincott Williams & Wilkins, Philadelphia